A Guide to Clinical Assessment & Professional Report Writing in Speech-Language Pathology

SECOND EDITION

A Guide to Clinical Assessment & Professional Report Writing in Speech-Language Pathology

SECOND EDITION

Edited by

Cyndi Stein-Rubin, MS, CCC-SLP, TSSLD, CTA-Certified Coach
Retired Lecturer and Clinical Supervisor
Department of Speech, Language, and Hearing Department
Brooklyn College of the City University of New York
Brooklyn, New York

Renee Fabus, PhD, CCC-SLP, TSHH
School of Health Technology and Management
Stony Brook University
Stony Brook, New York

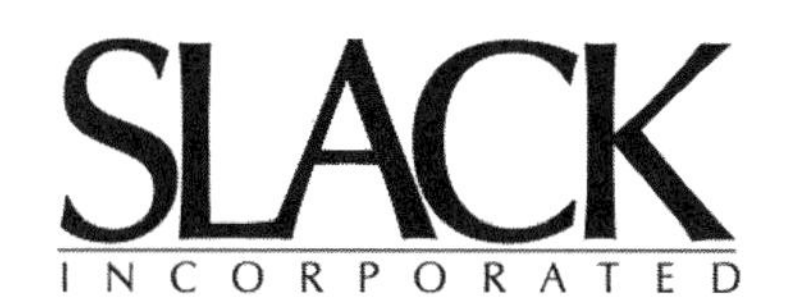

www.Healio.com/books

ISBN: 978-1-63091-372-4

The procedures and practices described in this publication should be implemented in a manner consistent with the professional standards set for the circumstances that apply in each specific situation. Every effort has been made to confirm the accuracy of the information presented and to correctly relate generally accepted practices. The authors, editors, and publisher cannot accept responsibility for errors or exclusions or for the outcome of the material presented herein. There is no expressed or implied warranty of this book or information imparted by it. Care has been taken to ensure that drug selection and dosages are in accordance with currently accepted/recommended practice. Off-label uses of drugs may be discussed. Due to continuing research, changes in government policy and regulations, and various effects of drug reactions and interactions, it is recommended that the reader carefully review all materials and literature provided for each drug, especially those that are new or not frequently used. Some drugs or devices in this publication have clearance for use in a restricted research setting by the Food and Drug and Administration or FDA. Each professional should determine the FDA status of any drug or device prior to use in their practice.

Any review or mention of specific companies or products is not intended as an endorsement by the author or publisher.

SLACK Incorporated uses a review process to evaluate submitted material. Prior to publication, educators or clinicians provide important feedback on the content that we publish. We welcome feedback on this work.

Published by: SLACK Incorporated
6900 Grove Road
Thorofare, NJ 08086 USA
Telephone: 856-848-1000
Fax: 856-848-6091
www.Healio.com/books

Contact SLACK Incorporated for more information about other books in this field or about the availability of our books from distributors outside the United States.

Library of Congress Cataloging-in-Publication Data

Names: Stein-Rubin, Cyndi, editor. | Fabus, Renee Laura, 1968- editor. | Preceded by (work): Stein-Rubin, Cyndi. Guide to clinical assessment and professional report writing in speech-language pathology.
Title: A guide to clinical assessment and professional report writing in speech-language pathology / [edited by] Cyndi Stein-Rubin, Renee Fabus.
Description: Second edition. | Thorofare, NJ : SLACK Incorporated, [2018] | Preceded by A guide to clinical assessment and professional report writing in speech-language pathology / Cyndi Stein-Rubin, Renee Fabus. Cilifton Park, NY : Cengage Learning, c2012. | Includes bibliographical references and index.
Identifiers: LCCN 2017048156 (print) | LCCN 2017048887 (ebook) | ISBN 9781630913731 (epub) | ISBN 9781630913748 (web) | ISBN 9781630913724 (pbk. : alk. paper)
Subjects: | MESH: Speech Disorders--diagnosis | Language Development Disorders--diagnosis | Medical records | Writing
Classification: LCC RC428.5 (ebook) | LCC RC428.5 (print) | NLM WL 340.2 | DDC 616.85/506--dc23
LC record available at https://lccn.loc.gov/2017048156

Printed in the United States of America.

Last digit is print number: 10 9 8 7 6 5 4 3

Dedication

This book is dedicated to the people who have shaped who I have become—my precious family and the countless clients, families, and students who I have coached, treated, taught, supervised, and mentored over the past 33 years.

Cyndi Stein-Rubin, MS, CCC, TSSLD-SLP, CTA Certified Coach

This book is dedicated to my students. Always remember to reach for the stars and never give up.

Renee Fabus, PhD, CCC-SLP, TSHH

Contents

Acknowledgments

I express my deep gratitude to my loving and devoted husband, Jeff, for his patience, support, and sense of humor—invaluable attributes in helping bring our work to fruition. I thank my beautiful sons, daughters-in-law, and grandchildren for their love, support, and inspiration. I would also like to acknowledge my wonderful parents, Ann and Raanan Wertheim (may my dad rest in peace), for instilling the values of education and developing a professional career in their children and for all the sacrifices they made along the way. Thank you to my wonderful parents-in-law for their constant interest and support in all of my endeavors. Special shout-outs to the contributors for their brilliant and dedicated work on this project and to my students who teach me more than anyone. Finally, I would like to thank my esteemed and accomplished partner in this work, Dr. Renee Fabus, for her scholarship and expertise in bringing this work to fruition.

—Cyndi Stein-Rubin, MS, CCC-SLP, TSSLD, CTA-Certified Coach

I thank all of our contributors for generously devoting their time to writing a chapter in our second edition of this text. This book would not have been possible without their dedication and diligence! I hope this book will prove to be a valuable resource for students, teachers, and novice and experienced clinicians in speech-language pathology. I would also like to acknowledge Lucille Nielsen-Rosander, who always provides excellent advice and guidance in all situations. Her students would agree that she was a first-class clinician, supervisor, and mentor in speech-language pathology. I aspire to have her knowledge and wisdom, combined with her sense of humor and approach to different situations.

—Renee Fabus, PhD, CCC-SLP, TSHH

About the Editors

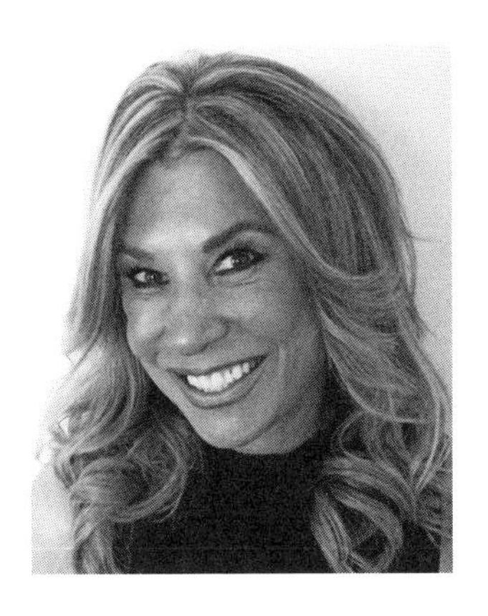

Cyndi Stein-Rubin, MS, CCC-SLP, TSSLD, CTA-Certified Coach is a retired full-time faculty member, lecturer, and clinical supervisor in the Department of Speech, Language and Hearing Department at Brooklyn College of the City University of New York (CUNY). She is a certified speech-language pathologist, professional life coach, and specialist in the field of human development. Cyndi Stein-Rubin was the recipient of the 2009 college-wide Award for Excellence in Teaching and has served on the committee for the past 4 years to select future award winners. Her area of expertise is in coaching and counseling students, clients, and families in the area of communication disorders, and her private practice focuses primarily on adults with disorders of fluency and voice. Cyndi Stein-Rubin delivers interactive and experiential workshops and presentations, drawing from fields such as psychology, counseling, and leadership. She lectures at universities, in the community, as well as internationally. She is the first author of a coauthored textbook, *A Guide to Clinical Assessment and Professional Report Writing in Speech-Language Pathology* (Cengage Learning, 2012). Her second book is *Counseling in Communication Disorders: Facilitating the Therapeutic Relationship*, coauthored by Beryl T. Adler.

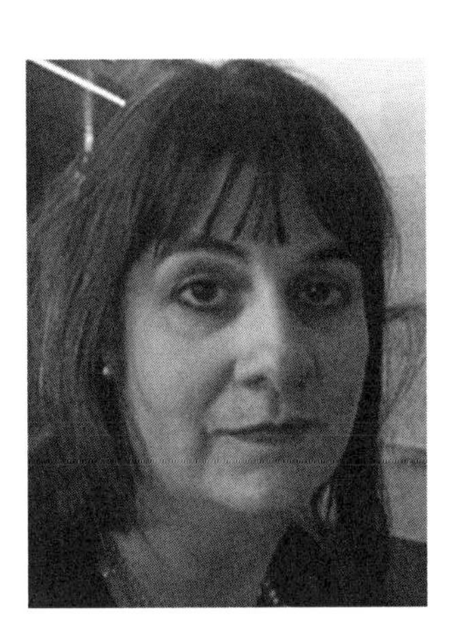

Renee Fabus, PhD, CCC-SLP, TSHH is an Associate Professor in the School of Health Technology and Management at Stony Brook University in New York. She received her bachelor's degree from New York University, her master's degree in speech-language pathology from Teachers College in New York, NY, and her PhD from Columbia University, also in New York. Dr. Fabus is a certified speech-language pathologist who has practiced in a variety of medical settings for 21 years. She has taught and supervised in programs in the New York City area and published in the areas of speech sound disorders, aphasia, dysphagia, and stuttering. She has served on various committees, boards, and editorial committees at the regional, state, and national levels.

Contributing Authors

Beryl T. Adler, MS, CCC-SLP, TSHH (Chapter 2)
Founding Partner/Clinical Supervisor
Adler, Molly, Gurland, LLC
Adjunct Lecturer
Department of Communication Arts and Sciences
Brooklyn College of the City University of New York
Brooklyn, New York

Diana Almodóvar, PhD, CCC-SLP, TSHH (Chapter 8)
Assistant Professor
Department of Speech-Language-Hearing Sciences
Lehman College of the City University of New York
Bronx, New York

Rochelle Cherry, EdD (Chapter 5)
Professor Emeritus
Brooklyn College of the City University of New York
Brooklyn, New York

Naomi Eichorn, PhD, CCC-SLP, TSSLD (Chapter 13)
Assistant Professor
School of Communication Sciences and Disorders
University of Memphis
Memphis, Tennessee

Dalia Elbaz-Pinto, MS, CCC-SLP, TSSLD (Chapter 15)
Speech-Language Pathologist
Clinical Supervisor
Department of Speech Communication Arts and Sciences
Brooklyn College of the City University of New York
Brooklyn, New York

Baila Epstein, PhD, CCC-SLP (Chapter 4)
Assistant Professor
Department of Speech Communication Arts and Sciences
Brooklyn College of the City University of New York
Brooklyn, New York

Elizabeth E. Galletta, PhD, CCC-SLP (Chapter 11)
Clinical Research Specialist, Speech Language Pathology
New York University Langone Health
Clinical Assistant Professor, Rehabilitation Medicine
New York University School of Medicine
New York, New York

Felicia Gironda, PhD, CCC-SLP (Chapters 6, 7)
Speech-Language Pathologist
Brookdale and Maimonides Medical Centers
Brooklyn, New York

Charles Goldman, MS, CCC-SLP (Chapter 1)
Board Certified Specialist-Fluency
Assistant Professor of Speech
Department of Communication Arts and Sciences
Brooklyn College of the City University of New York
Private Practice Specializing in Fluency Disorders
Brooklyn, New York

Gail B. Gurland, PhD, CCC-SLP, TSHH (Chapter 10)
Professor Emerita
Program in Speech-Language Pathology
Department of Speech Communication Arts and Sciences
Brooklyn College of the City University of New York
Brooklyn, New York

Patricia Kerman Lerner, MA, CCC-SLP, BCS-S (Chapter 14)
Clinical Assistant Professor
Department of Physical Medicine and Rehabilitation
New York University School of Medicine
New York, New York
Fellow, American Speech-Language-Hearing Association
Rockville, Maryland

Susan Longtin, PhD, CCC-SLP, TSHH (Chapter 9)
Associate Professor and Chair
Department of Speech Communication Arts and Sciences
Brooklyn College of the City University of New York
Brooklyn, New York

Klara Marton, PhD (Chapter 10)
Professor and Executive Officer
PhD Program in Speech-Language-Hearing Sciences
The Graduate School and University Center of the City University of New York
New York, New York
Department of Speech Communication Arts and Sciences
Brooklyn College of the City University of New York
Brooklyn, New York
Faculty of Special Education
Eotvos Lorand University
Budapest, Hungary

Laurie Michaels-Wilde, MS, CCC-SLP, TSSLD (Chapter 15)
Speech-Language Pathologist
Adler, Gurland, and Molly, LLC
Clinical Supervisor
Department of Speech Communication Arts and Sciences
Brooklyn College of the City University of New York
Brooklyn, New York

Susanna Musayeva, MS, CCC-SLP, TSSLD (Chapter 6)
Teacher of Speech Improvement
New York City Department of Education District 75 Citywide Speech Services
New York, New York

Dorothy Neave-DiToro, AuD, CCC-A (Chapter 5)
Assistant Professor
Brooklyn College of the City University of New York
Brooklyn, New York

Adrienne Rubinstein, PhD, CCC-A (Chapter 5)
Professor
Brooklyn College of the City University of New York
Brooklyn, New York

Natalie Schaeffer, DA, CCC-SLP (Chapters 3, 12)
Associate Professor
Clinical Supervisor
Director of Speech Laboratory
Department of Speech Communication Arts and Sciences
Brooklyn College of the City University of New York
Brooklyn, New York

Liat Seiger-Gardner, PhD, CCC-SLP (Chapter 8)
Associate Professor and Director of Graduate Students
Department of Speech-Language-Hearing Sciences
Lehman College of the City University of New York
Bronx, New York
PhD Program in Speech-Language-Hearing Sciences
The Graduate School and University Center of the City University of New York
New York, New York

Naomi Shualy, MS, CCC-SLP, TSSLD (Chapter 8)
Clinical Supervisor
Diana Rogovin Davidow Speech Language Hearing Center
Instructor
Brooklyn College of the City University of New York
Speech-Language Pathologist
Adler, Molly, & Gurland LLC
Brooklyn, New York

Tina M. Tan, MS, CCC-SLP, BCS-S (Chapter 14)
Supervisor
Pediatric Speech and Swallow Services
Department of Speech-Language Pathology
Rusk Institute of Rehabilitation Medicine
New York University Langone Medical Center
New York, New York

Amy Vogel-Eyny, MPhil (Chapter 11)
Speech-Language-Hearing Sciences
The Graduate School and University Center of the City University of New York
New York, New York

1

An Introduction to Assessment

A Diagnostic Philosophy in Speech-Language Pathology

Charles Goldman, MS, CCC-SLP

The Speech-Language Pathologist

About 45 years ago, the American Speech and Hearing Association, in the middle of an identity crisis, decided to change its name to the American Speech-Language-Hearing Association (ASHA; 2010) to account for the advancement in research, and our consequent enhanced understanding of the role of language development, in human communication. Along with this change came considerable debate. The title of *speech-language pathologist* (SLP) finally emerged as preferable to *speech therapist*, *speech correctionist*, *speech pathologist*, or *speech clinician*. The debate, although long since resolved, suggests that our predecessors believed that, despite our intentions for clarity, our field related to disorders of human communication could not easily be categorized by a single professional label.

We deal with the behavior of speech and language. Human behavior has always been at the center of psychology, and indeed many definitions of psychology reiterate this as its central provenance. There is no set of abilities more human than language-based communication, and there is no communication of greater concern to us than the communication used via our use of speech.

In dealing with behavior, psychologists study the thought and emotions that coexist with communication. An experienced and competent SLP always considers these aspects in his or her clinical contacts—so much so that the verbal behavior and the corresponding processes are inseparable. This is perhaps best encapsulated by the advice often offered by our more experienced elders in the profession: "Treat the whole person." No time in our clinical contact is as important as our initial evaluation, when we begin to form our opinions about the nature of a person's problems and the manner in which we might be able to help. Unless we can initially appreciate the clients in front of us in a way that includes their motivation, personality, and emotional reactivity, we are failing to fully understand the referral. In addition, familial, historical, and cultural factors need to be considered for accurate diagnostic impressions to be made and subsequent treatment plans to emerge. Familial contact in particular may be one of the most overlooked factors in a clinician's responsibility to treat the whole person (Rollins, 1987). With a child client, the parents are most often the providers and caretakers and the child is the dependent individual. With adults, often a significant other takes on an important caregiver role. Clients who have suffered unexpected illness or injury

Stein-Rubin, C., & Fabus, R. *A Guide to Clinical Assessment and Professional Report Writing in Speech-Language Pathology, Second Edition (pp 1-6).*

(e.g., stroke, traumatic brain injury) often find that they are dependent on specific family members. These caregivers are a most vital part of the interpersonal communicative circle of the client and as such need to be identified and addressed professionally to the same degree as the "targeted" client. In effect, a clinician beginning an evaluation with a child must assume that he or she is to treat two or three clients (i.e., the child and the child's parent or parents). Consequently, any person referred needs to be treated along with the relevant caregivers. Such thinking is essential for maximizing therapeutic outcomes.

As treatment proceeds, we continue to gather information about the behaviors and thoughts related to the communication issues revealed during the initial sessions. These treatment sessions are best perceived as a quest beginning with a more formal evaluation but always including evaluative elements in every subsequent treatment session. In doing so, we may better understand the client (and the client's communicative milieu), and we are better positioned to make adjustments to treatment rationales and methods.

The Integration of Cognitive, Physical, and Social-Emotional Factors

Speech and language behavior is part of typical growth and development for humans, and as such, we are unique in the animal world. However, we do share three areas of growth and development with the higher level animal kingdom: cognitive, physical, and social-emotional development (CPSED). It is only in human development that speech and language emerges from the combination of the three. In fact, all of the milestones in human speech and language development could also be assigned to one or more of the other areas, suggesting that it is only through our own study of human CPSED that we have come to understand typical milestones of speech and language behavior.

For an SLP conducting a diagnostic evaluation, the implication of this is critical. If we studied our clients' CPSED well enough, we would fully understand their communication behavior. Fortunately, many researchers have culled what may be considered the salient information from these areas of development and have suggested to us, through devices such as normative charts and communication disorder classification systems, usable information in the "speech-language category" of the human condition. As a clinical diagnostician, however, the task might be better approached if we were to uncover the CPSED factors for ourselves, individually, for each client we evaluate, without relying on the previously developed speech and language "lenses" of our predecessors. Nowhere is this philosophy more practically applied than during an initial clinical interview. Chapter 2 serves to expand on this viewpoint. Regardless of the potential referral problem, a clinician might best prepare for an interview with the understanding that CPSED must be investigated uniquely for each client and corresponding questions posed. It matters little whether the client is a 3 year old with a possible language delay or an adult with a recently acquired communication disorder. In either case, CPSED factors uniquely combine to shape the presenting problem and to influence the course of treatment one prescribes.

SLP as a Health Professional

An initial clinical evaluation by an SLP may lead to recommendations made to the client to seek other health professionals in conjunction with an SLP's treatment, as a condition for SLP treatment, or in lieu of SLP treatment. Especially in an era of increasing speech-language specialty certification, collaboration among other health professionals, educators, and involved "others" is almost always the best course of action.

When SLPs consider themselves "health professionals" instead of an SLP, they recognize that disorders of communication might need to be treated by multiple partners of varying training or disciplines. After all, if speech and language are the product of CPSED, then those health professionals who deal primarily with cognitive (e.g., psychologist, psychiatrist, teacher), physical (e.g., physician, occupational therapist, physical therapist), or social-emotional (e.g., psychologist, social worker, psychiatrist) issues may play an equal or even primary role in the treatment process. In other words, a diagnosing SLP who investigates a communication problem may not (depending on the individual client) take a primary role in the treatment for that client. In some cases, the presence of a significant speech-language disorder does not necessarily mean that the treating health professional should be an SLP. For example, a male adolescent who stutters mildly may be referred to you to help him manage his fluency control. In performing your evaluation, you discover that familial stress concerning a recent parental divorce is taking a heavy emotional toll on this client. Not only has his fluency control recently deteriorated, but his school grades have plummeted and he is turning to drugs for escape. An SLP who agrees to merely begin speech treatment is acting with little regard for the major life problems this young man faces. However, appealing to the individual and family caregivers to help this young man via counseling, substance abuse treatment, family therapy, or a combination of these approaches seems to be what is clinically most appropriate. In fact, accepting this individual as a client independently in your primary role as an SLP could be considered poor practice. However, those of us who have donned our "SLP blinders" may miss this greater role that an SLP should assume as a member of the health professions.

The Art of Active Listening

All people seeking an initial speech-language evaluation come to us with some version of a problem. As health professionals, we rarely resolve the referral issue by "fixing" the presenting problem, especially during an evaluation session. Because communication problems are behavioral in presentation, they are often complex in etiology. It is rare when we can offer resolution to a problem in a few easy steps or by offering some specific advice. What we can do most regularly in our work is to demonstrate to clients that we have an appreciation for their struggle and that we are making earnest attempts to see their problems as they do. This establishment of professional empathy is the way clinical trust begins. It must start from the very first diagnostic contact, and for it to be expanded and nurtured, it should be maintained throughout treatment. The single most important thing (and for most of us, a very difficult thing) a clinician can do is to listen. All of the diagnostic tools, approaches, tests, and procedures discussed in this book are secondary to our most fundamental activity. Listening is paramount because it sets the stage for empowering our clients to help themselves. The therapeutic process is about people garnering the resources in their lives toward the goal of self-help. The clinician is a guide along the way, sometimes offering the lead in the journey but always acknowledging that the trip has to be made by the client. The process of taking that journey with a knowledgeable and sensitive partner is the therapeutic process.

Our primary role, therefore, is not to make suggestions or give direction. This is not to say that these functions are unimportant or forbidden. They may, however, be overemphasized in our current "fix me" culture. The wise clinician makes suggestions and gives direction when in synch with verbal, and especially nonverbal, requests to do so. When Reik (1948) called for clinicians to "listen with their third ear," he may not have solely been providing aid to the practice of psychoanalysis. Perhaps all health professionals could be mindful of that suggestion. In effect, providing direction in a therapeutic journey that will result in your client's desired behavioral changes is often dependent on good timing from a clinician who is listening.

Near the end of an initial diagnostic evaluation, a client may ask direct questions regarding the course and nature of treatment (i.e., questions of prognosis). All too often, the beginning clinician is likely to fall back on a well intended and safe, but often meaningless, refrain: "It depends." This is frequently an unsatisfactory response that can become more twisted and misleading as one attempts to explain it further. The simple truth is that success in treatment always depends on many factors. A clinician may never be wrong in offering these words, but he or she is offering no new information, no synthesis of the information gleaned from the preceding evaluation, and no indication that he or she has begun to understand the problem from the perspective of the client(s). Instead of offering canned advice, why not review the factors involved with the client? In so doing, a mutual prognosis for treatment can be reached.

Even a beginning clinician forms opinions after spending a sizable amount of time interviewing, performing procedures, and administering tests. Your opinion regarding the information you have discovered is the way in which you earn your professional rewards. The novice clinician should become accustomed to stating opinions when it is opportune to do so. Although it may be true that you do not have the conviction of your opinions to the same degree you may have 10 years from now, you still owe it to your client to voice what you can with frank admissions of doubt if they exist, as well as with the emerging confidence you have developed in your clinical training and early professional experience.

In offering your honest opinion to a client, you are setting the stage for the respect and trust that may help shape all future therapeutic interactions. A client has sought you out to perform the evaluation, and the least you owe is an honest appraisal of the clinical picture. The prognosis for treatment and your evaluation of the severity of a presenting problem is dependent on the client's motivation, degree to which communication seems impaired, preliminary results of norm- and criterion-referenced tests and procedures, human and material resources that are available, support systems that can be tapped, and individual experience and knowledge of the clinician. All of these are factors that should be largely evident by the time a clinical opinion is offered. Review these factors with your client(s) and your therapeutic journey has begun in earnest.

Providing a Diagnostic Label

Sometimes SLPs perform evaluations for reasons secondary to helping clients deal with a presenting problem. Such evaluations are regularly performed under various circumstances to determine eligibility for services (Haynes & Pindzola, 2008). Common examples of these types of evaluations are those conducted by school systems to determine the presence of an educational disability and those conducted at the behest of an insurance company to determine reimbursement. In these circumstances, the SLP is usually bound by a finite set of classification entities that are predetermined. Although these evaluations are often the same evaluations we conduct when we respond to our clients' referral concerns, one end product of such evaluations may be a statement of eligibility or a classification label that is specific to the requirements of an outside source. The preceding are special evaluations with specific criteria involved. When more typical evaluations are performed, graduate students often ask, "In providing our opinion to our clients, do we always offer a diagnostic label?" This is a fairly complex issue that requires professional expertise, historical perspective, and pragmatic consideration.

ASHA was developed during the previous century, with stuttering a major concern of many of our founders. This one diagnostic entity, for example, is familiar to lay and professional people and is often what many today think of first when speech disorders are discussed. In addition, the disorder has roots that can be traced through thousands of years. In 1999, ASHA formed a task force on fluency terminology to define the disorder and related terms. Despite the best efforts of our professional leaders, no one definition for stuttering was discerned. It is likely that the disagreements among fluency experts arising from this document were so notable that a new task force on fluency terminology never convened; therefore, the original technical paper was rescinded in 2015. If we take the example of stuttering to suggest that the definition of a known and most researched diagnostic category can result in disagreement and confusion, it might lead us to consider the worth of classifying and labeling communication disorders at all. From a clinical perspective, a good argument can be made that the way a communication problem affects an individual is of most concern. The labeling of a problem may only confuse the client and his or her family and lead to assumptions that are untrue for specific individuals. Despite this clinical way of approaching the "labeling" question, there is much professional time and energy spent researching, defining, and redefining diagnostic entities. Stuttering is not unique in this regard. More recently, disorders such as autism, auditory processing, dyslexia, specific language impairment, Asperger's syndrome, learning disability, and sensory integration have been reconsidered due to their basic nature and the health professionals responsible for their diagnosis (ASHA, 2006).

All communication disorders are behavioral, and although some of them have been linked to genes and their influence, no disorders of communication are defined organically. Typical agents of physical disease (e.g., viruses, bacteria, chromosomal influence, mutant cell development) are generally not in the realm of discussion in diagnostic evaluations conducted by SLPs. Disorders of behavior, such as speech-language disorders, have to be defined behaviorally. This is often done by an agreed-on convention of criteria that is presented through research and study by the most influential members of the psychological community. This practice of defining disorders in this fashion is relatively new, dating back to the work of Robert Spitzer (Spiegel, 2005), when he originated the first edition of the *Diagnostic and Statistical Manual of Mental Disorders* (DSM) in the middle of the 20th century. This catalogue of disorders provides a scholarly basis on which trained health professionals may make a diagnosis. It was an attempt to reduce some of the subjectivity that previously went into the act of labeling a disorder that was not of physical origin or nature. To this day, the current fifth edition of the DSM (DSM-5) serves as a reference for practicing "mental" health professionals and consequently is published by the American Psychiatric Association (2013). Therefore, it may be initially surprising to some SLPs to find many disorders commonly encountered in our practice included in its tome. Some of these include receptive and expressive language disorder, autistic spectrum disorders, stuttering, and speech sound disorders. The inclusion of certain disorders and the exclusion of others are often strongly debated. For example, in the DSM-5, Asperger's syndrome was eliminated and included under the autistic spectrum disorders category (Wallis, 2009). For an SLP in particular, it is unclear to what the exact criteria for inclusion may be. For example, why is stuttering included, especially in view of the research evidence made directly linking it to genetic influences (Kang et al., 2010), but auditory processing disorders are absent? At least some DSM experts will argue that for a disorder to be included, there must be a high degree of agreement regarding diagnostic criteria among its contributors.

Perhaps the most important thing for an SLP to remember is that, when using a diagnostic category or label to describe a problem, you are doing no more than reiterating a list of agreed behaviors that comprise the disorder. This can well be a useful shorthand tool, but as we see with the example of the DSM, this method of categorizing what we learn about in individuals is subject to change as research and cultural understanding of the disorders change. Names and labels routinely go in and out of acceptance (e.g., think mental retardation vs. intellectual disability), and the list of symptoms that comprise these classifications change as we decide to categorize in concert with current societal and scientific thinking.

Disorders of communication involve multifactorial components and CPSED influences and are particularly subject to terminology revisions. A competent and active SLP needs to speak about findings using the latest and most agreed-on diagnostic-labeling entities. This helps establish clinical expertise and can also help create and maintain client trust. Moreover, when you share a diagnostic label with a client, it allows the client and his or her family to investigate corresponding literature and support groups and to conduct personal research involving the disorder, thereby increasing knowledge and enabling informed participation in the treatment process. The important caveat to this is to be sure that your client understands that being classified with the disorder is not synonymous with "having" the disorder. There is nothing physical that a client can have. A client can only display symptoms (i.e., behave in a certain way) that, under current classification systems, are most closely associated with a specific diagnostic entity.

An Investigative Rationale

When we conduct an evaluation to determine eligibility for services, we may often use a static assessment. In this approach to an evaluation, there may be a requirement to use a particular test or battery of tests or to adhere to some arbitrary or pre-established protocol. When we conduct an evaluation in a clinical problem-solving context, our ongoing interaction with the client is essential. This kind of interaction requires rapid clinical decision making and often greater skill in its execution. This investigative approach is a dynamic assessment and, although more challenging in nature, it is much more rewarding for both the client and clinician involved in the process (Westby, Burda, & Mehta, 2003).

A dynamic assessment begins with the first contact (often via the interview). The task at hand is to respond to the actions, questions, statements, concerns, and performance of the client(s) as effectively and efficiently as possible. It continues throughout the evaluation and is part of subsequent treatment sessions as well. An experienced and competent clinician realizes quickly that one cannot respond to every perceived client initiated notion. However, trust in your training and the development of your "clinical personality" will emerge and help guide you to respond to the most salient client behavior. The "art" of the evaluation is being able to selectively choose what to respond to and to do so in a way that furthers the mutual journey of clinical investigation and problem solving.

SLP graduate students often ask whether they should prepare a list of interview questions or a set of tasks and tests in advance of conducting an evaluation. In a static assessment, this may be routine, but in a dynamic assessment, it may hinder your listening abilities by setting off a checklist of activities that you may likely feel compelled to accomplish. Often such preparation seems to be a necessity for us (especially beginning clinicians) because of our discomfort and lack of experience with the dynamic assessment/listening process. To deny this is foolhardy, and this is why the most prudent approach may be to prepare for those questions or tasks. They can be developed in advance of the evaluation because they are solely based on the preliminary information you are likely to anticipate before you meet the client (i.e., age, nature of the communicative concern). If it were somehow possible to prepare for every eventuality during an assessment, a dynamic evaluation would not be necessary.

In effect, the questions asked and the tests and tasks presented that are not preplanned are what comprise the most significant part of the dynamic assessment. Therefore, a well-conducted dynamic assessment is a combination of interactions that are spontaneously choreographed in the interest of helping you investigate the referral problem presented. Ideally, a perfect dynamic evaluation is one in which all necessary queries are presented without superfluous investigation. The quest of the increasingly competent clinician is to get closer to this ideal as the practice of clinical art and science strive to be integrated during the course of a career.

The following chapters take you through the contributors' best guess of what you need to know that can be applied in varied clinical contexts during the investigation of myriad communication disorders affecting a diverse population of individuals in varied ways. We hope it will serve as an introduction to the graduate student and a worthwhile review for many clinicians. This knowledge is an essential part of your training and constitutes, in large measure, the crux of a dynamic evaluation. The application of this knowledge together with your developing clinical expertise and growing knowledge of your client are what constitute the art inherent in successful clinical work.

References

American Psychiatric Association. (2013). *Diagnostic and statistical manual of mental disorders* (5th ed.). Washington, DC: Author.

American Speech-Language-Hearing Association. (2006). Guidelines for speech-language pathologists in diagnosis, assessment, and treatment of autism spectrum disorders across the life span. Retrieved from http://www.asha.org/policy/GL2006-00049/

American Speech-Language-Hearing Association. (2010). History of ASHA. Retrieved from http://www.asha.org/about/history/

Haynes, W. O., & Pindzola, R. H. (2008). *Diagnosis and evaluation in speech-language pathology*. New York, NY: Pearson.

Kang, C., Riazuddin, S., Mundorff, J., Krasnewich, D., Friedman, P., Mullikin, J., & Drayna, D. (2010). Mutations in the lysosomal enzyme-targeting pathway and persistent stuttering. *New England Journal of Medicine, 362*, 677-685.

Reik, T. (1948). *Listening with the third ear: The inner experience of a psychoanalyst*. New York, NY: Farrar, Straus & Giroux.

Rollins, W. J. (1987). *The psychology of communication disorders in individuals and their families*. Englewood Cliffs, NJ: Prentice Hall.

Spiegel, A. (2005, January 3). The dictionary of disorder. *The New Yorker Annals of Medicine*. Retrieved from http://www.newyorker.com/magazine/2005/01/03/the-dictionary-of-disorder

Wallis, C. (2009, November 2). A powerful identity, a vanishing diagnosis. *The New York Times*. Retrieved from http://www.nytimes.com/2009/11/03/health/03asperger.html

Westby, C., Burda, A., & Mehta, Z. (2003). Asking the right questions in the right ways: Strategies for ethnographic interviewing. *The ASHA Leader, 8*, 4-17. Retrieved from http://leader.pubs.asha.org/article.aspx?articleid=2292396

2

Counseling and the Diagnostic Interview for the Speech-Language Pathologist

Cyndi Stein-Rubin, MS, CCC-SLP, TSSLD and Beryl T. Adler, MS, CCC-SLP, TSHH

Key Words

- already always listening
- attitude
- check in
- clarify your role
- clarifying
- clearing
- client's whole life
- co-creativity
- communication strengths
- counselor congruence
- denial
- design the alliance
- empathy
- empower
- expectations
- flow talk
- focused listening (Level II listening)
- global listening (Level III listening)
- grief
- internal listening (Level I listening)
- judgment
- language
- language of acknowledgment
- listening
- meta-view
- mind chatter
- naturally creative, resourceful, and whole
- nonverbal cues
- personal responsibility
- powerful questions
- preserve the client agenda
- process
- reflecting
- reframing
- summary probe
- willingness
- word traps

I. The Role of the Speech-Language Pathologist in the Counseling Process

The diagnostic interview is the first opportunity a speech and language pathologist (SLP)* or audiologist (AuD) has to meet with the parents, caregiver, and child with special needs, or with an individual who is seeking help for a speech, **language**, and/or hearing problem. It is essential to know how to relate, speak, listen, and gain the trust of the individual(s) seeking assistance. The first impressions made by the interviewer are often long-lasting. It is understandable that the interviewer, particularly a relatively new diagnostic

* Throughout the course of this chapter, the terms *interviewer, diagnostician, evaluator, speech clinician, clinician, therapist,* and *speech-language pathologist* (SLP) are used interchangeably.

Stein-Rubin, C., & Fabus, R. *A Guide to Clinical Assessment and Professional Report Writing in Speech-Language Pathology, Second Edition (pp 7-41).*

evaluator, would want to be recognized as someone who is knowledgeable and professional, compassionate and understanding, and self-confident yet willing to listen, as well as someone who can be trusted.

Parents seek us out as professionals for guidance and direction even though they may have their own opinions about the possible problems. The manner in which the evaluator welcomes, engages with, and listens to the family is of utmost significance. The initial phase of this relationship has a crucial impact on the direction the interview and therapy will take and on the family's response to the process. Therefore, it is essential to create a safe space for the family to share their thoughts, concerns, and fears about the future. Individuals with speech and language problems and their family members often come to us feeling lost; thus, it is at the heart of our professional responsibility to **empower** our clients and their families (Luterman, 2008a).

As we developed this chapter, we thought about our professional role and whether we are sensitive and open enough when communicating with our clients. As SLPs, we understand the physical, linguistic, and cognitive components of communication and the relevant terminology. However, we may avoid perpetuating the interpersonal piece and the honesty in genuine communication. We must be able to hear the feelings of our patients and be present to their struggle. Despite the scope of practice continually increasing the demand that we focus on the science of our profession, we must not forget the art of interpersonal communication. It is precisely the art and sensitivity that are invaluable; they are the catalysts in the healing process.

All human beings across cultures, races, and educational and economic levels share similar emotions. Despite cultural differences among individuals, there are more inherent parallels than differences. Although keeping cross-cultural differences in mind is important, it is far more productive to uncover what we, as individuals, all have in common. This creates a collaborative climate of you and me and what we can create—a climate of **co-creativity** (Whitworth, Kimsey-House, Kimsey-House, & Sandahl, 2007), which is discussed in greater detail later in the chapter. One crucial common denominator is that, at our core, we all want for each other. When a client and his or her family sit in front of us, it is crucial that we ask ourselves, "What do they want for themselves?" and "What do we want for them?"

Historically and traditionally, there have been questions about the role of the SLP in the counseling process. Is it appropriate for the SLP to counsel? Is it appropriate for the SLP to deal with the many feelings the potential clients experience? Previously, SLPs were encouraged to primarily discuss the facts and techniques related to the clients' challenges and our practice. The title speech-language "pathologist" implies that, through the techniques of our profession, we fix what is broken. A medical model of telling, explaining, and fixing, while avoiding the feelings of our clients, was at the forefront. We rarely addressed emotions. The feelings piece was relegated to psychologists, psychiatrists, and social workers. For the SLP, counseling was content centered, providing technical information only.

Content was something we as professionals could hold on to; it offered us a feeling of control. Relating subject matter was safe, predictable, structured; it is what we knew. In this way, we traditionally ended up avoiding a discussion about the client's feelings, which might include loss, pain, anger, and guilt. The open-ended nature of an emotionally charged discussion tended to intimidate and increase our feelings of insecurity in the diagnostic process. As a result, SLPs have frequently approached the role of counseling almost apologetically.

The reality is that our clients may become defensive, resistant, cry, or shut down. It is understandable that these situations are awkward for beginning diagnosticians, yet they are unavoidable when dealing with real human beings, and the ability to handle them when they arise is essential.

A close cousin to content-based counseling is telling and advising. It is far simpler to tell someone what to do than to call forth the answers from the individual. We, as professionals, tend to assume that the client comes to us for counsel in the form of advice. Ironically, the human tendency is to follow through on ideas that are born intrinsically rather than on those imposed on us from extrinsic sources. When we exclusively tell and advise our clients, we reinforce a relationship of dependency where the clients rely on us to rescue them from their circumstances (Luterman, 2008a).

Fortunately, our clinical role in the field of communication disorders has been evolving and changing. Our professional reality has been altered. Over the past 20 years, more universities have included counseling courses as part of their curriculum in speech and language therapy. The American

Speech-Language-Hearing Association (ASHA; 2006) has acknowledged the need to access parents' emotions:

> Content counseling is important for informational purposes, but emotional support and guidance through the grieving process also must be acknowledged and provided by audiologists. Furthermore, content counseling may not be successful with parents of newly identified hard of hearing children or deaf children until parents have opportunities to work through their emotions. Audiologists must acknowledge parents' feelings, which can be intense, as they engage themselves in providing emotional support and guidance through the grieving process. (ASHA, 2006, p. 9)

In addition, ASHA's Scope of Practice document includes counseling as part of the SLP's domains of responsibility: "Counseling individuals, families, coworkers, educators, and other persons in the community regarding acceptance, adaptation, and decision making about communication and swallowing" (ASHA, 2016).

The expansion and recognition of the SLP's role in the arena of counseling families of the communicatively impaired is due in great part to the work of David Luterman. Luterman's humanistic and family-centered approach to counseling has played a pivotal role in a slow-moving revolution toward infusing the human touch into the professions of speech pathology and audiology (Prizant, cited in Luterman, 2008a). The recent literature indicates that we, as communication professionals, are steadily forging new pathways in our clinical discipline as we incorporate a mental health perspective into the traditional content-based approach of the SLP. Accordingly, Geller and Foley (2009) pointed us to a reflective and affective orientation, challenging us to integrate mental health concepts into our professional expertise. They urged us to pay attention to our own as well as our client's internal affective states.

There have been two basic schools of thought in the counseling arena. One has been a directive approach based on content, informing, and advising and is results oriented. The other, a nondirective approach based on deep listening, validating, and connecting, is **process**-oriented, wherein the focus is on the relationship rather than on the goal. The nondirective or person-centered approach has its roots in Carl Rogers' (1951) branch of humanistic psychology.

Rogers (1951) highlighted the need for three critical ingredients to establish and maintain a successful therapeutic relationship: unconditional positive regard—"prizing the patient" and accepting him or her from a nonjudgmental, respectful stance; **empathy**—feeling the client's perspective as if you are truly viewing the situation standing in his or her shoes; and congruence—authenticity or genuineness where the clinician's words are aligned with internal observations and feelings, with emphasis placed on the continuous relationship.

As you read this chapter, you will notice several parallels across the aforementioned approaches: Carl Rogers' (1951) person-centered humanistic approach; David Luterman's (2008a) perspective on counseling; Geller and Foley's (2009) affective, reflective, and relational approach; and the coactive coaching model, an approach we introduce to you in the following section. Although a nondirective model forms the basis of this chapter, it is critical for the SLP to be skilled in both content and process. Providing content as well as suggestions is necessary when timed correctly and delivered with sensitivity. It is important to note that there are numerous other psychotherapy orientations to counseling, the resources for which are listed at the conclusion of this chapter.

The Importance of Addressing Emotions

The questions many of you may ask are, "What is our role and what is our responsibility as speech-language pathologists in the domain of emotions and counseling?" or "Is it within our ethical domain to deal with the emotions of our patients and their families?" You may say to yourself, "Who am I to tell these people what to do for their child, let alone how to feel?" or "Are they as frightened to hear the news as I am to give it?"

The reality is that we as professionals diagnose and treat human beings, not simply mouths or ears. Thus, we need to take into account the entire person (refer to Chapter 1 for a discussion of the interacting components of the whole person), as well as his or her family and surrounding environment. In counseling persons with communication disorders, we deal with life-altering situations, such as the news of a spouse who may never speak again, or of a child diagnosed with speech and language problems that may have an impact upon his or her future. Our clients and their families are human beings having a human experience and responding with normal human reactions to these difficult life challenges.

According to Luterman (2008a), not only is affective counseling within our domain, it is our responsibility to the client if we are to provide optimal treatment. Therefore, we, as SLPs, must be familiar with the various emotions a person with a communication disorder and his or her family may encounter in the grieving process. These reactions are cyclical and ubiquitous. We suggest that you refer to Chapter 3 of Stein-Rubin and Adler's (2016) textbook, *Counseling in Communication Disorders: Facilitating the Therapeutic Relationship*, for a more detailed discussion of the grieving cycle.

Throughout the years, we, as diagnosticians, have observed the reactions of clients and their families when a clinician overloads them with information that is likely to be perceived as stressful. The recipients of such overwhelming news, which is often the confirmation of their worst fears, tend to shut down. Under these conditions of information overload, clients and family members may have a "fight-or-flight" response. They may become defensive or resistant and struggle to absorb this information. The situation is often exacerbated when we, as professionals, present technical content and advice without regard for the individual's feelings. In contrast, there are those clients who seek to learn all they can at once, only to exhibit a delayed reaction. As clinicians, it is our responsibility to slow down the process of delivering information.

The Process

In light of the preceding discussion, the term *process* transcends several aspects of coaching and counseling clients. Just as we, as SLPs, are trained that diagnosis is an ongoing and dynamic process, we need to consider the emotional experience as a process as well. Thus, it is important that we provide the space for our clients to mentally and emotionally absorb information. The term *process* is referred to in the coactive coaching model in reference to joining with the client and meeting them where they are. The process approach to coaching focuses on the client's emotion, whether positive or negative, and encourages the client to go deeper into that feeling (Shirk, 2008).

Traditionally, as clinicians (particularly, as new clinicians), we strive to reach a definitive conclusion as efficiently as possible. Ironically, more is revealed in a clinical interview and counseling session when we approach the client from an authentically curious place. We must remain open to what is present in that moment. More is also learned over time when the partnership relationship is formed between the client and therapist. We need to trust in the process, provide the space and opportunity for our clients to process their emotions, and then get out of the way. As a result, our clients and their families will share, find their own way, and heal themselves. Attempting to take short cuts would be counterproductive and harmful.

Being Present

One of the biggest challenges to a clinician and, particularly, for a new counselor is the capacity to be present or fully attuned to the immediate moment, with a client or family's tears, pain, or other negative emotions. As caring individuals in a helping profession, our instinct is to cheer up our clients, make their sadness go away, and find them a "bright side." Although well intentioned, this "Pollyannaish" attitude implies that pain is taboo. This perspective, where any shred of negative emotion must be avoided, immediately alters the space, which serves as a container to hold the relationship (Geller & Foley, 2009). It is essential for the clinician to recognize these emotions and resist the urge to fix them, make them go away, or dodge them. It is only when the individual is given permission to fully experience his or her sadness or pain that he or she can move through the feeling and get down to the business of problem solving.

Oriah "Mountain Dreamer" House (1999) asks a relevant and powerful question in her poem, "The Invitation": "I want to know if you can sit with pain, mine or your own, without moving to hide it, fade it, or fix it."*

Clients and families have cried in our sessions. One cannot predict when this will occur. When it does happen, it may take us by surprise and cause us to freeze. It is not an unusual surprise that this encounter with a client may be the first time that he or she has let go and expressed fear or anguish. Clients have shared how their past attempts to express their emotions were met with reassurance by well-meaning family and friends. These confidants insisted that, "Things aren't that bad." These individuals advised our clients to "count their blessings," "appreciate what they have," or they simply changed the subject. As a result, our clients have conveyed the relief they experienced when they were given the space to lean into their emotion and the permission to release and express their pain.

Ironically, the being part is difficult for us as human beings; in reality, we behave more like human doings. It is in the being, rather than in the doing, that we

---

*From the poem "The Invitation" by Oriah "Mountain Dreamer" House from her book *The Invitation*, ©1999. Published by HarperOne, San Francisco, CA. All rights reserved. Printed with permission of the author. http://www.oriah.org

create the space for an evolving relationship to give our clients greater access to "self." The being part is what we might strive for to connect more fully to both our professional and personal lives.

When a client sheds tears and we feel uncomfortable, it is worthwhile to reflect on Oriah's question. Then, take her question a step further as we ask ourselves:

- "Why can't we sit with pain?"
- "Who is more uncomfortable and awkward with our client's tears—the client or ourselves?"
- "What can't we be with here and why?"

The more clients and families who cross our thresholds, and the greater the sphere of our experience in the profession, the more we realize that we must prepare for the reality that human mess is an integral and unavoidable part of humanness.

Geller and Foley (2009) proposed the following solution: "If professionals are trained to apply psychological constructs to their clinical relationships, they will become more reflective and less reactive to emotionally charged material." This challenge transcends therapeutic relationships and extends to our personal interactions as well. It is our hope that this chapter will help guide us toward trusting both ourselves and the process of human interaction. To empower our clients, we must develop the capacity to create a nonjudgmental space for their normal human emotions, including pain, **grief**, fear, and guilt.

Locus of Control

From passive victim to active agent.

—Manning (2009)

Central to the idea of client empowerment is the concept of imbuing clients with an internal locus of control. An internal as opposed to external locus of control means the client is secure in the feeling that the events in his or her life are within his or her power or ability to manage. People with an external locus of control believe that the events in their lives happen to them and that people do things to them. These are the individuals who will most likely be crying, "You are not going to believe what he did to me." People with an internal locus of control are more likely to believe that they have choice. Although they may not be able to control certain life circumstances, they are able to choose the way they react to those events. These self-empowered individuals have the capacity to notice their self-critical thoughts. They may then go on to challenge or dispute these destructive beliefs.

On the other hand, when positive things occur in their lives, individuals with an internal locus will more likely attribute these events to their skills, **attitude**, attributes, or choices they make (Manning, 2001). To facilitate our clients' external to internal shift, we need to provide the space for negative emotions and help our clients clarify and magnify their strengths. For additional information on locus of control, the reader is referred to Chapter 13 of this book.

Positive Psychology and a Strengths Perspective

Addressing weakness is important; however, positive psychologists emphasize that it is equally important, if not more so, to focus on and amplify strengths. As SLPs, we spend proportionately less time identifying and developing the strengths of our clients and their families. In contrast to "fixing weakness," by developing natural talents and strengths, we may achieve excellence. Moreover, once strengths are clarified, they may be used, indirectly, as a productive strategy to address weakness. According to Buckingham and Clifton (2001), we grow the most in areas of strength and slowest in areas of weakness. Nevertheless, human nature and society tends to encourage us to spend more time "fixing" what is deficient.

Take a moment to think about the last time someone expressed something positive about you. Compare how long-lasting the effects were compared with when you were criticized. Positive feedback tends to move right through us; we do not fully take it in. On the other hand, many of us hold on to and dwell on negative feedback or criticism.

Praise/Feedback

They don't need you to perform so they know how good YOU are; they need you to love them, so they know how good THEY are.

—(Source unknown)

The manner in which we provide praise or feedback is central to increasing self-esteem in ourselves and in others. Barbara Fredrickson (2009) discovered that individuals require a three-to-one ratio of positive to negative experiences or feedback to balance out the negative. In other words, for every one negative experience, we actively need to engage in three positive experiences to thrive. This revolutionary research has crucial implications when providing feedback to our clients and students. Although individuals require more positive than negative experiences to feel encouraged, a proportionately smaller degree of constructive responding is warranted. Negative feedback, when delivered with sensitivity and in a foundation of acknowledging the client's and family members' strengths, results in a positive response. Furthermore, the three-to-one ratio, which incorporates constructive feedback, solidifies trust and provides the receiver with the assurance that he or she is being given productive suggestions. Bear in mind that this ratio is an average and provides the concept of a proportion; it is not a fixed number.

Despite the importance of assuming a strengths perspective, as SLPs trained in the medical model, we may group clients under a generic label. This orientation assumes a deficits perspective, stripping our clients of their individuality, and they become the problem named. For example, one who stutters becomes the stutterer, and the human being is lost. Janice Fialka (1997) poignantly highlighted this sentiment in the following poem, written from a parent's perspective.

Advice to Professionals Who Must "Conference Cases"

Before the case conference,
I looked at my almost five-year-old son
and saw a golden-haired boy
who giggled at his baby sister's attempts to clap her hands,
who charmed adults by his spontaneous hugs and hellos,
who often became a legend in places visited

because of his exquisite ability to befriend a few special souls,
Who often wanted to play "peace marches"
And who, at the age of four,
went to the Detroit Public Library
requesting a book on Martin Luther King.

After the case conference,
I looked at my almost five-year-old son.
He seemed to have lost his golden hair.
I saw only words plastered on his face,
Words that drowned us in fear,
Words like:
Primary Expressive Speech and Language Disorder,
Severe Visual Motor Delay,
Sensory Integration Dysfunction,
Fine and Gross Motor Delay,
Developmental Dyspraxia and RITALIN now.

I want my son back. That's all.
I want him back now. Then I'll get on with my life.

If you could see the depth of this pain
If you feel this sadness
Then you would be moved to return
Our almost five-year-old son
who sparkles in sunlight despite his faulty neurons.

Please give us back my son
undamaged and untouched by your labels, test results,
descriptions and categories.
If you can't, if you truly cannot give us back our son
Then just be with us

quietly, gently, softly.

Sit with us and create a stillness
known only in small, empty chapels at sundown.
Be there with us
as our witness and as our friend.
Please do not give us advice, suggestions, comparisons or
another appointment. (That is for later.)

We want only a quiet shoulder upon which to rest our heads.

If you cannot give us back our sweet dream
then comfort us through this evening.
Hold us. Rock us until morning light creeps in.
Then we will rise and begin the work of a new day.

Source: From the book, *What Matters: Reflections on Disability, Community and Love* (2016) by Janice M. Fialka (Inclusion Press). www.danceofpartnership.com. To hear and watch a video of this poem, visit https://youtu.be/fXVBkaLAs80.

When we emphasize deficit, it affects not only the manner in which we view our clients, but the way in which we interact with them as well. This generates a self-fulfilling prophecy, or self-limiting belief, which indicates that labeling is disabling. The Social Model of Disability (Snow, 2007) maintains the position that it is society, rather than individuals with disabilities, that is disabled. This theory emphasizes the importance of altering society's perspective rather than striving to "fix" the client. Kathie Snow summarizes this view eloquently in the following excerpt:

> Nothing short of a paradigm shift in how we think about disability is necessary for change to occur. Disability, like ethnicity, religion, age, gender, and other characteristics, is a natural part of life. Some people are born with disabilities; others acquire them later in life. (And if we live long enough, many of us will acquire a disability through an accident, illness, or the aging process.)
>
> A disability label is not the defining characteristic of a person, any more than one's age, religion, ethnicity, or gender is the defining

characteristic. We must never use a disability label to measure a person's value or predict a person's potential. And we must recognize that the presence of a disability is not an inherent barrier to a person's success.

We do not need to change people with disabilities! We need to change ourselves and how we think about disability. When we think differently, we'll talk differently. When we think and talk differently, we'll act differently. When we act differently, we'll be creating change in ourselves and our communities. In the process, the lives of people with disabilities will be changed, as well.

Source: Excerpt from "A Gentle Revolution" by Kathie Snow (n.d.), as quoted from *Disability Is Natural*, www.disabilityisnatural.com. © Braveheart Press. Reprinted with permission.

An Inventory of Strengths

Martin Seligman (2002), the "father of positive psychology" (the science of happiness, human thriving, and flourishing) cited and described character strengths and virtues that are valued and ubiquitous across races, cultures, and religions. Seligman's work was born out of the discovery that the absence of negative emotion does not imply the existence of the positive state. For example, happiness is not defined as the absence of depression. This observation gave rise to positive psychologists seeking to systematically study and establish what was right with normal individuals as opposed to what was weak in patients with psychiatric disorders.

In his search for human attributes rather than human weakness, Seligman created a psychological manual of strengths to complement the *Diagnostic and Statistical Manual of Disorders*, the medical diagnostic handbook published by the American Psychiatric Association. Some of the strengths identified by Seligman (2002) include courage and valor, wisdom and the ability to see another's perspective, kindness and mercy, empathy, and leadership. Although our society is constantly in pursuit of perfection, one of the most universally prized character traits is genuineness and authenticity—the capacity to be real, the ability to be transparent.

The findings and concepts of this recently established branch of psychology mesh well with the needs of our profession. Each individual we encounter possesses a core of attributes, talents, and strengths. Part of our role is to call forth our clients and their family members to examine what has worked to get them to where they are today, despite their challenges. It is crucial that we then need to highlight those attributes, thereby giving our clients greater access to their individual core virtues. We therefore opt to view the clients' and family members' strengths rather than identifying them by their disorders.

To get in touch with your own strengths and personal attributes, we ask that you take a moment to write down three things that you like about yourself. It may help to call on several close family members or friends to provide an example of what they see as a unique force in you. Pay attention to the way you use that strength every day as you begin to claim it, own it, and further develop the talent. As we learn to appreciate our own strengths, we open the pathway for recognizing those of our clients.

1. ________________________________
2. ________________________________
3. ________________________________

How would shifting your lens from one of labeling a client to seeing the core strengths of the individual empower your clients and their families? How would it empower you? What will you say to a young boy who stutters when he claims, "I am not really a normal boy because a normal boy knows how to speak"? There are several roads you may take to respond to a client's statement such as this in a way that empowers him or her. There is no one correct response or answer.

When an individual shares an experience or emotion directly or indirectly, listening deeply without **judgment** and holding no agenda other than the client's makes the other individual feel fully witnessed and, as a result, empowered. A response that paraphrases and reflects back the message you hear behind the words is empowering for the client; he or she feels heard and valued (e.g., "It must be hard; you know just what you want to say but you can't say it when you want to."). In this way, we allow the client permission to be human (Manning, 2009)—a rare gift that we often do not make available, especially for ourselves. Once the client's feelings are validated and understood, we may then coach the client to **reframe** the event to the positive, to what works or has worked in the past, rather than focusing on what is weak. A strategy similar to the previous exercise may help the client shift his or her perspective. Eliciting the client's signature strengths may require prompting by coaching him or her through the exercise.

One way of drawing out an individual's strengths is by tapping into his or her core values. Values are the aspects of life that are important to a person:

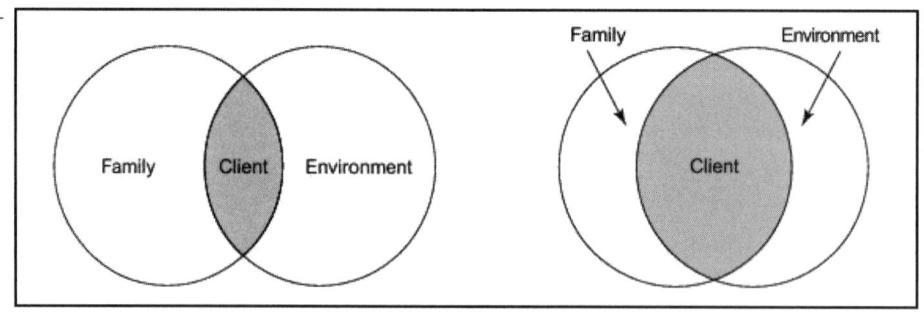

Figure 2-1. Impact of family and environment on client success.

experiences, activities, settings, goals, or relationships that the individual would not want to live without. The following **powerful questions** may help gain access to a client's signature strengths:

- What are you doing when you do not even notice the passage of time?

  ____

- Describe one outstanding experience or time in your life when you felt strong?

  ____

- How would your best friend describe you?

  ____

As you will see in the following section, it is critical to highlight and amplify the strengths for our clients as well as for their families. The previous exercise may be applied to counseling sessions and workshops with parents, spouses, and other family members.

The Role of the Family

By enrolling the family in the client's diagnosis and therapy, the entire structure of the clinical interaction is altered from solely the client to include the relationship with the family. In focusing on this relationship, we minimize the possibility of **denial** and resistance and empower the individuals to make productive decisions (Kalmanson & Seligman, 2006). To further facilitate the client's and family members' self-confidence, it is important to highlight the strengths of the team. Consistent with this, Luterman (2008a) noted that maternal self-esteem is the most positive prognostic indicator for children with literacy impairment.

The ideal collaborative alliance, in the best interest of the child, is between the clinician and family. If the feelings of family members are not honored, the likelihood of successful treatment is diminished. According to Napier and Whitaker (1978), the unit in human life with the most powerful dedication to growth is the family. They view the therapist as the "catalytic agent" who "unlocks" the family's own internal resources. The strengths of both the family and the child are viewed as pivotal factors in transformation.

The critical importance of the strengths of the family is further highlighted in the Hanen Centre training programs for parents, where parents' strengths in dealing with their children are specifically highlighted (Girolametto & Weitzman, 2006).

By listening to patients and family members of persons with disabilities, validating and valuing their views, we catalyze transformation in them and indirectly foster the clients' progress. We cannot underestimate the importance placed on the attention to the family as well as to a client's overall environment. Thus, we address the whole client and the **client's whole life** (Figure 2-1).

II. Developing the Therapeutic Relationship in Communication Disorders

For us to unify what we have proposed thus far, specific to the needs of our clients, it is our obligation to develop our own congruence. As noted earlier, **counselor congruence** implies an alignment between the intellectual and emotional components of self and the individual's actions. Congruence denotes that the person's actions are consistent with his or her core values; the individual is centered. For SLPs to achieve congruence, we must work on our own centering; hone our listening skills; sharpen our self-awareness; and have keener access to our own feelings, strengths, and core values. We must know who we are as we get to know who our clients are. As Maslow advised, "We must remember that knowledge of one's own deep nature is also simultaneously knowledge of human nature in general." It is only when counselors address and understand their own needs and are secure enough not to need to be the expert that they are fully present for the client (Luterman, 2008a).

For effective and compassionate interviewing/counseling, it is essential to develop the skills of **listening** and speaking in ways that will foster confidence in the people in need of our support and guidance. There is no room for judgment, self-righteousness, pressure, or arrogance in the clinical relationship. These attitudes form barriers between us and the people with whom we work. Our goal, on the other hand, is to create a safe alliance, not an adversarial one. Moreover, when we collaborate with our clients and their families, we can hear them more fully and learn more deeply. An equal and collaborative relationship creates the space for partnership, sharing, learning, and transformation. Thus, we become the catalysts in designing a powerful alliance. The power of counseling is in the relationship (Haynes & Pindzola, 2008; Whitworth et al., 2007).

Albert Murphy (1982) eloquently expressed this power as follows:

> Happiness in the noblest sense comes in large measure through helping relationships with others, stretching our professional resources and the resource of the mind and the heart. Every now and then something in our deeper selves enables us to realize that what truly counts. In life is not a matter of what is in you or what is in me but of what occurs between us. That divine spark of relationship may be the most fundamental life force of all. (p. 402)

As new evaluators, we may find that we fluctuate between our own fears of wanting to make a good impression on the family and the arrogance that may come with thinking that, as the professional, we have all the answers. This is a trap that detracts from the counseling process where compassion and understanding are essential.

Who are we as human beings sitting across from the family; how well do we know ourselves? How much have we done to develop our own congruence? To facilitate our own personal development as well as our clients' growth, we invite you to explore a coaching approach, mentioned previously, derived from the coactive coaching model (Whitworth et al., 2007).

Several hallmarks of the coactive coaching model include listening, curiosity, and the use of intuition. In addition, the cornerstones of the model encourage us to hold all human beings as **naturally creative, resourceful, and whole**, to **design the alliance** with our clients, to **preserve the client's agenda** at the forefront, and to address the client's whole life. (The last cornerstone, the client's whole life, was addressed previously in the background section of this chapter.) This previous belief of addressing the client's whole life supports all previous discussion referring to the importance placed on the involvement of the family and environment. We now take a look at the impact these assumptions and skills have on the counseling relationship.

The Client as Naturally Creative, Resourceful, and Whole

First, the model holds all human beings as naturally creative, resourceful, and whole (Whitworth et al., 2007); nothing broken and nothing to fix. All individuals possess inherent wisdom and solutions to many of their life problems. The coach or counselor trusts that the wisdom and solutions lie within the client. Intrinsic to this philosophy is the confidence that each person already carries the seeds for his or her own transformation and is therefore the expert on his or her own life. Similarly, we have learned from our experience that parents have a wealth of information about their children. It is our role to honor their accounts and to draw out this valuable content. Removing our "expert factor" becomes pivotal and transformative in fulfilling the mission of relationship. By trusting in the client's wisdom and the family's knowledge, we minimize dependency and foster empowerment. People may say they want advice; however, think about your response the last time you were being told or advised. How likely were you to own the behavior and follow through on this advice?

Many of us are familiar with the phenomenon of a self-fulfilling prophecy. Research in the areas of business and education has indicated that, when student or employee **expectations** are held high, performance increases. The same is true of the opposite: interacting with an individual as if he or she is incapable may diminish his or her ability to perform. If we subscribe to the core belief of the human capacity for change, we have faith in the inherent competence and resourcefulness of individuals and families.

Therefore, every one of us is naturally creative, resourceful, and whole. In addition, each clinician brings his or her unique style, gifts, and resources to the counseling relationship. The focus for each of us, in the counseling process, is to trust in our natural resources and in our inherent ability to connect with people. Like Rogers (1951), the coactive coaching approach "prizes the client" and believes in the power of human potential.

How does your paradigm shift when we do not have to be perfect? Take a few moments to reflect on the following questions in writing:

- What shifts when we are also held as naturally creative, resourceful, and whole?

____
____
____

- What changes when we trust in our ability to connect with people?

____
____
____

- What if we did not have to know everything?

____
____
____

- What difference would it make if we did not have to be perfect?

____
____
____

- How would the relationship look if our clients did not have to be perfect?

____
____
____

Designing the Alliance

Second, the co-active model advocates designing the alliance (Whitworth et al., 2007). What does this really mean?

The co-active coaching model places explicit emphasis on the designed alliance that is formulated between coach and client. This co-created relationship forms a container in which coaching/counseling occurs, similar to what is described by developmental theorists as a holding environment (Daloz, 1999). This holding environment created by the designed alliance provides a climate of trust between the coach and the client. This creative alliance is what makes the coaching approach so effective. Coaching is a co-creative relationship. Co-creativity means to create from another and to discover ourselves through each other (Whitworth et al., 2007).

As discussed in the earlier section "The Role of the Family," we design a co-creative alliance with our clients and also with their families. As coaches, we function like giant mirrors for our clients. There is an opportunity here for the coach and client to join together collaboratively for the sake of client growth. Both coach and client use all of their knowledge, resources, skills, and intuition to problem solve. In designing the alliance, we, as counselor/coach, remove the expert factor. Consequently, there is no authority figure and hence no dependence. The idea is to help the client connect to his or her own personal power as well as his or her own **personal responsibility**. This concept facilitates and supports our client to become part of the process of helping him- or herself.

In describing strong learning partnerships characterized by deep trust, adult educator Laurent Daloz (1999) said:

> To engender trust is central to any strong, nurturing relationship. Although the trust that characterizes an early relationship owes much of its strength to the ascribed authority of the teacher, more mature trust is sustained increasingly by the shared commitment of each partner. It must be constantly recreated. (p. 176)

As SLPs, we are skilled when it comes to establishing rapport. Once rapport is established, however, our focus shifts to the science component of the therapeutic relationship, and the relationship part may fade into the background. To preserve and develop the partnership relationship, it is not sufficient to welcome and make the client feel comfortable. Similar to all interpersonal interactions, the therapeutic relationship itself must be enriched and "recreated." As highlighted in the introduction to the chapter, the power that generates transformation (in both client and coach) is in the relationship. This power has a ripple effect. By continuously and consciously reflecting on our own and our client's internal worlds, we magnify trust and deepen the connection. This intimate connection benefits our clients and their families, intensifies our personal and professional gratification, and multiplies the impact of our clinical interactions exponentially.

Preserving the Client's Agenda

According to Luterman (2008a, 2000b), "The professional sets aside his agenda to engage in deep selfless listening to the client." It is crucial that we listen to our clients' voices, honor their accounts, and resist superimposing our theories upon their views. The co-active way underscores preserving the client agenda (Whitworth et al., 2007) at the forefront and supporting it. It is interesting that when one asks a clinician to predict what the client hopes to accomplish in therapy, the client's response is often inconsistent with the therapist's prediction. Asking the client to clarify goals and aspirations from the clinical process signifies respect, helps us glean critical information, and makes it more likely that the client will follow through. As Saleeby (2006) eloquently states, "The most reliable text cannot be found in the universal and abstract features of the theory; rather, it is contained within the story our clients will tell us about their lives." The client's agenda must consistently remain at the forefront with the coach supporting it throughout the relationship. When it comes to children with significant challenges such as autism spectrum disorders, we learn about their agenda by following their lead (The Hanen Centre, n.d.). It is important that we learn about the hopes and dreams of the family members and that we preserve their agenda as well.

One of the biggest challenges for the listener, coach, or counselor is to self-manage his or her own reactions, judgments, and internal comparisons (Whitworth et al., 2007). Psychologists and psychiatrists call the aforementioned phenomenon *projection*, or the tendency for an individual to subconsciously impose his or her needs, history, feelings, and views on what another person is expressing. How often have we wanted to intercede with a story or similar life situation and solution? Our mantra needs to be, "This is not about me." To free ourselves of judgment and to be truly open to what our client is telling us, we must constantly attempt to see things from the client's point of view and not through the lens of our own values, priorities, and experience.

We suggest that you take a few minutes to reflect on the following questions:

- How often have we, as professionals, found ourselves assuming the agenda with our clients?

  ____

  ____

- What opens up for us as clinicians when we ask our clients what they want to accomplish from the diagnostic meeting, rather than telling them what they should be doing?

  ____

  ____

- How might shifting the focus to the client's agenda alter the outcome?

  ____

  ____

To preserve the client's agenda and preclude judgment and an attachment to the outcome, the coach maintains a sincere curiosity about the client. Accordingly, curiosity and **focused listening** are major aspects of the co-active coaching environment.

Listening

To preserve the client's agenda and to truly hear what he or she needs, we must learn to listen well or to pay attention on a deep level. Listening is the foundation of the therapeutic relationship. The experience of truly being listened to is a powerful gift, partly because it is so rare. Taking the time to completely focus on another human being and make him or her feel heard has effects that are healing and transformative. For example, can you recall a favorite childhood relative such as an aunt, uncle, grandparent, or cousin who you considered special? Chances are it was because that person listened deeply to you, paid attention to you, and acknowledged who you were in the world.

Most people do not listen at a very deep level. Certainly, some individuals are inherently better listeners than others; it comes naturally to them. Fortunately, with practice, listening is a skill that can be developed and improved. As SLPs, we will frequently teach others how to listen and what to listen for, yet how often do we heed our own advice? Do we distinguish between listening and hearing? As professionals, it is our responsibility to develop our own congruence and enhance our own relationship skills, and thus we have devoted a chapter in our book, *Counseling for Communication Disorders: Facilitating the Therapeutic Relationship* to listening (Chapter 5 in Stein-Rubin & Adler, 2016). We encourage you to explore that work and develop and hone your listening skills. In the meantime, we invite you to take this opportunity to get curious about your listening skills and to discover what type of listener you are. Fill out the Listening Survey in Rebecca Shafir's book, *The Zen of Listening* (2000), score it, and examine the interpretation of your score.

When we listen to others, we tend to hear them through our own filters. Filters alter what we hear by imposing our own story on what the other individual is expressing. Our filters are the result of environmental, societal, experiential, emotional, and personality-based influences. These filters may occlude our ability to be fully present in our listening. Often, we think we are listening, yet we jump to conclusions or misinterpret what has been said. In certain instances, we are in mutual agreement and consequently perceive that we are aligned with each other. In contrast, another individual's comments and questions may stir up our own insecurities. In these instances, we hear something that could be an emotional trigger, our defenses come up, and we are gone. We are no longer fully present in our listening, and what the other individual is relating becomes all about us. It is challenging but crucial that we train ourselves in the capacity to make our mind blank in our mission to make the interaction all about them (Coach Training Alliance, 2005). Similarly, parents' listening is also affected by these dynamics. It has been said that parents have the capacity to listen for the first few minutes. As soon as the parents hear stressful news, they have figuratively left the room.

It is important to realize that each of us may bring subconscious information to a conversation. These thoughts may interfere with the original intentions of the speaker as well as with the listener's listening. In addition, sometimes we think we know where a conversation is going because a voice in our head takes the listening in that direction. Consequently, we react to the person as if we already know what he or she will say. This tendency has been effectively called **already always listening** (Landmark Worldwide, n.d.). This behavior also interferes with communication.

As we continue reading and developing our listening skills we may use these questions as a guide:

- How well have we learned to listen in our everyday lives?
- Are we able to tone down the many voices in our heads to truly hear what another person is saying?
- Do we succumb to a desire to interrupt, take over the conversation, or change direction without agreement or warning?
- Do we ask for clarification to better understand what another person is saying?
- How do we deal with silence and pauses? Do they make us uncomfortable, or do we view them as opportunities to invite a response?
- How frequently are we in a conversation when we suddenly realize that we have ignored what another person has said, changed the intent to meet our own, or have attempted to control the person's reaction?
- How often have we actually brought something to the conversation that was never there in the first place?
- How many times do we impose our judgments and opinions even when not asked?
- How often have we tried to fix rather than listen?
- Have we learned to be fully present?

Let us take a look at the three levels of listening identified and developed by the co-active coaching model (Whitworth et al., 2007). We briefly describe each of these three levels. Developing an awareness of and skill in the different levels will lead to greater presence and confidence in the counseling process and to effective communication.

Level I Listening (Internal Listening)

This level of listening is **internal listening** and has the spotlight on "me." It is our interpretation that everything spoken is about us and is thus egotistical in nature. **Level I listening** is full of **mind chatter**. Mind chatter refers to the ongoing dialogue in a person's head that distracts our focus and is full of judgment. Although our clients and their families are appropriately at Level I, it is not optimal for the diagnostic clinician to be at Level I Listening.

Level II Listening (Focused Listening)

The second level is focused listening and requires laser sharp concentration on the other party. In **Level II listening**, we listen to the words as well as to the meaning behind the words. When we are in Level II, we function as giant mirrors that reflect everything back to our clients. In this way, the client hears him- or herself more clearly. As the clinician develops focused listening, he or she learns to assume a meditative state, quiets mind chatter, uses silent pauses creatively, and becomes fully present to the client's words. To facilitate this mind-state, we suggest forming a mental image of "becoming blank": bundling up thoughts with a string and imagining placing them in a drawer. Then turn your attention back to the client (Coach Training Alliance, 2005).

Level III Listening (Global Listening)

Level III listening is **global listening** and means "listening" with all of your senses. At this higher and more integrated level of listening, the professional becomes aware of the shifts in client posture, changes in energy and mood, and even tuning into what is not verbalized. Level III Listening is what actors and actresses call "soft focus." This is taking in the atmosphere and energy all around the "bubble" that encapsulates you and the client. This is what Daniel Goleman (1995) referred to as the element of emotional intelligence, called *intuition*. When using your intuition and Level III listening, it is prudent to be aware of your gut reactions and at the same time to be tactful. The more experienced the student clinician becomes, the more confident he or she will be in expressing these intuitive hunches (e.g., "I get the feeling that …"; "I have a sense that …"). In addition, it is important to check these intuitive hits out with our clients with phrases such as, "How does that sound to you?"

Experiment with listening deeply at Level II and Level III in your everyday communicative interactions. Try it with the individual who cleans your workplace, the person behind the counter in the fast-food chain or bakery, your child, your colleagues, and your spouse or significant other. What do you notice about your listening? What is the impact of Level II and III Listening on your relationships?

Do we take the time to ask questions such as the following:

- "Let me see if I understand what you are saying …"
- "Do you mean …"
- "I'm not sure if I'm following your line of thinking …"

The following piece illustrates the transformative power of listening.

Please Listen

When I ask you to listen to me and you start giving advice you have not done what I ask.

When I ask you to listen to me and you begin to tell me why I shouldn't feel that way you are trampling on my feelings.

When I ask you to listen to me and you feel you have to do something to solve my problem, you have failed me, strange, as that might seem.

Listen! All I asked was that you listen. Not talk or do—just hear me.

And I can do for myself: I am not helpless. Maybe discouraged and faltering, but not helpless.

When you do something for me that I can and need to do for myself you contribute to my fear and weakness.

But, when you accept as a simple fact that I do feel what I feel, no matter how irrational, then I can quit trying to convince you and can get about the business of understanding what's behind this irrational feeling.

And when that's clear, the answers are obvious and I don't need advice.

Irrational feelings make sense when we understand what is behind them.

Perhaps that is why prayer works, sometimes for some people because G is mute, and He does not try to fix things. He just listens and lets you work it out for yourself.

So, please listen and just hear me. And, if you want to talk, wait a minute for your turn and; I will listen to you.

Source: Author unknown; as cited in Luterman, 2008a

There are several factors that influence our listening and communication. First is our judgment about what we observe and hear, second is the language we use and how it shapes our internal and external reality, and third is our expectations and preconceived notions about the people with whom we work.

Judgment

We are all human beings and, by nature, humans judge. We judge others on their appearance, on what they say, on their actions, and on their choices. In short, we tend to judge others on just about everything, and in turn, everyone else judges us. We suggest that you take a look (in the mirror) when you point your finger. Many of us have come to acknowledge that we also judge ourselves harshly. We may be our own harshest critics. Just as judging another has the effect of shutting down that individual, judging ourselves harshly will not serve us in the assessment process.

One of the most disturbing ways diagnosticians and clinicians judge relates to parental behavior. If a parent's response is tearful, we need to notice our own level of discomfort. If a parent's reaction is defensive, we may not realize that there is underlying grief or deep sorrow. There may be feelings of loss in response to a catastrophic change. When we listen on a deep level, we hear parents mourn the loss of their dream:

- The dream of a normal and perfect child; the child who does not meet their personal standard
- The dream of protecting that child from harm regardless of the circumstances
- The dream of who they were in this world as defined by their roles, which no longer fit or apply in the same way

The judgments we make as clinicians about family members often overlook their struggle with acceptance to bad news. The result is that we find ourselves judging their normal human responses to denial. Denial is a normal human coping mechanism for a trying situation whereby the individual does not psychologically "own" the problem or his or her grief. It is important to keep in mind that these responses are not exclusive to the parent–child relationship; they also apply to adult family members with communication disorders.

How often do we criticize parental behavior before we attempt to listen, assist, guide, and support them? How frequently do we reflexively shift into judgment mode when they do not carry out our recommendations? After all, how many of us have had the attitude, at one time or another, that since we are the professionals, we expect people to listen; they should listen. When our expectations are not fulfilled, we judge. What do those judgments really say about us?

Curiosity

One of the biggest antidotes to judgment is curiosity. If we remain open in our attitudes and authentically curious about the human being in front of us, we approach the entire diagnostic process from a more productive stance. It is almost impossible to maintain a genuinely curious attitude and to be judgmental at the same time.

By the same token, we could become really curious about ourselves and ask why we react in a particular way in a specific situation. For example, if a client or parent questions our diagnostic assessment, we may take it personally and react defensively. Instead, in that moment, it is important to ask ourselves what are we overacting to and why we are defending ourselves. Is this about our own insecurity or is it the fear that perhaps we might be wrong? It would be more productive to ask curious questions about what the other individual might be thinking and feeling. Their views and opinions are valuable resources for building the relationship and creating solutions together. Furthermore, on the basis of our clinical experience, we suggest that clinicians form a collaborative partnership, thus bridging the gaps formed by defensiveness, denial, and resistance. This co-creativity, or creating from each other, breaks down the walls that result from judgment and preconceived notions.

Evaluation Versus Judgment

This discussion would be incomplete if we did not distinguish between evaluating and judging. What is the difference between maintaining a judgmental vs. an evaluative attitude (Haynes & Pindzola, 2008)? The word *evaluative* denotes objectivity, whereas *judgment* implies subjectivity. In the word *evaluation*, there is spaciousness and possibility. When we adopt an evaluative stance, we are not sure exactly how things will turn out. While evaluating, we are moving in the direction of a means to an end and exploring possibilities. In contrast, judgment implies finality, restriction—a premeditated decision.

It is crucial for each of us to recognize the ways in which we judge others. Try the following exercise. Write five ways that you have judged others both personally and professionally. Describe the impact of each on the relationship.

1. ______________________________

____

2. ______________________________

____

3. ______________________________

____

4. ______________________________

____

5. ______________________________

____

Language

The language we use influences how people listen (Kegan, 2000). Our language discloses our judgments, attitudes, emotions, compassion, and sensitivity. When we tell a parent or patient to do something that we believe is important, the words we select to express the thought set up the entire listening process. The receiver of the message notices and hears everything through his or her own filters and may then be influenced by his or her own judgment. Therefore, the client's understanding of the evaluator's intended message depends on many factors.

Give this some thought: Does the language we use empower others and fill the space with possibility, or does it dictate to them and lead to a dead end? Does it accomplish the goal of collaboration between client and clinician? Furthermore, it is important to be mindful and sensitive to potential cultural differences that may exist. Does our language offend? This is expressed succinctly in the phrase, "speak without offending and listen without defending" (Landmark Worldwide, n.d.).

We also express our intention with the following:

- **Nonverbal cues**
  - Facial expressions
  - Body language
  - Suprasegmental aspects of communication give the message its color and melody:
    - Intonation
    - Timing
    - Stress

We learn a great deal about an individual's emotional state by listening to his or her voice.

At least 65% of communication is nonverbal (Owens, 2008). Sometimes there is a lack of congruence between verbal and nonverbal cues. According to Haynes and Pindzola (2008), sometimes the nonverbal cues may be more revealing. Thus, it is crucial to be mindful of our body positioning and facial expression while interacting with clients and families. A relaxed, stabilized body posture, inclined toward the client or reclined back, invites open communication and sharing. We must be conscious not to stand and talk down to family members who are seated when we are delivering information. When conversing with children, it is preferable to sit or bend down to meet them at eye level.

Word Traps

Let us examine language that may stir up defensiveness in others and in us. We refer to this vocabulary as **word traps**. Word traps are limiting phrases such as "I should" or "you should." Examine your internal response when you hear the word should. Does it offer options? Does *should* allow for possibility? In reality, when we think, listen, and speak in terms of should, we feel forced, pressured, and obligated. If *should* provokes these feelings in us, would it not ignite similar emotions in clients or family members? If taken to the next level, when we do not fulfill a *should*, we feel disappointed. Our disappointment may lead to feelings of guilt, which may then lead to anger and resentment. This sequence of emotions may occur with our clients and their families as well.

What shifts for you if we were to substitute *could* for *should* when speaking? Possibilities open up! We feel our locus of control move from one that is external to one that is internal (Manning, 2001). We then own and gain control over our situation. Most human beings react positively when they have a choice. Therefore, it is important that when we, as clinicians, speak to parents, we remove the pressure of *should* and provide the freedom of *could*.

Another frequent word trap is *but*. How many of you can recall a time you were given a compliment, followed by the word *but*? ("You did a very good job, but ..."). How did this affect your internal reaction to the compliment? Did it validate or deflate you? One alternative possibility to using the word but is to substitute and. For example, "I want to speak in public, but I am afraid." → "I want to speak in public and I am afraid." In the previous example, the *but* implied that because of fear, you will not proceed, whereas the *and* implied you will proceed despite the fear. We need to be mindful about our use of *but* when we communicate and then attempt to seek alternate words. Therefore, when listening to someone else and the inclination to say *but* arises, try saying "yes and ..." Expand on the other person's statement rather than making the client or student clinician wrong.

Take a moment to transform the following sentences by replacing *but* with *and*. Reflect on the resulting internal response.

- I want to visit my mother *but* she annoys me →
- I should treat my brother better *but* he's difficult →

A third word trap is the word *can't*. It is a word that may not have an alternative like *but* or *should*; however, it has a similar limiting impact. Because the term does not engender hope or possibility, it is best avoided in the clinical setting. On the other hand, when a client insists that he or she cannot perform a task, it is our job, as clinicians, to honor the difficulty the client is faced with when he or she is moving out of his or her comfort zone.

Many of us have a *can't* that is related to one of our fears. For example, you may say to yourself or out loud "I can't skydive," "I can't move to the next level in my career," or "I can't work and go to school at the same time." Take a moment to write down three *can't* statements related to your own fears.

1. ______________________________
   ____
2. ______________________________
   ____
3. ______________________________
   ____

Word Traps and Clinical Practice

Now, think about when we evaluate or counsel a client. He may say, "I can't do that," "It's too difficult," or "I'm afraid." Human beings rarely want to change what is familiar even if the known behavior is uncomfortable or unpleasant. Think about how challenging it is for any of us to make changes in our own behavior. Because it is difficult to relate to another person's fear, how easily do we fall into the trap of insisting that they can or that they should not be afraid? We may believe that these words are supportive. We must be cautious not to turn our persistence into their resistance. Alternative language to "yes you can" are questions such as "What are you willing to do?" and "What do you need to help you try?" This places the locus of control back within the client, thus empowering him or her to create the desired change.

The word **willingness** is part of the process. Our willingness to consider how we speak and how we listen, and the client's willingness to attempt change, is the road to partnership and collaborative learning, and it is at the heart of the counseling relationship.

It is worthwhile to coach our clients and their families in the art of using empowering language. Once rapport is engendered and the client achieves a level of trust, point out the client's use of self-sabotaging language or word traps (e.g., should, but, and can't). Support your clients and their families in teasing out and replacing their use of limiting language with words that encourage rather than discourage.

Negative words are difficult to take back once they are spoken. We need to be mindful of how we express ourselves rather than be reactive in our communication with clients. It is clear that the language we use and encourage in our counseling relationships, and the way in which these words are received, have the power to create either a partnership in problem solving or an adversarial situation that precludes growth.

The Language of Acknowledgment

Let us conclude with the **language of acknowledgment**. The term *acknowledgment* denotes "to recognize as being valid or having force or power" (Whitworth et al., 2007). It is more difficult to validate the positive than to highlight the negative in another individual. By the same token human beings have difficulty receiving and holding onto praise.

Acknowledging an individual highlights his or her internal strengths, thus fostering greater access to those gifts. Validating another individual is a courageous act. In many ways, it requires more courage than pointing out what is lacking. Acknowledgment involves being brave enough to step forward and authentically name what you see (The Coaches Training Institute, n.d.).

Acknowledging Versus Complimenting

The difference between complimenting and acknowledging is that a compliment is nonspecific and superficial. A true acknowledgment is direct and specific and reflects a tone of admiration.

Acknowledgment often validates how someone may be honoring another's core life values. For example:

Compliment: You are a good mother

Acknowledgment: I see how your child lights up when he sees you—it's apparent that the two of you have a special connection.

Notice the specific information in the acknowledgment as well as the admiration for the mother in relation to her child. Acknowledgment shows others who you know them to be in the world. There are three parts to an acknowledgment: (1) the statement, (2) how it resonates with the other individual, and (3) your observation of the other person's reaction. If your validation is authentic, it will resonate as true for the other. This will register in their facial expression and body language.

Clinical Suggestions for Family Members and Caregivers

As noted earlier in the chapter, it has been proven that in relationships and in organizations, focusing on the positive and on the strengths of the individual yield significantly higher results than dwelling on the negative. Although constructive criticism is necessary and has its place, society's tendency is to overlook the positive and focus on the negative. You may want to provide a family with an assignment that instructs them to deliver one acknowledgment per day, verbal or written, to a member of their family.

Acknowledgment has a positive physiological effect and influence on mood for the person receiving it as well as for the one delivering the validation. Therefore, delivering and receiving gratitude is healthy. Another suggestion is to ask each family member to write down when he or she observed the client display a unique strength. The family may then work together to create a "portrait" of the child that highlights his or her inherent talents (Cameron, 2007).

We invite you to answer the following questions:

- How generous and genuine are we with acknowledging others?
- How sincerely do we come across?
- How often do we hold back kind words?

What a shame to withhold kind words because validating others is a powerful builder of relationships. The benefits of acknowledgment in the diagnostic interview and in counseling sessions with clients and their families are clear. Experiment with acknowledgment in your everyday life and pay attention to the impact it has on others. Take a moment and let the client or family member know where he or she has a unique force or power and shine a light on it.

The deepest principle of human nature is the craving to be appreciated.

—William James

We would be remiss if we did not emphasize the importance of acknowledgment relating to "self." How easy and human it is for us to hold on to the negative. By doing this, we sabotage our best efforts. It is important to take the time to acknowledge ourselves for the strength, kindness, or resourcefulness that fostered our accomplishments. Take a few moments to acknowledge yourself for one thing today, allow time to take it in, write it down, and consider the kind of person you needed to be to say what you said, act as you did, or accomplish your task.

Assuming Personal Responsibility for Listening Judgments and Language

When we take personal responsibility for our listening, judgments, and language, we demonstrate our authenticity and self-awareness. We must be willing to acknowledge when we have tuned out, lost focus, or reverted back to Level I listening. We must be willing to own our misinterpretations and assumptions, and we must be confident enough to request clarification. We must be consistently aware of our judgments and whether they are interfering with our communication.

We must frame suggestions with the appropriate language (e.g., "May I offer a suggestion?" or "May I offer you some feedback?") so that we increase the client's or family member's feeling of control. When we ask permission to ask suggestions, we demonstrate that the client has power in the relationship. This further demonstrates that you, as the clinician or counselor, know your limits in the relationship and honor the client by respecting his or her boundaries (Whitworth et al., 2007).

Expectations

Listening, judgment, and language tie in with our expectations. As human beings, we weave webs of complexity from which escape is often difficult. We expect a great deal of our partners, families, children, students, patients and their families, and ourselves. On one hand, expecting the best in others fosters their growth. On the other hand, expectations may often be unrealistic. When we have unrealistic expectations, our resulting disappointments may negatively affect our relationships. On a daily basis, we are faced with our own personal and professional expectations, realistic and unrealistic, which are frequently thwarted. As disappointment sets in, so do judgment and attitude. These feelings show up in how we listen and in how we speak. How we handle the disappointments in all phases of our lives says a lot about who we are and how effective we will be as counselors.

The way we listen, the language we use, and the awareness of our judgments and expectations are essential in building the confidentiality and trust necessary to foster the therapeutic relationship. When you convey to parents that you are on their team by placing the child's best interest and agenda at the forefront, walls of resistance break down. Thus, the seeds for transformation are planted in the diagnostic process. When the client and family experience this connection, they leave feeling safe and hopeful, and they look forward to returning to the next phase of the therapeutic process.

III. The Diagnostic Interview and Postdiagnostic Conference

Although a clinical interview ought to resemble the flow and naturalness of a conversation, it differs from a dialogue in several crucial ways. As emphasized previously, the agenda of the client remains in the forefront. Therefore, the focus will be on the client and his or her problem and needs. Although we do not know specifically how the interview will conclude, our goal in the process is to uncover important information. Nevertheless, the more we are willing to wade into the unknown, without the security of a checklist, the quicker rapport will be established and the deeper the connection will be. Therefore, we recommend that to properly engage with the client and his or her family, you refer only occasionally to a prepared list of interview questions and refrain from writing copious notes during the interview process. Each facility may have its own template for the clinical interview. Do not be concerned about missing a question because you can check the template at the end to be sure your interview was complete. (See Appendix 2-A for samples of these interview forms at the end of the chapter.)

We have noticed that when we write, the clients and family members may lose focus and become somewhat uncomfortable. To manage this, we suggest the following:

- Prepare the client that we may be writing down some of the things said so that the client's ideas will be clear and so we will remember all of the information.
- Maintain consistent eye contact even when jotting down significant points.
- The clinician may ease up on note taking and use a tape recorder if the client and/or family member give verbal permission to do so.

The Interview (The Clinician's Tool Kit)

The information in this section is adapted and derived predominantly from the Coactive Coaching Model (Whitworth et al., 2007).

It is essential that the examiner is alert for and incorporates the information gained in the client/family interview with clinical assessment results. The clinician must pay attention to the following:

- Possible missing links in the diagnostic puzzle
- Client and family priorities and inconsistencies in:
  - Reports between each other's accounts
  - Incongruities between their oral reports and clinical data

Moreover, the clinician must note this conflicting information in the diagnostic report. To assist you in using a coaching approach during the clinical interview, we have included a list and description of coaching/counseling tools. The following toolkit will be helpful in the clinical interview and counseling process.

- **Reflecting** and **clarifying**
- **Summary probe**
- **Clearing**
- Powerful questions
- **Meta-view**
- Reframing
- Acknowledging
- Using silence

Reflecting and Clarifying

In reflecting, we simply mirror back to the client what he or she has just said. In this way, we act as a giant mirror and the client sees or hears him- or herself more clearly. It is striking what evolves from simply letting the individual hear his or her own words. This gives the client greater access to emotions and leads to client resourcefulness (Shirk, 2008). There are often revelations that appear for the client from this simple act. This act of reflecting also involves paraphrasing and interpreting the client's statement in our own words. This is generally more effective than simply repeating back what the client has said. For example:

Client: There are so many things to do and work on, schools to investigate, and I'm so tired.

Interviewer: It sounds like you feel overwhelmed.

Check in with the client when you reflect back or clarify what you heard, and be sure that the client agrees with your paraphrase. This further facilitates communication. If the client corrects you or disagrees, that serves as valuable feedback because it allows you a more representative picture about what he or she is feeling. Furthermore, if a client corrects reflection, this becomes an opportunity for the client to clarify his or her own thoughts and deepen self-discovery and serves as an invitation for you to proceed. Following are two possible dialogues that may result from checking in with the client. They illustrate how a quick confirmation from the client contributes to verifying your interpretation of the client's feeling.

Interviewer: Is that true?

Client: Yes, that's exactly how I feel; very overwhelmed.

Interviewer: So you feel very overwhelmed.

Client: Not really overwhelmed, more afraid than overwhelmed; scared.

Summary Probe

It is often a helpful transitional device to summarize, in your own words, what the client has told you. This is can be a tactful way to consolidate or steer the conversation back on track. It also provides the opportunity to use the client's thoughts to segue to the next topic and reinforces the depth of your listening both to yourself and to your client. This ensures that you have all of the information in the correct sequence and provides opportunity for more sharing. This tool makes the client feel truly heard. For example:

Clinician: Let me just back track for a minute here to be sure that I understand: You said that your child stuttered from about the age of 3 and became self-conscious about it this year in kindergarten? Is that right? Tell me more about that.

Clearing

Often people need to release their emotions (e.g., sadness, frustration, anger). Allow them some time to tell their stories, feel sorry for themselves, and release their negative emotions. Use your intuition to determine an individual's pressing need to vent and express his or her reactions to being unfairly targeted, feeling trapped, angry, frightened, and overwhelmed. Once people release the emotion, they are often more emotionally and cognitively ready to receive information.

Powerful Questions

Powerful questions are open-ended, curious, introspective, and thought-provoking questions. These inquiries prompt an individual to look deep inside and search for an authentic response. Do not be surprised if there is a silent pause following a powerful question. These are not the type of inquiries that people are accustomed to answering and often may require a deeper reflection. Try to limit your use of closed-ended, yes–no, or leading questions. When inquiries are leading, they have an underlying agenda of manipulating the client toward a particular type of response. Take care to preserve and not hijack the client's agenda. Here are some examples of curious powerful questions:

- What do you truly want?
- How will you know you received it?
- What about that is important to you?
- What's next?
- What else?
- What would that look like?
- What does "stuck" feel like?
- What will finishing that give you?
- How would it look if your life were balanced?
- What did you learn?
- What is getting in your way?
- What have you tried so far?
- What are you willing to do?
- What's working?
- What would you like to know that you don't know today?
- How does this (perspective) serve you?
- What would support you in accomplishing that?
- What have you done to get the job done so far?
- What is the cost?
- What is the benefit?
- What are you saying yes to?
- What are you saying no to?
- What is one more possible way of looking at this?
- How do you give your power away?

The following powerful questions illuminate and support the client's agenda and the designed alliance during the clinical interview:

1. What would you like to accomplish from today's session?
2. What is one important thing you are taking away today?

Meta-View

The meta-view assists the individual in gaining a perspective on his or her situation. This is another way of saying a "bird's-eye view." It is a miniature visualization exercise where you may ask the client to envision that he or she is taking a ride with you in a helicopter. Once the client is metaphorically high up in the air, ask, "Now what do see from here?" When you ask the client to look down and tell you what he or she sees now, the client's perspective will usually shift to a more empowered stance. You may hear the client respond with comments such as, "All of that does not look so important anymore," or "In the grand scheme of things, that does not look like such a big problem."

You may also suggest envisioning a trip into the future and looking back on this difficult time to help the client gain perspective on a difficult situation or dilemma. This may help the client project that things will fall into a rhythm and place and also highlight his or her potential accomplishments.

Reframing

Reframing relates in many ways to meta-view. Like meta-view, this tool helps the client to view the problem from another perspective. While meta-view brings the client to a metaphorically different vista, reframing helps the client redefine the problem into something positive. The client's view of reality may be causing him or her stress. Reframing shows the client that there are various points of view offering opportunity. Although there may be many perspectives that are true, reframing focuses on the fact that we always have choice. Thus, the premise is that all individuals possess the power to choose the way they view their situation.

Reframing a point of view provides the opportunity for the client to move from a position of being "stuck" or a victim into one of being in control. For example, helping the client alter his or her perspective may reduce the client's anxiety or guilt. You may offer a powerful question such as, "Your perspective is one point of view; what is another way you might look at this?" This may lead to a shift in paradigm for the client and consequently an epiphany best described as an intuitive "aha."

Readiness is an important marker for timing a reframe for any individual, and certainly for individuals with disabilities. An example of a reframe, made by a person who stutters, might be that stuttering has been an opportunity for personal growth and developing greater sensitivity to the needs of others. The reframe may also include that fact that many people who stutter have turned their limitations in a way to foster change in the lives of others with similar challenges.

Acknowledging

Please refer to Section II, specifically "The Language of Acknowledgment" on page 22.

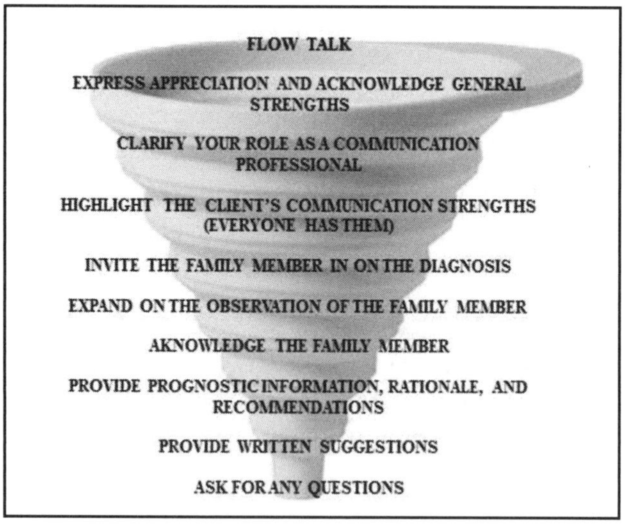

FLOW TALK
EXPRESS APPRECIATION AND ACKNOWLEDGE GENERAL STRENGTHS
CLARIFY YOUR ROLE AS A COMMUNICATION PROFESSIONAL
HIGHLIGHT THE CLIENT'S COMMUNICATION STRENGTHS (EVERYONE HAS THEM)
INVITE THE FAMILY MEMBER IN ON THE DIAGNOSIS
EXPAND ON THE OBSERVATION OF THE FAMILY MEMBER
AKNOWLEDGE THE FAMILY MEMBER
PROVIDE PROGNOSTIC INFORMATION, RATIONALE, AND RECOMMENDATIONS
PROVIDE WRITTEN SUGGESTIONS
ASK FOR ANY QUESTIONS

Figure 2-2. A framework for post-evaluation conference.

Using Silence

There are several types of silence. Silence is not only about being quiet or being still; there is silence with presence and silence with absence. When you are silent and fully present with other individuals, such as in group meditation, people feel connected; the silence is energized and supported. People in our culture are often uncomfortable with silence, assuming that the other individual is ill at ease. The reality is that we cannot assume that we know, what is going on in the other individual's heart and mind. There are infinite possibilities. For example, the person may simply be processing information, evaluating his feelings, or formulating a response. Just as we take care not to hijack a client's agenda, we must remember not to hijack the silence. We must honor one another's silence as an opportune time for thinking, reflecting, and learning. It is therefore important to refrain from projecting our own reactions onto our clients and making assumptions. When it comes to matters of silence, we need to take a step back and learn to trust in the process. We suspect you will come to learn that silence is your friend. It is in taking that creative pause that you make a space for the client to regroup and self-discover.

It is our hope that the previous coaching tools are useful in your communication with your clients and their families, and in all of your relationships. We suggest that you practice using your Level II and III listening whenever the opportunity presents itself and that you engage in both the use of powerful questions and providing acknowledgment in everyday interactions.

IV. The Post-Evaluation Toolkit

One of the most anxiety-provoking clinical situations for graduate students and novice speech clinicians is the post-evaluation conference. An inexperienced clinician agonizes over myriad issues that relate to both communicating the diagnostic results and making necessary recommendations to the parents. Additional factors often arise during the evaluation of which the family may not have been aware. For example, a child who was brought in for an articulation disorder that never resolved despite prolonged school-based speech therapy has been found to exhibit a significant receptive and expressive language disorder. Where does one begin?

We recommend the following general sequence of events in summing up the post-evaluation conference. The diagram in Figure 2-2 has been found to provide beginning clinicians with a framework that may prove to be supportive in a difficult situation.

The dialogue in a post-evaluation conference may be envisioned in the configuration of a funnel as the clinician moves from discussing most general to more specific information.

The following are the most important steps to include in the funnel:

- **Flow talk**
- Highlight positive attributes and general strengths
- **Clarify your role**
- Highlight **communication strengths**
- Enlist the family in the diagnosis
- Written recommendations
- Question and answer period
- One important take-away

Flow Talk

Do not underestimate the power of chitchat. "Flow talk" (Csikszentmihalyi, 1997), or casual conversation, often proves to be a soothing and humane transition in an otherwise stressful situation. This is an important part of your professional interaction with your client and his or her family.

Highlight Positive Attributes and General Strengths

After flow talk, the examiner moves into acknowledging the general personality or intellectual strengths of the client. For example, "It was a pleasure to meet and work with Suzy today. She has a delightful sense of humor and gives everything her best effort." After highlighting those general strengths, the clinician clarifies his role as a professional to the parent or client.

Clarify Your Role

The general public is not usually aware of the plethora of responsibilities woven into the fabric of the role of a SLP. It is important to explain that we do not simply treat a mouth. We find it helpful to relay that we are communication specialists and look at all aspects of spoken and written language. We look at numerous features of speech to include voice quality, pronunciation of sounds, and the fluent forward movement of speech.

Highlight Communication Strengths

At this juncture in the dialogue, the clinician may segue into the features of communication that he or she found to be areas of strength for this client. It is important to inform a parent that a child has much communication strength. For example, a child may present with a receptive and expressive language delay; however, he or she may also exhibit appropriate articulation, voice quality, and fluency. Furthermore, the oral peripheral examination may have been normal, exhibiting intact structures and function to support speech. One may always approach a situation from a position of strength and explain to the client and family that these positive features will serve the client well in therapy.

Enlist the Family in the Diagnosis

Following illumination of the client's areas of relative strength, the clinician may want to engage the client or family in sharing or reiterating their areas of concern or perception of the client's difficulty. We advise that you use the family or client's antecedents from the clinical interview and tie them into your own impressions to create a complete diagnostic description (Haynes & Pindzola, 2008). For example, "You mentioned earlier that when Jimmy relates the events of his day, you cannot always follow his account."

Approach the family members or client as naturally creative, resourceful, and whole and as having the answers to their own questions. It is important to remember that the parent is the expert on the child's life (Luterman, 2008b). In this way, we may elicit the diagnosis as well as suggestions collaboratively. For example, at the close of the post-evaluation conference, we suggest asking the client and/or family member what they noticed during the evaluation. You may be surprised at their insight. Their input may alleviate the pressure on the diagnostician to have to know everything and lessen the impact of possible bad news. This collaboration maximizes client and family openness, trust, and follow-through.

State what you observed about the client's areas in need of support using the family's antecedents. Discuss the general areas in need of support based on your formal and informal test results, then proceed to elaborate or move to the specific areas of difficulty. For example, a child may perform in the average range on the Test of Auditory Processing in all areas, with the exception of two: auditory comprehension and reasoning. Explain the purpose of the test and clarify that performance in most of the areas was at least average with the exception of two (which were below average). You might say something like, "In most of the skills that have been shown to support reading, she performed age-appropriately. She experienced difficulty in only two of seven subtests, where listening comprehension and responding to more abstract questions were involved." Be honest and authentic without providing excessive technical detail. Follow the parent's lead in providing additional specific information.

Once you summarize the issues to be addressed in therapy, check in with the family. For example, you may want to ask the family how this feedback fits with their gut feelings. Do the analysis and recommendations resonate for them? Does the information make sense? Typically, if they have been involved in the assessment and have been acknowledged for their observations and resourcefulness, they will maintain a positive attitude and be eager to initiate a collaborative effort toward remediation. We recommend that you provide a prognosis, how likely the client is to improve with or without therapy, with an associated rationale; for example, "Suzy is a bright and motivated child. She is fortunate to have a wonderful, supportive family. We anticipate that she will progress nicely in therapy." (For additional information on the importance of the family in the counseling and clinical process, please refer to Section I, "The Role of the Family" on page 14.

Provide Written Recommendations

Before dismissing your clients and their families, it is advisable to provide written recommendations on whether they are commencing therapy immediately. Aside from helping them, your suggestions empower the clients and families by providing them with immediate ways to support them in their situation. This mitigates feelings of being overwhelmed and helps to give them direction. Suggestions may include specific shared book reading activities with particular books; phonemic awareness exercises such as rhyme, songs, or finger plays; or initiating step one of a hierarchy of feared situations.

Question-and-Answer Period and Take-Away

Offer an opportunity for questions once the recommendations are made. This provides a lens through which the examiner may view the client or family member's interpretation of the process. In addition, the client's questions offer the examiner an opening to alleviate the client's unnecessary guilt and to offer additional support. Ask the client or family what is one important thing they are taking away with them from the evaluation process. This question serves to put the finishing bow on the first encounter. The question may also deepen the learning process and lend itself to the family feeling cared for and productive. Clients and families will never fail to surprise and delight you with their insights and responses, with their creativity and resourcefulness. Sit back and enjoy the ride!

Summary

We cannot overemphasize the importance of establishing the clinician–client relationship, which is a key factor in the success of the diagnostic evaluation. In addition, it is essential to have a counseling attitude as well as the tools to help improve the efficacy of treatment (Geller & Foley, 2009; Luterman, 2008a, 2008b).

Now that we have concluded the counseling and interviewing chapter, we are ready to take on the challenge of converting this information into professional report-writing format. We hope that the following chapter, "The Basics of Diagnostic Report Writing," will prove helpful in framing and executing the diagnostic report.

Appendix 2-A

Sample Diagnostic Pre-Interview Forms

Diagnosis: ______________________ *(Name, Address, Email, Phone, and Fax of Facility)*

Adult Case History Form

General Information

Name: ______________________ Date of Birth: ______________________

Address: ______________________ Phone: ______________________

City: ______________________ Zip: ______________________

Occupation: ______________________ Business Phone: ______________________

Employer: ____

Referred by: ______________________ Phone: ______________________

Address: ____

Family Physician: ______________________ Phone: ______________________

Address: ____

Single ☐ Widowed ☐ Divorced ☐ Spouse's Name: ______________________

Children (include names, gender, and ages):

______________________ ______________________

______________________ ______________________

______________________ ______________________

Who lives in the home?

______________________ ______________________

______________________ ______________________

What languages do you speak? If more than one, which one is your primary language? ______________________

____

Do you have eating or swallowing difficulties? If yes, describe. ______________________

____

____

List all medications you are taking. ______________________

____

____

Are you having any negative reactions to these medications? If yes, describe. ______________________

____

____

Describe any major surgeries, operations, or hospitalizations (include dates). ______________________

____

____

Today's Date: ______________________

Diagnosis: ______________________

Child Case History Form

General Information

Child's Name: ______________________ M/F: ______________________
Date of Birth: ______________________ Age: ______________________
Address: ______________________ Phone: ______________________
City: ______________________ Zip: ______________________
Does your child live with both parents? ______________________
Parent Name: ______________________ Age: ______________________
Parent Occupation: ______________________ Business Phone: ______________________
Parent Cell Phone: ______________________ Email: ______________________
Parent Name: ______________________ Age: ______________________
Parent Occupation: ______________________ Business Phone: ______________________
Parent Cell Phone: ______________________ Email: ______________________
Referred by: ______________________ Phone: ______________________
Address: ______________________
Pediatrician/Family Doctor: ______________________ Phone: ______________________
Address: ______________________
Dentist: ______________________ Phone: ______________________

Brothers and Sisters (include names and ages):
1. ______________________ Age: ______________________
2. ______________________ Age: ______________________
3. ______________________ Age: ______________________
4. ______________________ Age: ______________________

What languages are spoken in the home? ______________________

What languages does your child speak? ______________________

What languages does your child understand? ______________________

What is your child's dominant or primary language? ______________________

With whom does your child spend most of his or her time? ______________________

Describe your child's speech-language problem. ______________________

How does your child usually communicate (gestures, single words, short phrases, sentences)? ______________________

When was the problem first noticed? By whom? ______________________

Child Case History Form (continued)

Has the problem changed since it was first noticed? ______________________________
What do you think may have caused the problem? ______________________________
Are you able to understand your child when he or she speaks? Yes ☐ No ☐
Are others able to understand your child? Yes ☐ No ☐
Is your child aware of the problem? Yes ☐ No ☐
Is your child bothered by his or her speech or hearing problem? Yes ☐ No ☐
Does your child ever seem to ignore you when you speak to him or her? Yes ☐ No ☐
Does your child tend to avoid speaking situations? Yes ☐ No ☐

Have any other speech-language specialists seen your child? Who and when? What were their conclusions or suggestions? ______________________________

____

____

____

Have any other (physicians, psychologists, special education teachers, etc.) seen your child? If yes, indicate the type of specialist, when your child was seen, and the specialist's conclusions or suggestions. ____________

____

____

____

____

Are there any other speech, language, or hearing problems in your family or family history? If yes, please describe.

____

____

____

____

Health History

Mother's health condition during pregnancy: ______________________________

____

Full-term pregnancy? ______________________________
Unusual factors during delivery? ______________________________

____

Weight of your child at birth? ______________________________
Did your child require any special treatment? ______________________________

____

____

A. Immediately after birth? ______________________________

____

B. During the first few months? ______________________________

____

Child Case History Form (continued)

Medical History

Provide the approximate age at which your child suffered the following illnesses and conditions, if applicable.

Allergies ______	Asthma ______	Chicken pox ______
Colds ______	Convulsions ______	Croup ______
Dizziness ______	Draining ear ______	Ear infections ______
Encephalitis ______	German measles ______	Headaches ______
High fever ______	Influenza ______	Mastoiditis ______
Measles ______	Meningitis ______	Mumps ______
Pneumonia ______	Seizures ______	Sinusitis ______
Tinnitus ______	Tonsillitis ______	Other ______

Has your child had any surgeries? If yes, what type and when (e.g., tonsillectomy, adenoidectomy)? ______

Describe any major accidents or hospitalizations. ______

Is your child taking any medications? If yes, please list. ______

Have there been any negative reactions to medications? If yes, explain. ______

Developmental History

Was your child breastfed or bottle-fed? ______
Age at which your child was weaned? ______
Any feeding problems? If yes, explain. ______

Activity level of the baby? Excessive ☐ Average ☐ Below average ☐
Are there any chewing or swallowing problems (now or in the past)? ______
Did your child begin to eat table foods between ages 1 and 2 years? ______
Is there a history of excessive drooling? ______
When did you notice a reduction in the drooling? ______
Does your child use a pacifier? ______ Age? ______
Does your child suck his or her thumb? ______ Age? ______

Child Case History Form (continued)

Age at which the following took place?

Teething ______________________________

Crawling ______________________________

Sitting independently ______________________________

Feeding self ______________________________

Walking alone ______________________________

Toilet training ______________________________

Climbing stairs ______________________________

Riding a tricycle ______________________________

Riding a bicycle ______________________________

Scribbling with a crayon ______________________________

Drawing shapes/letters ______________________________

Cutting with scissors ______________________________

Putting together simple puzzles ______________________________

Stacking blocks ______________________________

How skillful is your child at dancing, throwing, and running?

Very skillful ☐ Skillful ☐ Average ☐ Awkward ☐ Very awkward ☐

Interaction and Play

Does (did) your child play frequently with children of his or her own age? ______________________________

Follower or leader? ______________________________

Fighting? ______________________________

Any teasing by playmates? ______________________________

For what reason? ______________________________

What games does your child prefer? ______________________________

Does your child play alone? ______________________________

Which parent plays most with your child? ______________________________

Which playmates play most with your child? ______________________________

Speech and Language Development

Did your child babble much as an infant? ______________________________ Age? ______

What were the first words spoken? ______________________________ Age? ______

Has your child put words together to form sentences? ______________________________ Age? ______

Were attempts made to teach your child to talk? ______________________________ Age? ______

Were gestures used in place of speech? ______________________________ Age? ______

Estimated size of vocabulary: Above average ☐ Average ☐ Below average ☐

Ability to construct sentences: Above average ☐ Average ☐ Below average ☐

Ability to produce sounds: Above average ☐ Average ☐ Below average ☐

Are there sounds your child is unable to produce or produces unclearly? ______________________________

____

Did your child ever tend to say words backward? ______________________________ Age? ______

Did your child ever tend to write words backward? ______________________________ Age? ______

Does your child read? ______________________________

How well does your child read? Above average ☐ Average ☐ Below average ☐

Does your child always understand when people speak to him or her? ______________________________

If not, when does your child have difficulty? ______________________________

Is your child quiet or talkative? ______________________________

Describe your child's response to sounds (e.g., responds to all sounds, responds to loud sounds only, inconsistently responds to sounds). Indicate date of latest audiological evaluation. ______________________________

____

Child Case History Form (continued)

Educational Development

Present school: ____________________ Teachers: ____________________
Present school grade: ____________________ Ever failed a grade? ____________________
School attendance: ____________________
Attitude toward school: ____________________
Subjects liked: ____________________
Names of schools attended: ____________________
____

Does your child receive special services? If yes, list the services and how long your child has been receiving the service.

____
____
____

Discipline

How is your child disciplined? ____________________
By whom? ____________________
What type of discipline is most effective? ____________________
Least effective? ____________________

Provide any additional information that might be helpful in the evaluation or remediation of your child's problem.

____
____
____
____
____
____
____
____
____
____

Today's Date: ____________________
Diagnosis: ____________________

Child Case History Form

Child's Name: ____________________ M/F: ____________________
Date of Birth: ____________________ Age: ____________________
Address: ____________________ Phone: ____________________
City: ____________________ Zip: ____________________
Does your child live with both parents? ____________________
Mother's Name: ____________________ Age: ____________________
Mother's Occupation: ____________________ Business Phone: ____________________
Mother's Cell Phone: ____________________ Email: ____________________
Father's Name: ____________________ Age: ____________________
Father's Occupation: ____________________ Business Phone: ____________________
Father's Cell Phone: ____________________ Email: ____________________
Referred by: ____________________ Phone: ____________________
Address: ____________________
Pediatrician/Family Doctor: ____________________ Phone: ____________________
Address: ____________________
Dentist: ____________________ Phone: ____________________

Brothers and Sisters (include names and ages):
1. ____________________ Age: ____________________
2. ____________________ Age: ____________________
3. ____________________ Age: ____________________
4. ____________________ Age: ____________________

What languages are spoken in the home? ____________________

What languages does your child speak? ____________________

What languages does your child understand? ____________________

What is your child's dominant or primary language? ____________________

With whom does your child spend most of his or her time? ____________________

Describe your child's speech-language problem. ____________________

How does your child usually communicate (gestures, single words, short phrases, sentences)? ____________________

When was the problem first noticed? By whom? ____________________

Child Case History Form (continued)

Has the problem changed since it was first noticed? ___
What do you think may have caused the problem? ___
Are you able to understand your child when he or she speaks? Yes ☐ No ☐
Are others able to understand your child? Yes ☐ No ☐
Is your child aware of the problem? Yes ☐ No ☐
Is your child bothered by his or her speech or hearing problem? Yes ☐ No ☐
Does your child ever seem to ignore you when you speak to him or her? Yes ☐ No ☐
Does your child tend to avoid speaking situations? Yes ☐ No ☐

Have any other speech-language specialists seen your child? Who and when? What were their conclusions or suggestions? ___

Have any other (physicians, psychologists, special education teachers, etc.) seen your child? If yes, indicate the type of specialist, when your child was seen, and the specialist's conclusions or suggestions. ___

Are there any other speech, language, or hearing problems in your family or family history? If yes, please describe.

Health History

Mother's health condition during pregnancy: ___
Full-term pregnancy? ___
Unusual factors during delivery? ___
Weight of your child at birth? ___
Did your child require any special treatment? ___

A. Immediately after birth? ___

B. During the first few months? ___

Child Case History Form (continued)

Medical History

Provide the approximate age at which your child suffered the following illnesses and conditions, if applicable.

Allergies ____________	Asthma ____________	Chicken pox ____________
Colds ____________	Convulsions ____________	Croup ____________
Dizziness ____________	Draining ear ____________	Ear infections ____________
Encephalitis ____________	German measles ____________	Headaches ____________
High fever ____________	Influenza ____________	Mastoiditis ____________
Measles ____________	Meningitis ____________	Mumps ____________
Pneumonia ____________	Seizures ____________	Sinusitis ____________
Tinnitus ____________	Tonsillitis ____________	Other ____________

Has your child had any surgeries? If yes, what type and when (e.g., tonsillectomy, adenoidectomy)? ______

____

____

Describe any major accidents or hospitalizations. ______________________

____

____

Is your child taking any medications? If yes, please list. ______________________

____

____

Have there been any negative reactions to medications? If yes, explain. ______________

____

____

Developmental History

Was your child breastfed or bottle-fed? ______________________

Age at which your child was weaned? ______________________

Any feeding problems? Is yes, explain. ______________________

____

Activity level of the baby? Excessive ☐ Average ☐ Below average ☐

Are there any chewing or swallowing problems (now or in the past)? ______________

Did your child begin to eat table foods between ages 1 and 2 years? ______________

Is there a history of excessive drooling? ______________________

When did you notice a reduction in the drooling? ______________________

Does your child use a pacifier? ______________________ Age? _____

Does your child suck his or her thumb? ______________________ Age? _____

Child Case History Form (continued)

Age at which the following took place?

Teething ____________________
Crawling ____________________
Sitting independently ____________________
Feeding self ____________________
Walking alone ____________________
Toilet training ____________________
Climbing stairs ____________________
Riding a tricycle ____________________
Riding a bicycle ____________________
Scribbling with a crayon ____________________
Drawing shapes/letters ____________________
Cutting with scissors ____________________
Putting together simple puzzles ____________________
Stacking blocks ____________________

How skillful is your child at dancing, throwing, and running?

Very skillful ☐ Skillful ☐ Average ☐ Awkward ☐ Very awkward ☐

Interaction and Play

Does (did) your child play frequently with children of his or her own age? ____________________
Follower or leader? ____________________
Fighting? ____________________
Any teasing by playmates? ____________________
For what reason? ____________________
What games does your child prefer? ____________________
Does your child play alone? ____________________
Which parent plays most with your child? ____________________
Which playmates play most with your child? ____________________

Speech and Language Development

Did your child babble much as an infant? ____________________ Age? _____
What were the first words spoken? ____________________ Age? _____
Has your child put words together to form sentences? ____________________ Age? _____
Were attempts made to teach your child to talk? ____________________ Age? _____
Were gestures used in place of speech? ____________________ Age? _____

Estimated size of vocabulary: Above average ☐ Average ☐ Below average ☐
Ability to construct sentences: Above average ☐ Average ☐ Below average ☐
Ability to produce sounds: Above average ☐ Average ☐ Below average ☐

Are there sounds your child is unable to produce or produces unclearly? ____________________
____

Did your child ever tend to say words backward? ____________________ Age? _____
Did your child ever tend to write words backward? ____________________ Age? _____
Does your child read? ____________________
How well does your child read? Above average ☐ Average ☐ Below average ☐

Does your child always understand when people speak to him or her? ____________________
If not, when does your child have difficulty? ____________________
Is your child quiet or talkative? ____________________

Describe your child's response to sounds (e.g., responds to all sounds, responds to loud sounds only, inconsistently responds to sounds). Indicate date of latest audiological evaluation. ____________________
____

Child Case History Form (continued)

Educational Development

Present school: ______________________ Teachers: ______________________

Present school grade: ______________________ Ever failed a grade? ______________________

School attendance: ______________________

Attitude toward school: ______________________

Subjects liked: ______________________

Names of schools attended: ______________________

____

Does your child receive special services? If yes, list the services and how long your child has been receiving the service.

____

____

____

Discipline

How is your child disciplined? ______________________

By whom? ______________________

What type of discipline is most effective? ______________________

Least effective? ______________________

Provide any additional information that might be helpful in the evaluation or remediation of your child's problem.

____

____

____

____

____

____

____

____

____

____

Today's Date: ______________________

Diagnosis: ______________________

GLOSSARY

Already always listening: Reacting to a person as if we already know just what he or she will say; a behavior that interferes with communication.

Attitude: How we handle the disappointments in all phases of our lives.

Check in: Verify whether the other individual agrees with your interpretation or ideas by asking him or her (e.g., "Does this feel right for you?").

Clarify your role: Relaying that speech-language pathologists are communication specialists and look at all aspects of spoken and written language and the functional way a human being understands and communicates.

Clarifying: Interview tool whereby the counselor interprets the client's account of his or her thoughts, ideas, and emotions in the counselor's own words.

Clearing: Allowing clients time to tell their story, feel sorry for themselves, and release their negative emotions.

Client's whole life: Refers to the importance placed on the involvement of the family and environment.

Co-creativity: To create in cooperation with another.

Communication strengths: Features of communication that are found to be areas of strength for this client.

Counselor congruence: An alignment between the intellectual and emotional components of the self and the individual's actions.

Denial: A normal human coping mechanism reaction to a trying situation in which the individual does not psychologically "own" the problem.

Design the alliance: Refers to the coach and the client joining together collaboratively for the sake of client growth.

Empathy: Identification with the thoughts, feelings, and attitudes of the client.

Empower: To give power, a greater sense of confidence, and self-esteem.

Expectations: The high standards we expect of ourselves or others in our lives that may often be unrealistic.

Flow talk: Casual conversation or "chit chat" that helps the clinician build a rapport with the client.

Focused listening (Level II listening): Listening to the meaning behind the client's words and reflecting everything back to the client.

Global listening (Level III listening): Listening with all of your senses and being aware of the shifts in the client's posture, changes in energy, mood, and tuning into what is not verbalized.

Grief: Deep sorrow, sadness, and feelings of loss in response to a catastrophic change.

Internal listening (Level I listening): Listening that is full of "mind chatter" and egotistical in nature because it involves interpreting what is spoken as being about oneself.

Judgment: Our attitude and reactions to disappointments in our lives.

Language: Our word selection, which can reveal our judgments, attitudes, emotions, compassion, and sensitivity toward the listener.

Language of acknowledgment: To recognize as being valid or having force or power

Listening: Paying attention on a deep level.

Meta-view: An interviewing/coaching tool that enables the client to gain a perspective on his or her situation.

Mind chatter: The ongoing dialogue in a person's brain that distracts his or her focus.

Naturally creative, resourceful, and whole: Coaching cornerstone of how all human beings are held; refers to all individuals possessing the inherent wisdom and solutions to many of their life problems.

Nonverbal cues: Facial expression and body language.

Personal responsibility: Refers to the responsibility of the clinician to provide affective counseling to the client so that treatment is optimal.

Powerful questions: Open-ended, curious, introspective, and thought-provoking questions.

Preserve the client agenda: Creating a climate where the client is valued and encouraged to focus on what is most meaningful to him or her, thus increasing clarity and access to strengths.

Process: A series of natural occurrences that produce change or development.

Reflecting: An interviewing tool in which the clinician acts as a giant mirror and repeats back to the client what he or she has just said, thereby providing the client with increased clarity on his ideas.

Reframing: A counseling tool that enables the client to redefine the problem into something positive.

Summary probe: An interview tool that is a tactful way to consolidate or steer the conversation back on track and also to gain clarification on the facts.

Willingness: A collaborative process that refers to our readiness to consider how we speak and listen, as well as the client's readiness to attempt change

Word traps: Commonly relied-on default phrases that limit possibility (e.g., "I/you should...").

References

American Speech-Language-Hearing Association. (2006). Roles, knowledge, and skills: Audiologists providing clinical services to infants and young children birth to 5 years of age. Retrieved from http://www.asha.org/policy/KS2006-00259

American Speech-Language-Hearing Association. (2016). Scope of practice in speech-language pathology. Retrieved from http://www.asha.org/policy/SP2016-00343/

Buckingham, M., & Clifton, D. (2001). *Now discover your strengths.* New York, NY: The Free Press.

Cameron, K. S. (2007). Building relationships by communicating supportively. In D. A. Whetten & K. S. Cameron (Eds.), *Developing management skills* (7th ed.). New York, NY: Prentice Hall.

Coach Training Alliance. (2005). Coach training accelerator. Boulder, CO: Author. Retrieved from http://www.coachtrainingalliance.com

Csikszentmihalyi, M. (1997). *Flow.* New York, NY: Basic Books.

Daloz, L. A. (1999). *Mentor: Guiding the journey of adult learners* (2nd ed.). San Francisco, CA: Jossey-Bass.

Fialka, J. (1997). Advice to professionals who must "conference cases." Retrieved from http://www.danceofpartnership.com

Fredrickson, B. (2009). *Positivity.* New York, NY: Crown Publishers/Random House.

Geller, E., & Foley, G. M. (2009). Expanding the "ports of entry" for speech-language pathologists: A relational and reflective model for clinical practice. *American Journal of Speech-Language Pathology, 18,* 1-14.

Girolametto, L., & Weitzman, E. (2006). It takes two to talk—the Hanen program for parents: Early language intervention through caregiver training. In R. McCauley & M. Fey (Eds.), *Treatment of language disorders in children* (pp. 77-103). Baltimore, MD: Paul H. Brookes Publishing.

Goleman, D. (1995). *Emotional intelligence.* New York, NY: Bantam Books/Dell.

Haynes, W. O., & Pindzola, R. H. (2008). *Diagnosis and evaluation in speech pathology* (7th ed.). Boston, MA: Allyn & Bacon.

Kalmanson, B., & Seligman, S. (2006). Process in an integrated model of infant mental health and early intervention practice. In G. M. Foley & J. D. Hochman (Eds.), *Mental health in early intervention: Achieving unity in principles and practice* (pp. 245-265). Baltimore, MD: Brookes.

Kegan, L. (2000). *How the way we talk can change the way we work.* San Francisco, CA: Jossey-Bass.

Landmark Worldwide. (n.d.). *Landmark Worldwide.* Retrieved from https://www.landmarkworldwide.com

Luterman, D. M. (2008a). *Counseling persons with communication disorders and their families* (5th ed.). Austin, TX: Pro-Ed.

Luterman, D. M. (2008b). *Sharpening counseling skills* [DVD]. Memphis, TN: Stuttering Foundation of America.

Manning, W. H. (2001). *Clinical decision making in fluency disorders.* Vancouver, Canada: Thomson/Delmar.

Manning, W. H. (2009). *Clinical decision making in fluency disorders* (3rd ed.). Clifton Park, NY: Cengage Learning.

Murphy, A. (1982). The clinical process and the speech-language pathologist. In G. Shames & E. Wiig (Eds.), *Human communication disorders* (pp. 386-402). Columbus, OH: Merrill.

Napier, A., & Whitaker, C. (1978). *The family crucible.* New York, NY: Harper & Row.

Oriah "Mountain Dreamer" House. (1999). "The invitation." In *The Invitation.* San Francisco, CA: HarperOne.

Owens, R. E. (2008). *Language development an introduction* (7th ed.) New York, NY: Pearson.

Rogers, C. (1951). *Client-centered therapy.* Boston, MA: Houghton Mifflin.

Saleeby, D. (2006). *The strengths perspective in social work practice* (4th ed.). New York, NY: Longman.

Shafir, R. Z. (2000). *The Zen of listening.* Wheaton, IL: Quest.

Seligman, M. (2002). *Authentic happiness.* New York: Free Press.

Shirk, A. (2008). *Foundations of the co-active approach to coaching* [draft]. San Rafael, CA: Coaches Training Institute.

Snow, K. (n.d.). Gentle revolution. *Disability Is Natural.* Retrieved from www.disabilityisnatural.com

Snow, K. (2007). *Counseling in communication disorders: A wellness perspective.* San Diego, CA: Plural Publishing Inc.

Stein-Rubin, C., & Adler, B. T. (2016). *Counseling in communication disorders: Facilitating the therapeutic relationship.* Thorofare, NJ: SLACK Incorporated.

The Coaches Training Institute. (n.d.). Retrieved from http://www.coactive.com

The Hanen Centre. (n.d.). *The Hanen Centre.* Retrieved from http://www.hanen.org

Whitworth, L., Kimsey-House, K., Kimsey-House, H., & Sandahl, P. (2007). *Co-active coaching—new skills for coaching people toward success in work and life.* Mountain View, CA: Davies-Black.

Additional Recommended Reading

Napier, A., & Whitaker, C. (1978). *The family crucible.* New York, NY: Harper & Row.

Yalom, I. D. (1980). *Existential psychotherapy.* New York, NY: Basic Books.

Yalom, I. D. (1989). *Love's executioner.* New York, NY: Basic Books.

Website Resources

Disability Is Natural: www.disabilityisnatural.com

Landmark Worldwide: www.landmarkworldwide.com

University of Pennsylvania Positive Psychology Center: http://ppc.sas.upenn.edu/

3

The Basics of Diagnostic Report Writing

Cyndi Stein-Rubin, MS, CCC-SLP, TSSLD and Natalie Schaeffer, DA, CCC-SLP

Key Words

- active voice
- background information
- colon
- comma
- complex sentence
- compound sentence
- embedded clause
- fragmented sentence
- gerund
- parallel structure
- parentheses
- passive voice
- positive statement
- preposition
- rambling sentence
- run-on sentence
- semicolon
- serial comma
- specific words
- transitional devices
- transitional element
- unnecessary words

The diagnostic report is a crucial document in our profession on many levels. First, it provides an analysis and synthesis of the information obtained through the client/family interview, assessment, and clinical intuition. Second, the diagnostic report is a venue for recommendations to be used in therapy. Third, clinical reports are a means of written communication among the clinician, other professionals (both within and outside of the domain of communication disorders), and outside facilities; clinical reports are also a source of communication between the evaluator and the client or family. Thus, the content must be expressed with the utmost accuracy and sensitivity. In addition, this document is frequently relied on as a basis for securing special services and for insurance reimbursement. Finally, the diagnostic report serves as a reflection of the professional integrity and competence of the speech-language pathologist (SLP) and of the facility from where the document is generated.

In view of the crucial role of the diagnostic report, one of the missions of this text is to provide support for students and student clinicians in this arena and to furnish a resource for instructors and supervisors who teach clinical report writing skills. Given the significance and complexity of this skill, it is no wonder that this task remains one of the most daunting for students and professionals in the speech-language profession. Moreover, because of the wide scope of our practice, opportunity for training students and clinicians in the process of clinical report writing is often limited. Furthermore, there is a paucity of textbooks and workbooks on diagnostic report writing in our

Stein-Rubin, C., & Fabus, R. *A Guide to Clinical Assessment and Professional Report Writing in Speech-Language Pathology, Second Edition (pp 43-64).*

field. Therefore, students may have to resort to their own devices in this area of considerable challenge and difficulty. The challenge is compounded related to the infusion of linguistically and culturally diverse clinicians in our profession. Accordingly, the first section of the chapter focuses on an overview of writing mechanics, grammatical usage, and stylistic pointers for report writing that are not only relevant, but crucial.

The second segment of this chapter emphasizes the **background information** or case history section of a report (i.e., the information delineated in the initial section of the diagnostic report). Background information refers to the portion of the diagnostic report that typically includes information such as pregnancy, health history, developmental milestones, education, occupation, and familial and social contexts. This topic is a natural continuation from Chapter 2, which addressed the client and family interview in which the examiner obtains the background information. Please refer to the questionnaires in the following chapters as well as to the forms included in Shipley and McAfee (2009) for assistance in outlining case history information.

This chapter progresses through a hierarchy, beginning with an inventory of grammatical rules. Follow-up exercises are supplied for hands-on application of these elements. The concluding portion of the chapter includes unrevised writing samples and corresponding edited versions of these excerpts. The modified examples are then followed by bullet points highlighting the pitfalls of the first version and guiding the reader through the modification process. Finally, we provide you with the opportunity to incorporate and apply the use of the grammatical concepts and technical information to create your own edited version of a practice sample. These final exercises give the writer an opportunity to integrate all phases of the hierarchy, which build on each other.

At the conclusion of the chapter, we call your attention to two rubrics that encompass formatting rules and provide key points to be included within each section of the diagnostic report. These rubrics may function as an overview before an evaluation, much like a road map for constructing the diagnostic report and as a checklist for editing the final product.

Whether you are a student, graduate clinician, practicing SLP, clinical supervisor, or instructor, it is our hope that this information will serve as a practical resource in enhancing written communication skills for diagnostic report writing in the profession.

Grammatical Rules and Usage

Table 3-1 defines the basic parts of speech and provides examples of their uses in sentences. These rules are relevant to the next section, which discusses the use of punctuation as it relates to parts of speech. For example, the use of **commas** and **semicolons** in sentences depends upon the writer's knowledge of parts of speech.

Punctuation and Grammatical Usage

In oral communication, we use the suprasegmentals of speech (intonation, pause, and stress) to add meaning and emphasis. In written communication, we depend on the use of linguistic markers or punctuation to help impart meaning. One of the primary missions of this chapter is to elucidate how to use punctuation correctly for the purpose of writing in the profession.

Comma

A comma is a punctuation mark that indicates a pause is needed in a sentence, as in the following examples.

Compound Sentence

A **compound sentence** is composed of two independent clauses connected by a conjunction (e.g., and, but, or, for, nor, so). Use a comma between two independent clauses in a compound sentence (i.e., two complete sentences connected by a conjunction). The comma is placed before the coordinating conjunction. For example:

Incorrect: The patient with aphasia had naming problems, he was able to communicate with his family.

Correct: The patient with aphasia had naming problems, but he was able to communicate with his family.

Complex Sentence

A **complex sentence** is one in which an incomplete sentence is dependent on the complete sentence that follows it. Use a comma to connect a dependent clause with an independent clause (i.e., to connect an incomplete sentence with a complete sentence). When a dependent clause with its marker (e.g., though, although, unless, after, before, once, as, whether, because, since, when, while, until, if) is at the beginning of the sentence, place

Table 3-1. Basic Parts of Speech With Definitions and Examples

Part of Speech	*Definition*	*Example*
Nouns	Nouns may be concrete, such as person, place, or thing, or abstract, such as a concept (e.g., *sincerity*).	The *client* was asked to read the *book* and answer the *clinician's* questions. He is a pillar of *sincerity*.
Proper nouns	Specific name of a person, place, or thing, such as *Susan*. Capitalize proper nouns.	*Brian's* performance was consistent across all assessment tasks.
Pronouns	Pronouns take the place of a noun. Like nouns, pronouns may function as the subject of a sentence or as the object of the sentence. In the second example, *she* is the subject and *him* is the object of the sentence. Examples of subject pronouns: *I, it, we, you, she, he, they* Examples of object pronouns: *it, me, you, us, him, her, them*	*He* (subject) exhibited difficulty elevating *his* (object) tongue. *She* led *him* into the examining room.
Articles	Articles include *a, an*, and *the*. They precede a noun or a noun phrase in a sentence.	*The* client maintained attention across all tasks presented.
Adjectives	Adjectives may describe a noun or pronoun.	Henry, a *delightful* 4-year-old boy, was referred to our center by his physician.
Verbs	Verbs are action words, such as *run* or *jump*, or a word that indicate a state of being, such as *is, are, was, were*, and *am*.	Ida *pointed* to the picture *named* by the clinician. Mathew *was naming* pictured objects.
Adverbs	Adverbs describe verbs. Many (although not all) end in *-ly*.	Mary walked *tentatively* into the examining room.
Conjunctions	Conjunctions are words that join parts of speech.	Susan labeled *and* described pictured objects.
• Coordinating	Examples of coordinating conjunctions: *and, but, for, because, unless, before, until, so that, since*	John sat down at the table, *but* he didn't play with the toys in front of him.
• Subordinating	Examples of subordinating conjunctions: *although, or, nor, so, yet*	*Although* Jimmy's score was one standard deviation below the mean, his performance was considered below average.
Prepositions	Prepositions are words that show a relationship between a noun and a pronoun (e.g., *in* the clinic). Prepositions also indicate space and time (e.g., *before* the session). Examples of prepositions: *at, by, on*	Kayla put the board *against* the wall and instructed the client to look *at* the pictures *on* the board.
Adapted from OWL Purdue Online Writing Lab, 2017 and The Writing Center at UNC, 2017.		

the comma between the dependent clause and the independent clause. For example:

Incorrect: Although the client understood the text he read aloud he pronounced the words incorrectly.

Correct: Although the client understood the text he read aloud, he pronounced the words incorrectly.

When a dependent clause and its marker come after the independent clause, it is not always necessary to use a comma. For example:

Incorrect: The client did not complete the language task, because he was tired.

Correct: The client did not complete the language task because he was tired.

Clauses That Qualify

Use a comma before a phrase that adds to or qualifies the original sentence. For example:

Incorrect: John had difficulty synthesizing a narrative usually when he spoke rapidly.

Correct: John had difficulty synthesizing a narrative, usually when he spoke rapidly.

Embedded Clauses

An **embedded clause** is one that can be removed from the sentence without changing the meaning of the sentence. Use a comma to mark off an embedded clause or added clauses. For example:

Incorrect: Laura a very conscientious child practiced her articulation homework every evening.

Correct: Laura, a very conscientious child, practiced her articulation homework every evening.

Transitional Element

A **transitional element** is a word, phrase, or sentence that connects a preceding topic to one that comes after it.

Use a comma after a transitional element (e.g., however, therefore, nonetheless, also, otherwise, finally, instead, thus, of course, above all, for example, in other words, as a result, on the other hand, in conclusion, in addition). For example:

Incorrect: The client was very distractible; therefore the evaluation was not completed.

Correct: The client was very distractible; therefore, the evaluation was not completed.

Serial Commas

Use **serial commas** when writing three or more items in a list in a sentence. Include the comma before the conjunctions *and* and *or*. For example:

Incorrect: The child had receptive, expressive and phonological problems.

Correct: The child had receptive, expressive, and phonological problems.

Do not use serial commas when writing only two parallel terms connected with a conjunction. For example:

Incorrect: The patient with aphasia had comprehension, and syntactical problems.

Correct: The patient with aphasia had naming and comprehension problems.

Use a serial comma along with numbers for a series of phrases. For example:

(1) Count the pills, (2) put them in a container, (3) cover the container, and (4) put it in the cabinet.

Semicolon

A semicolon is used to join two independent clauses (two complete sentences) when the clauses are not joined by a conjunction, especially when the sentences are closely related. For example:

Incorrect: Stuttering is a speech problem, it should not be ignored.

Correct: Stuttering is a speech problem; it should not be ignored.

Use semicolons in a complex enumeration of items (Example 1), or in a series that contains internal commas (Example 2).

Example 1: A number of questions remain unresolved: (1) whether beverages that contain caffeine are an important factor in heart disease; (2) whether such beverages can trigger arrhythmias; and (3) whether their arrhythmogenic tendency is enhanced by the presence and extent of myocardial impairment.

Example 2: We tested three groups: (1) low scorers, those who scored fewer than 20 points; (2) moderate scorers, those who scored between 20 and 50 points; and (3) high scorers, those who scored more than 50 points.

Colon

Use a **colon** to introduce a statement/paragraph or series. If the statement begins with a complete sentence, use a capital letter; otherwise, do not use a capital letter. For example:

Incorrect: He gave the following account: the client scored below the mean in the language test, and it was recommended that he begin speech and language therapy.

Correct: He gave the following account: The client scored below the mean in the language test, and it was recommended that he begin speech and language therapy.

Incorrect: He did the following tasks: (1) Completed the math test, (2) finished his homework, (3) read his novel for school, and (4) typed his paper.

Correct: He did the following tasks: (1) completed the math test, (2) finished his homework, (3) read his novel for school, and 3 (4) typed his paper.

Quotation Marks

Use quotation marks and punctuation marks correctly. The punctuation is placed inside the quotation marks. For example:

Incorrect: The clinician said, “Good job”.

Correct: The clinician said, “Good job.”

Parentheses

Parentheses are used to emphasize additional content, such as enclosing a brief explanation or an example. Sometimes commas might be a better choice.

Use parenthesis to set of nonessential material such as dates, clarifying information, or sources from a sentence. For example:

Incorrect: Grammatical punctuation as noted in the *Blue Textbook*, is used as a linguistic marker in written communication.

Correct: Grammatical punctuation (as noted in the *Blue Textbook*) is used as a linguistic marker in written communication.

Parentheses With Quotations

Put the period after the parentheses when using a quotation within parentheses in a sentence. For example:

The clinician told the student to give the client a reinforcer (e.g., "Good work").

Possession—Where to Put an Apostrophe

Singular: Mary's coat

More than one subject: Subjects' scores

Name ending with an s: Julius's or Julius' coat (be consistent)

Abbreviations

e.g., means "for example": Use e.g., to illustrate an example of more than one issue. For example:

M.G. produced numerous substitutions (e.g., w/r, n/m, t/s).

i.e., means "that is": Use i.e., to illustrate when the incident occurred once or with one issue. For example:

T.L. produced one articulatory error (i.e., w/r [M]).

Capitalization

Capitalize the first word of a quoted sentence (e.g., The client's mother stated, "He thinks faster than he speaks.").

Capitalize a proper noun (e.g., Beth Israel Hospital).

Capitalize a person's title when it precedes the name (e.g., Chairperson Smith).

Do not capitalize when the title is a description following the name (e.g., Mrs. Smith, the chairperson of the department, will address us at 10 a.m.).

Capitalize a title when used instead of a name (e.g., Will you help me with my reference list, Professor?).

Capitalize certain geographic terms (e.g., The client presented with regional dialect from the South.).

Capitalization Within Titles

Capitalize the first word of a title as well as all content words (nouns, verbs, adjectives, adverbs). Do not capitalize function words (but, as, if, and, or, nor, a, an, the, and prepositions of fewer than four letters [on, in]).

Capitalize federal or state titles when used as a name (e.g., He was evaluated at the Board of Education [BOE].).

Do not capitalize names of seasons unless they relate to the name of a semester (e.g., Fall semester; Spring semester).

Capitalize the names of specific course titles (e.g., Introduction to Phonetics).

Do not capitalize a broad area, such as mat (e.g., speech courses, as opposed to Speech 21).

Sentence Structure

Subject–Pronoun Agreement

The pronoun must reflect whether the noun is singular or plural. For example:

Incorrect: Everyone put on their coats.

Correct: Everyone put on his or her coat.

Subject–Verb Agreement

The verb must reflect whether the noun is singular or plural. For example:

Incorrect: The group are meeting tomorrow.

Correct: The group is meeting tomorrow.

Possession of a Verb With a Gerund (-ing)

A **gerund** is a verb form that ends in -ing; it is used as a noun in a sentence. For example:

John's practicing made a difference in his voice improvement.

Laura's coming late negatively impacted upon therapy.

Mom's reporting was very reliable.

Prepositions

A **preposition** is a word that shows a relationship between a noun and a pronoun (e.g., in the clinic; see Table 3-1). Do not end a sentence with a preposition. For example:

Incorrect: The client required material (homework) to study from.

Correct: The client required material from which to study.

Use of Who and Whom

Use the pronoun whom after a preposition. For example:

Incorrect: Who are you sending this client to?

Correct: To whom are you sending this client for an evaluation?

Use who if the person is not performing the action. Use whom if the person is performing the action. For example:

Incorrect: Amanda was the client whom was distractible during the evaluation.

Correct: Amanda was the client who was distractible during the evaluation.

Use of Active Voice

In the **active voice**, the subject is doing the action reflected in the sentence. In a sentence that expresses the **passive voice**, the subject is receiving the action. (The active voice is preferred.) For example:

Passive: The client was given 10 sentences by the clinician to practice at home.

Active: The clinician gave the client 10 sentences to practice at home.

Use of Positive Form

Use **positive statements** instead of negative ones. The former is clearer and more direct than the latter. For example:

Less desirable: His mother said he usually did not turn in his writing assignments on time.

Preferred: His mother said he usually turned in his writing assignments late (Strunk & White, 2000).

Use of Specific, Rather Than Vague, Words

Specific words provide more information and greater clarity than vague words. Use specific wording whenever possible (Strunk & White, 2000). For example:

Less desirable: After speaking his or her first word, a child quickly adds new words to his or her vocabulary.

Preferred: After speaking his or her first word, a child typically adds more than 20 new words to his or her lexicon each month, until it includes roughly 50 words.

Avoidance of Unnecessary Words

Use only those words that are necessary to convey your point; omit **unnecessary words** (Strunk & White, 2000). For example:

Less desirable: He said he was unaware of the fact that stuttering was treatable.

Preferred: He said he was unaware that stuttering was treatable.

Parallel Structure

A **parallel structure** indicates that a sentence consists of elements that are similar in grammatical form (parallel). For example:

Incorrect: The client's hobbies included swimming, reading, and to watch movies.

Correct: The client's hobbies included swimming, reading, and watching movies.

Fragmented Sentence

A **fragmented sentence** cannot stand by itself, as it is not a complete thought; that is, there is no subject–verb relationship. For example:

Incorrect: Some clients provided with therapy last week.

Correct: Some clients were provided with therapy last week.

Run-On Sentence

A **run-on sentence** is one in which two independent clauses are connected without punctuation to separate the clauses. For example:

Incorrect: He wasn't successful in therapy he didn't practice at home.

Correct: He wasn't successful in therapy; he didn't practice at home.

Incorrect: The client always came to therapy late he missed one-half of the session.

Correct: The client always came to therapy late; he missed one-half of the session.

Rambling Sentence

A **rambling sentence** contains many independent clauses and is too long. For example:

Incorrect: The client came to therapy, and she forgot to bring her homework, so she was very upset and began to cry, but the clinician calmed her down, and the client was able to produce the sounds correctly.

Correct: The client came to therapy, but she had forgotten her homework; she was very upset and began to cry. The clinician calmed her down, and the client produced the sounds correctly.

Paragraphs

Some of us struggle with configuring paragraphs in our written reports. Diagnostic reports in the profession are typically divided into general headings and subdivided further into subsections. Nevertheless, the need will arise to further partition content into paragraphs within each portion of the report. As in all writing, adhere to one idea for each paragraph. A paragraph should include an introductory statement or topic sentence that introduces the concept to be elaborated on further.

The next point to keep in mind is that the paragraph should be sufficiently developed. There is no hard-and-fast rule for the length of a paragraph, but if a paragraph is one-sentence long, it most likely has not been properly developed. Similarly, the visual appearance of the paragraph may be an indication that it is too lengthy. In that case, initiating a new paragraph may be appropriate.

As noted, a paragraph generally begins with an introductory sentence. To develop the paragraph, the writer provides additional supporting information, examples, observations relating to the topic sentence, and a concluding statement.

The development of a paragraph in a diagnostic report may be related to the following: (1) a logical sequence of events; (2) a statement of strengths followed by weaknesses; (3) a comparison of assessment results related to information from other parts of the evaluation (e.g., other testing instruments, the client interview); and (4) any other clear connection between the additional information and topic idea. The issues in the paragraph should tie into the target topic and relate to each other and to the main idea of the paragraph in a logical framework.

Notice in the following example how the topic sentence introduces the paragraph. The paragraph is developed by supporting the opening sentence with specific information such as assessment results, observations, and examples. A concluding statement is then provided. For example:

Clinical Impressions

Nancy presented with a moderate dysphonia characterized by strain, breathiness, noise, glottal attacks, and occasional phonation breaks. Nancy vocalized at the lower end of her pitch range (with limited pitch variation), squeezing her vocal folds at the ends of sentences. She spoke with a rapid rate and did not pause to replenish her breath supply; both behaviors contributed to the dysphonia. Resonance and vocal intensity were within normal limits. Informal and formal testing suggested that numerical values were consistent with the perceptual assessment of dysphonia (e.g., breathiness and vocal noise). Additionally, formal values confirmed informal results.

Let us now take a look at the factors that further clarify written communication.

Cohesion and Coherence

Written communication is different from oral communication on many levels. When reading printed text, one cannot rely on the communicator's prosody and body language to further clarify the intended message. In the case of written communication, one does not have the opportunity to ask questions or request clarification. Therefore, it is critical that the writer expresses information clearly and does not assume that the content is implicit.

In contrast, it is important that the written text is not redundant, that the sentences are to the point and not rambling, and that the reader may clearly follow the written train of thought. Written reports, as any other form of writing, should relay a cohesive and cogent message. One strategy for facilitating cohesion in writing is to ascertain that each sentence in the paragraph is tied to a central idea or premise. In addition, the writer wants to ensure that sentences are linked to each other in a logical manner.

Another way of creating cohesion and increasing the coherence of your document is through the use of pronouns or synonyms. When referring to an individual, concept, behavior, or test, the use of pronouns or synonyms within the same or a following sentence ensures that the reader follows the train of thought (OWL Purdue Online Writing Lab, 2017; The Writing Center at UNC, 2017). For example:

Evelyn exhibited difficulty following verbal directives. She required visual prompts to execute the task.

Evelyn's stuttering behavior was further characterized by the presence of secondary speech characteristics. These associated behaviors were characterized by limited eye contact, eye blinks, and facial tics.

Evelyn was distractible throughout the evaluation. Her distractibility was characterized by behaviors such as looking out of the window, fidgeting in her chair, and attending to and commenting on irrelevant visual details.

Another strategy to clarify and unify written content is using **transitional devices**, otherwise known as *connectives*, *cohesive devices*, or *ties*, within and between paragraphs. Cohesive ties are the "glue" that binds sentences together into a unit to form a whole paragraph or connect one paragraph to another. They are guides to alert readers that there is a relationship between various concepts or segments of your writing.

Transitional devices serve as verbal bridges and may be placed at the beginning of a sentence or further along in the sentence. For example:

Example 1: Jill identified all of the stimulus pictured items correctly. Nevertheless, her response time was delayed across all target items.

Example 2: Abe entered the examination room willingly and began to play with the toys. He cried, however, when his mother left the room.

Beginning a paragraph with a sentence that provides an overview of what will follow can also provide cohesion. The initial sentence summarizes and simplifies the main idea of the paragraph, and the sentences that follow provide greater detail. For example:

Example 1: Children with this disorder are more likely to have academic problems for several reasons. (Followed by sentences describing these reasons.)

Example 2: To address the problem, a three-step approach is recommended. (Followed by sentences describing each step.)

Example 3: Several factors may complicate diagnosis. (Followed by sentences explaining what these factors are.)

Example 4: Thomas has a long history of otitis media. (Followed by sentences summarizing this history.)

Using Transitions

As noted in the previous section, transitions enhance the clarity of your message by creating easy-to-follow ties between sentences, paragraphs, and the various sections of your diagnostic report. For example:

Although the findings appear to be valid, recent studies have shown conflicting results.

Anna's skills fell within normal limits; however, there was a significant discrepancy between her receptive and expressive linguistic scores on this test.

An effective transition uses words or phrases that show the kind of logical relationship you want to convey. Some transitional expressions, such as *similarly* or *in contrast*, express comparisons, whereas others, such as in sum, may relate a conclusion to an idea or to an inventory of assessment results. Refer to Table 3-2 for a classification of transitional expressions. The left column of the table indicates the kind of logical relationship the writer is trying to express. The second column of the table provides examples of words or phrases that express the logical relationship. Finally, the third column includes sample sentences for application of the transitional term.

Writing Professional Reports

Diagnostic reports in our profession are based primarily on a medical model, particularly when reporting background information such as health history and developmental data.

To further illustrate this point, imagine that you are in a physician's office after an examination, and the physician proceeds to recite your medical history into his Dictaphone machine. You may have noticed that the physician summarizes the data in a straightforward, succinct, and active voice. The doctor's sentences are straight to the point, do not ramble, nor do they circumvent the issue. The physician's use of the language and terminology is professional and formal, without the use exaggerated or emotional words or the embellishment of the facts. As they say in the police world, "The facts, just the facts." A diagnostic report reflects the use of a professional voice, not a voice engaged in conversation or relating a narrative.

For the report to maintain an objective stance, the writer does not assume that a client knows or does not know something, thinks or feels a certain way, or was

Table 3-2. Transitional Expressions and Sample Sentences

Logical Relationship	*Transitional Expression*	*Sample Sentences*
Similarity	also, in the same way, as such, just as, so too, likewise, similarly, consistent with, correspondingly, aligned with	Jennifer's performance on the Goldman-Fristoe Test of Articulation-2 was *aligned with* the examiner's observations during spontaneous speech.
Exception/contrast	but, however, in spite of, on the one hand, on the other hand, nevertheless, nonetheless, notwithstanding, in contrast, on the contrary, still, yet	The ENT physician recommended that John receive regular inoculations over the course of 1 year to treat his allergies; *however,* he did not follow through with the recommended treatment.
Sequence/order	first, second, third, next, then, finally	*First,* the client is asked to read a single word, and then to use it in a sentence. *Then,* the client is asked to read a paragraph aloud.
Time	after, afterward, at last, before, currently, at the same time, during, earlier, immediately, later, meanwhile, now, recently, simultaneously, subsequently, then	Mark received services in his preschool *followed by* private services obtained through an agency. Mark *subsequently* received speech-language services rendered by a school speech therapist.
Example	for example, for instance, namely, specifically, to illustrate	*Specifically,* Mary's higher aptitude for Numbers Backward supports her ability to use strategies to solve problems. *For example,* during the Numbers Backward task, Mary consistently verbally rehearsed the target items before responding.
Emphasis	even, indeed, in fact, of course, truly, it is noteworthy, it is important to note	Although Sharon's score fell within normal limits, *it is noteworthy* that she did not produce more than a maximum of two definitions for any of the 15 items presented.
Place/position	above, foregoing, adjacent, below, beyond, here, in front, in back, nearby, there	The *foregoing* difficulties were consistent with observations of Jose's behavior in the home setting.
Cause and effect	accordingly, consequently, hence, so, therefore, thus	Since the CASL is not standardized for bilingual individuals or for those older than 21 years old, exact scores are not reported. *Therefore,* the results were obtained for comparative purposes only.
Additional support or evidence	additionally, in addition, again, having said that, also, and, as well, besides, equally important, further, furthermore, in addition, moreover, then	Bobby's productions of /l/ in blends were distorted inconsistently or substituted by /r/ in some instances. *In addition,* Bobby devoiced word final consonant fricatives, stops, and affricates.
Conclusion/summary	finally, in a word, in brief, in conclusion, in the end, in the final analysis, on the whole, thus, to conclude, to summarize, in sum, in summary	*In sum,* Jane's speech intelligibility was significantly compromised secondary to her alterations in language form, differences in articulation as a result of Spanish-influenced English, and limited lexicon in the English language.

Table of transitional expressions adapted with permission from The Writing Center at UNC handout, "Transitions." Retrieved from http://writingcenter.unc.edu/tips-and-tools/transitions. Sample sentences created by chapter authors.

able or not able to complete a task. We may only state what is observed at the time and must avoid vocabulary that makes assumptions. For example, rather than state, "The client was not able to," write in direct-action terms what the client did or did not do—for example, "Susan did not label action pictures."

Although diagnostic reports are very different from other forms of written communication, they follow most of the same cardinal rules. Whenever possible, introduce your subject or paragraph. Next, substantiate your first "umbrella statement" with evidence, more detailed information, and/or examples. If possible, include a conclusion or summary statement to complete the paragraph.

Another important tool is to refer to the client by his or her name, alternating and varying the proper name throughout the text with use of the pronoun *he* or *she*. Other alternative terms for "the client" are "her son" or "his daughter" where applicable.

In addition, ideas should be organized, preferably in sequential order, in order of relevance; consolidated; and linked to each other. The importance of segueing between ideas applies to connections between paragraphs as well as between sentences. Use connective devices to link ideas. We will elaborate more on the use of connective devices later in this chapter.

When organizing case history and background information, state the positive information before the negative. For example, when discussing developmental milestones, state what was presented age appropriately before the delays, where applicable. For example, "All developmental milestones were reached age appropriately, with the exception of speech, which was delayed. X said his first word, 'Mama,' at age 17 months, and linked words together at age 30 months." It is also important to bear in mind to write the report in third person (e.g., "the examiner," "the clinician," or "the diagnostician," rather than using the first person "I"), and to keep tenses consistent.

To ensure a more polished report, we suggest using a thesaurus, a medical dictionary, and the Internet to aid in the use of a varied and professional terminology. Research the spelling, meaning, and purpose of the medication and/or treatment, and include a definition in parentheses. For example, "X suffered from recurring acute otitis media (infections of the middle ear)." It is our hope these suggestions and the following sample excerpts will ease the task of producing professionally written diagnostic reports.

Sample Reports and Modifications

The following excerpts from the Background Information sections of several diagnostic reports are presented in their raw, unrevised form. Following each original unrevised sample is the corresponding revised or corrected version. After each pair of examples are bulleted points that highlight the pitfalls of the first version. At the conclusion of the chapter, practice exercises are provided so that the reader may revise unedited samples.

Case History 1: Adult Voice

Original Version

Family/Social History

1. X lives in Forest Hills and gets along really well with her family.
2. She likes to play basketball and to surf and screams while she plays basketball.
3. X also said that she goes to a lot of social affairs such as weddings.
4. She reported that she first had a hoarse voice because she goes to many large parties.
5. She also felt that her neck and throat hurt and were dry so she drank water.
6. X thought her voice got worse because she yelled so much at the weddings and also because she doesn't get enough sleep.

Modified Version

Family/Social History

1. X currently resides in Forest Hills, New York, with her parents and two younger siblings, ages 12 and 8 years.
2. She enjoys close familial relationships and participates frequently in family activities and gatherings.
3. English is the only language spoken in the home setting.
4. X described herself as a social and athletic individual.
5. She competes in athletic sport activities and engages in large celebratory community functions on a regular basis.
6. X noted that she increases her vocal intensity while playing basketball and to overcome the loud background music at community affairs.
7. *See section on Voice/Medical History.*

Modifications

- Name both city and state in which the client resides; (compare Sentence 1 in original and modified versions).
- Information regarding vocal abuse would be more appropriately placed under Voice/Medical History rather than in Family/Social History (see Sentences 5 and 6 in original version; see Sentence 7 in modified version).

- Include complete information with respect to the home setting and its members; compare Sentence 1 in original version and modified version.
- Mention the language(s) spoken in the home (see Sentence 3 in modified version). Language is not noted in original version.
- Use formal rather than colloquial language (see Sentence 1 in original version and Sentence 2 in modified version) for comparison.
- Use introductory statements to introduce ideas, then follow up with specific information or examples (compare Sentence 1 in original version and Sentences 1, 2, and 3 in modified version).
- When information overlaps, you may refer to a previous section to avoid repetition (see reference to Voice/Medical History in Sentence 7 in modified version).
- Alternate use of the client's name and the pronoun *he* or *she* (Sentences 1 and 2 in modified version).

Case History 2: Preschool Language

Original Version

Birth and Developmental History

1. Mrs. Y had been ill with high blood pressure while pregnant with X.
2. Her doctor had required her to stay in bed for 3 months. X was delivered normally and had no health issues at birth.
3. He crawled at 6 months; walked at age 1 year; drank from a cup at age 1 year; and said his first word duck at 18 months.

Modified Version

Birth and Developmental History

1. Mrs. Y's pregnancy with X was unremarkable for the first two trimesters (through her sixth month).
2. In the third trimester of her pregnancy, Mrs. Y was diagnosed with perinatal preeclampsia (hypertension in pregnancy) and was consequently confined to bed rest for the duration of her pregnancy.
3. Mrs. Y's pregnancy with X subsequently progressed to term, and X was delivered through normal vaginal delivery weighing 6 lbs., 11 oz. at birth.
4. X's general health as a young infant was reportedly good. X was breastfed and weaned to a sippy cup at age 8 months.
5. No sucking, feeding, or swallowing problems were reported.
6. According to Mrs. Y, her son appropriately reached all developmental milestones with the exception of speech.
7. Although he reportedly cooed and babbled as an infant, he did not produce his first word, dada, until age 18 months.
8. Moreover, he did not begin to link words together to form two-word utterances until approximately age 2.5 years.

Modifications

- The introductory sentence should relate the positives before the negatives (compare Sentence 1 in original version to Sentence 1 in modified version).
- Use medical terminology for the medical conditions and define the terms in parentheses (compare Sentence 2 in original version to Sentence 2 and 3 in modified version).
- Specify the time of the medical condition during the pregnancy (Sentence 2 in modified version). Omitted in original version.
- Indicate whether the pregnancy was full term and the type of delivery, birth weight, and general postpartum infant health (Sentence 3 in modified version). Omitted in original version.
- Mention whether the infant was breastfed or bottle-fed (Sentence 3 in modified version). Omitted in original version.
- Note the presence or absence of sucking/feeding problems (Sentence 5 in modified version). Omitted in original version.
- Summarize typical developmental data in one sentence (Sentence 6 in modified version) rather than cite each milestone individually (Sentence 3 in original version).
- Mention individually only those milestones that are not typical (Sentence 8 in modified version).

Case History 3: Preschool-Age Language

Original Version

Health History

1. X had ear infections at ages 6, 8, 9, and 10 months and 1 year.
2. She took medication for ear infections.
3. At age 12 months, she had tubes put in both of her ears by her ENT physician.

Modified Version

Health History

1. Health history was positive for the presence of chronic otitis media (recurrent infections of the middle ear) from 6 through 12 months of age, and azithromycin, an oral antibiotic, was prescribed.
2. At 1 year of age, X's chronic serous effusion was treated by Dr. P, an ear, nose, and throat physician (ENT), with the surgical insertion of bilateral myringotomy tubes. The procedure took place at Beth Israel Hospital, New York City.
3. The tubes were removed in June (2010); last year; X's condition has reportedly resolved, and his hearing is currently within normal limits (WNL) (see enclosed ENT and audiological reports).
4. In addition, Dr. P continues to monitor the status of X's middle ear as well as his hearing.
5. Health history for the presence of high fevers, hospitalizations, or allergies was otherwise unremarkable, and X currently enjoys good health.

Modifications

- Medical terminology "was positive for the presence of" is useful for consolidating information and stating it directly (Sentence 1 in modified version).
- Summarize information wherever you see a trend rather than mention each item or age individually. (Compare Sentence 1 in original version to Sentence 1 in modified version).
- Use medical terminology wherever possible rather than colloquial terms; compare Sentence 1 in original version (e.g., "ear infection," "surgery in both ears") with Sentence 1 in modified version (e.g., "chronic otitis media"), and Sentence 2 in modified version (e.g., "surgical insertion of bilateral myringotomy tubes").
- Specify the name of the doctor and hospital and the location when possible; if unknown, state that the information was not available (Sentence 2 in modified version).
- Provide medical follow-up information if known (Sentence 4 in modified version).
- Include a closing sentence to indicate that you have highlighted all salient injuries, illnesses, hospitalizations, and so forth (Sentence 5 in modified version).

Case History 4: Adult With Aphasia

Original Version

Family/Social History

1. Mrs. Q lives with her husband and a full-time assistant.
2. She likes to watch Dancing With the Stars.
3. She also likes eating out with her husband and going to Broadway plays, museums, and traveling.
4. She gets fed up with her speech problem.
5. Mr. Q is upset with his wife's crying and bursts of anger.
6. He also would like her to speak up when she needs to go to the restroom.
7. He would like a speech therapist to teach her to do this.
8. Mr. Q also said he thought it would be a good idea to get psychological help.
9. They have been married for 45 years and have a daughter, son-in law, and four grandchildren who live in Florida.

Modified Version

Family/Social History

1. Mrs. Q lives with her husband, P, of 45 years and full-time live-in aid, Z.
2. English is the only language spoken in the home setting.
3. The Qs have one daughter, a son-in-law, and four grandchildren who reside in Tampa, Florida.
4. Mrs. Q reportedly enjoys reading the newspaper; traveling; going to the movies, Broadway plays, and museums; and dining in restaurants.
5. Her favorite television show is *Dancing With the Stars*.
6. When questioned as to how she perceives her speech, Mrs. Q conveyed that she was frustrated by her communication difficulties.
7. Mr. Q expressed his frustration with regard to his wife's emotional lability (a fluctuation of emotions more marked and intense than the existing circumstances might be expected to produce) characterized by inappropriate crying, bouts of anger, and use of foul language.
8. In addition, he expressed an interest in "training his wife" to verbally express or signal her toileting needs.

9. Mr. Q further relayed his desire to seek psychological support for his ability to cope with his wife's anger and frustration.

Modifications

- Pay attention to organization; stay on topic (Sentence 1 in modified version).
- Use varied references to the client, such as the client's name in addition to the pronoun *he* or *she* (all sentences throughout the document).
- Maintain a cohesive organization and avoid sudden shifts in topics (compare Sentences 1, 2, and 3 in original and modified versions).
- Use italics or quotation marks when referring to the specific name of something (e.g., *Dancing With the Stars*) and quotation marks when directly repeating an individual's statement (Sentence 5 and Sentence 8 in the modified version, respectively).
- Use formal language (entire document; see original and modified versions).

Practice Exercise

Please modify the following Medical/Health History derived from a client interview with a 25-year-old female with a previous diagnosis of autism.

Original Version

Medical/Health History

Q's medical history was remarkable. Q reported that she had been to the hospital twice. The first time Q had an accident and sprained her ankle in 2001. She was treated at St. James Hospital, Rye, NY, and wore a cast for a month. She was released the same day. The second incident occurred in 2006 because she had a seizure. She was treated at the above hospital overnight. Q thought the seizure was because of her hallucinations. She reported that she has been "Autistic" since first grade and has always had difficulties with communication and social skills. Q also said that other kids always teased and made fun of her. She stated that her past history does not bother her because she is only focused on the now and the future. She thinks she had hallucinations because of all the bullying from the other children.

She was prescribed a medication called risperidone for her seizures and hallucinations when her hallucinations and seizures occurred, and reportedly, has continued to take them since she still suffers from remembering negative things people say to her. There were no other health issues reported.

Original Version

Please revise the following unedited Medical/Health History of a 4-year-old boy with a phonological disorder.

Medical/Health History

Mrs. A said that her son X had a phenylketonuria (PKU) test. The test showed that her son had PKU right after he was born. He was in the hospital for about 7 days. The doctors were worried that he might have galactosemia, so they did blood tests and a spinal test. The results showed that he did not have galactosemia. X also had a lot of wax in his ear. His doctor cleaned out the wax on a regular basis. X is a mouth breather as noticed by his mother, and he snores in his sleep. He also had three ear infections. His mother did not remember in which ear or whether or not they were in both ears. He took antibiotics for the ear infections. He did not have any other health issues or incidents.

Diagnostic Report Guidelines

Style Sheet: Verify that you have followed every item on this checklist before submitting your report.

- Type your report in a Microsoft Word document (.doc or .docx).
- Page setup: Top and bottom margins should be 1" and left and right margins should be 1.25" (default).
- Use Times New Roman font, size 12, or Arial font, size 11, throughout the report.
- Use letterhead on the first page only.
- Number the pages at the center bottom beginning with page 2.
- Spacing: Type in single space and skip one line between paragraphs. Skip two lines before headings that begin with a Roman numeral.
- The first line of each paragraph should be indented .5" (default).
- Justify the body of all paragraphs.
- Leave one space between the punctuation mark ending the sentence and the beginning of the next sentence.
- Use italics for emphasis and use quotation marks to cite. (Punctuation is placed inside quotation marks.)

- Tables:
  - Place tables following the relevant section of text, not at the end of the document.
  - Number tables (e.g., **Table 1**) and bold the word *Table* and numbers.
  - Captions should be placed before tables and should be left-justified and bold.
  - Leave two spaces between the number of the table and the caption. For example:

    Table 1. Articulation errors exhibited on the Goldman-Fristoe Test of Articulation-2 (GFTA-2), Sounds-in-Words subtest.
  - Tables should be centered.
  - Headings within a table should be bold.
  - All cells that include numbers should be centered. (Position the cursor in the table. > Table Properties > Cell > Center.)
- If you are using phonetic symbols, use IPA font. You must embed the symbols into your document to ensure that they are readable from any compatible Word program.
  - To embed text in a Word 97–2004 document: Go to Tools > Options > Save > Check Embed TrueType fonts > OK
  - To embed text in a Word 2007 document: Click the Microsoft Office button > Word Options > Save > Check Embed fonts in the file > OK
- Proofread your report thoroughly.
- Save your report as a Microsoft Word document (.doc or .docx).
- Save at least one backup copy of your report.

Source: Diagnostic Report Guidelines created by Baila Epstein for use in the Diana Rogovin Davidow Speech and Hearing Center (DRDSHC) at Brooklyn College, CUNY.

Diagnostic Report

Include the following sections and the information pertaining to each item as applicable.

Speech-Language Evaluation

Client: ______________________ D.O.E.: ______________________
Address: ______________________ City, state, zip code: ______________________
Phone Number(s): ______________________ D.O.B.: ______________________
Parents (Full names of parents if a child is evaluated): ______________________
Diagnosis: ______________________

I. Reason for Referral

- State client's full name, age, and gender.
- Indicate whether the client is monolingual, bilingual, or multilingual. If the client is bi- or multilingual, indicate the languages spoken by the client.
- Note who referred the client.
- Explain the reason for referral.
- Indicate when the problem was first noticed.
- Give the full names of individuals who accompanied the client to the evaluation and their relationships with the client.
- List informants (e.g., family member interviewed during the evaluation, teacher contacted by phone).

II. Tests Administered/Procedures

- List the complete names of all tests administered and assessment procedures in the order in which they were conducted. Place abbreviations of test names in parentheses.
  - Interview
  - Audiological Screening
  - Oral-Peripheral Mechanism Examination
- Include the interview and informal testing (e.g., language sampling).
- Example of Administration Procedure List:
  - Parent Interview, Client Interview, Audiological Screening
  - Oral-Peripheral Mechanism Examination
  - Gray Oral Reading Tests-4 (GORT-4)
  - Test of Adolescent and Adult Language-3 (TOAL-3)
  - Informal Assessment of Oral Narrative Skills
  - Informal Assessment of Articulation, Voice, and Fluency

III. Background Information

Birth and Developmental History (if appropriate)

- Normal, premature, or complicated birth; birth weight
- Feeding/swallowing difficulties
- Achievement of developmental milestones

Diagnostic Report (continued)

Medical/Health History

- General state of health
- Hearing and vision
- Serious illnesses, injuries, hospitalizations, medications, allergies
- Previous evaluations by specialists and diagnoses

Family/Social History

- Family members: names, gender, ages
- Household members: names, gender, ages
- Languages spoken in the home and in other environments to which the client is regularly exposed. Indicate the frequency of use and reported proficiency for each language.
- Interaction with siblings
- Child's behavior and discipline used
- Attitude of family and friends toward the client's communication difficulties
- Social habits, hobbies, and interests
- Description of personality characteristics (e.g., leader, reticent)
- Social services received

Educational/Occupational History (if appropriate)

- Schools and educational programs attended and currently attending
- Ratio of teachers to students in educational setting
- Academic performance
- Interaction with peers
- Attitude of peers toward the client's communication difficulties
- Area of academic concentration and future career aspirations

Therapeutic History

- Type and time period of therapy
- Name and affiliation of provider
- Goals addressed and progress achieved
- Attitude of client and significant others toward therapy

IV. Clinical Observations

Introductory paragraph: Describe the client's general behavior, demeanor, ability to separate from significant other, cooperation, and attention.

Audiological Screening

- Type of sounds presented (e.g., pure tone)
- Presentation level (dB HL) and frequency (Hz) of sounds
- Lateral or bilateral presentation of sounds
- Results: pass or fail
    - Recommendation: If the client failed, was unable to be screened, or if inconsistent hearing abilities were reported, refer the client for a complete audiological evaluation.

Diagnostic Report (continued)

Oral-Peripheral Mechanism Examination

- Purpose of assessment
- Oral-peripheral features/abilities examined and findings (e.g., oral-facial symmetry, dentition, bilabial and lingual mobility, velopharyngeal movement, maintenance of air in oral cavity, condition of tongue and palate, diadochokinesis, ability to swallow various consistencies, etc.)

Order the subheadings for the following sections from the most to least important area of clinical concern.

Language Skills

Divide this section into formal and informal assessment by including subheadings, as follows:

Formal Assessment

Address the five components of receptive and expressive language: semantics, syntax, morphology, phonology, and pragmatics. For each measure, include the following:

- Complete name of the test with its abbreviation in parentheses
- Description of what the test purports to measure
- Description of the task and elicitation method (e.g., Alison was instructed to point to one of four pictures that corresponds with a spoken word.)
- Form of response (i.e., picture-pointing)
- Quantification of performance: standard score (mean = x, standard deviation = x), percentile rank, confidence interval, and an interpretation of these values.
    - If test scores are presented in table format, only repeat them in the body of a paragraph as necessary.
- Qualification of performance: description of behavior during testing (e.g., attention, request for repetition, delay in responding, eye contact).
- Summary statement: Summarize the client's performance on the test in one sentence.
- Indicate whether performance on the test corresponds with performance on other measures and information obtained during the interview.

Informal Assessment

Address the five components of receptive and expressive language: semantics, syntax, morphology, phonology, and pragmatics. For each measure, include the following:

- Purpose of the measure (e.g., to assess oral narrative skills)
- Description of the measure (e.g., oral storytelling task)
- Materials used (e.g., 29-page wordless picture book titled *Frog, Where Are You?* by Mercer Mayer)
- Elicitation method
- Form of response
- Quantification of performance: for example, percent correct, mean length of utterance (MLU), Narrative Scoring Scheme (NSS; Heilmann, Miller, Nockerts, & Dunaway, 2010)
    - Indicate what is considered typical based on normative data.
- Qualification of performance: description of behavior during testing (e.g., comprehension of instructions, initiation of conversation, turn-taking, topic maintenance)
- Summary statement: Summarize the client's performance on the task in one sentence.
- Indicate whether the results of informal assessment correspond with those from formal assessment and information obtained during the interview.

Diagnostic Report (continued)

Speech and Articulation/Phonological Skills

Divide this section into formal and informal assessments by including subheadings as shown under *Language Skills*.

- Include the same components (e.g., complete name of the test with its abbreviation in parentheses, what it purports to measure, etc.) as in formal and informal language assessments, as applicable.
- In quantifying performance during informal assessment, indicate what is considered typical based on normative data.
- If five or more articulation/phonological errors are exhibited, present the errors in a table and only mention the errors in the body of a paragraph as necessary.
- Phonemes should be typed in IPA font.
- Describe intelligibility in various speaking contexts.
- Quantify and qualify speech rate.
- Describe the results of stimulability assessment (trial therapy).

Voice and Vocal Parameters

Divide this section into formal and informal assessments by including subheadings as shown under *Language Skills*.

- Include the same components (e.g., complete name of the test with its abbreviation in parentheses, what it purports to measure, etc.) as in formal and informal language assessments, as applicable.
- Indicate whether the client's vocal quality, intensity, and resonance were within normal limits for his or her age, gender, and physical stature.
- In quantifying performance (e.g., s/z ratio, pitch), indicate what is considered typical based on normative data.
- State whether the results of formal testing (e.g., Multidimensional Voice Program Analysis) are aligned with findings from informal analysis (e.g., perceptual judgment of vocal quality during conversation).
- Describe the results of stimulability assessment (trial therapy).

Fluency

Divide this section into formal and informal assessments by including subheadings as shown under *Language Skills*.

- Include the same components (e.g., complete name of the test with its abbreviation in parentheses, what it purports to measure, etc.) as in formal and informal language assessments, as applicable.
- Indicate whether the client's fluency at the level of imitation through spontaneous speech was within normal limits.
- In quantifying performance during informal assessment (e.g., dysfluencies exhibited in conversation), indicate what is considered typical based on normative data.
- Describe the feelings and attitudes of the client and of significant others toward the client's fluency, as measured formally (e.g., Parent Attitudes Toward Stuttering Checklist) and as reported informally or inferred.
- State whether the results of formal testing (e.g., physical concomitants score on the Stuttering Severity Instrument-4) are aligned with findings from informal testing (e.g., physical concomitants exhibited during the client interview).
- Describe the results of stimulability assessment (trial therapy).

Diagnostic Report (continued)

V. Clinical Impressions

- Restate the client's full name, age, and gender.
- Provide summary of formal and informal findings.
- Provide prognosis with (and as appropriate, without) intervention and rationale.

VI. Recommendations (in list format)

State whether therapy is recommended; include the recommended number of weekly sessions, the client-to-clinician ratio, and the general goals of therapy.

A sample is as follows: *Individual speech therapy is recommended twice per week to increase Nathan's articulation skills with the following goals:*

A. Long-Term Goals
  1.
  2.

B. Short-Term Goals
  1.
  2.
    a.
    b.

C. Referrals recommended to client/parent (information/reports requested from client/parent).

D. Specific recommendations provided to client/parent.

(Name of clinician or clinical supervisor and credentials)
Speech-Language Pathologist

Source: Adapted from the Diana Rogovin Davidson Speech and Hearing Center (DRDSHC) at Brooklyn College, CUNY.

Conclusion

Adhere to the following points (where applicable) when writing diagnostic reports:

- Use professional language (medical, technical, and clinical terminology).
- Use formal rather than colloquial (conversational) language.
- State information in concise and direct sentences.
- Use the active voice (e.g., "The child spoke to the examiner"); avoid use of the passive voice (e.g., "The examiner was spoken to by the child").
- Refer to the client or family member by name or by the appropriate pronoun (he or she).
- Write the report in the third person (e.g., "the examiner," "the clinician," or "the diagnostician," rather than use the first person, "I").
- Introduce your report with the full name of the client (after the initial reference, you may revert to a first name, for example, in the case of a child).
- Conclude your diagnostic report summary with the full name of the client (e.g., in the section "Clinical Impressions").
- Use introductory sentences for new information or paragraphs whenever possible.
- Follow your introduction with more specific information.
- Write a concluding statement for each section or paragraph.
- Report information in a logical order (e.g., chronological order or order of importance, where applicable).
- State the positive information prior to the negative content whenever possible.
- Use terms such as *appeared*, *seemed*, *reported*, *reportedly*, *stated*, or *according to* __ when you are unsure whether the information provided is a factual.
- Use transitional devices to connect sentences, ideas, and paragraphs and maintain cohesion.
- When reporting health history, the phrases "were positive for the presence of __" or "negative for the presence of __" enhance cohesion of the report.
- Avoid use of subjective statements, emotional words, or exaggerations (e.g., extremely, very beautifully, terribly).

Practice Exercise 3-1

Revise the following sentences using the appropriate transitional devices selected from Table 3-2.

- X's developmental milestones were delayed by 1 year. The mother reported that X has made significant progress in his speech development over the past 6 months, and he is still not ready to attend a regular school.

  ____
  ____
  ____
  ____

- X noted that she communicates in English throughout her school day, but her pronunciation difficulties impede her ability to express her thoughts and ideas.

  ____
  ____
  ____
  ____

- X also explained that she has difficulty comprehending and responding to her instructor's questions. She reported that she requests repetition and clarification as needed.

  ____
  ____
  ____
  ____

- She attributed her vocal strain and hoarseness to increasing her vocal intensity over background noise during weddings. She associated her reduced vocal quality with lack of sleep.

  ____
  ____
  ____
  ____

Practice Exercise 3-2

In the content that follows, mark all the places in which you find the following:

1. Topic introduction
2. Alternative pronouns
3. Cohesive devices
4. Appropriate use of punctuation

- X's developmental milestones were age appropriate with the exception of speech. X said his first word at 2 years old. The mother reported that X has made significant progress in his speech development over the past six months; however, he is not ready to attend a regular school. It was determined that X requires further intervention, and that he receive speech-language therapy twice per week for 40-minute sessions.

Write the content under the appropriate label:

1. Topic introduction: ____________________
____
2. Alternative pronouns: ____________________
____
3. Cohesive devices: ____________________
____
4. Appropriate use of punctuation: ____________
____

Glossary

Active voice: The subject is doing the action reflected in the sentence.

Background information: Refers to the portion of the diagnostic report that typically includes information such as pregnancy, health history, developmental milestones, education, occupation, and familial and social contexts.

Colon: Used to introduce a statement/paragraph or series.

Comma: A punctuation mark that indicates a pause is needed in a sentence.

Complex sentence: A sentence in which an incomplete sentence is dependent on the complete sentence that follows it.

Compound sentence: A sentence composed of two independent clauses connected by a conjunction (e.g., and, but, or, for, nor, so).

Embedded clause: A clause that can be removed from a sentence without changing the meaning.

Fragmented sentence: A sentence that cannot stand by itself because it is not a complete thought; that is, there is no subject–verb relationship.

Gerund: A verb form that ends in *-ing*; used as a noun in a sentence.

Parallel structure: A sentence that consists of elements that are similar in grammatical form (parallel).

Parentheses: Used to provide additional content, such as enclosing a brief explanation or an example.

Passive voice: The subject receives the action in the sentence.

Positive statement: Stating information in the affirmative rather than in the negative provides greater clarity.

Preposition: A word that shows a relationship between a noun and a pronoun (i.e., in the clinic).

Rambling sentence: A sentence that contains many independent clauses and is too long.

Run-on sentence: A sentence in which two independent clauses are connected without punctuation to separate the clauses.

Semicolon: Punctuation used to join two independent clauses (two complete sentences) when the clauses are not joined by a conjunction, especially when the sentences are closely related; also used in serial constructions with internal commas.

Serial comma: Punctuation used when writing three or more items in a list in a sentence.

Specific words: Words that provide more information and greater clarity than vague words.

Transitional devices: Otherwise known as *connectives*, *cohesive devices*, or *ties*, these are used within and between paragraphs; cohesive ties are the "glue" that binds sentences together into a unit to form a whole paragraph or connect one paragraph to another.

Transitional element: A word, phrase, or sentence that connects a preceding topic to one that comes after it.

Unnecessary words: Words that are not necessary to convey your point; omit unnecessary words.

References

Heilmann, J., Miller, J., Nockerts, A., & Dunaway, C. (2010). Properties of the narrative scoring scheme using narrative retells in young school-age children. *American Journal of Speech-Language Pathology, 19*, 154-166.

OWL Purdue Online Writing Lab. (2017). Purdue University. Retrieved from http://owl.english.purdue.edu/sitemap

Shipley, K., & McAfee, J. (2009). *Assessment in speech-language pathology: A resource manual* (4th ed.). Clifton Park, NY: Delmar/Cengage Learning.

Strunk, W., Jr., & White, E. B. (2000). *The elements of style*. Needham Heights, MA: Allyn & Bacon.

The Writing Center at UNC. (2017). Tips and tools. Chapel Hill, NC: UNC College of Arts and Sciences. Retrieved from http://writingcenter.unc.edu/tips-and-tools

Additional Recommended Reading

American Medical Association. (2007). *American Medical Association manual of style: A guide for authors and editors* (10th ed.). Baltimore, MD: Williams & Wilkins.

American Psychological Association. (2010). *Publication manual of the American Psychological Association* (6th ed.). Washington, DC: Author.

The Guide to Grammar and Writing. (n.d.). Sentence fragments. Hartford, CT: CCC Foundation. Retrieved from http://grammar.ccc.commnet.edu/grammar/fragments.htm

Hegde, M. N. (2010). *A course book on scientific and professional writing for speech-language pathology* (4th ed.). Clifton Park, NY: Delmar/Cengage Learning.

ThoughtCo. (2017). Rambling and run-on sentences: Sentence fragments. Retrieved from https://www.thoughtco.com/rambling-and-run-on-sentences-1857155

4

Psychometrics for Speech and Language Assessment

Principles and Pitfalls

Baila Epstein, PhD, CCC-SLP

Key Words

- age-equivalent score
- alternate forms reliability
- concurrent validity
- confidence interval
- confidence level
- construct validity
- content validity
- correlation
- criterion-referenced test
- criterion-related validity
- grade-equivalent score
- inter-rater reliability
- intra-rater reliability
- measurement
- negative likelihood ratio
- nonstandardized test
- norm-referenced test
- normal distribution
- normative data (norms)
- percent exact agreement
- percentile (percentile rank)
- positive likelihood ratio
- practice effect
- predictive validity
- psychometrics
- qualification
- quantification
- raw score
- reliability
- reliability coefficient
- sensitivity
- specificity
- split-half reliability
- standard deviation
- standard error of measurement
- standard error of the difference between scores
- standard score
- standardization sample (normative sample)
- standardized test
- stanine
- test–retest reliability
- true score
- validity

As this book guides you through assessment of speech and language, you will be introduced to a vast array of **measurement** tools and procedures. Your knowledge of these measures will be clinically beneficial insofar as you can determine when and how to apply each one to your unique assessment experiences. To accomplish this task, you will need to understand the rationale for using particular measures and learn how to use them and interpret the results that they bear. Assessment also commonly requires the clinician to develop measures and determine how to evaluate performance when those measures are used. These aspects of assessment fall under the topic of **psychometrics**—the study of theories and techniques in the measurement (metrics) of psychological (psycho-) attributes. This chapter will acquaint you with fundamental principles and pitfalls to consider when

Stein-Rubin, C., & Fabus, R. *A Guide to Clinical Assessment and Professional Report Writing in Speech-Language Pathology, Second Edition (pp 65-89).*

making psychometric decisions in the assessment of speech and language skills.

Overview of Speech and Language Assessment

The primary goal of speech and language assessment is to determine whether a particular client requires intervention and, if necessary, to plan treatment based on the identified strengths and weaknesses of the individual. The clinician sets out to achieve this goal by measuring and describing the client's performance. Measurement is the assignment of numbers to attributes of objects according to rules (Stevens, 1946; Torgerson, 1958). Note that *attribute* in this definition conveys that measurement involves a particular characteristic of objects, not the objects themselves. We do not measure a person, but rather his or her speech and language abilities. The term *rules* refers to the explicit testing procedures that are used for measurement. Testing can be defined as a systematic procedure for observing or sampling behavior (Anastasi, 1988). The word *sampling* here indicates that tests can only measure a sample, or portion, of behavior in any given area. For example, one could measure an individual's reading comprehension skills in some, but not all, possible contexts. Clinicians can only observe snapshots of behavior. To make accurate clinical judgments, we must ensure that the samples we examine represent a client's typical behavior in everyday situations.

After measuring an individual's speech and language abilities, the clinician conveys the results of the assessment by describing the client's performance. A verbal description of an individual's behavior without numerical results is called **qualification** of performance. A clinician might report, for example, that Mr. Jackson exhibited poor ability to comprehend spoken, one-step directives. Verbal descriptions are informative, so why bother using numbers to describe a client's behavior? A drawback of qualification is that equally skilled clinicians may use similar terms to describe dissimilar behavior. This is because verbal descriptions are shaped by stylistic differences in communication and are prone to individual bias, or subjectivity. Because of this limitation, clinicians should use objective measures that provide numerical results, called **quantification**, in addition to providing qualification of behavior. An abundance of tests may be used for this purpose, and these tests can be dichotomized into those that are **standardized** and **nonstandardized**.

Standardized Versus Nonstandardized Tests

When procedures for administration and scoring of a test are identical for each individual tested, the test is considered standardized. Because the measurement procedures are consistent across examiners, one can assume that differences in performance reflect differences in the ability being measured rather than differences in testing conditions. There are four primary benefits of using standardized tests, which may be classified as objectivity, quantification, communication, and economy (Nunnally & Bernstein, 1994). Objectivity means that a test finding is verifiable by other testers rather than based on one tester's perception or guesswork. Quantification, as defined above, refers to the numerical results provided by standardized measures. These numerical results summarize performance and ease comparison of results across subtests of standardized tests. Communication refers to the exchange of assessment results among professionals. Using standardized measures facilitates the sharing of test results among clinicians who are familiar with particular standardized tests. Lastly, once standardized tests are developed, they save clinicians the time and resources that would otherwise be needed to subjectively evaluate individuals. This advantage is referred to as *economy*.

Norm-Referenced Versus Criterion-Referenced Tests

Many standardized tests have **normative data**, or **norms**, that enable the examiner to compare an individual's performance with that of other people from the same population. These tests are called **norm-referenced tests**. Test developers derive norms by employing professionals to administer a newly designed test to a large number of people. The individuals tested are collectively referred to as the **standardization**, or **normative**, **sample** and should represent the people for whom the test is intended. For example, a test may have a standardization sample of 5- to 18-year-old monolingual, English-speaking children who are receiving general education in the United States. Following test administration, the professionals score the test using identical procedures. This process yields norms that describe the performance of the population for whom the test was designed. Norms are often useful when we want to compare an individual's performance with that of a standardization sample on whatever ability a test measures. The norms serve as a frame of reference in determining whether a client performed similar to others from his or her population. Examples of frequently used norm-referenced tests in speech and language assessment include the Goldman-Fristoe Test of Articulation-3 (GFTA-3; Goldman & Fristoe, 2015); the Preschool Language Scale-5 (PLS-5; Zimmerman, Steiner, & Pond, 2011); the Stuttering Severity Instrument-4 (SSI-4; Riley, 2009); and the Boston Diagnostic Aphasia Examination-3 (BDAE-3; Goodglass, Kaplan, & Barresi, 2000), among numerous other tests that are mentioned in this book.

In many testing situations, norm-referenced testing may be unfeasible or inappropriate. For example, norms might not be available for an examinee who speaks a particular dialect or whose cultural background does not match that of a standardization sample of a particular test (Taylor & Anderson, 1988; Terrell, Arensberg, & Rosa, 1992). Norm-referenced testing would also be inappropriate for an individual with intellectual disability because the client could not be matched with a normative sample on the basis of either chronological or mental age (Salvia & Ysseldyke, 1991; Snyder-McLean & McLean, 1988). A discussion of appropriate testing methods for these populations does not fall within the scope of this chapter. Readers are referred to Caesar and Kohler (2007) for a discussion of this topic.

There are other situations in which norms are not appropriate for test interpretation. As a general example, if we are interested in whether someone is a competent driver, the performance of other drivers is irrelevant. Now, consider this scenario. Amy attends a school in a district characterized by low levels of academic performance. Within her school district, she scored in the top 10% of children at her grade level on a reading comprehension achievement test. Amy's score indicates that she is capable of comprehending written text at an age-appropriate level, but this may not be true relative to national norms (Walsh & Betz, 1990). It may be more informative in this case to know whether Amy has mastered certain reading comprehension abilities, as opposed to how she comprehends relative to other children in her school district.

When the goal of assessment is to determine whether a person can perform a certain task rather than how the person performs relative to others, the clinician may opt to use a **criterion-referenced test** (Glaser, 1963; Glaser & Klaus, 1962). Measures designed by clinicians to informally assess specific abilities of their clients in a particular domain are criterion-referenced. Standardized tests can also be criterion-referenced.

Norm- and criterion-referenced tests differ in the test items used to obtain scores and in the way that the scores are presented and interpreted. Whereas norm-referenced test items are selected to differentiate individuals, criterion-referenced test items are intended to cover the content of a specific area. Norm-referenced test scores must be presented in a standardized form in contrast to criterion-referenced test scores, which may be provided in the form of **raw scores** or percentages. In norm-referenced testing, the examinee's score is compared to a group of scores obtained by the standardization sample; in criterion-referenced testing, the examinee's score is compared with either a score or set of scores that are referred to as *criterion levels, cutoffs*, or *performance standards* (McCauley, 1996). These scores are used to distinguish mastery vs. nonmastery of a skill or content. How are these scores determined? Logically, test developers must use empirical data on group performance to select appropriate cutoffs. Therefore, although tests are traditionally classified as either norm- or criterion-referenced, these types of testing overlap because we typically use the performance of others as a frame of reference—either explicitly (norm-referenced) or implicitly (criterion-referenced; Messick, 1975).

Another assessment scenario in which criterion-referenced testing is advisable is when the clinician is seeking information regarding specific abilities or behaviors. This often applies during an initial evaluation when the clinician is interested in (a) examining a particular skill to confirm a diagnosis or (b) identifying therapy goals, tasks, stimuli, and settings that would be suitable for the client (Hutchinson, 1988; McCauley & Swisher, 1984b). Over the course of therapy, the clinician might wish to know whether the client has acquired specific skills that have been targeted in treatment. Norm-referenced tests are not designed to assess progress over a period of therapy. For instance, a clinician might devote several months of speech-language intervention to target one area of expressive morphology that is tested by only three items on a language test. Most likely, scores on the second administration of the test would not adequately capture progress that has been achieved. To track a client's progress over the course of treatment, criterion-referenced measures that have been designed to assess the ability of interest should be used.

Table 4-1. Key Features of and Differences Between Standardized and Nonstandardized Tests and Norm- and Criterion-Referenced Tests

Standardized Tests	*Nonstandardized Tests*
• Require uniform procedures for administration and scoring • Offer the benefits of objectivity and quantification of performance, facilitate communication of test results, and are often time-saving	• May involve individualized procedures for administration and scoring • Are appropriate alternatives for testing populations for whom standardized testing is not suitable • Generally provide a more natural assessment of communication
Norm-Referenced Tests	***Criterion-Referenced Tests***
• Are standardized • Compare an individual's performance to that of other people from the same population • Include test items that are intended to differentiate individuals • Typically focus on broad content • Performance must be presented as standardized scores for meaningful interpretation	• May or may not be standardized • Determine mastery of a skill or content • Address content in a specific area • Include test items that are intended to cover content in a domain • Performance can be presented as raw scores for meaningful interpretation

To conform with standards of evidence-based practice, clinicians who develop criterion-referenced tests should refer to data from peer-reviewed sources to determine the skills and knowledge that should be demonstrated at a particular age. A summary of guidelines for test development provided by the Standards for Educational and Psychological Testing (American Educational Research Association, American Psychological Association, & National Council of Measurement in Education, 1985), which may be applied to the design of criterion-referenced measures, is provided by McCauley (1996). Clinicians might also benefit from reviewing Vetter's (1988) proposed techniques for the development of informal, criterion-referenced measures.

Examples of some published criterion-referenced measures that are commonly used in speech and language assessment include the Hodson Assessment of Phonological Patterns-3 (HAPP-3; Hodson, 2004) and the Rossetti Infant-Toddler Language Scale (Rossetti, 1990). Informal criterion-referenced measures that are commonly used in the assessment of speech and language skills include mean length of utterance (Brown, 1973); type-token ratio (Templin, 1957); maximum phonation time (Colton & Casper, 1990); percentage of intelligible words (Weiss, Gordon, & Lillywhite, 1987); and percentage of consonants correct (Shriberg, Austin, Lewis, McSweeny, & Wilson, 1997; Shriberg & Kwiatkowski, 1982), among many others.

All norm-referenced tests are standardized, whereas criterion-referenced tests may or may not be standardized. Nonstandardized tests do not involve the use of uniform procedures for test administration and scoring. Tests created by clinicians to assess specific knowledge or skills demonstrated by their clients are nonstandardized, criterion-referenced measures.

Despite their advantages, standardized tests are not always appropriate tools for the assessment of communication skills. Communication is an individualized social process and is therefore inherently incompatible with the scripted, one-size-fits-all approach of standardized testing. Moreover, many standardized tests are designed to assess a particular communication skill in isolation, such as the assessment of expressive syntax apart from semantic and pragmatic abilities. This one-dimensional approach detracts from the naturalness of the examinee's communication. There is always a trade-off in using standardized tests, and they should be supplemented or replaced by nonstandardized tests as appropriate.

Because evaluation of speech and language commonly requires both standardized and nonstandardized testing, these forms of assessment are complementary. Regardless of their differences, both types of testing should be planned and executed with careful attention to the psychometric principles and pitfalls detailed in what follows. Before proceeding to the next topic, look at Table 4-1 to review some of the key points covered in this section on standardized, nonstandardized, and norm- and criterion-referenced tests.

Test Characteristics

What makes a "good" measure? Two of the most critical gauges of a test's quality are the **reliability** and **validity** of its scores. Reliability is the degree to which a test measures an attribute in a manner that is repeatable. Reliability is therefore sometimes referred to as *repeatability* or *replicability*. Validity denotes the degree to which evidence supports that a test measures what it is intended to measure.

Reliability

Just as repeated measurements of a piece of furniture should bear identical results, scores from repeated administration of a test should be quite similar, or reliable. There are two main assumptions underlying the concept of reliability (Walsh & Betz, 1990). First, any individual tested has a fixed quantity of the attribute being measured at the time of testing. For example, a client presumably has a given number of words in his or her receptive vocabulary at a specific time of assessment. If this quantity could be determined with 100% accuracy, it would be a **true score**. The second assumption is that every measurement includes some error. A score on a test or test item therefore includes two components: the client's hypothetical true score on whatever has been measured and some error of measurement. This is commonly expressed as follows:

$$X = T + E$$

Observed Score = True Score + Error

In this equation, X symbolizes the observed score, T is the true score, and E refers to the error. The observed score alone is of no use, as it could be highly inaccurate if there is a large contribution of error to the above equation. In other words, we cannot determine how accurate a score is unless we know how inaccurate it is likely to be (Rust & Golombok, 1989). The size of error can be estimated and conveyed as a **reliability coefficient** (r_{xx}). This measure tells us the proportion of variability in a group of observed scores that reflects true scores (i.e., true individual differences) rather than error.

All published tests are obligated to report reliability coefficients, including how they were calculated. This information is provided in a test manual. To select tests appropriately, you will need to understand several types of reliability and know how to interpret reliability coefficients. Clinicians and test developers who design assessment measures must know the formulas for calculating reliability and are referred to Pedhazur and Schmelkin (1991) for a detailed discussion of this topic.

Test–Retest Reliability

There are multiple techniques for measuring reliability. This section focuses on those most commonly used in the field of speech and language assessment. One type of reliability reflects the stability of the measure and is referred to as **test–retest reliability**. This measure requires two administrations of a particular test, referred to as a *test* and *retest*, to the same individuals. The time interval between the test and retest should be planned to avoid or reduce the influence of previous testing on performance, known as the **practice effect**. This effect is the result of increased knowledge or familiarity due to repeated exposure to the same test. There is no universal recommendation for the appropriate gap in time between the test and retest because this will depend on the nature of the test being used. This method of measuring reliability produces two scores for each individual: a score at time one and a score at time two. The relationship between the two sets of scores, called a **correlation** (r), is represented by a reliability coefficient (r_{xx}). You can expect all tests to have a test–retest reliability coefficient between 0 and 1. A correlation of 1 indicates perfect reliability and is obtained when examinees achieve identical scores on the test and retest. This rarely occurs. If the test–retest correlation is 0, the test has no reliability whatsoever, and its results are meaningless. Higher reliability coefficients are, of course, better.

Alternate Forms Reliability

In some cases, examinees are likely to exhibit practice or experience effects, such as differences in motivation, on the second administration of a test. This would result in disparate performance between the test and retest and would artificially reduce the size of the correlation between the test and retest scores, yielding a low reliability coefficient. To circumvent this problem, a method called **alternate forms reliability** may be used. Two equivalent forms of a test are created and each form is administered to the same group of individuals. The correlation between the two sets of scores is the reliability coefficient. Alternate forms reliability, also known as *parallel* or *equivalent forms reliability*, is one measure that informs us of the internal consistency of a test.

Split-Half Reliability

Reliability can also be estimated by randomly splitting a test into two halves and determining the relationship between the two sets of half-scores. The correlation between the scores on the two halves provides an estimate of the reliability of each half-test. A simple calculation derived from the Spearman–Brown formula (Thorndike, Cunningham, Thorndike, & Hagen, 1991) is then applied to estimate the reliability of the entire test. This method bears a measure called **split-half reliability**, which reflects the internal consistency of the test.

Two additional estimates of reliability that are commonly used to express the internal consistency of a test are Cronbach's alpha (Cronbach, 1951) and the Kuder-Richardson Formula 20 (KR-20; Kuder & Richardson, 1937). Both of these methods yield reliability coefficients that are mathematically equivalent to the average value of the reliability coefficients that would be obtained for all possible combinations of test items when split into two half-tests. This is the estimate we would derive if we computed the split-half reliability of a test, then randomly divided the test items into another set of halves, calculated the split-half reliability again, and continued doing this repeatedly until we computed all possible split-half estimates of reliability. Cronbach's alpha is used to estimate the reliability of scores for continuous test data as well as for rating scales with response alternatives such as *always*, *sometimes*, and *never*. The KR-20 is analogous to Cronbach's alpha but is used for test items with dichotomous choices, such as yes–no responses. Both Cronbach's alpha and the KR-20 provide reliability estimates that reflect the homogeneity of test items.

Inter- and Intra-Rater Reliability

Test–retest reliability, alternate forms reliability, and split-half reliability are generally suitable measures for standardized tests that have objective scoring procedures. How does one calculate the reliability of measures that are characterized by reduced objectivity? This pertains, for example, to rating scales for assessment of vocal quality and to measures of narrative writing. Different examiners are likely to arrive at different scores for these measures, especially if the specifications for scoring are vague. Even when using a clearly delineated scoring system, two independent examiners may disagree on scores. This might apply when testing involves judging a number of complex variables, as in the assessment of conversational skills. Score discrepancies among raters may also result from differences in their training, as well as personal biases. By calculating the correlation among examiners' sets of scores on a measure, **inter-rater reliability** can be determined. This measure tells us if there is general agreement among scores derived by different examiners.

Inter-rater reliability indicates if the raters were consistent in their measurements, but they could be consistently inaccurate. This measure of reliability should therefore be supplemented by information that tells us about the accuracy of the measure. Suppose two examiners are counting disfluencies as a child produces an oral narrative. Both raters count five disfluencies in total. If this procedure is repeated for a number of children and the raters consistently count the same number of disfluencies per child, the procedure they are using will have perfect reliability, a correlation of 1. It is quite possible, though, that the two raters identified different types of disfluencies and, therefore, did not agree on the specific disfluencies exhibited. To factor in concurrence among raters, a reliability measure called **percent exact agreement** (PEA; Haynes & Pindzola, 2007; Sheard, Adams, & Davis, 1991) can be computed, as follows:

$$\frac{\text{No. of Agreements}}{\text{No. of Agreements} + \text{No. of Disagreements}} \times 100 = \text{percent exact agreement}$$

The formula for PEA tells us the number of behaviors that were judged the same across raters. This method could also be used by one clinician to determine the consistency of the clinician's measurements over repeated scoring of a sample, a measure referred to as **intra-rater reliability**. Because PEA, as well as other percentage of agreement measures, does not account for the contribution of chance agreement to the total agreement score, it should be used and reported with caution (Hayes & Hatch, 1999). Alternative methods for estimating inter- and intra-rater reliability that avoid this problem by using correlation measures are described by Schiavetti and Metz (2006).

Inter- and intra-rater reliability are also useful measures for determining the reliability of scores on standardized tests. When these tests require open-ended responses (i.e., sentence construction tasks) as opposed to close-ended responses (i.e., multiple-choice questions), discrepancies among and within scorers may arise. A high level of inter- or intra-rater reliability indicates that the scoring system for the test is reliable.

How Are Reliability Coefficients Interpreted?

Some error creeps into all measurements; therefore, scores from two administrations of the same test to a particular individual are likely to be somewhat different. We need to know what proportion of the difference, or variance, among observed scores reflects a difference in the true score (i.e., what we are testing) as opposed to error variance. From a reliability coefficient of .90, we know that 90% of the variance is attributable to the true score and only 10% is error variance.

What is the minimum reliability coefficient for a test to be considered of good quality? This depends on the type of reliability estimated and how the test will be used. We expect reliability coefficients for measures of internal consistency (e.g., alternate forms and split-half reliability) to be higher than those for test–retest reliability because the latter one is more volatile due to the passage of time between the test and retest. The following guidelines apply to alternate forms and split-half reliability, as well as to several other measures of internal consistency: Tests with high-stake outcomes, in which case the lives of individuals may be seriously affected by the results, should have reliability coefficients of at least .90 (Nunnally & Bernstein, 1994). Several researchers (Aiken, 1991; Rosenthal & Rosnow, 1991; Weiner & Stewart, 1984) have suggested that reliability coefficients should be .85 or higher when scores on a measure are used to make clinical decisions. When scores are used for research purposes (i.e., examining group differences), reliability coefficients of .80 are adequate (Nunnally & Bernstein, 1994).

The standards for evaluating reliability coefficients in estimating test–retest reliability are less straightforward because various factors must be considered, including the duration between the test and retest, learning that occurred between the test administrations, and the ability under examination (Charter, 2003). Standards for inter-rater reliability coefficients are also less definitive. Charter advised the adoption of higher standards for inter-rater reliability relative to internal consistency reliability. Salvia, Ysseldyke, and Bolt (2007) recommended using reliability coefficients greater than .90 for test–retest and inter-rater reliability.

Different types of reliability measures usually yield different coefficients for the same test, so it is important to take note of both the reliability coefficient and the formula by which it was calculated. Also, bear in mind that reliability coefficients for a particular test pertain only to the standardization sample of that test and can only be generalized to individuals who match the sample. Lastly, for a correlation to be meaningful, the probability level for the statistical result must be less than .05 ($P < .05$), which means that there is less than a 5% chance that the observed relationship is due to chance alone. When multiple correlational analyses are performed for a particular measure, it is appropriate to use a probability of $P < .01$ or $P < .001$ to control for the likelihood of observing a significant relationship merely because multiple statistical tests are being conducted.

Standard Error of Measurement

Once the reliability coefficient of a measure is known, it is helpful to estimate the relative size of the error (E) vs. the true score (T) in the $X = T + E$ equation for a specific individual tested. How close is Sharon's observed test score on expressive vocabulary to her true score, for instance? Because some error impinges on all measurements, the true score is only hypothetical. If Sharon took a particular test an infinite number of times, a hypothetical distribution of scores would be obtained. The mean (M), or arithmetic average, of the distribution would be Sharon's true score. The spread of scores around the mean is expressed as the **standard error of measurement** (SEM). The following formula is used to derive the SEM:

$$\text{SEM} = \text{SD of the test } \sqrt{1 - r_{xx}}$$

In this equation, SD refers to the **standard deviation**, which is a measure of the average variability in a set of scores. The SD is computed on the basis of the mean of the data set and is expressed in the same units as the scores. The preceding formula shows that the SEM is dependent on the SD of the test and the reliability coefficient of the test scores. Tests that have large SD units will have larger SEMs than tests with small SD units, even if their reliability coefficients are equal. Therefore, the magnitude of the SEM cannot be used independently as an index of reliability (Urbina, 2004).

Using the SEM reported in a test manual, test examiners can derive the upper and lower limits of a range, called a **confidence interval**, around a person's observed score. The confidence interval is used to estimate the likelihood that the person's true score falls within a range of the observed score. This estimation is performed by computing the following formula:

$$\text{Confidence interval for true score} = \text{Observed score} \pm \text{SEM}$$

Different **confidence levels** are used to construct confidence intervals depending on the desired level of

Table 4-2. Relationship Between Confidence Levels and Confidence Intervals as Applied to a Standard Score of 8 (M = 10; SD = 3) on the Sentence Comprehension Subtest of the CELF-5 for Children Aged 7;0 (Years;Months) to 7;11

A	*B*	*C*	*D*
Confidence Level	**Standard Score Points Derived From the SEM**	**Subtest Standard Score ± B**	**Confidence Interval (= C)**
68%	1	8 ± 1	7 to 9
90%	2	8 ± 2	6 to 10
95%	3	8 ± 3	5 to 11

certainty in the precision of the test. This is illustrated in Table 4-2, which includes data for children between the ages of 7;0 (years;months) and 7;11 on the Sentence Comprehension subtest of the Clinical Evaluation of Language Fundamentals-5 (CELF-5; Wiig, Semel, & Secord, 2013). On the basis of the SEM, the number of standard score points that should be used to create confidence intervals has been computed and is provided for the 68%, 90%, and 95% confidence levels. After selecting a confidence level, the examiner constructs a confidence interval by adding and subtracting from the examinee's standard score the number of points that correspond to the confidence level.

Notice that using the 68% confidence level provides a confidence interval that is narrow, indicating good test precision, but there is a 32% chance that the confidence interval does not include the true score (100% – 68% = 32%). That is a high risk. The 90% and 95% confidence levels provide wider bands of scores and are therefore less precise, but they are also less risky. The interpretation for the 95% confidence interval in this example is as follows. Chances are 95/100 that the client's true score on this measure falls within the range of 5 to 11 (Urbina, 2004).

Conventionally, the 95% confidence level is used, which means that there is a 5% chance that the examinee's true score does not fall within the confidence interval. When critical decisions such as classification, eligibility, or placement are made based on test outcomes, a high confidence level should be adopted to ensure more certainty in the measure (Walsh & Betz, 1990). If an observed score falls below a cutoff for normality and the confidence interval extends into the average range, caution should be exercised in interpreting the results. In such a case, error in the measure may be masking performance that is within normal limits.

There are two basic reasons for constructing and reporting confidence intervals. One reason is that confidence intervals call attention to the fact that, due to measurement error, test scores are less precise than one might expect for numerical results. Therefore, when major clinical decisions are made on the basis of test results, measurement error, as conveyed by the SEM, should be strongly considered. Confidence intervals are also essential when comparing two or more scores obtained by the same individual on various subtests or parts of a test battery. For example, a clinician may seek to determine whether the difference in scores obtained by an examinee on receptive and expressive language subtests is statistically significant, or unlikely to have occurred by chance. Many test manuals provide tables that present data based on a statistic called the **standard error of the difference between scores**, or SE_{diff}. Using the SE_{diff}, confidence intervals can be derived to ascertain whether differences between test scores are significant in view of measurement error (Urbina, 2004).

To review, a reliability coefficient expresses the degree to which the results of a measure are repeatable and the SEM signifies the amount of error in the measure. A test with a high amount of measurement error is likely to have reduced reliability. Before using a test, check the test manual for reliability coefficients and the SEM. A high reliability coefficient and a low SEM indicate that the scores of a measure are reliable.

Low levels of reliability may not be due to the nature of a test or ability measured only; they may relate to the population for which a test is intended. For example, infants and young children often demonstrate shorter attention span, more susceptibility to fatigue, and less motivation to fulfill tasks relative to school-age children. As a result, tests designed for these populations sometimes have relatively low levels of reliability (Aiken, 1998).

Validity

A test that is reliable measures some characteristic consistently. This does not mean that the test measures what it was designed to measure, which is expressed by the term *validity*. It is possible for a test to be valid for one purpose and invalid for another purpose. Therefore, a test must be validated for each proposed interpretation of the data that it yields (Messick, 1989). For example, a test may be valid for the purpose of answering the question, "Do the results suggest that the examinee has a language impairment?" but may be invalid for obtaining other diagnostic information such as, "What are the examinee's deficient areas?" (Merrell & Plante, 1997).

Can a test be reliable but not valid? Sure, it can. Imagine that you purchased a ruler that should be 12 inches long and that has 12 marks for inches but was mistakenly manufactured as 13 inches long. Each time you measure an object with the ruler, you will obtain the same result, but it will be incorrect. The ruler is reliable because it yields consistent results, but it is not valid because it does not accurately measure length (Walsh & Betz, 1990). Next question: Can a test that is not reliable be valid? No. Logically, a test that is valid will bear consistent results to some degree. Usually, reliability and validity are a matter of degree, not an all-or-none property. There are various methods of establishing validity. The main types of validity that are critical for speech and language assessment are discussed in the following sections.

Content Validity

As mentioned earlier in this chapter, we cannot measure an individual's communication skills in all possible contexts; we can only sample behavior using a limited number of test items. The content of a test should represent all test items that could possibly be used to assess the ability that is being measured. We want a test to have **content validity** so that we can generalize a client's performance on a test to all possible test items, or situations, that fall within the domain measured. To establish content validity, the dimension that the test items are meant to measure must be specified. This is usually based on the judgment of test developers and experts who are well versed on the ability of interest. A test developer may then convene a panel of clinicians with expertise in the area of assessment to scrutinize and rate the appropriateness of each test item. In brief, careful test construction and expert judgment are the foundations of content validity.

Content validity is usually determined qualitatively rather than quantitatively because the way in which a measure lacks validity is more important than the degree to which this applies. For example, if a test of auditory comprehension largely reflects memory abilities, the bias of memory must be considered.

Criterion-Related, Concurrent, and Predictive Validity

Another type of validity considers whether a new measure is associated with a separate, existing measure, or criterion, of the same ability. If new measure A of phonological processing is correlated with an independent measure of phonological processing (B), the criterion (measure A) has **criterion-related validity**. This type of validity includes two other measures of validity: **concurrent validity** and **predictive validity**. When scores on measures A and B are obtained from the same individuals concurrently, or at approximately the same time, concurrent validity can be determined. Scores on the new test of phonological processing should correlate with those of an existing test that is widely regarded as a valid measure of this ability. Realize that the old and new tests can correlate even if neither test measures phonological processing. For this reason, concurrent validity is never an adequate measure of validity on its own. Predictive validity can be measured by determining whether performance on a new measure predicts future performance on a test with established validity that will be administered to the same normative group.

Construct Validity

The most straightforward way to determine whether a test measures what its developers claim it measures is through **construct validity** (Walsh & Betz, 1990). The term *construct* refers to the theoretical ability or characteristic that is being measured, which generally, cannot be measured directly. An individual's reading comprehension, for example, is not directly observable. We can design tests that we think measure reading comprehension indirectly. On the basis of our knowledge and intuitions about reading comprehension, we hypothetically construct variables that underlie this ability. Through construct validation, data are gathered to support the notion that performance on a particular test is actually a reflection of reading comprehension.

Here is how construct validation is performed. First, test developers precisely define the construct of interest and specify hypotheses on how and to what degree the construct is related to other variables. As a basic example, assume it is postulated that reading comprehension is associated with receptive vocabulary. A test would be designed with a focus on measuring reading comprehension so that differences in performance on the test mainly result from differences in the construct rather than from extraneous factors. As part of test construction, the reliability of the test is then determined. Next, research studies would be performed to examine the relationship between the test and the variable that is presumably related to the construct, which is receptive vocabulary in this case. These studies should reveal that individuals show similar performance on the newly designed test of reading comprehension relative to a measure of receptive vocabulary. A correlational method, which looks for an association between measures, is one appropriate way to measure the hypothesized relationship between the construct and other variables.

If a high correlation, or strong relationship, exists between the measures of reading comprehension and receptive vocabulary, this suggests that each of the measures is valid for its intended purpose. A low correlation, or weak relationship, between the two measures indicates that either one or both tests may not be valid. In fact, if the predicted relationship between the measures is not found, it may be due to an invalid measure, an incorrect hypothesis, or both.

How Are Validity Coefficients Interpreted?

Guidelines for the interpretation of validity coefficients vary across fields based, in part, on the complexity of the constructs under examination and on how precise we expect our measurement techniques to be (Furr & Bacharach, 2014). The most widely adopted guidelines for interpreting correlation coefficients in the behavioral sciences are those of Cohen (1988), who classified the magnitude of effect sizes as follows: Those of .10 are small, those of .30 are medium, and those of .50 are large (pp. 77-81). Hemphill (2003) reviewed several large studies in psychology and suggested the following guidelines: Correlations below .20 are small, correlations between .20 and .30 are medium, and correlations greater than .30 are large. Generally, validity coefficients are much smaller than reliability coefficients.

To recap, two gauges of a test's quality are its reliability and validity. Information on these test characteristics must be reported in a test manual and it is imperative that clinicians consider this material prior to using a test. Published reviews on the reliability and validity of numerous language and articulation tests and screeners are disappointing and underscore the importance of being an educated consumer of commercially available tests (McCauley & Swisher, 1984a; Sturner et al., 1994). Further guidance in this area is provided by Hutchinson (1996) in his description of 20 questions related to test use and interpretation that examiners should seek to answer when reviewing a test manual to determine the psychometric adequacy of a test.

Some clinicians fail to consider whether their self-designed measures are reliable and valid, and this is a grave error. Consider the assessment of fluency, which often includes calculations of stuttering moments, such as percentage of syllables stuttered. These calculations are dependent on the evaluator's trained ear, and inter-rater judgments among even seasoned clinicians may be disparate (Cordes & Ingham, 1994). Therefore, video recording of diagnostic sessions is advisable to permit reliability checks within and across raters. The same principle applies to the assessment of voice based on perceptual judgments, which are subjective and may therefore be plagued by limited reliability. An extensive literature review of studies involving voice quality judgments revealed a large degree of variability in inter- and intra-rater reliability across studies (Kreiman, Gerratt, Kempster, Erman, & Berke, 1993). Kent (1996) reviewed studies on auditory-perceptual judgments in clinical practice and research related to five communication disorders: stuttering, aphasia, dysarthria, apraxia of speech, and voice disorders. He noted the vulnerability of auditory-perceptual judgments in these areas to error and bias, which threaten the reliability and validity of these measures, and provided suggestions to improve auditory-perceptual methods of measurement.

At this point, you may think that a clinician merely needs to examine the reliability and validity of an instrument to address the question, "What is a good measure?"; however, there are additional considerations. Obviously, your choice of a particular measure should be driven by the clinical problem that you are attempting to solve. Studies (e.g., Records & Tomblin, 1994) that have examined the decision-making process of American Speech-Language-Hearing Association (ASHA)-certified clinicians indicate that test selection is considerably influenced by subjective criteria such as the clinician's familiarity with tests. Regrettably, test selection is also commonly determined by the availability of tests in the clinician's setting and financial considerations related to the cost of tests. Test selection should instead be dictated by a clinician's theoretical perspective on how to assess knowledge or skills in a particular area and should be supported by objective, data-based, psychometric analyses. In addition, a good measure is one that suits the client and the testing situation. In selecting a measure, the evaluator's task is to consider the psychometric adequacy of a measure in relation to the client undergoing testing and the testing environment. This topic will be elaborated upon later in this chapter in a discussion on multicultural considerations in assessment.

To summarize the preceding section:

- The quality of a test should be judged by evaluating the following types of reliability and validity, as appropriate:
  - Reliability
    - Test–retest reliability
    - Alternate forms reliability
    - Split-half reliability: Cronbach's alpha, KR-20
    - Inter- and intra-rater reliability
  - Validity
    - Content validity
    - Criterion-related validity
    - Concurrent validity
    - Predictive validity
    - Construct validity
- Clinicians should examine the reliability and validity of their self-designed measures.
- Confidence intervals, which are calculated based on the SEM, should be reported with the results of a speech and language evaluation.

Measurement Error

Recall that there will be some degree of error in all assessments, and it must be quantified whenever possible. Measurement error in test scores may be attributed to five main sources (Lyman, 1978): time influence, test content, the testing situation, the examiner, and the examinee.

Time influence refers to variability in performance on a particular test from one administration to the next. Sometimes, examinees recall answers that they provided on previous administrations of a test, and this causes them to respond differently than they would have otherwise responded. In other cases, errors result from the individual practicing specific test items between test administrations. When score differences between repeated administrations of the same test are due to the examinee's changed abilities in the area of interest, changes in test scores reflect true variance as opposed to error variance.

A second type of error variance pertains to the content of the test items, which are only a sample of the possible items that could be used to measure performance. If the test items are not representative of the knowledge or skills under examination, scores on the test may be skewed. You can probably relate to this type of error variance if you have experienced taking an exam that disproportionately covered the small amount of course material that you had not studied well.

The testing situation is another possible source of error variance. An environment that is noisy, excessively cold or warm, or intimidating to the examinee may detract from test performance. The examiner may introduce error variance if he or she incorrectly administers a test or scores a test inaccurately. For instance, if an examiner repeats a question on a test that disallows repetition of test items, measurement error may be generated. Examiners are obligated to restrict this type of error by familiarizing themselves with the standardized procedures governing the administration and scoring of the tests that they use. Nonstandardized measures should likewise be administered with careful attention to testing practices that might distort test results. Providing feedback that reflects a judgment on the accuracy of a response, for example, should typically be avoided because it might influence an examinee's behavior and thereby introduce error variance.

Lastly, let us consider the examinee as a source of error variance. Misbehavior, illness, fatigue, or a lack of motivation on the examinee's part during testing may introduce error into an observed score. These factors sometimes constitute a reason to reschedule testing, or minimally, to report their potential impact on test outcomes.

To reiterate, some degree of error is inevitable in the testing process. This obligates examiners to follow three approaches to curb measurement error:

1. Be thoroughly informed and well practiced in the administration and scoring of tests before using them.
2. Construct test items for informal measures so that they fairly assess the knowledge or ability of interest.
3. Carefully consider testing conditions to optimize the examinee's performance.

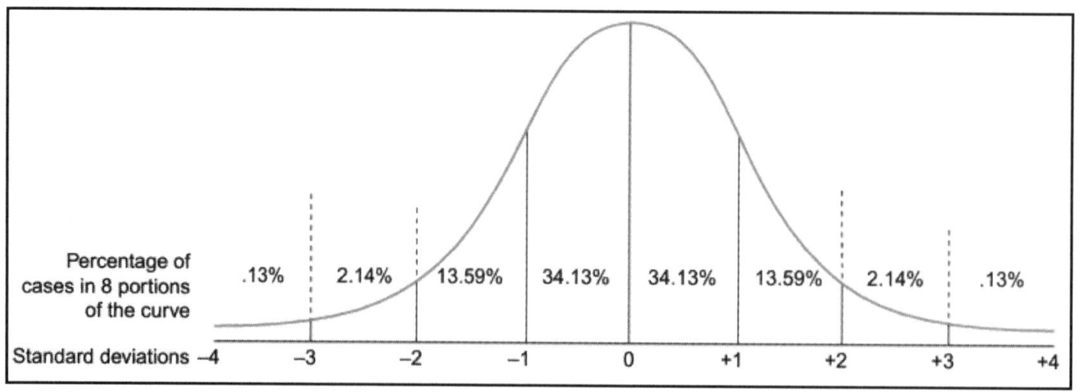

Figure 4-1. Characteristics of scores from a large sample of people.

Instrumental Measurement of Speech and Language

Some dimensions of speech and language cannot be measured solely through behavioral observations. A clinician who suspects insufficient velopharyngeal closure during speech might opt for aerodynamic assessment to measure air pressure, airflow, and air volume in the vocal tract. Oral pressure-sensing tubes to assess air pressure, a pneumotachograph for measurement of airflow, and spirometers for assessment of lung volumes are a few of the instruments available to clinicians. Evaluation of voice disorders may involve computerized measurement of acoustic parameters, such as jitter and shimmer, which correspond with the perceptual identification of hoarseness (Baken & Orlikoff, 2000). Assessment of dysphagia commonly involves instrumental measurement because behavioral observation cannot be used to examine all aspects of the swallowing process (Logemann, 1998). In recent years, instrumental measurement has been expanded to include computerized assessment of various speech and language skills that have traditionally been evaluated through behavioral observations.

Professionals sometimes mistakenly place blind faith in their equipment. Regardless of how sophisticated your instruments are, exercise caution in collecting and interpreting the numerical results that they provide. Be sure to calibrate instruments prior to use (ASHA, 2016; Principle of Ethics II). It is advisable to collect several measures of a parameter and to compare the results across measurements. When using a computerized program that evaluates an examinee's performance against a normative group, ensure that the examinee matches the normative sample.

Dealing With Data

You made an educated decision to use a particular test and administered the test. Now you are confronted with the challenge of handling the test results. To meet this challenge, you will need a basic understanding of statistical concepts in testing. This requires a discussion of the following terms: the **normal distribution**, raw scores, **standard scores**, **percentiles**, **stanines**, and **age**- and **grade-equivalent scores**.

The Normal Distribution

Scores from a large sample of people typically have several characteristics, which are illustrated in Figure 4-1. Most of the scores cluster around an average, or mean, value, represented by a single peak. The mean is referred to as a *measure of central tendency* because it represents the tendency of most scores within a normal population to fall near the center of the distribution rather than along the tails of the distribution. Both sides of the mean are symmetrical; they are mirror images. Some scores are very high and others are very low. These properties describe the normal distribution, often referred to as the *normal bell-shaped curve*. When examining group data, it is important to describe the extent to which individual scores in the distribution vary from one another, which is called *variability*. One of the most commonly used measures of variability is the SD. As described earlier in this chapter, the SD is a measure of the average distance of scores from the mean of the scores in the distribution. The cases of all individuals in a particular sample fit under the curve. Different proportions of cases fall in each interval under the curve and they directly correspond to the SD of scores, as follows.

- ~68% of cases in the sample fall within 1 SD (from -1 to +1) from the mean

- ~95% of cases in the sample fall within 2 SD (from -2 to +2) from the mean
- ~99.7% of cases in the sample fall within 3 SD (from -3 to +3) from the mean

Consider a test that has a mean of 100, an SD of 15, and normally distributed scores in its normative sample. To compare a client's score on this test to the mean, the score must be expressed in SD units as a standard score. Each SD corresponds with a standard score, as follows. One SD above the mean = 100 (mean) + 15 (1 SD), 2 SD above the mean = 100 + 2(15), and so on. For negative SD values, 1 SD below the mean = 100 – 15 (1 SD), 2 SD below the mean = 100 – 2(15), and so on.

Examine Figure 4-1 and note that the percentages of the normal distribution that lie under each portion of the curve are shown. Typically, most of the normative sample (34.13% + 34.13% = 68.26%) achieves a score that is within 1 SD from the mean. What proportion of the population is likely to obtain a score that is between -1 to -2 SD from the mean? Only 13.59%. An even smaller percentage of individuals (2.14%) are likely to score from -2 to -3 SD from the mean. This figure should offer you an understanding of how norm-referenced tests enable examiners to place an examinee's score somewhere along the normal curve to determine whether the individual has performed typically. If a client achieved a standard score of 90 on a test with a mean of 100 and an SD of 15, you would readily know that the client's performance falls within the average range because a large percentage of the normative sample, approximately 68%, scored within the same range. In contrast, a score of 65, which is greater than -2 SD from the mean, is obtained by a very small percentage of the normative sample and would be cause for concern.

Many clinicians agree that the cutoff at which a score becomes abnormal is -2 SD. There are dissenting opinions, however, regarding the point within the -1 to -2 SD range at which clinical concern becomes warranted. Arbitrarily, some clinicians adopt a cutoff of -1.25 SD, whereas others opt for a cutoff of -1.5 SD. When a test is used to help determine whether a child has a particular disorder, the selection of a cutoff should be made with reference to how children with the disorder of interest actually score on the test. For instance, a clinician who would like to use -1.5 SD as a cutoff to identify a child as language impaired should examine whether the test that he or she wishes to administer offers evidence that children in this category, but not children with typical language skills, are likely to score -1.5 SD or lower on the test. The application of arbitrary cutoff score criteria across multiple norm-referenced language tests for the identification of language impairment is not adequately supported by the data provided in test manuals (Spaulding, Plante, & Farinella, 2006).

The rampant misapplication of arbitrary cutoff scores across tests is probably due in part to state or local administrative regulations that dictate cutoff scores on standardized tests to determine eligibility for speech and language services regardless of the test administered. Failure to consider extant data to identify an appropriate cutoff score for a particular test violates the standards for evidence-based practice, as outlined by ASHA (2005):

> In making clinical practice evidence-based, audiologists and speech-language pathologists ... evaluate prevention, screening, and diagnostic procedures, protocols, and measures to identify maximally informative and cost-effective diagnostic and screening tools, using recognized appraisal criteria described in the evidence-based practice literature.

Now, we move on to discuss the types of scores that are commonly used in standardized testing.

Raw Scores

Step 1 in managing the results of a standardized test is grading the test according to its scoring system. This commonly involves counting the number of correct, or incorrect, responses or allotting points based on how much each test item is worth and then summing the points. This process yields a raw score, which is exactly what the term denotes; it is preliminary and must be further "processed" to be meaningful. For example, knowing that David answered 20 questions correctly is hardly helpful, nor is it useful to know that he answered 70% of the items on a test correctly. We do not know whether these values are good or poor without a frame of reference. If we know how other individuals with a similar background as David performed on the test, we have a basis for comparison. As explained earlier, test developers obtain this information by having professionals administer a test to a standardization sample. The characteristics of the scores for the sample, called *norms*, enable comparison of one person's test score to those of other people from the same population. On the basis of norms, raw scores from any examinee can be converted into a score that indicates how the individual performed relative to the standardization sample. This type of score is the standard score mentioned earlier.

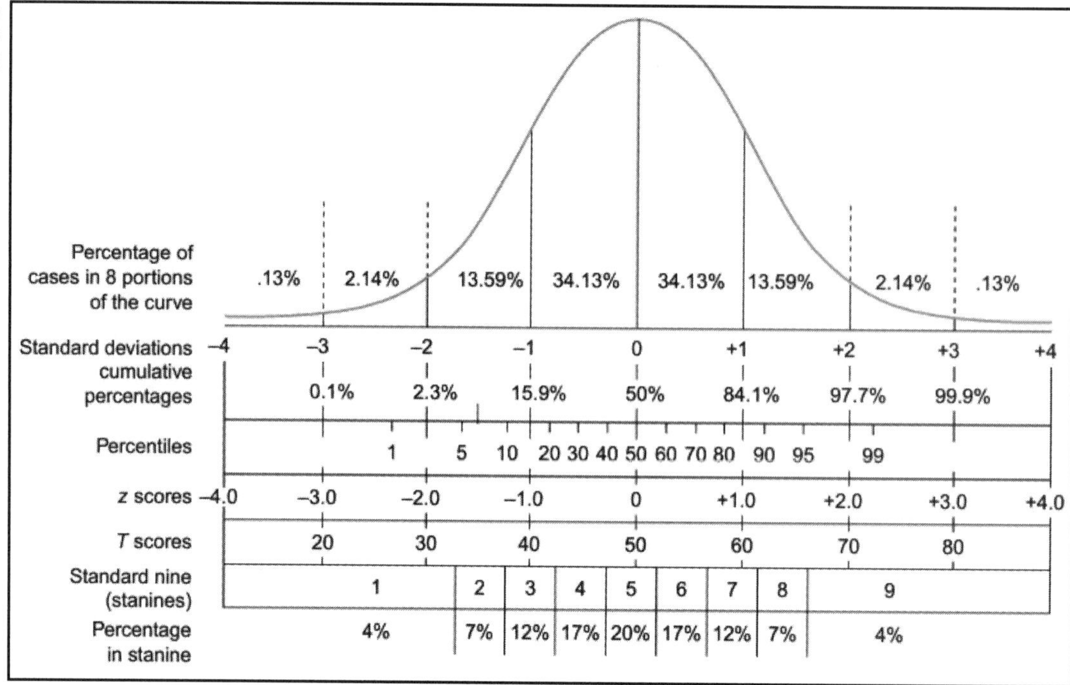

Figure 4-2. Illustration of how *z* and *T* scores relate to the normal distribution.

Standard Scores

A standard score tells us the distance between an individual's score and the mean of the sample in SD units. There are two basic types of standard scores, the *z* score and the *T* score, and both assume that the data of interest are normally distributed. A *z* score has a mean of 0 and an SD of 1. Typically, *z* scores range from -3 to +3. Figure 4-2 illustrates how *z* scores and *T* scores relate to the normal distribution. As shown, *z* scores are equivalent to SDs for a normal distribution. A *z* score of -2, for instance, corresponds with an SD of -2.

The calculation to transform a raw score into a *z* score is simple. First, the mean of the raw scores obtained by the standardization sample, or an age-group of the sample, on a test is subtracted from the examinee's raw score, then the number derived is divided by the SD of the test. Generally, test manuals provide tables that can be used to convert raw scores into standard scores. Imagine that, on a test that has a mean of 100 and an SD of 15, an individual obtains a standard score of 89. Place this score along the normal distribution. One SD below the mean is equivalent to a score of 85 (100 – 15 = 85). Although the examinee's standard score is below the mean, it is within the average range.

To avoid using negative numbers and decimal points in standard scores, *T* scores have been developed. *T* scores have a mean of 50 and an SD of 10. To compute a *T* score, a raw score is first converted to a *z* score. Then, the *z* score is multiplied by 10 and 50 is added. Figure 4-3 shows an example of how *z* scores and *T* scores are calculated.

Percentiles

Remember that raw scores are not directly interpretable. If the mean and SD of a test are known, *z* scores and *T* scores can be immediately interpreted. Another procedure for converting raw scores into a number that is meaningful involves percentiles, also referred to as *percentile ranks*. A percentile indicates the percentage of people in the standardization sample whose raw scores fall at or below a particular raw score. For example, if 20% of the individuals in a standardization sample obtained raw scores at or below 18, the score of 18 would correspond to the 20th percentile.

Percentiles are derived based on a cumulative frequency distribution. This means that, for each raw score on a test, the percentage of individuals with scores at and below that score is calculated. For example, the cumulative percentage of scores for a raw score of 20 includes all percentages for raw scores of 0 through 20. The score at the center of the distribution is the median, and an equal number of scores lie above and below this score. The median is equivalent to the 50th percentile. A score considerably above the 50th percentile is above average, whereas a score significantly below the 50th percentile is below average.

Raw score = 25, Mean = 20, *SD* = 10

$$z = \frac{\text{Raw Score} - \text{Mean}}{SD} \qquad z = \frac{25 - 20}{10} = \frac{5}{10} = .5$$

$$T = 10z + 50 \qquad T = 10(.5) + 50 = 55$$

Figure 4-3. An example of how *z* and *T* scores are calculated.

Note in Figure 4-2 that most of the scores, and thus many percentile ranks, in a normal distribution are in the vicinity of the mean, rather than at the upper and lower extremes of the curve. If one compares two raw scores that differ by 10 points, the percentile difference between the scores will be relatively wide if the scores are close to the mean and narrow if they are far from the mean. When comparing an individual's performance on two administrations of a test, realize that small differences in raw scores may correspond to large differences in percentiles if the percentiles lie close to the mean.

Suppose an adolescent obtained a raw score of 32 on a test of expressive syntax. Using the table in the test manual that is appropriate for the examinee's age and gender, you would be able to determine the percentile to which this score corresponds. Assume the corresponding percentile is 68. This indicates that the examinee scored as well as or better than 68% of the standardization sample. This score is clearly within the average range. You can look at Figure 4-2 to estimate the SD to which this percentile corresponds. If your answer is .5 SD, your estimate is accurate. What is considered a clinically significant, or atypical, percentile? As shown in Figure 4-2, a percentile of 10 is slightly greater than 1 SD below the mean. If you opt for the criterion that a score greater than or equal to -1.25 SD is clinically significant, a percentile at or below this number would be cause for concern.

Percentiles are commonly used to interpret test scores because they are readily understood by both professionals and laypeople. A limitation of percentiles is that differences between them do not represent absolute differences between scores; they depend on where the scores fall in the normal distribution, as noted earlier.

Stanines

Another type of standard score that is sometimes used in speech and language assessment is the stanine, which is an abbreviation for *standard nine*. Stanines have a mean of 5, an SD of approximately 2, and range from 1 to 9 (see Figure 4-2). Table 4-3 demonstrates how raw scores are easily converted to stanines. First, the raw scores from a standardization sample are ordered from lowest to highest. Then the lowest 4% of scores are assigned a stanine of 1, the following 7% of scores are assigned a stanine of 2, the next 12% receive a stanine of 3, and so forth. In contrast to *z* scores, *T* scores, and percentiles, stanines can only be single-digit numbers and are therefore sometimes preferred for ease of interpretation. Many test manuals include tables to convert raw scores into stanines.

Table 4-3. Assignment of Stanines to Percentages of a Standardization Sample

Stanine	*Percentage of Sample*	*Cumulative Percentage of Sample*
1	4	4
2	7	11
3	12	23
4	17	40
5	20	60
6	17	77
7	12	89
8	7	96
9	4	100

Age- and Grade-Equivalent Scores

Standardized tests commonly provide tables that can be used to equate an examinee's raw score with an age or grade using age- and grade-equivalent scores. For instance, if a 7-year-old child's raw score on a test of expressive vocabulary equals the median raw score of 6-year-olds in the standardization sample, the child's age-equivalent score would be 6 years. Does this indicate that the child is delayed in expressive vocabulary? We could not readily answer this question without knowing about the normal variability around the mean for 7-year-olds on the particular test administered. Standard scores convey this information, but equivalent scores do not. This is the most critical limitation of equivalent scores. Moreover, equivalent scores are misleading because they suggest that the distance between the individual's age-equivalent score and his or her chronological age equals the amount of time by which the individual is delayed. This would suggest that the child just described has a 1-year delay in expressive vocabulary. Likewise, a 16-year-old who obtains an age-equivalent score of

15 years might be viewed as having a 1-year delay in this area. This may be highly inaccurate. It is possible that these children are not functioning 1 year below the normal range of variability in the standardization sample of the test; age-equivalent scores are based on a single raw score and do not account for normal variability. Furthermore, it may be inferred that the client's functioning is equivalent to his or her age equivalency (i.e., the 7-year-old is functioning as a 6-year-old). This inference is misguided because the strategies employed during the exam and the types of errors demonstrated by the 7-year-old child may not match those of the average 6-year-old in the normative sample (Salvia & Ysseldyke, 1991).

There are two additional factors that are unaccounted for by equivalent scores. First, the 1-year difference for the 7-year-old may have resulted from scoring incorrectly on 10 or more items, whereas for the 16-year-old, the difference may be due to errors on only a couple of items. This is because it takes fewer errors for an older examinee to obtain a particular difference between his chronological age and age-equivalent score relative to a younger examinee. According to classical test theory, a larger number of observations included in a calculation generally yields a more reliable result than a smaller number of observations. Consequently, the reliability for age-equivalent scores is likely to diminish with age (McCauley & Swisher, 1984b; Salvia & Ysseldyke, 1991). Second, there are inequalities in the rate of development, and differences in behavior from year to year shrink dramatically from infancy to adulthood. Therefore, if a child is delayed by 1 year, the significance of the delay greatly depends on the age of the child tested; this information is not expressed by equivalent scores (Urbina, 2004). An additional psychometric drawback of age-equivalent scores is that they may be indirectly estimated by interpolating between two ages for which normative data are provided or by extrapolating from available data to older or younger ages (McCauley & Swisher, 1984b; Salvia & Ysseldyke, 1991).

Grade-equivalent scores are derived by identifying the grade level or fraction of a grade level in a standardization sample that matches the test taker's performance. If we say that a child scored at the fifth-grade level on a test of written language, this means that the child's performance corresponds with the average performance of fifth graders in the standardization sample. Grade-equivalent scores are beset with the same aforementioned disadvantages as age-equivalent scores. Furthermore, matching performance to a grade level erroneously assumes that there is uniformity in the content and mastery of school curricula across the schools, school districts, and states that comprise a standardization sample (Urbina, 2004).

Grade-equivalent scores are also deceptive because they mask the fact that we generally expect to find greater progress in achievement in the early grades of elementary school relative to middle or high school grades. This means that a 1-year difference between one's school grade and grade-equivalent score during the early grades is much more significant than it is during the high school years. Lastly, grade-equivalent scores are sometimes mistakenly interpreted as reflecting the mastery of content or ability at a particular grade level. A third grader who performs at the sixth-grade level on a reading comprehension test might be described as having mastered sixth-grade reading comprehension abilities. This interpretation is overreaching; the score merely indicates that the child performed significantly above grade level. Similarly, if a second grader achieves a grade-equivalent score of 3.8 (third grade, eighth month), this does not mean that the child scored correctly on the same test items as the average third grader in the standardization sample; there may be qualitative differences between the second grader's performance and that of the average third grader (Urbina, 2004).

Age- and grade-equivalent scores remain widely used despite the misconceptions that they engender because they are readily understood by professionals and laypeople. The preceding discussion, however, should prompt us to question whether equivalent scores are readily misunderstood and whether they should be abandoned. The American Psychological Association (1974) has advised test publishers to discontinue publishing equivalent scores in test manuals. Some state departments of education require use of equivalent scores for documenting eligibility of services (Lawrence, 1992). This is unfortunate. When use of equivalent scores is mandated, clinicians would be wise to supplement these scores in an evaluation report with a judicious interpretation.

Let us review the various types of test scores that have been described here. Raw scores are the initial scores obtained from test results and are not directly interpretable. Converting raw scores to standard scores (such as *z* scores, *T* scores, and stanines) and to percentiles enables us to describe an examinee's performance relative to norms. You might be wondering which of these scores should be documented in an evaluation report. Independently, raw scores

Box 4-1. Summary of Performance on the PPVT-4 (see Figure 4-4 on page 82)

The PPVT-4 was administered to assess A.T.'s receptive vocabulary. On this test, four colored pictures are presented on each page, and the examinee is required to identify the picture that is labeled by the examiner. A.T. achieved a standard score of 77, mean (M) = 100, standard deviation (SD) = 15, which is slightly greater than -1.5 SD from the mean. This score corresponds to a percentile of 6, indicating that A.T. scored as well as or better than 6% of the children included in the standardization sample of this test. A.T.'s performance is below the average range and suggests that his receptive vocabulary is moderately deficient. Table 4-4 summarizes A.T.'s scores on the PPVT-4.

are not informative and should not be included in a report. Standard scores and percentiles communicate similar information in different ways. To facilitate the reader's understanding of test results, it is advisable to include both types of scores in an evaluation report. Confidence intervals are also important to document because they remind us to consider measurement error when interpreting test scores. A checklist of the essential psychometric components to include in an evaluation report is provided in the appendix of this chapter.

Figure 4-4 shows the front cover page of the *Peabody Picture Vocabulary Test, Fourth Edition* (PPVT-4; Dunn & Dunn, 2007) Record Form. We will use this form to demonstrate how to interpret and report the different types of scores covered in the preceding section. Box 4-1 and Table 4-4 demonstrate how the results of this test might be provided in an evaluation report. You will see that whereas the standard score and percentile should be described in the text of the report, other types of scores can be summarized in a table or omitted, as appropriate.

Interpretation of Test Data

Now you have the bedrock knowledge to derive and understand a variety of test scores. It would be sufficient to merely list the scores in a diagnostic report if the scores could make clinical decisions, but they cannot. You, the clinician, bear the responsibility of interpreting test data accurately. To do so, consider the purpose of norm-referenced tests. Most

Table 4-4. Results of the PPVT-4 (M = 100; SD = 15)

Standard Score	*95% Confidence Interval*	*Percentile*	*Stanine*
77	71 to 85	6	2

norm-referenced tests are designed to answer a yes–no question (Muma, 1978): Did the examinee perform within normal limits in a particular area? The answer to this question will depend on the criterion you adopt for your cutoff score, as discussed earlier. A question commonly asked by clinicians is which standard scores correspond to the labels *mild, moderate, severe,* and *profound* that may be used to describe the severity of a communication disorder? There is no straightforward answer to this question, and the answer may justifiably depend on what is being measured. For example, you might decide that a score corresponding to -1.5 SD on a test of receptive vocabulary signals a mild deficit and interpret the same score on a test of expressive syntax as indicative of a moderate deficit. Such a judgment might reflect personal or societal perspectives on the value of a particular skill.

Diagnosis Based on Test Results

Beyond choosing descriptors for test scores, some clinicians ask how to select a diagnostic label, such as language-learning disorder, based on the results of a test. Beware of this error. It is never acceptable to adopt a diagnostic label solely based on the results of one test. A diagnosis is formulated by synthesizing information from a case history, informally collected observational data, and ideally, from the results of several tests. When the purpose of testing is to identify a particular impairment, the clinician should select a test based on evidence of its diagnostic accuracy, which is how accurately the test identifies the diagnostic categories of examinees (Dollaghan, 2004). For a test to have diagnostic accuracy, it must show adequate **sensitivity** and **specificity**. A sensitive test seldom fails to identify a particular disorder in an examinee. Mathematically, sensitivity is the ratio of people who test positive on a measure to those examinees with the disorder. A specific test rarely identifies an examinee as having a disorder when he or she does not have the disorder. This is mathematically equivalent to the proportion of people who test negative on a measure to those examinees without the disorder. Data on the sensitivity and specificity of a test should be, but are often not,

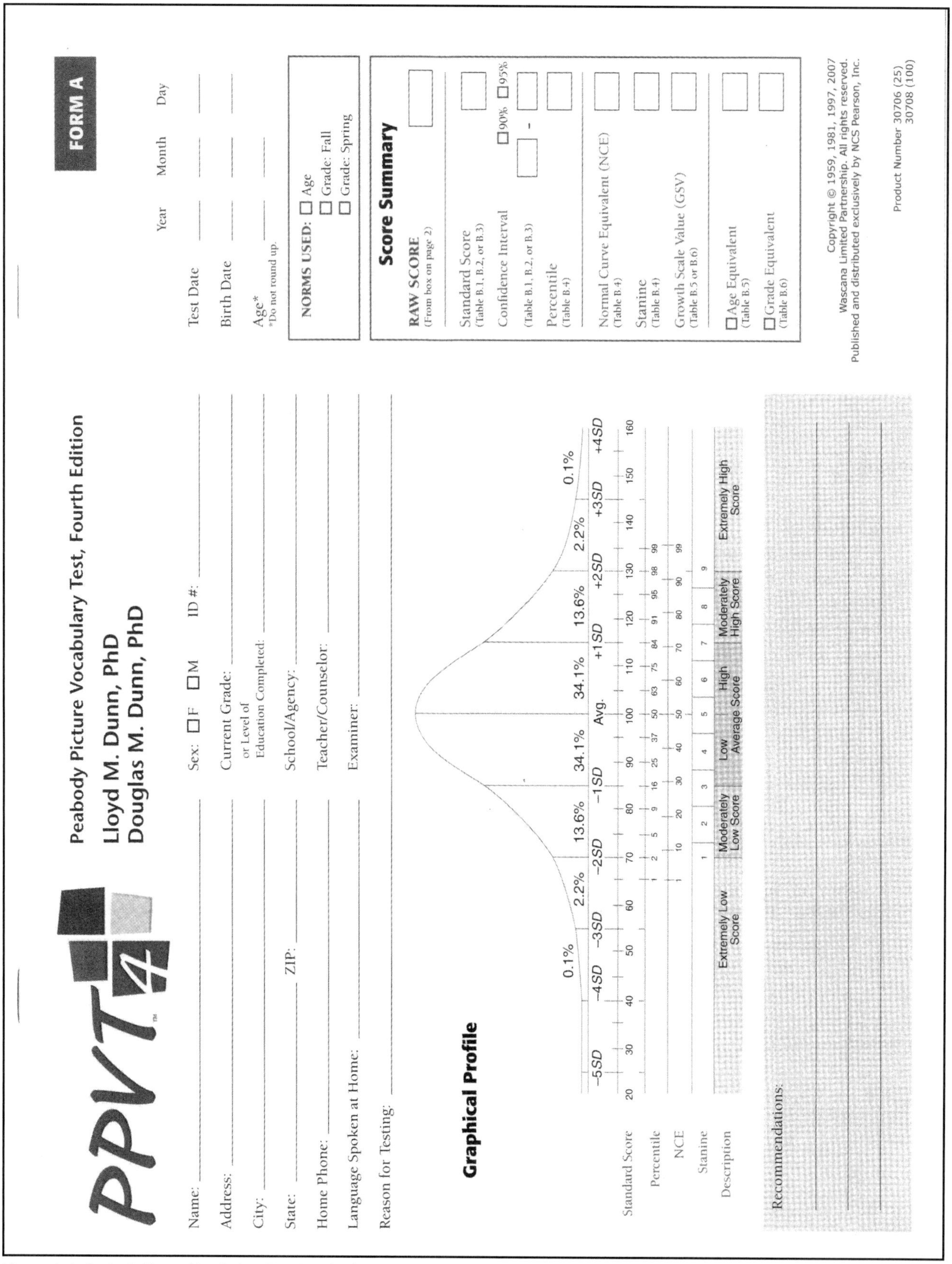

PPVT™ 4

Peabody Picture Vocabulary Test, Fourth Edition

Lloyd M. Dunn, PhD
Douglas M. Dunn, PhD

FORM A

Name: ______ Sex: ☐F ☐M ID #: ______

Address: ______ Current Grade: ______ or Level of Education Completed: ______

City: ______

State: ______ ZIP: ______ School/Agency: ______

Home Phone: ______ Teacher/Counselor: ______

Language Spoken at Home: ______ Examiner: ______

Reason for Testing: ______

	Year	Month	Day
Test Date	___	___	___
Birth Date	___	___	___
Age*	___	___	

*Do not round up.

NORMS USED: ☐ Age ☐ Grade: Fall ☐ Grade: Spring

Score Summary

RAW SCORE (From box on page 2) ☐

Standard Score (Table B.1, B.2, or B.3) ☐

Confidence Interval ☐90% ☐95% (Table B.1, B.2, or B.3) ☐ - ☐

Percentile (Table B.4) ☐

Normal Curve Equivalent (NCE) (Table B.4) ☐

Stanine (Table B.4) ☐

Growth Scale Value (GSV) (Table B.5 or B.6) ☐

☐Age Equivalent (Table B.5) ☐

☐Grade Equivalent (Table B.6) ☐

Graphical Profile

0.1% | 2.2% | 13.6% | 34.1% | 34.1% | 13.6% | 2.2% | 0.1%

−5SD | −4SD | −3SD | −2SD | −1SD | Avg. | +1SD | +2SD | +3SD | +4SD

Scale	Values
Standard Score	20 30 40 50 60 70 80 90 100 110 120 130 140 150 160
Percentile	1 2 5 9 16 25 37 50 63 75 84 91 95 98 99
NCE	1 10 20 30 40 50 60 70 80 90 99
Stanine	1 2 3 4 5 6 7 8 9
Description	Extremely Low Score; Moderately Low Score; Low Average Score; High Average Score; Moderately High Score; Extremely High Score

Recommendations:

Product Number 30706 (25)
30708 (100)

Figure 4-4. *Peabody Picture Vocabulary Test, Fourth Edition (PPVT-4).* (Copyright © 2007 Wascana Limited Partnership. Published and distributed exclusively by NCS Pearson, Inc. Reproduced with permission. All rights reserved. "PPVT" is a trademark of Wascana Limited Partnership.)

provided in test manuals (Spaulding et al., 2006). In evaluating the diagnostic accuracy of a measure used for identification of a particular impairment, a recommended criterion for "good" sensitivity or specificity is 90% to 100%, and a criterion for "fair" sensitivity or specificity is 80% to 89% (Plante & Vance, 1994).

An alternative method for evaluating a test's diagnostic accuracy can be performed by computing **positive** and **negative likelihood ratios** (Dollaghan, 2004). These measures reflect the degree of confidence in the accuracy of test scores in classifying impaired examinees as impaired (positive) and typical examinees as typical (negative). Relative to sensitivity and specificity, positive and negative likelihood ratios are less affected by the characteristics of the standardization sample of a test. According to Dollaghan, accurate diagnoses are likely if a test's positive likelihood ratio is greater than 10 and its negative likelihood ratio is less than 0.2. An application of this method to the evaluation of diagnostic accuracy for the Structured Photographic Expressive Language Test—Preschool-2 (SPELT-P-2; Dawson, Eyer, & Fonkalsrud, 2005) is described in an article by Greenslade, Plante, and Vance (2009).

Planning Intervention Goals Based on Responses to Test Items

Many clinicians are not content with the binary (yes, there is a problem/no, there is not) outcome of norm-referenced tests and, therefore, overanalyze test results and plan treatment goals based on correct and incorrect responses to particular test items. This approach has been criticized because of its psychometric limitations and failure to adhere to standards for evidence-based practice (McCauley & Swisher, 1984b; Merrell & Plante, 1997; Plante & Vance, 1994). One key problem with planning therapy goals based on responses to test items is that standardized tests are not designed to identify the specific items within a domain that are difficult for an examinee. Remember that tests only sample behavior and often include just a few items to assess performance in any specific area. An individual's ability in a given area should not be determined on the basis of a few test items that he or she may have managed to pass or happened to fail. Delineating therapy objectives based on individual test responses may lead to an inaccurate representation of an examinee's clinical profile. Moreover, norm-referenced tests do not tap all of the knowledge or abilities that may need to be targeted in intervention. Lastly, norm-referenced tests are not validated for the objective of planning intervention goals based on responses. The aforementioned limitations do not indicate that errors on a test should not be examined altogether; the message is not to overanalyze errors. Let us consider an appropriate method for error analysis.

Error Analysis

Examiners commonly score knowledge-based items on a right-or-wrong basis. As a consequence of this unidimensional approach, the diagnostician may lose a wealth of information. The first step in error analysis is classifying the types of errors within and across tests. For example, it may be noted that an examinee used prepositions incorrectly in 4 out of 12 responses on a test of oral sentence construction. This finding means probe further; center your testing spotlight on the examinee's ability to produce prepositions at various levels of complexity and in various contexts. This can be accomplished through informal measures, such as narrative language sampling, and by using a variety of clinician-created measures.

Error analysis is more appropriate and informative when applied to test items that are open-ended rather than close-ended. This is because examinees may guess the answers to close-ended questions when they are unsure of their responses and, as a result, their responses may not accurately reflect their abilities. For example, examinees are more likely to correctly guess the picture that corresponds with a spoken vocabulary word from among four choices than they are likely to correctly guess the definition of an unknown word. For this reason, error analysis for close-ended responses should be curbed. A case in which error analysis is completely unwarranted is when extremely low scores are obtained on a test. In fact, a percentile at or near 1 should prompt the examiner to question whether the test was suitable for the client altogether.

Cultural Considerations

Thus far, this chapter has focused on psychometric procedures for evaluating the abilities, or behavior, of individuals. An examinee's behavior must be evaluated against the backdrop of his or her culture. This requires careful consideration of an examinee's culture when considering the psychometric adequacy of all assessment measures and procedures.

Assessment tools are culture-bound; they reflect aspects of the culture in which they originate, including knowledge, values, and communication strategies

(Greenfield, 1997). Because culture pervades human behavior (Anastasi, 1988), assessment tools cannot be designed as culture-free. There are three primary issues that prevent the application of norm-referenced measures across cultures: content bias, linguistic bias, and disproportionate representation in standardization samples (Laing & Kamhi, 2003).

When test materials and procedures are based on the assumption that children have been exposed to similar concepts and world experiences, the test contains content bias. Many tests are constructed based on the concepts and knowledge used in White, middle-class contexts (Washington, 1996) and therefore, non-White, lower- or upper-class examinees may not be as familiar with the test content as examinees from the White, middle-class population. Likewise, picture stimuli may be appropriate test items for examinees from particular geographic regions. A picture of a taxi on a test of vocabulary for children might be an unfair test item for a child raised in a rural area, for example. Language or dialectal differences between the examiner and examinee may introduce linguistic bias into the administration of standardized tests. As noted earlier in this chapter, the standardization sample must represent the population to which the child will be compared. To achieve representativeness, national census data are typically used alongside demographic information to determine the number of examinees from different racial/ethnic groups that should comprise the normative sample. Even when an examinee is represented proportionately in a standardization sample, the test may not be relevant or appropriate for the examinee (Hutchinson, 1996). For example, consider the case of Sofia, a bilingual child whose dominant language is Spanish. Even if Sofia is represented in the normative sample of a language test by some percentage of bilingual children, her test scores might be artificially low if the majority of the normative sample consists of children whose primary language is English.

The problems of content bias, linguistic bias, and disproportionate representation in standardization samples may lead to the over- or under-identification of speech and language problems in culturally and linguistically diverse (CLD) populations (Stockman, 2000; Wilson, Wilson, & Coleman, 2000). To avoid contaminating standardized test results with cultural bias, the tester should determine whether the examinee matches the standardization sample of a particular test. An inviolable rule of psychometrics is that norm-referenced tests are only appropriate for examinees comparable to the individuals who comprise the normative sample.

Regrettably, school administrators commonly mandate the use of standardized tests for the assessment of bilingual children suspected of having speech and language impairments despite the paucity of nonbiased, norm-referenced measures in languages other than English (Langdon & Cheng, 2002; Peña, Iglesias, & Lidz, 2001). School-based clinicians who confront this challenge are encouraged to review the recommended practices of the Individuals With Disabilities Education Act (IDEA, 2004) and ASHA's (2004) guidelines for the assessment of CLD individuals. When legislation of a school district clashes with these recommendations, school-based clinicians should lobby their state education departments to modify assessment requirements.

How about using tests that are reliable and valid for CLD populations? There is no such thing. The testing process itself, including the situation and client-clinician interaction, is culturally biased. To assess a CLD individual, the clinician must be familiar with the language, culture, settings, materials, and interaction patterns of the CLD client. Criterion-referenced measures that reflect this knowledge are commonly more suitable than norm-referenced measures for the purpose of determining whether a CLD client is language impaired (Battle, 2002). Alternative assessment procedures, such as language sampling and ethnographic interviewing (Battle, 2002; Crago & Cole, 1991; Kayser & Restrepo, 1995; Mattes & Omark, 1991; Westby, 1990), as well as dynamic assessment (Goldstein, 2000; Gutiérrez-Clellen & Peña, 2001; Peña et al., 2001; Ukrainetz, Harpell, Walsh, & Coyle, 2000), are also commonly appropriate to include in the assessment of individuals from CLD populations.

Whether the clinician is administering a norm- or criterion-referenced test or is following an alternative assessment method, the potential influences of both the examiner's culture and the examinee's culture on test performance should be considered. In some cases, the cultural disparity between a client and clinician may constitute a reason to refer the client to a clinician who is culturally better suited to evaluate the client. This type of referral is appropriate as long as it is not rooted in any form of discrimination (ASHA, 2016; Principle of Ethics I).

Finally, we come to one of the most key caveats for dealing with assessment results. The interpretation, communication, and clinical application of test results should be considered within a context that accounts for all relevant information about the examinee (Maloney & Ward, 1976). A collection of test scores may be meaningless and, worse, misleading if it is not accompanied by pertinent medical, familial, cultural, educational, and social information. This body of information can be culled from interviews and naturalistic observation.

Summary

After reading this book, you will be equipped with a hefty toolbox of measures for the assessment of speech and language. Be careful. Each tool is comparable to a double-edged sword. If used properly, a tool has tremendous utility for facilitating increased understanding of a client's strengths and weaknesses. If misused, a measure can be harmful by providing inaccurate information that may hamper a client's prospects for remediation. The challenge of becoming a master diagnostician is hinged on your ability to integrate knowledge of psychometrics and communication disorders with sound judgment and professional integrity.

This chapter introduced you to essential concepts of psychometrics in the assessment of speech and language. The importance of both qualifying and quantifying client performance was emphasized. Norm- and criterion-referenced tests were differentiated and psychometric parameters for gauging the quality of a test, including various measures of reliability and validity, were explained. Even superior tests are prone to measurement error, as represented by the SEM, and you are now prepared to evaluate estimates of the amount of error in a measure. Common types of scores generated by tests, including raw scores, standard scores, percentiles, stanines, and age- and grade-equivalent scores, were detailed. As noted, these scores are only meaningful when interpreted judiciously in the context of other clinically significant information pertaining to the client's personal history and present level of functioning. In addition, this chapter described measures of diagnostic accuracy, including sensitivity, specificity, and positive and negative likelihood ratios, which should be examined when a test is used to identify a disorder. Lastly, the chapter has underscored that the measures and testing process in the assessment of speech and language skills must be tailored to the cultural background of both the examinee and the examiner.

Table 4-5. Results of the SPELT-P-2 (M = 100; SD = 15)

Standard Score	*95% Confidence Interval*	*Percentile*
83	71 to 95	16

Sample Data for a Practice Exercise

Rebecca is a 4;3-year-old girl who attends a regular education preschool. She was referred for a speech-language evaluation because her classroom teacher reported that she has difficulty expressing herself and that she commonly demonstrates grammatical errors. As part of her evaluation, Rebecca was administered the SPELT-P-2 (Dawson et al., 2005). The purpose of this test is to identify children aged 3;0 to 5;11 who may have problems expressing morphologic and syntactic structures. For every test item, one or two color photographs are presented, and the examiner provides verbal prompts to elicit responses with targeted morphologic and syntactic structures. Use the data in Table 4-5 to write a one-paragraph summary of Rebecca's performance on this test.

Appendix 4-A

Psychometric Checklist for Evaluation Reports in Speech and Language Assessment

Measures

Standardized Tests

- ☐ Provide the full name of the test, followed by its acronym.
- ☐ Describe what the test measures.

Nonstandardized Tests

- ☐ Describe the task and what it was designed to assess.

Results

Quantify performance: Provide the following scores along with an interpretation for each one.

- ☐ Standard score with the mean and standard deviation of the test in parentheses
- ☐ Percentile
- ☐ Confidence interval and corresponding confidence level

Qualify Performance

- ☐ Describe performance using modifiers such as *above average, high-average, average, low-average,* or *below average* or describe a deficit using the terms *mild, moderate, severe,* or *profound.*
- ☐ Provide examples of correct or incorrect responses for illustrative purposes (e.g., Taylor omitted obligatory morphological endings, as demonstrated in the following productions: *Yesterday, we* **walk** *to the park* and *These girls are* **play** *ball.*)
- ☐ Describe the client's behavior during testing (e.g., distractible, inattentive, cooperative)

Summary

- ☐ Summarize the client's overall performance on the test.
- ☐ Relate performance on the test to performance on other measures or observations of the same abilities.

Glossary

Age-equivalent score: The median raw score for a particular age.

Alternate forms reliability: The consistency between the sets of scores from two equivalent forms of a test that are administered to the same group of individuals.

Concurrent validity: The degree to which performance on a measure correlates with performance on a similar, previously validated measure when both measures are used at the same time (i.e., concurrently).

Confidence interval: The upper and lower limits of a range around a person's observed score used to estimate the likelihood that the person's true score falls within a range of the observed score.

Confidence level: A level used to construct a confidence interval according to the desired level of certainty in the precision of a test.

Construct validity: The degree to which a measure reflects the ability of interest, or construct.

Content validity: The degree to which a measure comprises items that represent all test items that could possibly be used to assess the ability under examination.

Correlation (r): A statistical relationship between two or more variables.

Criterion-referenced test: A test designed to determine whether an individual can perform a certain task without direct reference to how the individual performs relative to others.

Criterion-related validity: The degree to which a newly developed measure of a particular ability is correlated with an independent measure of the same ability.

Grade-equivalent score: The median raw score for a particular grade.

Inter-rater reliability: The consistency among examiners' sets of scores on a measure, which indicates if there is general agreement among scores derived by different examiners.

Intra-rater reliability: The consistency of an examiner's measurements over repeated scoring of a sample.

Measurement: The assignment of numbers to attributes of objects according to rules.

Negative likelihood ratio: A measure of diagnostic accuracy that indicates the degree of confidence in the finding that an individual classified as typical by a test does not have the disorder under examination.

Nonstandardized test: A test that does not involve the use of uniform procedures for test administration and scoring.

Norm-referenced test: A standardized test that provides normative data that enable the examiner to compare an examinee's performance to that of a standardization sample.

Normal distribution: The distribution of a set of data that clusters around the mean, resembling a bell-shaped curve.

Normative data (norms): Data that characterize the performance of a defined population on a particular measure.

Percent exact agreement: A method of computing the number of behaviors that were judged the same across raters to determine the reliability of scoring.

Percentile (percentile rank): A value that indicates the percentage of people in the standardization sample whose raw scores fall at or below a particular raw score.

Positive likelihood ratio: A measure of diagnostic accuracy that indicates the degree of confidence in the finding that an individual classified as disordered by a test has the disorder under examination.

Practice effect: The influence of previous testing on performance measures resulting from increased knowledge or familiarity with repeated exposure to the same or similar test.

Predictive validity: The degree to which performance on a new measure predicts future performance on a test with established validity that will be administered to the same normative group.

Psychometrics: The study of theories and techniques in the measurement (metrics) of psychological (psycho-) attributes.

Qualification: A verbal or written description of an individual's performance or behavior without numerical results.

Quantification: Numerical results that describe an individual's performance or behavior.

Raw score: A test score computed by counting the number of correct, or incorrect, responses or by allotting points based on how much each test item is worth and then summing the points.

Reliability: The degree to which a test measures an attribute in a manner that is repeatable; replicability.

Reliability coefficient (r_{xx}): A measure that tells us an estimate of the proportion of variance in a group of observed scores that reflects true individual differences rather than error.

Sensitivity: A measure of a standardized test's diagnostic accuracy based on the ratio of individuals who test positive for a particular disorder to those examinees with the disorder.

Specificity: A measure of a standardized test's diagnostic accuracy based on the ratio of individuals who test negative for a particular disorder to those examinees without the disorder.

Split-half reliability: The degree to which a measure has internal consistency, as estimated by randomly splitting a test into two halves and determining the relationship between the two sets of half-scores.

Standard deviation (SD): A measure of the average distance of scores from the mean of the scores in the distribution.

Standard error of measurement (SEM): The standard deviation of measurement errors that would be obtained from numerous repeated administrations of a test to an individual.

Standard error of the difference between scores (SE_{diff}): A statistical method of deriving confidence intervals to ascertain whether differences between test scores are significant in view of measurement error.

Standard score: A score that indicates the distance between an individual's score and the mean of the sample in standard deviation units.

Standardization sample (normative sample): The group of individuals to whom a test under development is administered to derive normative data.

Standardized test: A test that requires the use of uniform procedures for administration and scoring.

Stanine ("standard nine"): A standard score that has a mean of 5, an SD of approximately 2, and a range from 1 to 9.

Test–retest reliability: The degree to which a measure is stable, as estimated by determining the consistency of scores between two administrations of a particular test to the same individuals.

True score: A hypothetical score reflecting the ability under examination if the ability could be determined with one hundred percent accuracy.

Validity: The degree to which evidence supports that a test measures what it is intended to measure.

References

Aiken, L. R. (1991). *Psychological testing and assessment* (7th ed.). Boston, MA: Allyn & Bacon.

Aiken, L. R. (1998). *Tests and examinations.* New York, NY: Wiley.

American Educational Research Association, American Psychological Association, & National Council on Measurement in Education. (1985). *Standards for educational and psychological testing.* Washington, DC: American Psychological Association.

American Psychological Association. (1974). *Standards for educational and psychological tests.* Washington, DC: Author.

American Speech-Language-Hearing Association. (2004). Knowledge and skills needed by speech-language pathologists and audiologists to provide culturally and linguistically appropriate services. Retrieved from http://www.asha.org/policy/ks2004-00215.htm

American Speech-Language-Hearing Association. (2005). Evidence-based practice in communication disorders [Position Statement]. Retrieved from https://www.asha.org/policy/PS2005-00221/

American Speech-Language-Hearing Association. (2016). Code of ethics. Retrieved from https://www.asha.org/Code-of-Ethics/

Anastasi, A. (1988). *Psychological testing* (6th ed.). New York, NY: Macmillan.

Baken, R. J., & Orlikoff, R. F. (2000). *Clinical measurement of speech and voice* (2nd ed.). San Diego, CA: Thomson Learning/Singular.

Battle, D. (2002). Language development and disorders in culturally and linguistically diverse children. In D. Bernstein & E. Tiegerman-Farber (Eds.), *Language and communication disorders in children* (pp. 354-386). Boston, MA: Allyn & Bacon.

Brown, R. (1973). *A first language, the early stages.* Cambridge, MA: Harvard University Press.

Caesar, L. G., & Kohler, P. D. (2007). The state of school-based bilingual assessment: Actual practice versus recommended guidelines. *Language, Speech, and Hearing Services in Schools, 38,* 190-200.

Charter, R. A. (2003). A breakdown of reliability coefficients by test type and reliability method and the clinical implications of low reliability. *Journal of General Psychology, 130,* 290-304.

Cohen, J. (1988). *Statistical power analysis for the behavioral sciences* (2nd ed.). Hillsdale, NJ: Erlbaum.

Colton, R. H., & Casper, J. K. (1990). *Understanding voice problems: A physiological perspective for diagnosis and treatment.* Baltimore, MD: Williams & Wilkins.

Cordes, A. K., & Ingham, R. J. (1994). The reliability of observational data: 2. Issues in the identification and measurement of stuttering events. *Journal of Speech and Hearing Research, 37,* 279-294.

Crago, M., & Cole, E. (1991). Using ethnography to bring children's communicative and cultural words into focus. In T. M. Gallagher (Ed.), *Pragmatics of language: Clinical practice issues* (pp. 99-132). San Diego, CA: Singular.

Cronbach, L. J. (1951). Coefficient alpha and the internal structure of tests. *Psychometrika, 16,* 297-334.

Dawson, J., Eyer, J. A., & Fonkalsrud, J. (2005). *Structured photographic expressive language test—Preschool* (2nd ed.). Dekalb, IL: Janelle.

Dollaghan, C. (2004). Evidence-based practice in communication disorders: What do we know, and when do we know it? *Journal of Communication Disorders, 37,* 391-400.

Dunn, L. M., & Dunn, D. M. (2007). *Peabody picture vocabulary test* (4th ed.). San Antonio, TX: Pearson Assessments.

Furr, R. M., & Bacharach, V. R. (2014). *Psychometrics: An introduction* (2nd ed.). Thousand Oaks, CA: Sage.

Glaser, R. (1963). Instructional technology and the measurement of learning outcomes. *American Psychologist, 18,* 519-521.

Glaser, R., & Klaus, D. J. (1962). Proficiency measurement: Assessing human performance. In R. Gagne (Ed.), *Psychological principles in systems development* (pp. 419-476). New York, NY: Holt, Rinehart, & Winston.

Goldman, R., & Fristoe, M. (2015). *Goldman–Fristoe test of articulation* (3rd ed.). San Antonio, TX: Pearson.

Goldstein, B. (2000). *Cultural and linguistic diversity resource guide for speech-language pathologists.* San Diego, CA: Singular.

Goodglass, H., Kaplan, E., & Barresi, B. (2000). *Boston diagnostic aphasia examination* (3rd ed.). Philadelphia, PA: Lippincott Williams & Wilkins.

Greenfield, P. M. (1997). You can't take it with you: Why ability assessments don't cross cultures. *American Psychologist, 52,* 1115-1124.

Greenslade, K. J., Plante, E., & Vance, R. (2009). The diagnostic accuracy and construct validity of the Structured Photographic Expressive Language Test—Preschool: Second Edition. *Language, Speech, and Hearing Services in Schools, 40,* 150-160.

Gutiérrez-Clellen, V., & Peña, E. (2001). Dynamic assessment of diverse children: A tutorial. *Language, Speech, and Hearing Services in Schools, 32,* 212-224.

Hayes, J. R., & Hatch, J. A. (1999). Issues in measuring reliability: Correlation versus percentage of agreement. *Written Communication, 16,* 354-367.

Haynes, W. O., & Pindzola, R. H. (2007). *Diagnosis and evaluation in speech pathology* (7th ed.). Boston, MA: Allyn & Bacon.

Hemphill, J. F. (2003). Interpreting the magnitude of correlation coefficients. *American Psychologist, 58,* 78-79.

Hodson, B. (2004). *Hodson assessment of phonological patterns* (3rd ed.). Austin, TX: Pro-Ed.

Hutchinson, T. (1988, Spring). Coming changes in speech and language testing. *Hearsay: Journal of the Ohio Speech and Hearing Association,* 10-13, 27.

Hutchinson, T. A. (1996). What to look for in the technical manual: Twenty questions for users. *Language, Speech, and Hearing Services in Schools, 27,* 109-121.

Individuals With Disabilities Education Act of 2004, Pub. L. No. 108-446, 118 Stat. 2647 (2004).

Kayser, H., & Restrepo, M. (1995). Language samples: Elicitation and analysis. In H. Kayser (Ed.), *Bilingual speech-language pathology: An Hispanic focus* (pp. 265-286). San Diego, CA: Singular.

Kent, R. (1996). Hearing and believing: Some limits to the auditory-perceptual assessment of speech and voice disorders. *American Journal of Speech-Language Pathology, 5*(3), 7-23.

Kreiman, J., Gerratt, B. R., Kempster, G. B., Erman, A., & Berke, G. S. (1993). Perceptual evaluation of voice quality: Review, tutorial, and a framework for future research. *Journal of Speech and Hearing Research, 36,* 21-40.

Kuder, G., & Richardson, M. (1937). The theory of the estimation of test reliability. *Psychometrika, 2,* 151-160.

Laing, S. P., & Kamhi, A. (2003). Alternative assessment of language and literacy in culturally and linguistically diverse populations. *Language, Speech, and Hearing Services in Schools, 34,* 44-55.

Langdon, H. W., & Cheng, L. L. (2002). *Collaborating with interpreters and translators.* Eau Claire, WI: Thinking Publications.

Lawrence, C. (1992). Assessing the use of age-equivalent scores in clinical management. *Language, Speech, and Hearing Services in Schools, 23,* 6-8.

Logemann, J. A. (1998). *Evaluation and treatment of swallowing disorders.* Austin, TX: Pro-Ed.

Lyman, H. B. (1978). *Test scores and what they mean* (3rd ed.). Englewood Cliffs, NJ: Prentice-Hall.

Maloney, M. P., & Ward, M. P. (1976). *Psychological assessment: A conceptual approach.* New York, NY: Oxford University Press.

Mattes, L., & Omark, D. (1991). *Speech and language assessment for the bilingual handicapped.* Oceanside, CA: Academic Communication Associates.

McCauley, R. J. (1996). Familiar strangers: Criterion-referenced measures in communication disorders. *Language, Speech, and Hearing Services in Schools, 27,* 122-131.

McCauley, R. J., & Swisher, L. (1984a). Psychometric review of language and articulation tests for preschool children. *Journal of Speech and Hearing Disorders, 49,* 34-42.

McCauley, R. J., & Swisher, L. (1984b). Use and misuse of norm-referenced tests in clinical assessment: A hypothetical case. *Journal of Speech and Hearing Disorders, 49,* 338-348.

Merrell, A., & Plante, E. (1997). Norm-referenced test interpretation in the diagnostic process. *Language, Speech, and Hearing Services in Schools, 28,* 50-58.

Messick, S. A. (1975). The standard problem: Meaning and values in measurement and evaluation. *American Psychologist, 30,* 955-966.

Messick, S. (1989). Meaning and values in test validation: The science and ethics of assessment. *Educational Researcher, 18,* 5-11.

Muma, J. (1978). *Language handbook: Concepts, assessment, intervention.* Englewood Cliffs, NJ: Prentice-Hall.

Nunnally, J., & Bernstein, I. (1994). *Psychometric theory* (3rd ed.). Columbus, OH: McGraw-Hill.

Pedhazur, E. J., & Schmelkin, L. P. (1991). *Measurement, design, and analysis.* Hillsdale, NJ: Erlbaum.

Peña, E., Iglesias, A., & Lidz, C. (2001). Reducing test bias through dynamic assessment of children's word learning ability. *American Journal of Speech-Language Pathology, 10,* 138-154.

Plante, E., & Vance, R. (1994). Selection of preschool language tests: A data-based approach. *Language, Speech, and Hearing Services in Schools, 25,* 15-24.

Records, N. L., & Tomblin, J. B. (1994). Clinical decision making: Describing the decision rules of practicing speech-language pathologists. *Journal of Speech and Hearing Research, 37,* 144-156.

Riley, G. D. (2009). *Stuttering severity instrument for children and adults* (4th ed.). Austin, TX: Pro-Ed.

Rosenthal, R., & Rosnow, R. L. (1991). *Essentials of behavioral research: Methods and data analysis* (2nd ed.). New York, NY: McGraw-Hill.

Rossetti, L. (1990). *Rossetti infant-toddler language scale.* East Moline, IL: Linguisystems.

Rust, J., & Golombok, S. (1989). *Modern psychometrics: The science of psychological assessment.* New York, NY: Routledge.

Salvia, J., & Ysseldyke, J. E. (1991). *Assessment* (5th ed.). Boston, MA: Houghton Mifflin.

Salvia, J., Ysseldyke, J., & Bolt, S. (2007). *Assessment in special and inclusive education* (10th ed.). Boston, MA: Houghton Mifflin.

Schiavetti, N., & Metz, D. E. (2006). *Evaluating research in communicative disorders* (5th ed.). Boston, MA: Allyn & Bacon.

Sheard, C., Adams, R. D., & Davis, P. J. (1991). Reliability and agreement of ratings of ataxic dysarthric speech samples with varying intelligibility. *Journal of Speech and Hearing Research, 34*, 285-293.

Shriberg, L. D., Austin, D., Lewis, B. A., McSweeny, J. L., & Wilson, D. L. (1997). The Percentage of Consonants Correct (PCC) metric: Extensions and reliability data. *Journal of Speech, Language, and Hearing Research, 40*, 708-722.

Shriberg, L. D., & Kwiatkowski J. (1982). Phonological disorders III: A procedure for assessing severity of involvement. *Journal of Speech and Hearing Disorders, 47*, 256-270.

Snyder-McLean, L., & McLean, J. E. (1988). Sociocommunicative competence in the severely/profoundly handicapped child: Assessment. In D. E. Yoder & R. D. Kent (Eds.), *Decision making in speech language pathology* (pp. 64-65). Philadelphia, PA: Decker.

Spaulding, T. J., Plante, E., & Farinella, K. A. (2006). Eligibility criteria for language impairment: Is the low end of normal always appropriate? *Language, Speech, and Hearing Services in Schools, 37*, 61-72.

Stevens, S. S. (1946). On the theory of scales of measurement. *Science, 103*, 667-680.

Stockman, I. (2000). The new Peabody Picture Vocabulary Test—III: An illusion of unbiased assessment. *Language, Speech, and Hearing Services in Schools, 31*, 340-353.

Sturner, R. A., Layton, T. L., Evans, A. W., Heller, J. H., Funk, S. G., & Machon, M. W. (1994). Preschool speech and language screening: A review of currently available tests. *American Journal of Speech-Language Pathology, 3*, 25-36.

Taylor, O. L., & Anderson, N. B. (1988). Communication behaviors that vary from standard norms: Assessment. In D. E. Yoder & R. D. Kent (Eds.), *Decision making in speech-language pathology* (pp. 84-85). Philadelphia, PA: Decker.

Templin, M. (1957). *Certain language skills in children*. Minneapolis: University of Minneapolis Press.

Terrell, S. L., Arensberg, K., & Rosa, M. (1992). Parent–child comparative analysis: A criterion-referenced method for the nondiscriminatory assessment of a child who spoke a relatively uncommon dialect of English. *Language, Speech, and Hearing Services in Schools, 23*, 34-42.

Thorndike, R. M., Cunningham, G. K., Thorndike, R. L., & Hagen, E. P. (1991). *Measurement and evaluation in psychology and education* (5th ed.). New York, NY: Macmillan.

Torgerson, W. S. (1958). *Theory and methods of scaling*. New York, NY: Wiley.

Ukrainetz, T., Harpell, S., Walsh, C., & Coyle, C. (2000). A preliminary investigation of dynamic assessment with Native American kindergartners. *Language, Speech, and Hearing Services in Schools, 31*, 142-154.

Urbina, S. (2004). *Essentials of psychological testing*. Hoboken, NJ: Wiley.

Vetter, D. K. (1988). Designing informal assessment procedures. In D. E. Yoder & R. D. Kent (Eds.), *Decision making in speech-language pathology* (pp. 84-85). Philadelphia, PA: Decker.

Walsh, W. B., & Betz, N. E. (1990). *Tests and assessment* (2nd ed.). Englewood Cliffs, NJ: Prentice-Hall.

Washington, J. (1996). Issues in assessing the language abilities of African American children. In A. Kamhi, K. Pollock, & J. Harris (Eds.), *Communication development and disorders in African American children: Research, assessment, and intervention* (pp. 35-54). Baltimore, MD: Brookes.

Weiner, E. A., & Stewart, B. J. (1984). *Assessing individuals: Psychological and educational tests and measurement*. Boston, MA: Little, Brown.

Weiss, C. E., Gordon, M. E., & Lillywhite, H. S. (1987). *Articulatory and phonologic disorders*. Baltimore, MD: Williams & Wilkins.

Westby, C. (1990). Ethnographic interviewing. *Journal of Childhood Communication Disorders, 13*, 110-118.

Wiig, E. H., Semel, E., & Secord, W. A. (2013). *Clinical evaluation of language fundamentals* (5th ed.). San Antonio, TX: Pearson.

Wilson, W., Wilson, J., & Coleman, T. (2000). Culturally appropriate assessment: Issues and strategies. In T. Coleman (Ed.), *Clinical management of communication disorders in culturally diverse children* (pp. 101-128). Boston, MA: Allyn & Bacon.

Zimmerman, I. L., Steiner, V. G., & Pond, R. E. (2011). *Preschool language scales* (5th ed.). San Antonio, TX: Pearson.

5

Audiological Screening in the Speech-Language Evaluation

Rochelle Cherry, EdD; Adrienne Rubinstein, PhD, CCC-A; and Dorothy Neave-DiToro, AuD, CCC-A

Key Words

- audiogram
- audiometric configuration
- auditory processing disorder
- cochlear hearing loss
- cochlear implant
- complete audiological evaluation
- conditioned play audiometry
- conductive hearing loss
- FM system
- frequency
- intensity
- mixed hearing loss
- neural hearing loss
- otitis media with effusion
- otoacoustic emissions
- otoscopic inspection
- ototoxic drugs
- peripheral hearing loss
- pure-tone air conduction hearing screening
- retrocochlear hearing loss
- reverberation
- sensorineural hearing loss
- sensory hearing loss
- signal-to-noise ratio
- site of lesion
- speech banana
- tinnitus
- tympanogram
- tympanometry
- vertigo

Introduction

Properly identifying hearing loss is critical for both the adult as well as child population with whom speech-language pathologists (SLPs) work. For example, adults with undetected hearing loss might be mistakenly labeled as being unresponsive, cognitively impaired, or confused. A child with a hearing loss can be erroneously diagnosed, for example, as being on the autistic spectrum or having attention-deficit/hyperactivity disorder (ADHD), auditory processing difficulties, or cognitive impairment. In addition, when audiologists are not available at a site, it is the SLP to whom their partners in interprofessional practice (e.g., teachers, physicians, nursing personnel, psychologists, occupational and physical therapists, and social workers) may turn for clarification about hearing-related issues. It is therefore incumbent on the SLP to have sufficient knowledge and understanding of concepts related to the screening, testing, and treatment of hearing loss as well as its implications on speech, language, and academic performance. The SLP is often the first professional in a position to identify the possibility of hearing impairment as the cause of, or a contributing

Stein-Rubin, C., & Fabus, R. *A Guide to Clinical Assessment and Professional Report Writing in Speech-Language Pathology, Second Edition (pp 91-112).*

Table 5-1. Classification of Degree of Hearing Loss

Range	*Classification*
-10 to 15 dB HL	Hearing within normal limits
16 to 25 dB HL	Hearing within normal limits (adults) Slight hearing loss (children)
26 to 40 dB HL	Mild hearing loss
41 to 55 dB HL	Moderate hearing loss
56 to 70 dB HL	Moderately severe hearing loss
71 to 90 dB HL	Severe hearing loss
>90 dB HL	Profound hearing loss

factor in, the delayed development or impaired performance of a client. Awareness of the potential of hearing loss and its implications and knowledge of appropriate screening techniques can make the difference between an appropriate or inappropriate referral, as well as the difference between a correct or incorrect diagnosis and subsequent treatment. The American Speech-Language-Hearing Association (ASHA) recommends that hearing screenings be included as part of every comprehensive speech-language evaluation (ASHA, n.d.). This chapter summarizes information critical to the SLP regarding hearing loss in general and screening of hearing loss in particular.

Prevalence and Incidence of Hearing Loss

The incidence of hearing loss varies with age. The National Institute of Deafness and Other Communication Disorders has established that approximately 17,000 infants and toddlers are identified with hearing loss each year, making it among the most common birth defects (Cherry, 2011). More than 30 million Americans aged 12 years and older have bilateral hearing loss, and if unilateral hearing losses are included in the estimates, the number rises to more than 48 million (Lin et al., 2013). It has been reported that in the adolescent population of the United States, one in six have high-**frequency** hearing loss, and this loss is often attributed to noise exposure (Sekhar et al, 2016). The incidence of hearing loss increases with each passing decade. Among individuals in their 40s, it is estimated at 12.9%, rises to 28.5% for those who are in their 50s, 44.9% for individuals in their 60s, and 89.1% for individuals in their 80s (Barber & Lee, 2015).

Table 5-2. Classification of Type of Hearing Loss

Type of Hearing Loss	*Classification*
Conductive hearing loss	Pathologies originating in the outer and/or middle ear (e.g., impacted cerumen, otitis media, otosclerosis)
Sensory or **cochlear hearing loss**	Pathologies originating in the inner ear (e.g., Meniere's disease, hearing loss induced by noise exposure, ototoxic drugs, viruses/bacteria, and/or genetic influences)
Neural or **retrocochlear hearing loss**	Pathologies originating in the eighth nerve (e.g., vestibular schwannoma, auditory neuropathy/dyssynchrony)
Mixed hearing loss	Pathologies that affect both the conductive and sensorineural parts of the ear

Classification of Hearing Loss

Peripheral hearing loss is characterized by an obstruction in the transmission of the auditory signal through the outer/middle/inner ears and/or eighth nerve. (Damage to the auditory system beyond the eighth nerve is called an **auditory processing disorder**.) A peripheral hearing loss may be classified along several dimensions including degree (severity) of hearing loss and the type of loss (site of damage). The classification of degree of loss may be described as slight, mild, moderate, moderately severe, severe, or profound. Table 5-1 summarizes the ranges in dB HL (decibels hearing level) for each of the preceding labels. The level at which hearing loss begins is more stringent in children because adults are more likely able to compensate for some reduction in hearing due to their prior knowledge of language and experiences. Therefore, the category of "slight" hearing loss from 16 to 25 dB HL, is generally reserved for children and is considered within normal limits for adults. This issue is discussed in more detail later in the chapter. Classification of the loss based on the site of the damage appears in Table 5-2.

Impact of Hearing Loss on Speech and Language

The critical role of hearing in oral communication in general, and the development of speech and language in particular, cannot be overstated. The impact of hearing loss on speech perception and listening ability, as well as speech and language development, varies depending on factors such as the following:

- Degree of loss: The greater the loss, the greater the impact. This is discussed in greater detail later in the chapter.
- **Audiometric configuration** (shape of the hearing loss on the **audiogram**): The patient's thresholds are plotted on an audiogram (pictorial representation of hearing). Sounds are presented at particular frequencies that represent where the majority of speech information falls (250 to 8000 Hz) and the **intensity** level (decibel level in dB HL) at which they hear the sounds recorded on the audiogram. The degree of hearing loss can be the same at all frequencies (flat). Alternatively, the configuration can be greater in the high frequencies (sloping) or greater in the low frequencies (rising). A hearing loss greater in the higher frequencies interferes more with speech understanding than one that is greater in the low frequencies. More spoken consonants are represented in the high frequencies, whereas spoken vowels tend to have more energy in the low frequencies.
- Age of onset: Congenital (acquired at birth) and prelinguistic (occurring before age 3 years) hearing loss would have a greater adverse effect than one acquired after language is learned (postlingual) because of the critical age for language learning.
- Age of individual: A decline in the speed of central auditory processing and cognition in the aging population has been noted in the literature (Anderson, White-Schwoch, Parbery-Clark, & Kraus, 2013; Füllgrabe, Moore, & Stone, 2015; Getzmann, Gajewski, & Falkenstein, 2013).
- **Site of lesion** (location of the damage): A conductive hearing loss mainly causes sensitivity problems (i.e., once the talker speaks louder, the effects of the hearing loss are generally overcome). A **sensorineural hearing loss**, which affects the inner ear and/or eighth nerve, causes both problems of sensitivity and clarity, with a sensory hearing loss associated with fewer problems in clarity than a neural one.
- Number of ears affected: A hearing loss in one ear (unilateral) typically has less impact than a bilateral hearing loss. A unilateral hearing loss is most challenging when the speaker is on the side of the impaired ear and the listener is in a poor acoustic environment, such as in a noisy room, or is trying to identify the source of a sound.
- Presence of concomitant disorders: Those who are otherwise typically developing will be less affected than those who present with additional impairments (e.g., visual or cognitive issues).
- Speed and type of intervention: The earlier a hearing loss is treated, the faster the child's language development and subsequent academic achievement. Both the hearing assistance technology chosen and other habilitative decisions regarding therapy play a crucial role in the success of the intervention.
- Family involvement: The commitment and support of the family in (re-)habilitative efforts are pivotal. Empathic support of family members is important not only with children, but also in the rehabilitation of adults with hearing impairment. Socioeconomic status (Ching et al., 2013a) and maternal educational level have also been correlated with improved outcomes (Ching et al., 2013b).
- The listening environment: This impacts communication success not only for those with unilateral losses, as noted earlier, but even more so for those who are bilaterally impaired. The intensity (strength of the sound) of the speech in relation to competing sounds (i.e., **signal-to-noise ratio**—the ratio of the intensity of the desired sound to the background noise) and the degree of **reverberation** (echo) interfere with communication among not only those with hearing loss (Neuman, Wroblewski, & Rubinstein, 2009), but also those with learning and attention problems; developmental disabilities in areas of speech, language, and reading; and second-language learners (Crandell, Smaldino, & Flexer, 2005). Even children who are typically developing are adversely affected by noise and reverberation, especially younger children (Neuman, Wroblewski, Rubinstein, & Hajicek, 2009).

Clients With a History of Previous Audiometric Evaluation

In cases where a client arrives to the SLP with audiometric information already in hand, these findings must be interpreted to determine the implications of the loss on speech recognition and the goals of therapy. A gross estimate of the relationship between the audiometric results and the perception of speech sounds can be determined by plotting the patient's

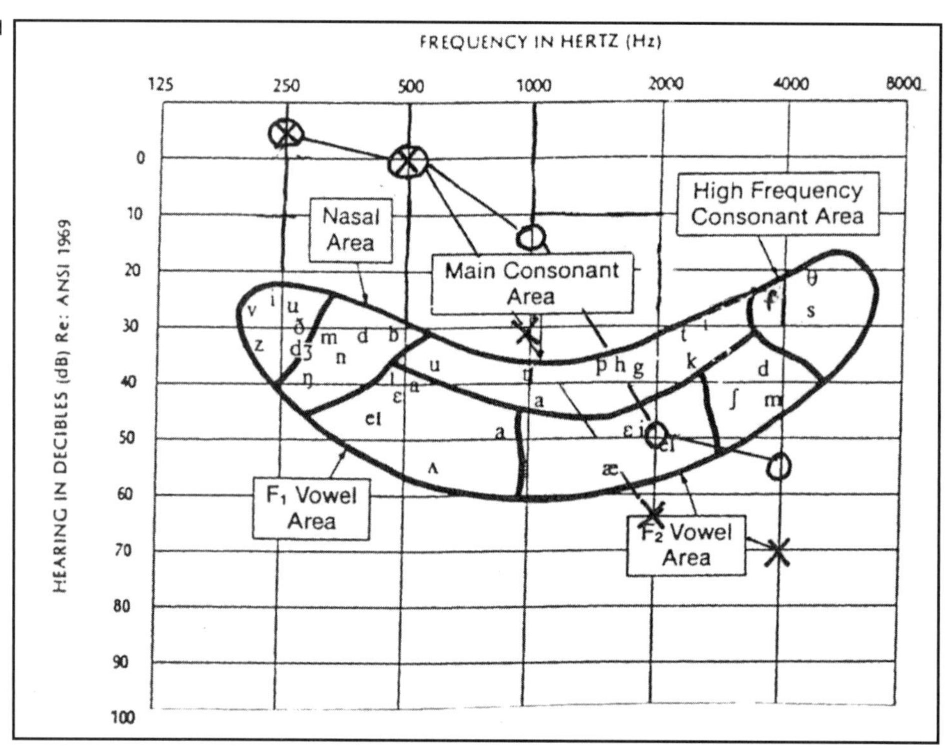

Figure 5-1. Speech banana. (Adapted from Cherry, 1997.)

audiometric results on an audiogram with a superimposed **speech banana**. The audiogram is the chart that depicts hearing ability. Figure 5-1 is an illustration of a speech banana and corresponding audiogram. The speech banana was developed by taking an audio sample of a speech stimulus at an overall normal conversational level, and analyzing the frequency composition and intensity for each phoneme. For example, the /f/ consonant phoneme is a relatively soft sound of about 25 dB HL, with a concentration of energy around 4000 Hz. The phonetic or orthographic symbol for this sound will be placed on the audiogram at that location. Vowels, on average, are much stronger in intensity and lower in frequency, as can be seen by their locations on the audiogram. Some sounds may appear at more than one frequency because they have more than one area of frequency concentration. After the phonemes are placed on the audiogram, a line is drawn to surround all of the symbols. The shape that is created resembles a banana.

When the pure-tone results are added to the audiogram with the speech banana, one can identify which phonemes will not be audible by noting those that are found above the line formed by connecting the pure-tone thresholds symbols (O for the right ear and X for the left ear). For example, the pure-tone threshold at 4000 Hz is 70 dB HL for the left ear and 55 dB HL for the right ear. The /f/ sound, which has a signal strength of 25 dB HL during normal conversation, would not be audible in either ear.

In the event that a child is being evaluated with hearing loss as the presenting cause of the language delay, there will also be a particular focus on the habilitation history (e.g., when loss was diagnosed and/or when intervention began, use of hearing aids, **cochlear implants** [surgically implanted devices to access sound], other hearing assistive technology such as **FM systems** [wireless electronic devices], previous speech-language therapy, etc.). For any client, including an adult who is being evaluated for a speech or language impairment, the issue of rehabilitative hearing history must be explored even if the hearing loss is only an ancillary problem.

Speech and Language Characteristics Associated With Hearing Loss

The speech and language characteristics that are affected by hearing loss vary across a number of factors. The impact on children vs. adults is obviously a critical factor, and thus, these two populations are reviewed separately.

Pediatric Population

Delays due to hearing impairment have been documented in vocabulary development, grammatical and conversational skills, literacy, and speech production activities of children with hearing loss. The severity of the speech and language impairments found in these children is variable depending upon the factors previously cited. In the case of children, whether the loss was acquired prelingually or postlingually is particularly critical.

Specifically, the common problems found in children with hearing impairments are as follows:

- Vocabulary: Some children with hearing impairment tend to have reduced receptive and expressive vocabulary, difficulty with multiple meanings (write/right), and problems with figurative language (Culbertson, 2007; Tye-Murray, 2007). Some more recent studies, however, suggest that many children with mild-to-moderate hearing loss and timely treatment perform as well as their normal hearing peers (Moeller, Tomblin, Yoshinaga-Itano, McDonald, & Jerger, 2007).
- Grammar (syntax): Some children with hearing impairment tend to use shorter and simpler sentences, overuse specific sentence patterns (subject–verb–object) even when inappropriate, infrequently use adverbs and conjunctions, and incorrectly use irregular verb tense (Culbertson, 2007). Koehlinger, Van Horne, and Moeller (2013) examined the spoken-language skills of young children (3- and 6-year-olds) with mild-to-moderately severe hearing loss. All but three of the children wore hearing aids. They found that the children with hearing loss lagged behind their normal hearing peers in grammatical aspects of language.
- Conversational skills (pragmatics): Some children with hearing impairment demonstrate a more limited knowledge of the rules of conversation (how to change a topic or end a conversation). In addition, they have a limited use of communication repair strategies, which may affect their understanding of what someone else has said (Tye-Murray, 2007).
- Literacy: Some children with hearing impairment have difficulty with reading comprehension, writing, and phonological processing, though many children with hearing impairment are normal readers (Moeller et al., 2007). Even children with mild-to-moderate hearing loss who use hearing aids have been shown to be poorer spellers than their counterparts with normal hearing (Park, Lombardino, & Ritter, 2013).
- Speech production: Children with mild-to-moderate hearing loss tend to have fewer errors and more intelligible speech than children with more severe hearing problems (Eisenberg, 2007), with most errors in the production of high-frequency consonants (/s/, /ʃ/, /tʃ/) and blends (Culbertson, 2007). Some children with more severe hearing loss have historically demonstrated poor intelligibility, nonstandard voice quality, and problems correctly producing vowels, as well as consonants, a pattern referred to as *deaf speech* (Hedge & Maul, 2006).

Today, with earlier identification and treatment and using newer technologies (digital hearing aids and cochlear implants), the outcomes for children born with hearing loss have significantly improved. Cochlear implantation and accompanying speech and language therapy have increased the opportunities for congenitally deaf children to learn alongside their peers in a mainstream classroom (Dunn et al., 2014). Several studies have shown that children using cochlear implants acquire speech in the same pattern as normal hearing children, and with a greater proficiency than children with the same degree of hearing loss who use hearing aids (Blamey, Barry, & Jacq, 2001; Yoshinaga-Itano, Baca, & Sedey, 2010). With early implantation and long-term use, it has been shown that prelingually deaf children, adolescents, and young adults who received implants before age 7 years often reach the speech intelligibility performance within the range of their counterparts with normal hearing (Montag, AuBuchon, Pisoni, & Kronenberger, 2014). Although the speech and language delays of a specific child with a hearing loss are impossible to predict, Anderson and Matkin (2007) developed a chart describing the possible impact of different degrees of hearing loss on the understanding of speech and language, social skills, and projected educational accommodations needed. An adapted version of this chart appears in Appendix 5-A.

Adult and Geriatric Population

Adults who develop hearing loss will experience little or no effect on expressive skills, although their hearing losses will affect their speech perception. In addition, issues that may be noticed include straining to hear, responding inappropriately, dominating conversations, and difficulty hearing in group or noisy situations. Patients often report being frustrated or embarrassed about not understanding what is being said. Untreated hearing loss has been correlated with withdrawing from social situations, and depression, and is often reported as a burden for family, friends, and coworkers. In addition, it has also been linked to cognitive decline (Lin et al., 2011, 2013). Lin et al. (2013) conducted a long-term study involving 1984 participants in the age range of 70 to 79 years. Results indicated a greater risk for cognitive decline for the participants with hearing loss. Despite the issues surrounding untreated hearing loss, many hearing aid users delay obtaining aids up to 10 years after they are first diagnosed as having a hearing loss (Davis, Smith, Ferguson, Stephens, & Gianopoulos, 2007). **Tinnitus** is also commonly reported in the adult population (Ng, Archbold, Harrigan, & Mulla, 2015). Tinnitus is the perception of sound in the absence of external stimuli. It is often described by patients as a ringing, buzzing, roaring, clicking, or hissing sound in one or both ears. Occasional tinnitus does not necessarily warrant a referral, but if a patient reports persistent tinnitus, a referral for a **complete audiological evaluation** is advised.

Most adults with hearing loss will also benefit from appropriate hearing assistance technology. Many of the earlier difficulties associated with using amplification, such as that of a whistling hearing aid (feedback) or the perception of the annoying sound of the person's own voice (occlusion effect), have been addressed through better feedback management technology and more comfortable hearing aid fittings, such as those that are open (unplugged). Whereas means to improve performance in noisy environments is still an area of intense investigation, technology to facilitate the comfortable use of amplification in these environments has been met with greater success.

Significant advancements in hearing aid technology have also allowed for smaller, more cosmetically appealing aids. Many newer models of hearing aids allow the wearer to control their hearing aids with a smart phone and allow for the streaming of music and phone calls. Hearing aid users also have the option of using a remote microphone or their smart phone to hear speech presented at a distance.

Specific Parameters for Screening

ASHA's (2016) scope of practice for speech-language pathology includes screening individuals for hearing loss. Although audiologists perform the bulk of the testing procedures to evaluate peripheral hearing loss (through a comprehensive battery of hearing testing), included within the SLP scope of practice is the assessment of the following:

- The presence of hearing loss through **pure-tone air conduction hearing screening** (a short test of several individual frequencies at one intensity) and self-assessment screening scales (such as the Hearing Handicap Inventory for the Elderly (see Appendix 5-B)
- Outer and middle ear function through **otoscopic inspection**, where the ear canal and eardrum are examined with a light source, and screening **tympanometry**, a procedure to check mobility of the middle ear system

Guidelines for Pure-Tone Screening

The ASHA published guidelines for audiological testing vary based on the specific age group (ASHA, n.d.). The pediatric guidelines for hearing screening are divided into newborns and infants (0 to 6 months), infants and toddlers (6 to 36 months), preschoolers (3 to 5 years), and school-age children (5 to 21 years). Regulations regarding the screening protocols and referral timelines vary by state. This chapter is geared toward the protocols for screening beginning with preschool age. For children whose developmental age does not match their chronological age, the screening technique should be consistent with the child's developmental abilities. For children younger than 3 years or for those who cannot be conditioned for the pure-tone screening, **otoacoustic emissions** (OAEs) may be considered, and a referral to an audiologist is indicated. Evoked OAEs are low-level, typically inaudible sounds produced by the outer hair cells (OHC) of the cochlear in response to sound. OAE testing involves a small probe being inserted in the ear canal. The probe produces an acoustic stimulus that travels through the outer and middle ear to the OHC and measures the response of the OHC to the stimulus. The presence of OAEs indicates normal peripheral hearing or no greater than a mild (or in some cases moderate) hearing loss. It is important to note that OAEs only assess up to the OHC and are not a substitute for a hearing test.

Rationale for Pure-Tone Screening

All individuals being evaluated for a speech and/or language problem should have a pure-tone hearing screening if they have not had an audiological evaluation by a licensed audiologist within 6 months for children under age 5 years or within 1 year for older children and adults. This is especially critical for children due to the profound adverse effects of hearing impairment on the development of speech, language, and later academic achievement, as noted previously. The auditory channel is the main vehicle for speech and language input. Because there is a critical period for language learning, an optimal channel during that period is essential. Children do not have the benefit of prior knowledge by which they could fill in missing linguistic information lost due to a hearing loss. They need all of the details of the auditory input. If an adult hears "two cat_" and misses the morphological marker, he or she can easily figure it out from the redundancy in language. A child, however, needs to learn the morphological markers and cannot afford to miss them. In this example, the problem is exacerbated by the fact that permanent hearing loss tends to be sensorineural, with greater loss in the high frequencies; the /s/ phoneme has energy in the high frequencies and is one of the weaker sounds. The effect on morphology is just one example. It is easy to predict how vocabulary acquisition, grammar, and articulation ability would also be affected. It should be kept in mind that, even though a child has passed the newborn hearing screening, subsequent screenings are warranted to confirm results and rule out later acquisition of hearing loss. In addition, newborn hearing screenings are not designed to identify slight or mild hearing loss.

Ruling out a hearing loss in adults, although not as critical, is also important. A clinician who does not correctly identify the presence of a hearing loss in an adult may draw flawed conclusions, leading to an incorrect diagnosis. For example, one of the authors once observed an adult being evaluated for aphasia who did not respond appropriately to several test items because she did not hear it correctly rather than due to brain damage. As a result, the degree of impairment due to aphasia was initially assumed to be more significant than was the case. Another example is the older patient who may be judged inappropriately as more confused or withdrawn than is the case because of difficulty hearing.

Administration Procedure for Pediatric Pure-Tone Screening

Procedures for the pure-tone hearing screening should include the following:

- Appropriate infection control. According to the American Academy of Audiology (AAA; n.d.b) guidelines for pure-tone testing, equipment and any contaminated surfaces require cleaning and disinfecting after every physical contact with the patient. The use of either disposable acoustically transparent earphone covers for standard earphones or disposable insert earphone tips is recommended. Handwashing between patients and disinfecting tables and chairs and any toys used during testing for children is also recommended. In addition, if the SLP comes into contact with the client's hearing aid, he or she must be mindful of the importance of disinfecting the aid (Bankaitis, 2002). Proper infection control is imperative as individuals with compromised immune systems are particularly susceptible to opportunistic infections (AAA, n.d.b).
- Calibrated pure-tone audiometer in a quiet room. A biological check of the audiometer must be performed before testing, which includes a listening check by the clinician. According to ASHA, the listening check should be performed by an individual with known normal hearing thresholds at each test frequency at an intensity level that is at least 10 dB HL below the prescribed screening level (e.g., 10 dB HL for screening conducted at 20 dB HL; ASHA, n.d.). This will also confirm that the acoustic environment is quiet enough and allows for the detection of the sounds presented. This is especially critical in cases in which the 500 Hz frequency is incorporated into the testing protocol.
- Clear and simple instructions.
  - For young children: A common strategy is to give the child a block and have him or her hold it near one ear. A sample of instructions should be given as follows: "You are going to get to wear these special earphones. After I put them on, wait and listen. You will hear a sound, like a beep or a whistle. As soon as you hear the sound, drop the block in the bucket. The sounds may be very soft, so listen carefully. Do you have any questions?" Very young children may be told, "You are going to be like an airplane pilot. Listen for a tiny birdie in the sky."
  - For older children and adults: Instructions may be as follows: "You are going to hear a series of tones. Raise your hand when you hear the tone or think you hear the tone."
- Placement of earphones: The red earphone is placed on the right ear and the blue earphone on

the left. Jewelry or glasses should be removed if they interfere with earphone placement (when supra-aural earphones are used). If insert earphones are being used, otoscopy should first be performed to ensure a clear ear canal, and proper insertion of earphones should ensured. Instructions should always be given before placing earphones.

- Positioning: Although there are advantages to facing the child and viewing facial expressions while testing, one must be careful to avoid giving any cues if such a position is chosen.
- Choice of task: Most preschoolers can be tested successfully using a portable audiometer and a technique referred to as **conditioned play audiometry**. In this technique, the child is taught to provide a play response (e.g., putting a block in a bucket) upon hearing a sound. A minimum of two conditioning (practice) trials are recommended. The clinician may assist the child in the appropriate action at first. When the child is able to perform the task independently, the test will begin. By age 5 years, many children can perform the screening task like adults by raising their hand. In either case, social praise should be included to maintain the response by the child.
- Screening under earphones: Excessive ambient noise or physiologic noise from the child while performing hearing screenings is a major concern because it has the potential to mask the presented tones (particularly 500 Hz and below). As stated previously, a quiet room is needed and the clinician must first conduct a biologic check to ensure that tones presented can be detected. 1000, 2000, and 4000 Hz (at 20 dB HL for children, 25 dB HL for adults) are standard frequencies included in a screening. When testing adolescents and adults, it is preferable to add 6000 Hz (and 8000 Hz) due to increased noise exposure and its effect on high frequencies (Sekhar et al., 2016; Serpanos, Senzer, Renne, Langer, & Hoffman, 2015). However, it should be noted that, when presented higher frequency tones, insert earphones are preferable due to a high false-positive rate with standard earphones. At least two presentations at each frequency per ear are necessary to ensure reliability. Using a continuous tone or pulsed tone (1 to 2 seconds long) usually will not affect the clinical test results, although a pulsed tone is sometimes perceived as easier to identify and is advantageous if the person complains of tinnitus (ringing in the ear).
- Pass–fail/referral criteria: In the absence of responses, at one or more frequencies, attempt to reinstruct/recondition or reposition the earphones, and then rescreen before referring. The screening is not passed and a referral should be made if there are no responses at one or more of the test frequencies in either ear, or if the patient cannot be trained reliably to perform the task (ASHA, n.d.). It is recommended that children who fail the screening should be referred for a medical and/or an audiological evaluation (ASHA, n.d.).
- Results of the screening are recorded on a form, as shown in Figure 5-2, by placing a check or X in each box depending on whether the tone was heard. For adults, ASHA recommends using a 25-dB HL tone at the same frequencies as for children and the same referral for a complete audiological evaluation if they do not respond at this level at any frequency in either ear.

Avoiding Pitfalls in Pure-Tone Screening

To ensure success during the screening of young children in particular, several pitfalls must be avoided or overcome:

- Failure to get the earphones on the child: Placing the earphones on the parent first often does not impress the reluctant child at all. Taking an earphone off the headset and placing it near the ear at first with a louder tone to make it audible can sometimes accustom the child to the task, at which point he or she may be willing to have the earphones placed by or even on the ear. Some children may prefer insert earphones if they are available because they look less cumbersome, although supra-aural earphones have the advantage that they can be placed more quickly.
- Failure to choose a conditioning stimulus level that is sufficiently audible to the child: The decision should be based on informal observation before testing and information from the parents, although parental report can be unintentionally misleading at times. Keep in mind that soft speech is about 30 dB HL, and normal conversation is about 50 dB HL. To condition for a screening, 40 dB HL at 1000 Hz is generally a good place to start. If the child does not respond, a louder tone can be used for training.

Name: ______________________ Date: ______________

Date of Birth: _________________ Examiner: ___________

	500 Hz	**1000 Hz**	**2000 Hz**	**4000 Hz**
Right				
Left				

Screening Level: __________ dB HL

Pass: _____ Refer: _____

Figure 5-2. Audiometric screening form.

- Failure to communicate the task: Initially, the clinician may coax the child by physically helping him or her make the desired motor response. Because this is only a screening procedure, it is not expected that the clinician should spend an inordinate period of time trying to condition the child. Depending on time availability and the importance of the screening information at the time of the evaluation, the clinician may try to simplify the task at first by using a verbal direction as the stimulus (e.g., "Put the block in!") while the child learns to wait until she or he hears something and is then instructed what to do. If the child understands this, he or she can then be instructed to do the same thing when hearing the tone.
- Failure to choose an appropriate task: Putting a block in a bucket or a ring on a peg is generally acceptable, but occasionally, children may not engage in the task unless it is more interesting to them, such as putting pieces into a puzzle. Conversely, the task should not be so interesting that it distracts the child from attending to the sounds. Some children in this age group can be tested using conventional audiometry, which requires the child to raise a hand when he or she hears the sound (tone).
- Failure to reinforce the response appropriately: Following the correct response, the child should be reinforced enthusiastically. Verbal praise or clapping is usually sufficient.
- Failure to use appropriate timing in the presentation of the stimulus: The clinician must not present the stimuli in a set pattern or the child will learn to respond at the appropriate time for the signal without needing to hear it. Varying the timing between signal presentations is essential for valid results.
- Inadvertently giving a cue that the stimulus was just presented: Common errors include letting the child see the clinician pressing the stimulus bar or looking up each time a sound is presented. A child who is facing away from the clinician should be checked for inadvertent cues from other sources, such as the reflection from a one-way mirror. In addition, the clinician should not ask the child if he or she heard the sound after every stimulus.

Some of these issues may also come into play when testing adults with cognitive challenges.

Rationale and Guidelines for Tympanometry Screening

Tympanometry is an objective procedure used to determine the mobility of the middle ear (compliance), air pressure of the middle ear, and volume of the ear canal. ASHA recommends that young children (up to 6 years) and others at risk for **otitis media with effusion** (OME) (inflammation with fluid in the middle ear) should be screened using tympanometry (ASHA, n.d.). OME has the potential to cause medical problems; hearing loss; balance (vestibular) problems; issues with behavior; ear discomfort; and possible speech, language, and learning deficits (Rosenfeld et al., 2016). In addition, a child may have OME and pass a pure-tone screening. Therefore, a hearing screening cannot rule out the presence of OME. The AAA (n.d.a) lists several risk factors for OME, including children with craniofacial anomalies (cleft lip or palate), infants and young children enrolled in multichild day care settings, Native American heritage, or those with Down syndrome.

The ASHA screening guidelines includes screening individuals for middle ear disease using tympanometry and otoscopic inspection (ASHA, n.d.). There are several screening tympanometers commercially available that are easy to use, will automatically indicate pass–fail status as well as plot a **tympanogram**, and report specific results. Unfortunately, many SLPs do not routinely include tympanometry in their standard practice. In light of this, the Colorado Department of Education (2004) recommended at least including a 500-Hz tone for children from preschool through fifth grade if tympanometry is not available.

Procedure for Tympanometry

ASHA recommends visual inspection of each ear, using a lighted or video otoscope to rule out any contraindications before performing the procedure (e.g., impacted cerumen, draining or pressure equalization tubes; ASHA, n.d.). Tympanometry should be performed as follows:

- After seating the child near the tympanometer, perform otoscopy.
- Give instructions:
  - "I am going to take a funny picture of your ear. Sit as still as possible." The child may be told to watch the picture being taken or can be focused on another interesting toy or video while the procedure is taking place.
- Offer a reinforcer; the prospect of a sticker is often sufficient.
- Use a low-frequency probe tone (e.g., 220 Hz) and a positive-to-negative air pressure sweep to produce the tympanogram.
- Assess the results and referral. Assessment includes the location of the peak on the x-axis (estimate of middle ear pressure), the size of the ear canal volume, as well as the height and shape (width) of the tympanogram (estimate of compliance).
  - Immediate medical referral: This is indicated with evidence of ear drainage, ear canal obstruction (e.g., cerumen or foreign object), ear canal volume greater than 1.0 cm^3 accompanied by a flat tympanogram (which is consistent with a perforation or a patent pressure equalizing tube), and if the child fails a rescreening.
  - Rescreening: This is recommended within 6 weeks for children if their compliance (flexibility of the tympanic membrane/middle ear system) is less than 0.3 mmhos or tympanic width greater than 200 daPa, suggesting a conductive mechanism that is potentially stiffer than the norm.

Key Clinical Interview Questions

The purpose of the interview questions is to determine whether a hearing loss should be suspected, what might be the cause, and what are the implications. For example, a child with a history of ear infections may be affected by a fluctuating hearing loss that may not be manifested at the time of screening. The number and types of questions raised will vary if the client is a child or adult or if hearing loss is the main cause of the speech-language problem or an ancillary one.

History of Hearing Loss

- Do you suspect a hearing loss, and if so, which ear(s)?
- Have you had a recent hearing test, and if so, do you have or know the test results?
- Do you attribute a hearing loss to any factor?
- Is there any significant medical history, such as:

 - Frequent ear infections?
 - Family history of hearing loss?
 - Other medical problems?
 - Noise exposure?
 - **Ototoxic drugs** (drugs that are damaging to the ear)?
 - Problems during pregnancy or delivery (for a child)?
 - Results of newborn hearing screening (for a child)?
- Do you suffer from a sensation of moving or spinning (**vertigo**) or ringing in your ears (tinnitus)?
- At what age was the hearing loss identified (child)?
- Describe your child's developmental milestones (child).
- How is the child performing in school (child)?
- Is the child receiving any services (child)?
- What are the results of other developmental evaluations (child)?

(Re)habilitative History

- What amplification devices have been used in the past?
- At what age(s) were they introduced?
- What amplification or other assistive devices are currently being used?
- How successful is your hearing technology (e.g., problems, benefits)?

Sample Case History 1

Mrs. X arrived at our center with her 6-year-old daughter, Ann Marie, at the recommendation of Ann Marie's teacher. Mrs. X reported that Ann Marie does not speak as clearly as other children her age. In addition, her teacher noted that she appears to daydream frequently and often does not answer questions appropriately. Mrs. X does not suspect a hearing loss; however, she did report a history of frequent ear infections. Ann Marie's birth history was unremarkable, and developmental milestones were within normal limits with the exception of speech production, according to her mother. Her medical history also revealed a history of seasonal allergies, for which she is being treated. Ann Marie has an older brother with no reported speech, language, or hearing problems.

Sample Procedures Chosen to Administer

Any child who is referred due to a speech and/or language problem should be given a pure-tone hearing screening for each ear at least at 1000, 2000, and 4000 Hz. Given the high rate of otitis media in the population, a tympanometric screening is also advisable. In the example of Ann Marie, the history of frequent ear infections and seasonal allergies emphasizes the need for a middle ear screening. Before any tympanometric screening is performed, it is important to check each ear via otoscopy to rule out interference of cerumen with the probe tube and to observe the shape of the ear canal to facilitate appropriate insertion.

Sample Audiological Section Written in a Diagnostic Report

Ann Marie did not pass a hearing screening presented at 20 dB HL, and at 1000, 2000, and 4000 Hz in either ear. She also did not pass a tympanometric screening, which is consistent with her history of recurrent otitis media. A complete audiological evaluation followed by a medical referral to an ear, nose, and throat physician, if warranted, was therefore recommended.

Sample Case History 2

Mrs. Y arrived at our center with her 2.5-year-old only child, Jason, due to concerns about his speech development. She reported that he is only using a few words that are difficult to understand. Mrs. Y reported that she does not suspect a hearing loss because he responds when the doorbell or telephone ring. In addition, Jason did pass his newborn hearing screening, and Mrs. Y reported no history of ear infections. She noted a progressive hearing loss in one of his first cousins, although she did not have any further details about it. Mrs. Y reported no other developmental delays, and the remaining medical history was unremarkable.

What results might you expect from the audiological screening and why?

Appendix 5-A. Relationship of Hearing Loss to Listening and Learning Needs

Possible Impact on the Understanding of Language and Speech	*Possible Social Impact*	*Potential Educational Accommodations and Services*
	16- to 25-dB HL Hearing Loss	
• Impact of hearing loss that is approximately 20 dB HL can be compared with the ability to hear when index fingers are placed in the ears • Child may have difficulty hearing faint or distant speech. At 16 dB HL, a student can miss up to 10% of speech signal when the teacher is at a distance greater than 3 feet • A 20 dB HL or greater hearing loss in the better ear can result in absent, inconsistent, or distorted parts of speech, especially word endings (s, ed) and unemphasized sounds • Percent of speech signal missed will be greater whenever there is background noise in the classroom, especially in the elementary grades when instruction is primarily verbal and younger children have greater difficulty listening in noise • Young children have the tendency to watch and copy the movements of other students rather than attending to auditorily fragmented teacher directions	• May be unaware of subtle conversational cues, which may cause the child to be viewed as inappropriate or awkward • May miss portions of fast-paced peer interactions that could begin to have an impact on socialization and self-concept • Behavior may be confused for immaturity or inattention • May be more fatigued due to extra effort needed for understanding speech	• Noise in typical classroom environments impede the child from having full access to teacher instruction. Will benefit from improved acoustic treatment of classroom and sound-field amplification • Favorable seating necessary • May often have difficulty with sound/letter associations and subtle auditory discrimination skills necessary for reading • May need attention to vocabulary or speech, especially when there has been a long history of middle ear fluid • Depending on loss configuration, may benefit from low power hearing aid with personal FM system • Appropriate medical management is necessary for conductive losses • In-service on impact of "minimal" 16- to 25-dB HL hearing loss on language development, listening in noise and learning, required for teacher
	26- to 40-dB HL Hearing Loss	
• Effect of a hearing loss of approximately 20 dB HL can be compared with the ability to hear when index fingers are placed in the ears • A 26- to 40-dB HL hearing loss causes greater listening difficulties than a "plugged ear" loss • Child can "hear" but misses fragments of speech, leading to misunderstanding • Degree of difficulty experienced in school will depend on the noise level in the classroom, distance from the teacher, and configuration of the hearing loss, even with hearing aids • At 30 dB HL, can miss 25% to 40% of the speech signal • At 40 dB HL, may miss 50% of class discussions, especially when voices are faint or speaker is not in line of vision	• Barriers begin to build with negative impact on self-esteem as child is accused of "hearing when he or she wants to," "daydreaming," or "not paying attention" • May believe he or she is less capable because of difficulties understanding in class • Child begins to lose ability for selective listening, and has increasing difficulty suppressing background noise, causing the learning environment to be more stressful • Child is more fatigued due to effort needed to listen	• Noise in typical class will impede the child from full access to teacher instruction • Will benefit from hearing aid(s) and use of a desktop or ear-level FM system in the classroom • Needs favorable acoustics, seating, and lighting • May need attention to auditory skills, speech, language development, speechreading, and/or support in reading and self-esteem • Amount of attention needed typically related to the degree of success of intervention prior to 6 months of age to prevent language and early learning delays • Teacher in-service on impact of a 26- to 40-dB HL hearing loss on listening and learning to convey that it is often greater than expected

(continued)

Appendix 5-A. Relationship of Hearing Loss to Listening and Learning Needs (continued)

Possible Impact on the Understanding of Language and Speech	*Possible Social Impact*	*Potential Educational Accommodations and Services*
26- to 40-dB HL Hearing Loss (continued)		
• Will miss unemphasized words and consonants, especially when a high-frequency hearing loss is present • Often experiences difficulty learning early reading skills such as letter–sound associations • Child's ability to understand and succeed in the classroom will be substantially diminished by speaker distance and background noise, especially in the elementary grades		
41- to 55-dB HL Hearing Loss		
• Consistent use of amplification and language intervention before age 6 months increases the probability that the child's speech, language, and learning will develop at a normal rate. Without amplification, the child may understand conversation at a distance of 3 to 5 feet if sentence structure and vocabulary are known • The amount of speech signal missed can be 50% or more with 40-dB HL loss and 80% or more with 50-dB HL loss • Without early amplification, the child is likely to have delayed or disordered syntax, limited vocabulary, imperfect speech production, and flat voice quality • Addition of a visual communication system to supplement audition may be indicated, especially if language delays and/or additional disabilities are present • Even with hearing aids, child can "hear" but may miss much of what is said if the classroom is noisy or reverberant • With personal hearing aids alone, the ability to perceive speech and learn effectively in the classroom is at high risk • A personal FM system to overcome classroom noise and distance is typically necessary	• Barriers build with negative impact on self-esteem as child is accused of "hearing when he or she wants to," "daydreaming," or "not paying attention" • Communication will be significantly compromised with this degree of hearing loss if hearing aids are not worn • Socialization with peers can be difficult, especially in noisy settings such as cooperative learning situations, lunch, or recess • May be more fatigued than classmates due to effort needed to listen	• Consistent use of amplification (hearing aids + FM) is essential • Needs favorable classroom acoustics, seating, and lighting • Consultation/program supervision by a specialist in childhood hearing impairment to coordinate services is important • Depending on early intervention, success in preventing language delays, special academic support will be necessary if language and educational delays are present • Attention to growth of oral communication, reading, written language skills, auditory skill development, speech therapy, and self-esteem likely • Teacher in-service required with attention to communication access and peer acceptance

(continued)

Appendix 5-A. Relationship of Hearing Loss to Listening and Learning Needs (continued)

Possible Impact on the Understanding of Language and Speech	*Possible Social Impact*	*Potential Educational Accommodations and Services*
56- to 70-dB HL Hearing Loss		
• Even with hearing aids, child will typically be aware of people talking around him or her, but will miss parts of words said, resulting in difficulty in situations requiring verbal communication (both one-to-one and in groups) • Without amplification, conversation must be very loud to be understood; a 55-dB HL loss can cause a child to miss up to 100% of speech information without functioning amplification • If hearing loss is not identified before age 1 year and appropriately managed, delayed spoken language, syntax, reduced speech intelligibility, and flat voice quality is likely • Age when first amplified, consistency of hearing aid use, and early language intervention strongly tied to success of speech, language, and learning development • Addition of visual communication system often indicated if language delays and/or additional disabilities are present • Use of a personal FM system will reduce the effects of noise and distance and allow increased auditory access to verbal instruction • With hearing aids alone, ability to understand in the classroom is greatly reduced by distance and noise	• If hearing loss was late-identified and language delay was not prevented, communication interaction with peers will be significantly affected • Children will have greater difficulty socializing, especially in noisy settings such as lunch, cooperative learning situations, or recess • Tendency for poorer self-concept and social immaturity may contribute to a sense of rejection; peer in-service is helpful	• Full-time, consistent use of amplification (hearing aids + FM system) is essential • May benefit from frequency transposition (frequency compression) hearing aids depending on loss configuration • May require intense support in development of auditory, language, speech, reading, and writing skills • Consultation/supervision by a specialist in childhood hearing impairment to coordinate services is important • Use of sign language or a visual communication system by children with substantial language delays or additional learning needs may be useful to access linguistically complex instruction • Note-taking, captioned films, etc. often are needed accommodations • Teacher in-service required
≥ 71-dB HL Hearing Loss		
• The earlier the child wears amplification consistently with concentrated efforts by parents and caregivers to provide rich language opportunities throughout everyday activities and/or provision of intensive language intervention (sign or verbal), the greater the probability that speech, language, and learning will develop at a relatively normal rate	• Depending on the success of intervention in infancy to address language development, the child's communication may be minimally or significantly affected • Socialization with hearing peers may be difficult	• There is no one communication system that is right for all hard-of-hearing or deaf children and their families • Whether a visual communication approach or auditory/oral approach is used, extensive language intervention, full-time consistent amplification use, and constant integration of the communication practices into the family by 6 months of age will highly increase the probability that the child will become a successful learner

(continued)

Appendix 5-A. Relationship of Hearing Loss to Listening and Learning Needs (continued)		
Possible Impact on the Understanding of Language and Speech	*Possible Social Impact*	*Potential Educational Accommodations and Services*
	≥ 71-dB HL Hearing Loss (continued)	
• Without amplification, children with 71- to 90-dB HL hearing loss may only hear loud noises about 1 foot from the ear • When amplified optimally, children with hearing ability of 90 dB HL or better should detect many sounds of speech if presented from close distance or via FM • Individual ability and intensive intervention before 6 months of age will determine the degree that sounds detected will be discriminated and understood by the brain into meaningful input • Even with hearing aids, a child with a 71- to 90-dB HL loss will typically be unable to perceive all high pitch speech sounds sufficiently to discriminate them, especially without the use of FM • The child with hearing loss greater than 70 dB HL may be a candidate for cochlear implant(s), and the child with hearing loss greater than 90 dB HL will not be able to perceive most speech sounds with traditional hearing aids • For full access to language to be available visually through sign language or cued speech, family members/caretakers must be involved in the child's communication mode from a very young age	• Children in general education classrooms may develop greater dependence on adults due to difficulty perceiving or comprehending oral communication • Children may be more comfortable interacting with deaf or hard-of-hearing peers due to ease of communication • Relationships with peers and adults who have hearing loss can make positive contributions toward the development of a healthy self-concept and a sense of cultural identity	• Children with late-identified hearing loss (i.e., after 6 months of age) will have delayed language • This language gap is difficult to overcome, and the educational program of a child with hearing loss, especially those with language and learning delays secondary to hearing loss, requires the involvement of a consultant or teacher with expertise in teaching children with hearing loss • Depending on the configuration of the hearing loss and individual speech perception ability, frequency transposition aids (frequency compression) or cochlear implantation may be options for better access to speech • If an auditory/oral approach is used, early training is needed on auditory skills, spoken language, concept development, and speech • If culturally deaf emphasis is selected, frequent exposure to deaf American sign language users is important • Educational placement with other signing students who are deaf or hard of hearing (special school or classes) may be a more appropriate option to access a language-rich environment and free-flowing communication • Support services and continual appraisal of access to communication and verbal instruction is required • Note-taking, captioning, captioned films, and other visual enhancement strategies are necessary; training in pragmatic language use and communication repair strategies is helpful • In-service of general education teachers is essential

(continued)

Appendix 5-A. Relationship of Hearing Loss to Listening and Learning Needs (continued)		
Possible Impact on the Understanding of Language and Speech	*Possible Social Impact*	*Potential Educational Accommodations and Services*
	Unilateral Hearing Loss	
• Child can "hear" but can have difficulty understanding in certain situations, such as hearing faint or distant speech, especially if the poor ear is aimed toward the person speaking • Will typically have difficulty localizing sounds and voices using hearing alone • The unilateral listener will have greater difficulty understanding speech when the environment is noisy and/or reverberant, especially when the normal ear is toward the overhead projector or another competing sound source and poor-hearing ear is toward the teacher • Exhibits difficulty detecting or understanding soft speech from the side of the poor-hearing ear, especially in a group discussion	• Child may be accused of selective hearing due to discrepancies in speech understanding in quiet vs. noise • Social problems may arise as child experiences difficulty understanding in noisy cooperative learning or recess situations • May misconstrue peer conversations and feel rejected or ridiculed • Child may be more fatigued in classroom due to greater effort needed to listen if class is noisy or has poor acoustics • May appear inattentive, distractible, or frustrated, with behavior or social problems sometimes evident	• Allow the child to change seat locations to direct the normal hearing ear toward the primary speaker • Student is at 10 times greater risk for educational difficulties as children with two normal hearing ears. One-third to one-half of students with unilateral hearing loss experience significant learning problems • Children often have difficulty learning sound/letter associations in typically noisy kindergarten and grade 1 settings • Educational and audiological monitoring is warranted • Teacher in-service is beneficial • Typically will benefit from a personal FM system with low gain/power or a sound-field FM system in the classroom, especially in the lower grades • Depending on the hearing loss, may benefit from a hearing aid in the impaired ear or a hearing aid the crosses the signal to the normal hearing ear
	Mid-Frequency or Reverse Slope Hearing Loss	
• Child can "hear" whenever speech is present but will have difficulty understanding in certain situations • May have difficulty understanding faint or distant speech, such as a student with a quiet voice speaking from across the classroom • The "cookie bite" or reverse slope listener will have greater difficulty understanding speech when the environment is noisy and/or reverberant, such as a typical classroom setting • A 25- to 40-dB HL degree of loss in the low- to mid-frequency range may cause the child to miss approximately 30% of speech information, if unamplified; some consonant and vowel sounds may be heard inconsistently, especially when background noise is present • Speech production of these sounds may be affected	• Child may be accused of selective hearing or "hearing when he or she wants to" due to discrepancies in speech understanding in quiet vs. noise • Social problems may arise as the child experiences difficulty understanding in noisy cooperative learning situations, lunch, or recess • May misconstrue peer conversations, believing that other children are talking about him or her • Child may be more fatigued in the classroom setting due to greater effort needed to listen • May appear inattentive, distractible, or frustrated	• Personal hearing aids are important but must be precisely fit to hearing loss • Child likely to benefit from a sound-field FM system, a personal FM system, or assistive listening device in the classroom • Student is at risk for educational difficulties • Can experience some difficulty learning sound–letter associations in kindergarten and first grade classes • Depending on degree and configuration of loss, child may experience delayed language development and articulation problems • Educational monitoring and teacher in-service warranted

(continued)

Appendix 5-A. Relationship of Hearing Loss to Listening and Learning Needs (continued)		
Possible Impact on the Understanding of Language and Speech	*Possible Social Impact*	*Potential Educational Accommodations and Services*
High-Frequency Hearing Loss		
• Child can "hear" but can miss important fragments of speech • Even a 26- to 40-dB HL loss in high-frequency hearing may cause the child to miss 20% to 30% of vital speech information if unamplified • Consonant sounds /t/,/s/, /f/, /th/, /k/, /sh/, /ch/ likely heard inconsistently, especially in the presence of noise • May have difficulty understanding faint or distant speech, such as a student with a quiet voice speaking from across the classroom, and will have much greater difficulty understanding speech when in low background noise and/or reverberation is present • Many of the critical sounds for understanding speech are high-pitched, quiet sounds, making them difficult to perceive. The words: cat, cap, calf, and cast could be perceived as "ca," word endings, possessives; plurals and unstressed brief words are difficult to perceive and understand • Speech production may be affected • Use of amplification often indicated to learn language at a typical rate and ease learning	• May be accused of selective hearing due to discrepancies in speech understanding in quiet vs. noise • Social problems may arise as the child experiences difficulty understanding in noisy cooperative learning situations, lunch, or recess • May misinterpret peer conversations • Child may be fatigued in the classroom due to greater listening effort • May appear inattentive, distractible, or frustrated • Could affect self-concept	• Student is at risk for educational difficulties • Depending on onset, degree, and configuration of loss, child may experience delayed language and syntax development and articulation problems • Possible difficulty learning some sound–letter associations in kindergarten and first grade classes • Early evaluation of speech and language skills is suggested • Educational monitoring and teacher in-service is warranted • Will typically benefit from personal hearing aids and use of a sound-field or a personal FM system in the classroom • Use of ear protection in noisy situations is imperative to prevent damage to inner ear structures and resulting progression of the hearing loss
Fluctuating Hearing Loss		
• Of greatest concern are children who have experienced hearing fluctuations over many months in early childhood (multiple episodes with fluid lasting ≥ 3 months) • Listening with a hearing loss that is approximately 20 dB HL can be compared to hearing when index fingers are placed in the ears • This loss or worse is typical of listening with fluid or infection behind the eardrums • Child can "hear" but misses fragments of what is said. Degree of difficulty experienced in school will depend on the classroom noise level, distance from the teacher, and current degree of hearing loss	• Barriers begin to build with negative impact on self-esteem as the child is accused of "hearing when he or she wants to," "daydreaming," or "not paying attention" • Child may believe he or she is less capable due to difficulties understanding in class • Typically poor at identifying changes in own hearing ability • With inconsistent hearing, the child learns to "tune out" the speech signal	• Impact is primarily on acquisition of early reading skills and attention in class • Screening for language delays is suggested from a young age • Ongoing monitoring for hearing loss in school, communication between parent and teacher about listening difficulties, and aggressive medical management is needed • Will benefit from sound-field FM or an assistive listening device in class • May need attention to development of speech, reading, self-esteem, or listening skills • Teacher in-service is beneficial

(continued)

Appendix 5-A. Relationship of Hearing Loss to Listening and Learning Needs (continued)		
Possible Impact on the Understanding of Language and Speech	*Possible Social Impact*	*Potential Educational Accommodations and Services*
Fluctuating Hearing Loss (continued)		
• At 30-dB HL, can miss 25% to 40% of the speech signal • A child with a 40-dB HL loss associated with "glue ear" may miss 50% of class discussions, especially when voices are faint or the speaker is not in the child's line of vision • Child with this degree of hearing loss will frequently miss unstressed words, consonants, and word endings	• Children are judged to have greater attention problems, insecurity, and distractibility and may have issues with self-esteem • Tend to be nonparticipative and distract themselves from tasks; often socially immature	

Comments:

Please consider indicated items in the child's educational program:

_____ Teacher and class staff in-service and seating close to teacher (preferential seating)
_____ Hearing monitoring at school every _____ months
_____ Amplification monitoring by class staff on a daily basis
_____ Contact your school district's audiologist
_____ Protect ears from noise to prevent further hearing loss
_____ Educational support services/evaluation
_____ Screening/evaluation of speech and language
_____ Note-taking, use of smart pen technology, closed captioned films, visuals
_____ FM system trial period
_____ Educational consultation/program supervision by specialist(s) in hearing loss
_____ Regular contact with other children who are deaf or hard of hearing
_____ Periodic educational monitoring such as October and April teacher/student completion of paper-based screening tools such as the Screening Instrument For Targeting Educational Risk (SIFTER) or the Listening Inventory For Education (LIFE).

NOTE: All children require full access to teacher instruction and educationally relevant peer communication to receive an appropriate education.

Distance, noise in classroom, and fragmentation caused by hearing loss prevent full access to spoken instruction. Appropriate acoustics, use of visuals, FM amplification, sign language, notetakers, communication partners, etc. increase access to instruction. Needs periodic hearing evaluation, rigorous amplification checks, and regular monitoring of access to instruction and classroom function (monitoring tools at https://sifteranderson.com/uploads/Relationship_of_Hearing_Loss__Listening__Learning_Need_1_per_pg.pdf).

Adapted with permission from Anderson, K. L., & Matkin, N. D. (2007). Relationship of degree of hearing loss, listening and learning needs. Available from *Supporting Success for Children with Hearing Loss*, http://successforkidswithhearingloss.com

Appendix 5-B. Hearing Handicap Inventory for the Elderly (HHIE)

Instructions: The purpose of this questionnaire is to identify difficulties you may be experiencing because of impaired hearing.

Please check the clear box that best describes your experience.

Item	*Hearing Handicap Inventory for the Elderly*	*Yes (4 points)*	*Sometimes (2 points)*	*No (0 points)*
E1	Does a hearing problem cause you to feel embarrassed when you meet new people?			
E2	Does a hearing problem cause you to feel frustrated when talking to members of your family?			
S1	Do you have difficulty hearing when someone speaks in a whisper?			
E3	Do you feel handicapped by a hearing problem?			
S2	Does a hearing problem cause you difficulty when visiting friends, relatives, or neighbors?			
S3	Does a hearing problem cause you to attend religious services less often than you would like?			
E4	Does a hearing problem cause you to have arguments with family members?			
S4	Does a hearing problem cause you difficulty when listening to TV or radio?			
E5	Do you feel that any difficulty with your hearing limits or hampers your personal or social life?			
S5	Does a hearing problem cause you difficulty when in a restaurant with relatives or friends?			
	Total Points of Items With Letter Indications E1 Through E5:			
	Total Points of Items With Letter Indications S1 Through S5:			
	Total Raw Score: __ (Sum of all points E+S)			

Interpreting the Raw Score

0 to 8 = 13% probability of hearing impairment (no handicap/no referral)

10 to 24 = 50% probability of hearing impairment (mild-moderate handicap/refer)

26 to 40 = 84% probability of hearing impairment (severe handicap/refer)

For the item column, E = emotional aspect of hearing loss and S = social impact of hearing loss.

Adapted with permission from Ventry, I., & Weinstein, B. (1983). Identification of elderly people with hearing problems. *American Speech-Language-Hearing Association, 25*(7), 37-42.

Summary

The audiological screening is a critical part of the speech-language assessment because a hearing impairment may be a contributing factor, if not the cause, of the delayed development or impaired performance of a client. The SLP is often the first professional in a position to identify a hearing impairment, and these skills are included in ASHA's (2016) "Scope of Practice for Speech-Language Pathologists." The recommended protocol should include pure-tone screening for both children and adults, and tympanometric screening for populations at risk for otitis media. For both preschool and school-age children, the screening is not passed if they do not respond at 20 dB HL at any test frequency in either ear (ASHA, n.d.). For adults, ASHA recommends using a 25-dB HL criterion at the same frequencies. Referral for a complete audiological evaluation is recommended if the screening is not passed.

Glossary

Audiogram: A chart representing a person's hearing ability, with frequency in hertz on the horizontal axis, and intensity in decibels on the vertical axis. The thresholds of hearing are plotted separately for each ear using different symbols (a red circle for the right ear and a blue x for the left).

Audiometric configuration: Change in amount of hearing loss with changes in frequency, as represented on the audiogram.

Auditory processing disorder: Difficulties in the processing of auditory information in the central nervous system.

Cochlear hearing loss: Pathology originating in the inner ear.

Cochlear implant: A surgically implanted electronic device that provides access to sound for individuals with severe to profound hearing impairment.

Complete audiological evaluation: A battery of tests designed to determine the amount of hearing loss in each ear, the location of the damage causing the loss, and the impact on speech understanding.

Conditioned play audiometry: A technique often used with children to determine hearing loss in which the child is taught to provide a play response (e.g., putting a block in a bucket) upon hearing a sound.

Conductive hearing loss: A pathology originating in the outer and/or middle ear.

FM system: A wireless electronic device consisting of a microphone that transmits a signal from the speaker to the listener (receiver/loudspeaker). It is meant to compensate for the deleterious effects of distance, noise, and reverberation.

Frequency: The rate of vibration of a sound in cycles per second or hertz, perceived as pitch.

Intensity: The amplitude of sound measured in decibels, perceived as loudness.

Mixed hearing loss: A pathology originating in both the conductive and sensorineural parts of the ear that cause a loss in hearing.

Neural hearing loss: A loss of hearing originating in the eighth nerve.

Otitis media with effusion: Inflammation of the middle ear with fluid.

Otoacoustic emissions (OAEs): Evoked OAEs are low-level, typically inaudible sounds produced by the OHCs of the cochlear in response to sound, which can be used for screening purposes.

Otoscopic inspection (otoscopy): The process of inspecting the ear canal and tympanic membrane (eardrum) using a tool consisting of a light source and magnifier.

Ototoxic drugs: Drugs that can cause damage to the ear and to hearing ability (e.g., certain antibiotics, loop diuretics, salicylates).

Peripheral hearing loss: A loss in hearing due to damage anywhere from the outer ear through the eighth nerve.

Pure-tone air conduction hearing screening: A pure-tone test that involves the ability to hear sound at a single intensity. A person who cannot hear at the predetermined passing intensity level does not pass the screening and must be referred for further diagnostic testing.

Retrocochlear hearing loss: Pathologies originating in the eighth nerve.

Reverberation: The continuation of a sound after the original sound has stopped. It occurs in an enclosed space, which causes echoes when sound is reflected off the walls.

Sensorineural hearing loss: A loss of hearing originating in the inner ear or the eighth nerve.

Sensory hearing loss: A loss of hearing originating in the sensory portion (hair cells) of the inner ear.

Signal-to-noise ratio: The ratio of the intensity level of a desired sound to the intensity level of the background noise, expressed in decibels. When the signal is 10 dB HL more than the noise, for example, the signal to noise ratio would be +10 dB HL.

Site of lesion: Location(s) where the damage occurs in the auditory system.

Speech banana: The sounds of speech in terms of their relative intensity and frequency composition plotted on an audiogram form the shape of a banana.

Tinnitus: Sensation of ringing or buzzing in the ear, which can be due to many underlying pathologies.

Tympanogram: A chart on which the tympanometric results are plotted showing the mobility of the middle ear, estimated air pressure of the middle ear, and volume of the ear canal.

Tympanometry: A procedure used to determine the mobility of the eardrum and the status of the middle ear system.

Vertigo: Type of dizziness in which there is a sense of moving or spinning, related to the balance system in the inner ear.

References

American Academy of Audiology. (n.d.a). Audiologic guidelines for the diagnosis & treatment of otitis media in children. Retrieved from https://www.audiology.org/publications-resources/document-library/audiologic-guidelines-diagnosis-treatment-otitis-media

American Academy of Audiology. (n.d.b). Infection control task force. Retrieved from https://www.audiology.org/publications-resources/document-library/infection-control-audiological-practice

American Speech-Language-Hearing Association. (n.d.). Childhood hearing screening. Retrieved from https://www.asha.org/Practice-Portal/Professional-Issues/Childhood-Hearing-Screening/

American Speech-Language-Hearing Association. (2016). Scope of practice in speech-language pathology. Retrieved from http://www.asha.org/policy/SP2016-00343

Anderson, K. L., & Matkin, N. D. (2007). Relationship of degree of hearing loss, listening and learning needs. Retrieved from https://sifteranderson.com/uploads/Relationship_of_Hearing_Loss__Listening__Learning_Need_1_per_pg.pdf

Anderson, S., White-Schwoch, T., Parbery-Clark, A., & Kraus, N. (2013). A dynamic auditory-cognitive system supports speech-in-noise perception in older adults. *Hearing Research, 300*, 18-32.

Bankaitis, A. U. (2002). What's growing on your patients' hearing aids? A study gives you an idea. *The Hearing Journal, 55*, 48-54.

Barber, S. J., & Lee, S. R. (2015). Stereotype threat lowers older adults' self-reported hearing abilities. *Gerontology, 62*, 81-85.

Blamey, P. J., Barry, J.B., & Jacq, P. (2001). Phonetic inventory of development in young cochlear implant users six years post-operation. *Journal of Speech Hearing Research, 44*, 73-79.

Cherry, R. (1997). An integrated approach to aural rehabilitation. Seminars in Hearing. *Aural Rehabilitation with Adults, 18*, 167-184.

Cherry, R. (2011). The importance of hearing and listening in language development. In S. Levey & S. Polirstok (Eds.), *Language development and differences*. Thousand Oaks, CA: Sage.

Ching, T. Y., Dillon, H., Hou, S., Zhang, V., Day, J., Crowe, K., & Flynn, C. (2013a). A randomized controlled comparison of NAL and DSL prescriptions for young children: Hearing-aid characteristics and performance outcomes at three years of age. *International Journal of Audiology, 52*(Suppl. 2), S17-S28.

Ching, T. Y., Dillon, H., Marnane, V., Hou, S., Day, J., Seeto, M., & Zhang, V. (2013b). Outcomes of early-and late-identified children at 3 years of age: Findings from a prospective population-based study. *Ear and Hearing, 34*, 535-552.

Colorado Department of Education. (2004). *Standard practices for audiology services in the schools*. Denver, CO: Author.

Crandell, C., Smaldino, J., & Flexer, C. (2005). *Sound field amplification: Applications to speech perception and classroom acoustics* (2nd ed.) New York, NY: Thompson Delmar Learning.

Culbertson, D. (2007). Language and speech for the deaf and hard of hearing. In R. L. Schow & M. A. Nerboone (Eds.), *Introduction to audiologic rehabilitation* (pp. 197–244). Boston, MA: Pearson Education.

Davis, A., Smith, P., Ferguson, M., Stephens, D., & Gianopoulos, I. (2007). Acceptability, benefit and costs of early screening for hearing disability: A study of potential screening tests and models. *Health Technology Assessment, 11*, 1-294.

Dunn, C. C., Walker, E. A., Oleson, J., Kenworthy, M., Van Voorst, T., Tomblin, J. B., & Gantz, B. J. (2014). Longitudinal speech perception and language performance in pediatric cochlear implant users: The effect of age at implantation. *Ear and Hearing, 35*, 148-160.

Eisenberg, L. S. (2007). Current state of knowledge: Speech recognition and production in children with hearing impairment. *Ear and Hearing, 28*, 766-772.

Füllgrabe, C., Moore, B. C., & Stone, M. A. (2015). Age-group differences in speech identification despite matched audiometrically normal hearing: Contributions from auditory temporal processing and cognition. *Frontiers in Aging Neuroscience, 6*, 347.

Getzmann, S., Gajewski, P. D., & Falkenstein, M. (2013). Does age increase auditory distraction? Electrophysiological correlates of high and low performance in seniors. *Neurobiology of Aging, 34*, 1952-1962.

Hedge, M. N., & Maul, C. A. (2006). *Language disorders in children: An evidence based approach to assessment and treatment*. Boston, MA: Pearson Allyn & Bacon.

Koehlinger, K. M., Van Horne, A. J. O., & Moeller, M. P. (2013). Grammatical outcomes of 3-and 6-year-old children who are hard of hearing. *Journal of Speech, Language, and Hearing Research, 56*, 1701-1714.

Lin, F. R., Metter, E. J., O'Brien, R. J., Resnick, S. M., Zonderman, A. B., & Ferrucci, L. (2011). Hearing loss and incident dementia. *Archives of Neurology, 68*, 214-220.

Lin, F. R., Yaffe, K., Xia, J., Xue, Q., Harris, T., & Purchase-Helzner, E. (2013). Hearing loss and cognitive decline in older adults. *Journal of the American Medical Association Internal Medicine, 173*, 293-299.

Moeller, M. P., Tomblin, J. B., Yoshinaga-Itano, C., McDonald, C., & Jerger, S. (2007). Current state of knowledge: Language and literacy of children with hearing impairment. *Ear and Hearing, 28*, 740-753.

Montag, J. L., AuBuchon, A. M., Pisoni, D. B., & Kronenberger, W. G. (2014). Speech intelligibility in deaf children after long-term cochlear implant use. *Journal of Speech, Language, and Hearing Research, 57*, 2332-2343.

Neuman, A., Wroblewski, M., & Rubinstein, A. (2009). Effects of noise and reverberation on speech recognition of children with cochlear implants. Poster presented at the Conference on Implantable Auditory Prostheses, Lake Tahoe, NV, July 14, 2009.

Neuman, A., Wroblewski, M., Rubinstein, A., & Hajicek, J. (2009). Combined effects of noise and reverberation on sentence reception of normal hearing children and adults. Poster presented at the American Academy of Audiology Convention, Dallas, TX, April 3, 2009.

Ng, Z. Y., Archbold, S., Harrigan, S., & Mulla, I. (2015). Conspiring together: Tinnitus and hearing loss. British Tinnitus Association. Retrieved from http://www.acufenichefare.it/wp-content/uploads/2016/01/BTA-TEF-Conspiring-Together-FINAL.pdf

Park, J., Lombardino, L. J., & Ritter, M. (2013). Phonology matters: A comprehensive investigation of reading and spelling skills of school-age children with mild to moderate sensorineural hearing loss. *American Annals of the Deaf, 158*, 20-40.

Rosenfeld, R. M., Shin, J. J., Schwartz, S. R., Coggins, R., Gagnon, L., Hackell, J. M. & Poe, D. S. (2016). Clinical practice guideline otitis media with effusion (update). *Otolaryngology–Head and Neck Surgery, 154*(Suppl. 1), S1-S41.

Sekhar, D. L., Zalewski, T. R., Beiler, J. S., Czarnecki, B., Barr, A. L., King, T. S., & Paul, I. M. (2016). The sensitivity of adolescent hearing screens significantly improves by adding high frequencies. *Journal of Adolescent Health, 59*, 362-364.

Serpanos, Y. C., Senzer, D., Renne, B., Langer, R., & Hoffman, R. (2015). The efficacy routine screening for high-frequency hearing loss in adults and children. *American Journal of Audiology, 24*, 377-383.

Tye-Murray, N. (2007). *Foundations of aural rehabilitation* (3rd ed.) Clifton Park, NY: Delmar.

Ventry, I., & Weinstein, B. (1983). Identification of elderly people with hearing problems. *American Speech-Language-Hearing Association, 25*(7), 37-42.

Yoshinaga-Itano, C., Baca, R. L., & Sedey, A. L. (2010). Describing the trajectory of language development in the presence of severe to profound hearing loss: A closer look at children with cochlear implants versus hearing aids. *Otology & Neurotology, 31*, 1268-1274.

Website Resources

Alexander Graham Bell Association for the Deaf and Hard of Hearing: www.agbell.org
American Academy of Audiology: www.audiology.org
American Society for Deaf Children (ASDC): www.deafchildren.org
American Speech-Language-Hearing Association (ASHA): www.asha.org
Audiology Online: www.audiologyonline.com
Centers for Disease Control and Prevention, Hearing Loss in Children: www.cdc.gov/ncbddd/hearingloss/facts.html
Educational Audiology Association: https://edaud.org
Gallaudet University: www.gallaudet.edu
Hands and Voices: www.handsandvoices.org
Hearing Loss Association of America: www.hearingloss.org
HelpKids Hear: www.helpkidshear.org
Listen-Up: www.listen-up.org
National Association of the Deaf (NAD): www.nad.org
National Institutes on Deafness and Other Communication Disorders (NICDC): www.nidcd.nih.gov
National Technical Institute for the Deaf (NTID): www.ntid.rit.edu
Project REAL: www.projectreal.niu.edu/projectreal
U.S. Department of Education: www.ed.gov

6

Assessment of the Oral-Peripheral Speech Mechanism

Renee Fabus, PhD, CCC-SLP, TSHH; Felicia Gironda, PhD, CCC-SLP; and Susanna Musayeva, MS, CCC-SLP, TSSLD

Key Words

- afferent
- alveolar ridge
- apraxia
- buccal
- buccoversion
- Class I malocclusion
- Class I occlusion
- Class II malocclusion
- Class III malocclusion
- cleft palate
- deciduous (shedding) teeth
- diadochokinesis
- distoversion
- dysarthria
- efferent
- faucial pillars
- fistula
- frenum
- functional anomaly
- infraverted
- labiodentals
- labioversion
- linguadentals
- linguaversion
- macroglossia
- macrognathia
- malocclusion
- mesioversion
- microdontia
- microglossia
- micrognathia
- occlusion
- open bite
- oral-peripheral examination
- overbite
- overjet
- permanent teeth
- prognathia
- ptosis
- reflexes
- structural anomaly
- submucous cleft
- supernumerary teeth
- supraverted
- tongue thrust
- tongue-tie
- torsiversion
- underbite
- velopharyngeal closure

Introduction

The **oral-peripheral examination** (also termed *oral facial examination* or *speech mechanism examination*; Johnson-Root, 2015) is an assessment of the anatomical and functional integrity of the structures that support speech and swallowing, and it is an essential part of a complete speech, language, and swallowing evaluation. This part of the diagnostic assessment is administered to clients of all ages, from infancy through adulthood. It is important to note that the oral-peripheral

Stein-Rubin, C., & Fabus, R. *A Guide to Clinical Assessment and Professional Report Writing in Speech-Language Pathology, Second Edition (pp 113-130).*

examination is usually performed after obtaining case history information about the client (e.g., the client's medical history). The clinician can obtain information about the client's ability to follow directions and communicate his or her wants and needs. Sometimes, the clinician is the person to first become aware of any possible neurological deficits based on the results of the oral-peripheral examination. If so, the speech-language pathologist (SLP) is responsible for making appropriate referrals after the evaluation. The purposes of examining the speech mechanism are to observe the efficiency of the client's sensory and motor functions of the cranial nerves for speech and swallowing, and to identify **structural** and **functional anomalies** that may contribute to a speech or swallowing disorder. Some examples of published tests and materials that contain oral-peripheral assessment protocols are the Clinical Assessment of Oropharyngeal Motor Development in Young Children (Robbins & Klee, 1987), the Structural/Functional Battery of Oral-Motor Tasks (Wertz, 1985), the Dysarthria Profile (Robertson, 1982), the Dysarthria Examination Battery (Drummond, 1993); the Frenchay Dysarthria Assessment (Enderby, 1983), Orofacial Myofunctional Evaluation With Scores (Felício & Ferreira, 2008), Robbins-Klee Oral Speech Motor Protocol (Robbins & Klee, 1987), and the Dworkin-Culatta Oral Mechanism Examination and Treatment System (Dworkin & Culatta, 1980). Hegde and Freed (2013), Hegde and Promoville (2017), Shipley and McAfee (2015), and this chapter have sample oral-peripheral examination forms. Additionally, when performing evaluations on clients suspected of having a motor speech disorder or dysphagia, the SLPs will assess the cranial nerves for speech and swallowing. Hence, motor speech disorder evaluations and clinical bedside examination forms contain the necessary information for an oral-peripheral examination. For example, there is a motor speech disorder evaluation template and clinical swallowing evaluation on the American Speech-Language-Hearing Association (ASHA) Portal, which contains all of the necessary elements for an oral-peripheral examination (http://www.asha.org/Practice-Portal/Templates). In addition, Swigert (2010) provides information about the various types of **dysarthria**, site of lesion, impact of functioning, and assessment forms using the International Classification of Functioning, Disability and Health (World Health Organization, 2001) as a comprehensive framework for assessing dysarthria. Refer to the references section at the end of this chapter for additional resources. SLPs may choose to create their own oral-peripheral form based on the population they are assessing (e.g., child vs. adult), setting of employment (e.g., university clinic vs. outpatient rehabilitation center), and of course, their knowledge of the anatomy and physiology of the speech and swallowing mechanism.

Minimal materials required to perform an examination of the oral-peripheral mechanism include sterile gloves, a penlight, a tongue depressor, a mirror, and a stopwatch. Other materials that may be used, depending on the client's age and abilities, include a glass of water, lollipops, bubbles, and sterile cotton swabs/gauze. When conducting an oral-peripheral examination, examiners should follow standard infection control precautions, including washing their hands with soap and warm water for at least 15 seconds, both before putting sterile gloves on both hands and also after removing the gloves. The disposal of the materials used into a nonmedical waste bin should be immediate, and no materials should remain in the testing area (Johnson-Root, 2015; Shipley & McAfee, 2009, 2015). Students and novice clinicians are encouraged to practice or role-play with others because the oral-peripheral examination is the most "hands-on" procedure the clinician has to learn and master with some degree of tactile agility. During role-play, the students or novice clinicians may wish to practice stating the overall purpose of the exam and instructions for each task, then record their observations as they are conducting the examination. At first, students will perceive this experience as uncomfortable, but with more experience and knowledge, novice clinicians will become comfortable with the purpose of the examination and why it is a necessary component of any speech-language and swallowing evaluation.

The components of a comprehensive assessment, which can take from 15 to 30 minutes to perform by an experienced SLP, are described in this chapter. At first, however, depending on their personality, coordination, and dexterity, it may take students or novice clinicians longer to conduct this examination. When determining which of these components to include in an assessment of a particular client, and in planning how long the testing may require, it is also important to take into consideration the age of the client, the etiology and nature of the disorder, and the information that can be derived from specific oral-peripheral procedures (Duffy, 2013; Freed, 2012; Webb, 2017). The novice clinician may face some challenges when first performing the examination, including providing an overall explanation of the examination, stating the instructions for the different tasks, and feeling comfortable being in close proximity to the client. The clinician should have a strong understanding of the exam's purpose and what he or she needs to ascertain from the examination. Throughout the examination, the clinician will make many observations pertaining to different aspects of the speech and swallowing mechanism; it is important to be well organized and to self-manage overwhelming emotions. As the clinician acquires experience, he or she will become increasingly aware that individual variations in structure and function are typically exhibited and are not necessarily indicative of speech or swallowing deficits.

Finally, to fully assess the structural and functional integrity of the speech and swallowing mechanism, the clinician must have a solid understanding of both the anatomy and physiology of the face and neck and how it changes over time, as well as familiarity with the bones, cartilages, and muscles that comprise the speech and swallowing mechanism. Additionally, the clinician should have a comprehensive understanding of neuroanatomy, cranial nerves and their function, motor pathways, and upper and lower motor neuron damage. The reader is directed to Bhatnager (2013); Fuller, Pimentel, and Peregoy (2012); Mayo Clinic (1998); Seikel, Drumright, and Seikel (2013); Seikel, King, and Drumright (2010); Webb (2017); and Zemlin (2000) for excellent reviews of this material. Swigert (2010) provides a notable description about upper and lower motor neuron damage. A brief overview of the cranial nerves is provided here because it is critical that the clinician know the name and sensory or motor function of each of the cranial nerve that subserve speech and swallowing and thereby understand the deeper neurological processes underlying the oral behaviors observed.

Cranial Nerves

There are 12 pairs of cranial nerves (CNs). Our focus will be on the six CNs that are critical for speech and swallowing. CNs are classified by name and Roman numeral. For example, the fifth CN is named the *trigeminal nerve* and is referred to as *CN V*. CNs transmit sensory information from the periphery toward the central nervous system (**afferent** or sensory), carry impulses away from the central nervous system to the periphery to initiate muscle movement (**efferent** or motor), or serve both sensory and motor functions (mixed). CNs innervate ipsilateral (same side as nuclei) or contralateral (opposite side from nuclei) structures. Additionally, some nerves provide bilateral (ipsilateral and contralateral) innervation. Table 6-1 provides a summary of the type, innervations, and function of CNs for speech and swallowing assessed in the oral-peripheral examination.

Infant Reflexes

Examination of CN function of neonates and infants is achieved through observation of the child at rest (e.g., facial symmetry), in spontaneous activities (e.g., crying), and by evaluating oral **reflexes** gently. Oral reflexes are involuntary stereotypical motor movements that occur in response to sensory stimulation. They are present at birth and become integrated as the child's nervous system develops (Table 6-2). An absence of oral reflexes at birth or their persistence beyond the age at which they are expected to be integrated raises questions about the integrity of the child's nervous system and necessitates further evaluation by a pediatric specialist or a pediatric neurologist (Johnson-Root, 2015; Morris & Klein, 2000; Sheppard, 1995; Shipley & McAfee, 2015).

Assessment, Parameters, and Instructions for Completing an Oral-Peripheral Examination

An oral-peripheral examination typically begins with an assessment of the external and most visible structures, such as the face, and is completed with an examination of the internal and least visible structures, including the velum. A comprehensive oral-peripheral examination protocol is provided in Appendix 6-A, and the components of the oral-peripheral examination are described in the following sections. The form used during the oral-peripheral examination is not important, but the goal should be a thorough assessment of the oral structures and their functions. As previously mentioned, some published oral-peripheral examination assessments include those by Dworkin and Culatta (1980) and Robbins and Klee (1987). Other sample oral-peripheral assessment forms are provided in motor speech disorders, dysphagia and speech sound disorder textbooks, and the ASHA portal (see additional resources at the end of the chapter).

Included in this section are the name of each physical structure to assess, instructions on how to assess structural integrity, instructions on how to assess function (both motor and sensory as appropriate), and possible interpretations of observations and findings (which is unique to this chapter), such as the potential

Table 6-1. Cranial Nerves Involved in the Oral-Peripheral Assessment

Cranial Nerve (CN)	*Type*	*Innervation*	*Function*
CN V: trigeminal	Mixed	Bilateral	Sensory: face, head, and oral structures (gums, teeth, hard and soft palate), and anterior two-thirds of the tongue Motor: muscles of mastication (chewing)
CN VII: facial	Mixed	Partially bilateral and partially ipsilateral	Sensory: taste for the anterior two-thirds of the tongue and nasopharynx Motor: muscles of facial expression, stapedius muscle, and lacrimal and salivary glands (submandibular and sublingual)
CN VIII: vestibulocochlear	Sensory	Bilateral	This nerve has two divisions: the vestibular nerve for equilibrium and the cochlear nerve for hearing
CN IX: glossopharyngeal	Mixed	Bilateral	Sensory: oropharynx, tonsils, soft palate, and touch and taste for the posterior one-third of the tongue and carotid body Motor: pharyngeal constrictor muscles, stylopharyngeus muscle, and salivary glands (parotid)
CN X: vagus	Mixed	Bilateral	Sensory: pharynx, larynx, trachea, bronchi, abdomen, and carotid body Motor: soft palate (except tensor tympani), pharyngeal constrictors, larynx, cardiac muscles, and muscles of respiration and digestion
CN XI: spinal accessory	Motor	Contralateral	Motor: muscles of the neck (sternocleidomastoid and trapezius)
CN XII: hypoglossal	Motor	Contralateral	Motor: all intrinsic and extrinsic muscles of the tongue except for the palatoglossus muscle

Adapted from Mayo Clinic, 1998; Webb, 2017; Wilson-Pauwels, Akesson, & Stewart, 1988; Wilson-Pauwels, Stewart, Akesson, & Spacey, 2013.

Table 6-2. Oral Reflexes of the Newborn

Reflex	*How Clinician Should Elicit the Reflex*	*Infant's Reaction*	*Function*
Phasic bite	Touch the child's lips and gums	Rhythmic opening and closing of the jaw	Disappears by 9 to 12 months
Rooting	Stroke the child's cheek or angle of the mouth	Head turns in the direction of stroking and mouth opens	Disappears by 6 months; may persist if child is breastfed
Suck-swallow	Touch the child's lips	Rhythmic sucking (firm approximation of lips and vertical tongue movement) and swallowing	Emerges by 6 months; brought under voluntary control by 9 to 12 months
Gag	Stroke the posterior aspect of the child's tongue with a gloved finger	Mouth opens widely, tongue protrudes, and pharyngeal constrictors contract	Persists through adulthood for about 60% of people

Adapted from Johnson-Root, 2015; Morris & Klein, 2000; Shipley & McAfee, 2015.

effects of any structural and functional anomalies noted, on speech and swallowing function. Finally, at the end of this section, because the clinician must be aware that a referral to experts outside the field of speech-language pathology may be necessary, we provide examples of some situations when referral to other professionals is warranted. In addition, CNs are referenced when relevant, and there is a Selected Resource section, including web, book, and journal resources, at the end of the chapter that follows the format of a neurologic oral structure examination.

Face

Assessing Facial Structural Integrity

The clinician should note the overall head size, shape of the face, facial symmetry, and spacing of facial features (e.g., eyes). This can be completed during an introductory conversation.

Assessing Facial Functional Integrity

Facial Motor Integrity

Facial muscle integrity should be evaluated first at rest. The clinician should note any abnormal observations, such as flattening of the nasolabial folds (creases that extend from either side of the nostrils to the corners of the mouth), drooping of the angles (corners) of the lips, and **ptosis** (drooping of the eyelid). To evaluate rate, strength, and range of motion of muscles of facial expression, the clinician should instruct the client to wrinkle his or her forehead, frown, pucker, smile, bare teeth, and close his or her eyes tightly (Swigert, 2010; Webb, 2017).

Facial Sensory Integrity

The clinician may choose to perform sensory testing on the client. To test for this, the clinician instructs the client that he or she is going to examine the client's ability to feel touch on the face. The client's eyes should be closed. The clinician strokes only the center of the client's face, not the periphery (Webb, 2017). The clinician places a cotton swab/gauze in the three divisions on both sides of the face: ophthalmic, maxillary, and mandibular (above the eyebrows, above the upper lip toward the cheek and between the lower lip and the chin; Webb, 2017). The client is instructed to indicate on which side of the face the clinician has applied pressure (Duffy, 2013; Webb, 2017). Additionally, lingual sensitivity should be assessed if chewing and swallowing are a concern.

Interpretation of Findings

The size, shape, and symmetry of the facial structures should be assessed. Anomalies may affect speech and swallow function and may be indicative of a syndrome. For example, wide-set eyes, ptosis, midface retrusion, **prognathia**, and **malocclusion** (Class III, described later) is characteristic of Apert syndrome, whereas ptosis, zygomatic aplasia (underdevelopment of the cheek bones), **micrognathia**, and underdevelopment of the ear occur in Treacher Collins syndrome. These anomalies can affect breathing, feeding, and articulation (Fuller et al., 2012; Zemlin, 2000).

Examination of symmetry of the face at rest and movements of the facial muscles permits assessment of the integrity of CN VII, the facial nerve. Ipsilateral flattening of one nasolabial fold, an inability to close one eye, drooping of one of the angles of the lips, and an inability to frown on one side of the forehead is indicative of unilateral peripheral CN VII nerve damage such as in Bell palsy (idiopathic rapid onset of weakness on one side of the face). When the client can frown on both sides of his or her forehead but the nasolabial fold is flattened and the angle of the lip is drooping, a facial nerve lesion has occurred within the central nervous system. Ptosis is indicative of CN III, oculomotor nerve damage. CN V, the trigeminal nerve, carries sensory information from the face, head, and oral structures to the central nervous system. Decreased sensitivity to touch is consistent with damage to this nerve.

Head and Neck

Assessing Head Support

The clinician should note head posture at rest and drooping of the head or shoulder.

Assessing Neck Muscle Function

The clinician should assess the function of the sternocleidomastoid and trapezius muscles, which are innervated by the accessory CN (CN XI). Function of the trapezius muscles can be assessed by instructing the client to shrug both shoulders while the clinician places light pressure on each shoulder. Integrity of function of the sternocleidomastoid can be evaluated by instructing the client to rotate his or her head to the side while the clinician lightly resists the movement by placing a hand on the client's neck (Duffy, 2013; Webb, 2017).

Interpretation of Findings

Drooping of the shoulder, a weak shoulder shrug, or reduced head-turning suggest damage to the accessory CN (CN XI). Damage to CN XI can negatively affect speech loudness by compromising breath support and adversely affect resonance by altering the configuration of the vocal tract.

Lips

Assessing Labial (Lip) Structural Integrity

The clinician should observe the client's lips at rest for structure, symmetry, posture (closed and open), and condition. The clinician should note evidence of a cleft lip and should describe its type (unilateral or bilateral) and extent (notch or complete splitting of the lip to the nares [nostrils] of the cleft). Observation of drooling should also be noted.

Assessing Labial Functional Integrity

Labial range of motion and labial closure and seal are examined. Labial strength of movement against resistance is examined with a tongue depressor.

Labial Range of Motion

The clinician should instruct the client to protrude and retract his or her lips. This may be accomplished by asking the client to pucker and smile (CN VII) or instructing the client to produce /u/ and /i/. These movements may be evaluated in isolation and then in repeated rapid sequence. Ask the client to open and close his or her lips rapidly. Slow, labored movement or a reduced range of motion should be noted.

Labial Closure and Seal

Labial closure is assessed by asking the client to purse his or her lips. Labial seal can be assessed by instructing the client to approximate his or her lips and puff out his or her cheeks. The clinician should assess the strength of the labial seal by evaluating the client's ability to maintain puffed cheeks while resisting gentle external pressure achieved by the client tapping on or gently squeezing one cheek and then both cheeks. This task also assesses **buccal** strength and integrity of the velopharyngeal seal (described later).

Interpretation of Findings

Dry lips may indicate dehydration. Structural anomalies such as the presence of abnormal tissue growth or a cleft will warrant referral to a physician. Habitual mouth posture is indicative of whether a client tends to breathe through the mouth or nose. Mouth breathing is generally attributed to low muscle tone; blocked passage of the nasopharynx by enlarged tonsils or adenoid tissue; or temporary congestion of the nasal cavity caused by allergies, swollen sinuses, nasal polyps, or small benign masses (Kummer, 2014; Shipley & McAfee, 2015).

Further assessment by an otolaryngologist may be warranted to confirm the cause of the open mouth posture and to implement any necessary treatment.

Swallowing of saliva requires the development of both oral sensation to detect saliva and adequate muscle movements to swallow it. Drooling is normal during development of the neuromuscular system and teething. Drooling beyond age 3 years or excessive drooling can be indicative of reduced sensitivity of the oral mechanism that compromises the child's ability to detect the presence of saliva or poor control of oral secretions due to neuromuscular deficits (Morris & Klein, 2000). Adults who have difficulty managing saliva may have decreased speech intelligibility or dysphagia.

Reduced labial range of motion occurs as a result of damage to the facial nerve (CN VII) and affects articulation and swallowing (Duffy, 2013; Swigert, 2010). Speech intelligibility is negatively affected by compromised lip closure for bilabial phonemes, lip rounding for glides and back vowels, and lip spreading for front vowels (see Chapter 7). A weak labial seal can cause anterior spillage of food, liquid, and saliva during oral intake as well as limitations producing bilabial phonemes (Duffy, 2013; Swigert, 2007).

Mandibular Structure and Function

Assessing Mandibular Structural Integrity

The clinician should examine the size of the mandible (jaw) in relation to the upper part of the face and how low the jaw hangs at rest (Duffy, 2013).

Assessing Mandibular Functional Integrity

The clinician should assess the range, speed, and accuracy and symmetry of jaw movements (CN V). To do this, the clinician should ask the client to slowly open his or her mouth. Any deviation of the jaw upon opening should be noted. To assess mandibular strength, the clinician should instruct the client to maintain a closed jaw in opposition to light downward pressure exerted on the mandible by the clinician. Any opening of the jaw should be documented (Duffy, 2013; Swigert, 2010; Webb, 2017). Additionally, the client should be instructed to lateralize his or her jaw against resistance. The client is asked to move his or her jaw to one side and hold it in position as the clinician attempts to move the jaw toward the center (Webb, 2017).

Interpretation of Findings

An undersized (micrognathic) or oversized (**macrognathic**) mandible may be noted. The presence of either abnormal mandibular development may be indicative of a syndrome. Both presentations can negatively affect articulation by altering tongue placement relative to dentition. Additionally, micrognathia can interfere with infant feeding as the tongue may be relatively large compared with the jaw, leaving little space in the oral cavity for sucking and swallowing (Duffy, 2013).

Deviation of the jaw to the side at rest or during movement and decreased bite strength are consistent with damage to the trigeminal nerve (CN V). Damage to CN V can affect articulation and mastication (chewing) of food (Duffy, 2013).

Dentition

The teeth are contained within the alveoli of the maxillae and mandible. They are used to produce **labiodentals**, **linguadentals**, and fricatives (Bauman-Waengler, 2012; Bernthal, Bankson, & Flipsen, 2013). There are four types of teeth: incisors, cuspids, bicuspids, and molars. Teeth are used for mastication and for the production of speech sounds including labiodentals (contact between the lower lip and teeth) and linguadentals (contact between the tongue tip and the upper and lower front teeth). Eruption of the **deciduous** or **shedding teeth** (also known as *milk* or *baby teeth*) begins between 6 and 9 months of age and continues until 2 to 3 years old, while **permanent teeth** (the second set of teeth) appear between 6 and 12 years of age (Ash & Nelson, 2003). There are 20 deciduous teeth in the mouth of a child, which are then replaced, or exfoliated, by 32 permanent teeth (Ash & Nelson, 2003; Seikel et al., 2010, 2013).

Axial Orientations

There are several distinct orientations of individual teeth: **torsiversion** (tooth is rotated or twisted on its long axis); **labioversion** (tooth leans forward, toward the lips); **linguaversion** (tooth leans inward, toward the tongue); **buccoversion** (molars lean outward, toward the cheek); **distoversion** (tooth leans away from the midline, along the arch); and **mesioversion** (tooth tilts toward the midline between the two central incisors). A tooth that is **infraverted** does not make occlusal contact with its pair in the opposite arch, above or below it, and a tooth that is **supraverted** extends too far into the oral cavity. Both situations can result in an **open bite** (Seikel et al., 2010, 2013; Zemlin, 2000).

Dental Occlusion and Malocclusion

Occlusion is defined as the complete meeting of the upper and lower teeth; a **Class I occlusion** refers to the normal relationship between upper and lower dental arches in which the first molars of the mandibular arch are advanced ahead by one-half tooth of the maxillary molars. For further discussion and illustration of malocclusions, please refer to Seikel and colleagues (2010, 2013) and Zemlin (2000).

Types of Malocclusions

There are three types of malocclusions, or misalignment of teeth:

1. **Class I malocclusion** (neutrocclusion): This occurs when the dental arches are properly aligned at the molars, but individual anterior teeth are misaligned. If the upper incisors project horizontally beyond the lower incisors by a few millimeters, **overjet** results. If the upper incisors project vertically, hiding the lower incisors, **overbite** results. Similarly, if the lower incisors project vertically beyond the upper incisors, **underbite** results (Zemlin, 2000).
2. **Class II malocclusion** (distocclussion): With this type of malocclusion, the mandible is set back. The first mandibular molars are retracted by at least one tooth from the first maxillary molars. This condition may be caused due to retrognathia (retruded mandible) and micrognathia (undersized mandible; Zemlin, 2000).
3. **Class III malocclusion** (Mesioclussion): With this type of malocclusion, the mandible is jutting forward. The first mandibular molar is advanced at least one tooth beyond the first maxillary molar. This malocclusion is characteristic of prognathia (protruded mandible) and macrognathia (oversized mandible; Zemlin, 2000).

Examining Dental Structural and Functional Integrity

Dental Alignment

The clinician should examine the alignment of the client's dentition by asking the client to bite down and smile.

Dental Decay

The clinician should ask the client to open his or her mouth to evaluate the client's general oral hygiene and the condition of dentition.

Interpretation of Findings

It is important to note any dental anomalies or dental malocclusions that may negatively impact speech production. For example, malocclusions, missing teeth, **supernumerary teeth** (teeth in excess of the normal number), and **microdontia** (teeth that are smaller than appropriate for the dental arch) may compromise adequate precision in the production of labiodentals, linguadentals, and alveolar phonemes, as well as efficient mastication of solids before the initiation of swallowing. Labioversion or other axial orientations could be a result of **tongue thrust** or thumb-sucking (Hall, 2000).

The health of the teeth and oral mucosa should be noted. A referral to a dentist is warranted when dental decay, anomalies, or malocclusion are noted. Baby bottle tooth decay, also known as *early childhood caries*, or "bottle rot," occurs when babies are given sweetened liquids from a baby bottle for prolonged periods of time. Poor oral hygiene is also a primary risk factor for the development of aspiration pneumonia because food particle residue allows a buildup of bacteria that can be aspirated with saliva (Langmore, Terpenning, & Schork, 1998).

If a client is wearing dentures, the clinician should note whether the maxillary (top) and/or mandibular (bottom) dentures are worn and whether they are full (all teeth are missing) or partial (only some teeth are missing). The clinician should also note goodness of fit. Poorly fitting dentures can impact speech intelligibility by affecting precision of articulation and compromise mastication of food. The reader is referred to Zemlin (2000) and Seikel et al. (2010, 2013) for a detailed and illustrated review of malocclusions and axial orientations.

Tongue

Assessing Lingual (Tongue) Structural Integrity

Lingual Surface

The clinician should examine the size, surface, color, completeness, and symmetry of the tongue at rest (CN XII). Attention should be paid to the smoothness of the lateral margins of the tongue. The presence of furrows that give the tongue a corrugated appearance should be noted. In addition, it is important to note extraneous lingual movements when the tongue is at rest. These movements, called *fasciculations*, are caused by involuntary small contractions of small bundles of muscle fibers under the surface of the tongue.

Frenum

The clinician should instruct the client to elevate his or her tongue tip to the **alveolar ridge**. The clinician should then inspect the **frenum** (also known as the *frenulum*), which is a thin band of tissue that attaches the inferior surface of the tongue to the floor of the oral cavity.

Assessing Lingual Functional Integrity

Lingual Range of Motion

To assess lingual range of motion, the clinician should instruct the client to protrude and then elevate and depress the tongue. The client should rotate his or her protruded tongue in a clockwise and counterclockwise direction. The clinician should note the rate and range of tongue motion as well as whether lingual movements are accompanied by compensatory jaw movements.

Lingual Strength

The clinician should evaluate lingual strength by instructing the client to protrude his or her tongue. The clinician should create resistance against the protruded tongue by pressing the flat side of the tongue depressor first against the midline of the tongue and then against the lateral margins of the tongue.

Interpretation of Findings

Microglossia and **macroglossia** describe a tongue that is too small or too large relative to the mandible, respectively. These presentations rarely affect articulation. The presence of transient lingual papillitis (pimples on the tongue) may be caused by physical or chemical irritation. A grayish tongue may reflect paralysis (Johnson-Root, 2015; Shipley & McAfee, 2015). Tinting is commonly symptomatic of precancerous lesions including leukoplakia (white patches), erythroplakia (red patches), and erythroleukoplakia (mixed red and white patches). Timely referral to a physician such as an otolaryngologist is warranted if any of these lesions are observed.

Absence of part of the tongue may have resulted from surgical excision (glossectomy). Loss of tongue tissue may compromise articulation, oral preparation, and oral transit during the swallow.

In the majority of cases, presentation of a short frenum, also referred to as **tongue-tie** or *ankyloglossia*, will not negatively affect articulation. However, in some cases, articulation of lingua-alveolars and even lingua-dental consonants may be compromised by reduced tongue movement. The surgical intervention to eliminate tongue-tie is called *frenulectomy* and is typically performed by an ear, nose, and throat physician (Johnson & Jacobson, 2007).

Asymmetry, decreased rate and range of tongue movement, reduced tongue strength, and deviation of the tongue upon protrusion are consistent with hypoglossal nerve damage (CN XII). Lingual fasciculations (one of the many physical findings present in dysarthias, such as amyotrophic lateral sclerosis and Parkinson disease), furrows, and atrophy may also be present (Duffy, 2013). A referral to a neurologist is necessary if any of these features are present. Damage to CN XII can compromise articulation, oral preparation, and oral transit phases of swallowing. The client who presents with weakness on both sides of the tongue may have a bilateral lesion to CN XII (Webb, 2017). On the other hand, a client who presents with decreased lingual tone will have a lower motor neuron lesion and a client with increased lingual tone will have an upper motor lesion (Webb, 2017). Webb (2017) also suggests examining the tongue tip, blade, and back of the tongue by instructing the client to produce different sounds (e.g., /t/, /y/ and /k/).

Jaw movements accompanying tongue movements are expected in young children until age 8 to 11 years (Cheng, Murdoch, Goozée, & Scott, 2007). After that age, the tongue no longer requires external stability provided by the jaw and demonstrates independent movement from the jaw.

Diadochokinesis

Labial and lingual motility can be evaluated by measuring the **diadochokinetic** syllable rate. This is a measure of how quickly the client can accurately produce a series of rapid sound sequences. Both the alternating motion rate (AMR; speed of repetitions of a series of the same syllable such as /pʌ, pʌ, pʌ/) and sequential motion rate (SMR; speed of repetitions of a series of different syllables such as /pʌ, tʌ, kʌ/) can be evaluated.

To calculate the AMR, the clinician should instruct the client to repeat series of /pʌ, pʌ, pʌ/, /tʌ, tʌ, tʌ/, and then /kʌ, kʌ, kʌ/ as fast as possible. The AMR is determined by how long it takes the client to produce 20 repetitions of the same syllable (e.g., /pʌ/, /tʌ/, or /kʌ/). Alternatively, the AMR can be calculated as the number of times the client can produce /pʌ/, /tʌ/, or /kʌ/ in a predetermined period of time. The SMR is determined by how long it takes the client to produce 10 repetitions of syllables in sequence (/pʌ, tʌ, kʌ/). The SMR can also be determined by the number of times the client can produce /pʌ, tʌ, kʌ/ in a given period of time. For young clients and clients who exhibit difficulty producing /pʌ, tʌ, kʌ/, the clinician should ask the client to rapidly repeat "buttercup" or "pattycake" rather than /pʌ, tʌ, kʌ/ (Haynes & Pindzola, 2008). Production of each series should be repeated three times. Typically, the best performance over the three trials of the task is documented. The client's AMRs and SMRs can be compared with norm-referenced data that is available from Duffy (2013) and Fletcher (1972). Please refer to Appendix 6-B for instructions.

Interpretation of Findings

Slow diadochokinetic rates and irregular rhythm of productions are indicative of a motor speech disorder such as **apraxia** or dysarthria. Apraxia of speech is characterized by an impaired ability to plan, position, and order the articulators for volitional speech production (Freed, 2012). The SMRs of clients with apraxia may be slow, syllables may be produced out of order, or inconsistent substitution of other sounds for target phonemes may be observed. Additionally, isolated movements may be better than those attempted in sequence. Dysarthria results from weakness or incoordination of the muscle movements for speech. There are several types of dysarthria depending on the site of lesion. Refer to any of the motor speech disorder textbooks cited in the references (Duffy, 2013; Freed, 2012; Swigert, 2010). The characteristics of AMRs and SMRs depend on the type of dysarthria that the participant exhibits. For example, clients with flaccid dysarthria present with slow and regular AMRs, while clients with ataxic dysarthria have AMRs that are also slow but irregular (Freed, 2012).

Hard Palate

Assessing Structural Integrity of the Hard Palate

The clinician should inspect the contour and width of the client's hard palate. The clinician should also note the presence of any **fistulas**, scars, or discoloration of the hard palate. A blue tinge or translucent zone (zona pellucida) along the midline of the hard palate should be noted (Johnson-Root, 2015; Shipley & McAfee, 2015).

Cleft Palate/Fistula

The clinician should note the presence and type of a **cleft palate** (a birth defect that occurs when tissues of the palate fail to fuse during early fetal development) and note the presence of a fistula (an opening in the palate). Careful examination of the palate of children with Apert syndrome and Treacher Collins syndrome is warranted as these children are at a higher risk for the development of a cleft palate (Hegde & Promoville, 2017; Kummer, 2014; Shipley & McAfee, 2015).

Interpretation of Findings

A high and narrow palate may negatively affect articulation of palatal sounds. A blue line along the midline of the palate is indicative of a **submucous cleft** (a separation in the bone or muscles of the palate with intact mucosal covering; Kummer, 2014; Shipley & McAfee, 2015). Clefts, fistula, and other structural abnormalities require evaluation by a physician.

Soft Palate

Assessing Velar (Soft Palate) Structural Integrity

The clinician should ask the client to open his or her mouth and then observe the configuration of the soft palate and uvula (tissue that projects posteriorly and downward from the velum). The presence of a cleft or fistula should be noted. If a bifid (split) uvula is observed, this may also indicate the presence of a submucous cleft (Hall, 2000). If the uvula deviates to the side, a neurological impairment may be present (Duffy, 2013).

Assessing Velopharyngeal Functional Integrity

Velopharyngeal closure separates the nasal cavity from the oral cavity. It is achieved by the simultaneous elevation and retraction of the soft palate (velum) and anterior movement and medialization of the walls of the nasopharynx. This separation occurs for all oral sounds but not for nasal sounds. The velum is innervated primarily by the glossopharyngeal nerve (CN IX; Wilson-Pauwels et al., 1988, 2013). The integrity of velopharyngeal function can be assessed without instrumentation in three ways. Any anomalies should be further assessed using nasometry or nasal endoscopy (Kummer, 2014).

Velopharyngeal Function Using Mirror

The clinician should hold a mirror under the client's nares and instruct the client to produce nasal phonemes (the sounds /m/, /n/, and /ŋ/) and then produce oral consonants (the remaining consonants). If velopharyngeal closure is adequate, the mirror will become foggy during production of the nasal phonemes and minimally foggy during production of oral consonants. If velopharyngeal closure is inadequate, a foggy mirror will be noted during production of oral phonemes, as well as nasal phonemes (Hardy, 1983; Johnson-Root, 2015; Shipley & McAfee, 2015). This may be due to velopharyngeal incompetence resulting from compromised elevation of the velum due to damage to the glossopharyngeal nerve (CN IX) or velopharyngeal insufficiency (inadequate tissue to achieve closure of the velopharyngeal port; Hardy, 1983; Johnson-Root, 2015; Shipley & McAfee, 2015).

Velopharyngeal Function by Closing Nares

Closure of the nares will eliminate nasal resonance from speech sounds. The clinician should gently pinch the client's nares closed during production of non-nasal sounds. Closure of the nares will eliminate nasal resonance from sounds. The quality of non-nasal sounds produced with and without closure of the nares should be compared. Another way to assess nasality is to use a straw or listening tube (which serves to amplify the sound) to listen for hypernasality and nasal emission during client production of oral sounds (Kummer, 2014).

Interpretation of Findings

A change in quality resulting from closing the nares during production of non-nasal sounds would indicate compromised velopharyngeal closure. This is because manual occlusion of the nares is serving the valving function normally performed by the velum closing. This may result from velopharyngeal incompetence or velopharyngeal insufficiency (Duffy, 2013; Hardy, 1983; Kummer, 2014).

Phonation of /a/

The clinician should instruct the client to stick out his or her tongue and produce /a/ while the clinician exerts light pressure on the blade of the client's tongue with a tongue depressor. A small penlight should be used to illuminate oral structures. The clinician should observe the symmetrical movement of the uvula at the onset of phonation, which should last at least 10 seconds across all age groups (Duffy, 2013). Additionally, the client may be instructed to sustain /a/ and note the time in seconds during three trials.

Kummer (2014) describes a detailed pediatric intraoral examination that includes having the child say /æ/ (as in "hat") and stick the tongue out and down as far as possible, looking for the following:

- Oral cavity size
- Position of the tongue tip relative to the alveolar ridge
- Presence of a fistula
- Signs of a submucous cleft
- Position of the uvula during phonation

- Size of the tonsils
- Signs of upper airway obstruction

Interpretation of Findings

Inadequate velopharyngeal closure is associated with hypernasality (a nasal quality to oral speech sounds), nasal emissions (sound escapes from the nose during speech; Kummer, 2014), and nasal regurgitation of food and liquids during oral intake (Hardy, 1983). Hypernasality is one of the many physical findings that can occur in dysarthias such as myasthenia gravis and pseudobulbar palsy (Duffy, 2013; Kummer, 2014).

Additional Procedures

There are some additional procedures that a clinician may choose to perform during the oral-peripheral exam depending on the client's age, cognitive skills, and mental status.

Screen the Swallow

There are published swallowing screen and assessment measures available. A list of the published swallowing assessments is provided in the References section. The clinician can observe the client swallow his or her saliva and liquid (if the client is not NPO [nothing by mouth]). The clinician can then ask the client to reswallow while the clinician places his or her fingers midline on the client's throat, under the chin (palpation). The clinician then observes the excursion and timing of the rise and fall of the client's larynx to determine whether the swallow is delayed or incomplete (Duffy, 2013; Johnson-Root, 2015). The clinician will observe for any clinical signs of aspiration. For a complete discussion of swallowing, please refer to Chapter 14.

Interpretation of Findings

Note the presence or absence of lingual protrusion. The presence of lingual protrusion is indicative of a tongue thrust during swallowing (protruded tongue during swallowing), also known as a *reverse swallow pattern*. On the re-swallow, note the presence and speed of laryngeal elevation and motility. Absence, delay, or incompleteness are symptoms of dysphagia (Duffy, 2013; Johnson-Root, 2015). Please refer to Chapter 14 for a detailed description of the processes of deglutition.

Assess the Gag Reflex

The clinician can ask the client to open his or her mouth and protrude the tongue. The clinician can then exert gentle pressure at the level of the **faucial pillars** (folds of tissue at the lateral margins of the posterior oral cavity that join the velum and with the base of the tongue) with a tongue depressor (Freed, 2012). A reflexive protrusion of the tongue, elevation of the soft palate, and anterior movement of the pharyngeal wall may be observed. This task can also be used to assess velopharyngeal closure (Kummer, 2014).

Interpretation of Findings

Testing a client's gag reflex may yield a strong, weak, or absent response, none of which necessarily reflects either the integrity of the glossopharyngeal nerve (CN IX) that mediates the gag reflex (Johnson & Jacobson, 2007) or the integrity of the client's pharyngeal swallow (Wilson-Pauwels et al., 1988, 2013). Care should be taken not to elicit reverse peristalsis (vomiting), especially in small children (Morris & Klein, 2000).

Apraxia and Dysarthria

If the SLP is evaluating an adult with a possible diagnosis of a motor speech disorder, he or she may choose to assess for nonverbal oral apraxia (e.g., "stick out your tongue") or apraxia of speech (repeat words of increasing syllable length and complexity), ask the client to count from 1 to 20, and read the "Rainbow or Grandfather Passage" to perceptually evaluate the five speech production components (respiration, phonation, prosody, articulation, and resonance; Freed, 2012). Additional materials used to assess speech rate and intelligibility can be found in Shipley and McAfee (2009, 2015) and Bleile (2015). Clinicians may choose to assess a client's intelligibility in multisyllabic words with consonants and vowels in different positions in addition to reading a passage. The stimuli for this potential task could be found in word dictionaries (e.g., Blockcolsky, 1990; Blockcolsky, Frazer, & Frazer, 1998).

Instructions for Assessing Various Age Groups

As we stated earlier, clinicians conduct oral-peripheral examinations on all clients; however, there are modifications to consider depending on the client's age, medical condition, cognition, and level of cooperation. Not all approaches apply to all clients.

Instructions for Assessing Young and Difficult-to-Test Children

Completing an oral-peripheral examination on young children or children who are difficult to test can be challenging mainly because these children may become frustrated and display difficulty following directions. Some strategies can be implemented to facilitate their successful participation in the evaluation (Bauman-Waengler, 2012; Bleile, 2015; Johnson-Root, 2015; Kummer, 2014):

- Obtain information from a parent or guardian about how to motivate the child to participate in various tasks before the evaluation. For example, find out about the child's favorite TV shows, characters, or toys. Use this knowledge to maintain the child's attention and cooperation during the assessment. Older children may benefit from a short explanation of each procedure.
- Sit at eye level with the child.
- Incorporate games into the evaluation to elicit spontaneous movements of oral structures (e.g., use blowing bubbles to assess labial rounding).
- Encourage the child to look inside the clinician's oral cavity with or without the penlight.
- Conduct the oral motor exam on the child's doll. Pretend that the child's doll whispers instructions for completing assessment tasks into the clinician's ear (e.g., "Dora the Explorer wants you to open your mouth wide").

Use a lollipop or applesauce as a cue for the child to move his or her lips or tongue in a certain direction. Always check with the parent regarding any allergies first. Simplify instructions depending on the child's age. Instruct the younger child to imitate the clinician performing movements with his or her articulators.

Instructions for Assessing Difficult-to-Test Adults

When the client has difficulty following the clinician's verbal directions due to comprehension deficits, cognitive impairment, or a language barrier, the clinician can use the following methods to facilitate the client's participation (Duffy, 2013; Johnson-Root, 2015):

- Enlist the client's trust by engaging in a brief conversation that inquires about the client's health and mention how this examination will help.
- Model facial expressions and labial and lingual positions for the client to imitate.
- Use gentle tactile cues to the facial area.
- Set up a mirror to provide visual feedback to the client.
- Explain the purpose of each task thoroughly.

Findings That May Indicate the Need for Referrals to Other Professionals

Structural and functional anomalies in the speech and swallow mechanism may need to be assessed by other professionals (Johnson & Jacobson, 2007).

Facial asymmetry, ptosis, rigid or reduced facial tone, decreased sensitivity to light touch to the face, asymmetry of the nasolabial fold or drooping of the corner of the lips, lingual deviation, uvular asymmetry, fasciculations of the tongue, and abnormal elevation of the velum are examples of conditions that indicate peripheral or central nerve damage. If a client demonstrates any of these conditions, referral to a neurologist is warranted. A short lingual frenulum that interferes with function; enlarged tonsils or adenoids and open mouth posture at rest; mouth breathing; poor condition or deviant structure of the hard or soft palate; discoloration of the oral pharynx; sores in the oral cavity that will not heal; or the appearance of leukoplakia, erythroplakia, or erythroleukoplakia should be examined by an otolaryngologist. Restricted range of jaw motion, pain in the temporomandibular joint, poor dental hygiene, dental abnormalities, and the presence of malocclusions should be assessed by a dentist and/or orthodontist.

Sample Case History and Oral-Peripheral Section

This section includes a case history, rationale for oral-peripheral exam, writing rubric for oral-peripheral section, and the oral-peripheral section of the diagnostic report.

Case History

A child attended a speech-language evaluation session. The mother reported that her son's speech was delayed and that he has limited expressive language skills. He communicates with few words (mostly one-syllable) and his speech is unintelligible.

Rationale for Procedure

The SLP will conduct an oral-peripheral examination as outlined in this chapter and especially examine oral structure and functional integrity and articulatory diadochokinetic rates.

Outline for the Oral-Peripheral Section of Diagnostic Report on Speech Mechanism

- Introduce this section in the traditional manner, stating what type of examination was informally conducted and the rationale.
- Provide a general overview of your findings in terms of structure and function to support speech.
- Note the structure of head, jaw, and facial symmetry.
- Discuss an informal assessment of velopharyngeal movement upon /a/ phonation.
- Note the condition of other structures when the client opens his or her mouth for the previous assessment (e.g., hard and soft palate, uvula, tongue, tonsils, and dentition).
- Note oral mobility for opening and closing the oral cavity; note symmetry.
- Note whether the client maintained air in the buccal cavity against resistance (which further corroborates velopharyngeal function).
- Describe bilabial mobility for protrusion and retraction of the lips.
- Describe lingual mobility for elevated, depressed, lateralized, and circular movements.
- Describe jaw movements.
- Note specific CN functioning.
- Describe informal assessment of diadochokenesis in isolation and in sequence
- Note presence of tongue thrust pattern where applicable.
- Provide appropriate referrals (e.g., orthodontist, otolaryngologist) at the conclusion of the report in the section on recommendations if necessary.

Oral-Peripheral Section of the Diagnostic Report

An oral-peripheral exam was conducted on 09/01/09. The client exhibited good head and neck support. No facial asymmetry was noted. Facial and articulatory sensitivity was within normal limits (WNL). Labial and lingual structural integrity was WNL. Labial and lingual functional integrity was reduced. The client exhibited reduced labial retraction and protrusion and lingual protrusion and depression. The jaw was WNL. Dental condition was good. The client exhibited a Class I occlusion and dental axial orientation was good. The palate was in good condition. The uvula was present in midline and elevated with /a/ production. The tonsils were present and not enlarged. Articulatory diadochokinesis for AMR and SMR was WNL. On the basis of the results of the oral-peripheral examination, the CNs for speech and swallowing were functioning normally.

Practice Exercise for Writing the Oral-Peripheral Examination Section of the Diagnostic Report

Using the previous instructions from the chapter, including the outline and sample case history report, use the following case history information to construct a well-written oral-peripheral examination report.

Case History Exercise

A.B., a 53-year-old woman, was seen for a speech and language evaluation after being diagnosed with Parkinson disease. A.B. was cooperative, and her adult son served as her concerned and reliable informant. Her medical history consisted of a recent diagnosis of Parkinson disease and a previous stroke. During the oral-peripheral assessment, the client was alert and oriented x4 (person, place, time, and situation). She sat upright and maintained a good sitting posture. She did not have sensation on the right side of her face, had facial drooping on the right side, and had difficulty puckering and smiling (with labial drooping on the right side). She had difficulty protruding her tongue and lateralizing it. Labial and lingual strength was reduced. Mandibular movements were good. Buccal strength was reduced on the right side of her face. Palatal functions were WNL. Her vocal intensity was reduced upon /a/ phonation and during conversational speech. Her vocal quality was breathy and hoarse at times. Diadochokinetic rates were reduced both in isolation and in sequence.

Exercise: Write the oral-peripheral section of the diagnostic report and include information about CN functioning in your write-up.

Summary

When conducting an assessment of the oral-peripheral mechanism, the clinician must thoroughly examine all of the oral-peripheral structures and functions described in this chapter, collecting and interpreting a broad range of clinical information expediently. The examination by an experienced clinician can provide both diagnostic information and indications for therapy. As clinicians acquire experience, they will become increasingly aware that structural anomalies are typically exhibited and do not necessarily impair speech or swallowing functions. It is therefore essential that novice clinicians maximize their opportunities to practice conducting this examination on individuals with normal speech mechanisms, strengthening their frame of reference for normal variations and providing a basis of comparison for abnormal findings.

Appendix 6-A

Sample Oral-Peripheral Examination Form

Facial Characteristics: ____________________

Head and Neck Support: ☐ WNL ☐ Abnormal

Comments: ____________________

Lips

Symmetry: ☐ WNL ☐ Abnormal
Posture: ☐ Open ☐ Closed
Purse: ☐ WNL ☐ Abnormal
Retract: ☐ WNL ☐ Abnormal
Protrude: ☐ WNL ☐ Abnormal
Strength: ☐ WNL ☐ Abnormal

Comments: ____________________

Jaw

Symmetry: ☐ WNL ☐ Abnormal
Size: ☐ WNL ☐ Abnormal
Open: ☐ WNL ☐ Abnormal
Close: ☐ WNL ☐ Abnormal
Strength: ☐ WNL ☐ Abnormal
Lateralize: ☐ WNL ☐ Abnormal

Comments: ____________________

Dentition

Condition: ☐ WNL ☐ Abnormal
Occlusion: ☐ Mesioclusion ☐ Distoclusion ☐ Overbite
Overjet: ☐ Underbite

Comments: ____________________

Tongue

Condition: ____________________
Frenulum: ☐ WNL ☐ Short
Protrude: ☐ WNL ☐ Abnormal
Elevate: ☐ WNL ☐ Abnormal
Depress: ☐ WNL ☐ Abnormal
Lateralize: ☐ WNL ☐ Abnormal
Strength: ☐ WNL ☐ Abnormal

Comments: ____________________

Palate

Condition: ____________________
Contour: ☐ WNL ☐ Abnormal
Velopharyngeal Closure: ☐ WNL ☐ Abnormal
Uvula: ☐ WNL ☐ Abnormal
Tonsils: ☐ Present ☐ Absent ☐ Enlarged

Comments: ____________________

Diadochokinesis

pʌ, pʌ, pʌ (20 reps in _ sec) ☐ WNL ☐ Abnormal
tʌ, tʌ, tʌ (20 reps in _ sec) ☐ WNL ☐ Abnormal
kʌ, kʌ, kʌ (20 reps in _ sec) ☐ WNL ☐ Abnormal
pʌ, tʌ, kʌ (20 reps in _ sec) ☐ WNL ☐ Abnormal

Dry Swallow: ☐ WNL ☐ Abnormal

Additional Measures:

Sensation for cotton swab/gauze

Ophthalmic Division: ____________________
Maxillary Division: ____________________
Mandibular Division: ____________________
Lingual Sensation: ____________________

Reflexes: Gag: ☐ Strong ☐ Weak (Reduced) ☐ Absent

Appendix 6-B

Instructions for Measuring Diadochokinetic Rate

Materials needed: stopwatch, worksheet, and pencil.

1. First, model all of the tasks with the child, asking the child to listen to you say the sounds, then to repeat the sounds along with you, then to try it alone. Substitution words can be adapted for children who stutter—ask the child to listen to you say "buttercup" and "patty cake," repeat the words along with you, then to try them alone.
2. When finished practicing, instruct the child to wait until you say "go," then to start and keeping saying the sound as fast as he or she can until you say "stop."

Table 6-B-1. Norms for Syllable Production in Seconds, by Age

Age	*pʌ*	*tʌ*	*kʌ*	*fʌ*	*lʌ*	*pʌtə*	*pʌkə*	*tʌkə*	*pʌtəkə*
6 mean	4.8	4.9	5.5	5.5	5.2	7.3	7.9	7.8	10.3
SD	0.8	1.0	0.9	1.0	0.9	2.0	2.1	1.8	3.1
7 mean	4.8	4.9	5.3	5.4	5.3	7.6	8.0	8.0	10.0
SD	1.0	0.9	1.0	1.0	0.8	2.6	1.9	1.8	2.6
8 mean	4.2	4.4	4.8	4.9	4.6	6.2	7.1	7.2	8.3
SD	0.7	0.7	0.7	1.0	0.6	1.8	1.5	1.5	2.1
9 mean	4.0	4.1	4.6	4.6	4.5	5.9	6.6	6.6	7.7
SD	0.6	0.6	0.7	0.7	0.5	1.6	1.5	1.7	1.9
10 mean	3.7	3.8	4.3	4.2	4.2	5.5	6.4	6.4	7.1
SD	0.4	0.4	0.5	0.5	0.5	1.5	1.4	1.2	1.5
11 mean	3.6	3.6	4.0	4.0	3.8	4.8	5.8	5.8	6.5
SD	0.6	0.7	0.6	0.6	0.6	1.1	1.2	1.3	1.4
12 mean	3.4	3.5	3.9	3.7	3.7	4.7	5.7	5.5	6.4
SD	0.4	0.5	0.6	0.4	0.4	1.2	1.5	1.1	1.6
13 mean	3.3	3.3	3.7	3.6	3.5	4.2	5.1	5.1	5.7
SD	0.6	0.5	0.6	0.5	0.5	0.8	1.5	1.3	1.4

Scores represent time, in seconds, required for 20 repetitions of single syllables, 15 repetitions of bisyllables, and 10 repetitions of /pʌ, tʌ, kʌ/.

Reprinted with permission from Fletcher, S. G. (1972). Time-by-count measurement of diadochokinetic syllable rate. *Journal of Speech and Hearing Disorders, 15*, p. 765.

Data Collection Worksheet

Sound Repetitions	pʌ × 20	tʌ × 20	kʌ × 20	pʌ, tʌ, kʌ × 10
Time Lapsed in Seconds				
+ or – SD				

3. With each series, have the stopwatch ready to time the child. Say "go" and simultaneously start the watch; stop the child and the stopwatch after 20 repetitions of pʌ and write down the number of seconds on the stopwatch. Reset the watch and repeat the process for tʌ and kʌ. For /pʌ, tʌ, kʌ/, stop after 10 repetitions.
4. Compare the amount of time in seconds that it took the child to complete each task with the norms by age as originally measured by Fletcher (1972), reproduced in Table 6-B-1.
5. Calculate the number of standard deviations (SDs) the child is above (slower rate) or below (faster rate) these norms. For example, the mean and SD for a 7-year-old child for 10 repetitions of /pʌ, tʌ, kʌ/ as measured by Fletcher (1972) was 10.0 seconds with an SD of 2.6 seconds. If the child being tested took 14.2 seconds to complete the sequence, the number of SDs above the norm would be 1.6 [14.2 – 10.0 = 4.2; 4.2 ÷ 2.6 = 1.6].

Glossary

Afferent (or sensory): Transmit sensory information toward the brain or nerve cell body.

Alveolar ridge: The boney ridge in the maxillary bone behind the upper anterior dentition.

Apraxia: Impaired capacity to program the position of speech musculature and the sequencing of muscle movements for the volitional production of sounds.

Buccal: Pertaining to the cheek portion of the human face.

Buccoversion: Molars tilt toward the cheek.

Class I malocclusion: A normal orientation of the molars occurring with variations in the anterior parts of the upper and lower dental arches.

Class I occlusion: A normal relationship between upper and lower dental arches in which the first molar of the mandibular arch is one-half tooth advanced of the maxillary molar.

Class II malocclusion: The mandible is retracted because the first mandibular molars are retracted at least one tooth from the first maxillary molars, giving the appearance of a receding chin.

Class III malocclusion: The mandible is protruded because the first mandibular molar is advanced further than at least one tooth beyond the first maxillary molar.

Cleft palate: A birth defect that results when tissues of the palate fail to fuse during early fetal development; can vary from a complete separation of the skin and bone of both the hard and soft palate to partial defects.

Deciduous (shedding) teeth: Milk (or baby) teeth that begin to erupt between 6 and 9 months of age.

Diadochokinesis: The ability to alternate diametrically opposite muscular actions (of the articulators).

Distoversion: A tooth leans away from the midline, along the arch.

Dysarthria: A motor speech production impairment caused by central or peripheral nervous system involvement of one or more of the speech subsystems of respiration, phonation, resonance, articulation, or prosody.

Efferent (or motor): Mediate impulses away from the brain and cell body.

Faucial pillars: Folds of tissue at the lateral margins of the posterior oral cavity that join the velum with the base of the tongue.

Fistula: An opening in the palate, sometimes occurring after surgery from poor wound healing.

Frenum: A thin band of tissue connecting the inferior surface of the tongue to the floor of the oral cavity.

Functional anomaly: Refers to the use and coordination of anatomical components.

Infraverted: Tooth does not make occlusal contact with its pair in the opposite arch, above or below it.

Labiodentals: Contact between the lower lip and teeth.

Labioversion: Tooth tilts toward the lips.

Linguadentals: Contact of the tongue tip between the upper and lower front teeth.

Linguaversion: Tooth tilts toward the tongue.

Macroglossia: Tongue considered too large for the size of the client's oral cavity.

Macrognathia: Large jaw.

Malocclusion: Misalignment of teeth.

Mesioversion: Tooth tilts toward that midline between the two central incisors.

Microdontia: Teeth that are smaller than appropriate for the dental arch.

Microglossia: Tongue considered too small for the size of the client's oral cavity.

Micrognathia: Small jaw.

Occlusion: The complete meeting of the teeth of the upper and lower dental arches.

Open bite: Upper and lower anterior teeth are unable to approximate, with a visible space between them.

Oral-peripheral examination (oral facial examination; speech mechanism examination): An assessment of the structural and functional integrity of the structures used for speech production.

Overbite: A small part of the lower teeth are observable.

Overjet: The upper incisors project beyond the lower incisors vertically by a few millimeters.

Permanent teeth: Second set of teeth that develop and remain throughout life.

Prognathia: A protruded mandible.

Ptosis: Drooping of the eyelid.

Reflexes: Involuntary responsive motor movements

Structural anomaly: Refers to skeletal, muscular, nerve, and tissue anatomical components.

Submucous cleft: A defect in the muscles of the soft palate only.

Supernumerary teeth: Additional teeth to the normal number.

Supraverted: Tooth that extends too far into the oral cavity.

Tongue thrust: The pattern of swallowing in which the tongue is protruded forward during swallowing.

Tongue-tie: Describes a short or restricted lingual frenum.

Torsiversion: The tooth is rotated or twisted on its long axis.

Underbite: Upper and lower posterior teeth are unable to approximate.

Velopharyngeal closure: The separation of the nasal cavity from the oral cavity by movement of the velum superiorly and posteriorly and by the construction of the pharyngeal wall around the velum.

References

Ash, M. M., & Nelson, S. J. (2003). *Wheeler's dental anatomy, physiology, and occlusion* (8th ed.). Maryland Heights, MO: Saunders Elsevier.

Bauman-Waengler, J. A. (2012). *Articulatory and phonological impairments.* New York, NY: Pearson Higher Education.

Bernthal, J., Bankson, N. W., & Flipsen, P., Jr. (2013). *Articulation and phonological disorders.* New York, NY: Pearson Higher Education.

Bhatnager, S. (2013). *Neuroscience for the study of communication disorders.* Baltimore, MD: Lippincott Williams & Wilkins.

Bleile, K. M. (2015). *Manual of articulation and phonological disorders. Infancy through adulthood* (3rd ed.; Clinical Competence Series). Clifton Park, NY: Delmar Cengage Learning.

Blockcolsky, V. (1990). *Book of words: 17,000 words selected by vowels and diphthongs.* Tucson, AZ: Communication Skill Builders.

Blockcolsky, V., Frazer, J. M., & Frazer, D. H. (1998). *40,000 selected words organized by letter, sound, and syllable.* Tucson, AZ: Communication Skill Builders.

Cheng, H. Y., Murdoch, B. E., Goozée, J. V., & Scott, D. (2007). Physiologic development of tongue-jaw coordination from childhood to adulthood. *Journal of Speech, Language, and Hearing Research, 50*, 352-360.

Drummond, S. (1993). *Dysarthria examination battery.* Tucson, AZ: Communication Skill Builders.

Duffy, J. R. (2013). *Motor speech disorders: Substrates, differential diagnosis and management* (3rd ed.). St. Louis, MO: Elsevier Mosby.

Dworkin, J. P., & Culatta, R.A. (1980). *Dworkin-Culatta oral mechanism examination.* Nicholasville, KY: Edgewood Press.

Enderby, P. (1983). *Frenchay dysarthria assessment.* Austin, TX: Pro-Ed.

Felício, C. M., & Ferreira, C. L. (2008). Protocol of orofacial myofunctional evaluation with scores. *International Journal of Pediatric Otorhinolaryngology, 72*(3), 367-375.

Fletcher, S. G. (1972). Time-by-count measurement of diadochokinetic syllable rate. *Journal of Speech and Hearing Disorders, 15*, 763-770.

Freed, D. B. (2012). *Motor speech disorders: Diagnosis and treatment* (2nd ed.). Clifton Park, NY: Delmar Cengage Learning.

Fuller, D. R., Pimentel, J. T., & Peregoy, B. M. (2012). *Applied anatomy & physiology for speech-language pathology & audiology.* Baltimore, MD: Lippincott Williams & Wilkins.

Hall, P. K. (2000). The oral mechanism. In J. D. Tomblin, H. L. Morris, & D. C. Spriesterbach (Eds.), *Diagnosis in speech-language pathology* (2nd ed.). San Diego, CA: Singular.

Hardy, J. C. (1983). *Cerebral palsy.* Englewood Cliffs, NJ: Prentice Hall.

Haynes, W. O., & Pindzola, R., H. (2008). *Diagnosis and evaluation in speech pathology* (7th ed.). Boston, MA: Allyn & Bacon.

Hegde, M. N. & Freed, D. (2013). *Assessment of communication disorders in adults.* San Diego, CA: Plural.

Hegde, M. N. & Promoville, F. (2017). *Assessment of communication disorders in children.* San Diego, CA: Plural.

Johnson, A. F., & Jacobson, B. H. (2007). *Medical speech-language pathology* (2nd ed.). New York, NY: Thieme Medical.

Johnson-Root, B. (2015). *Oral-facial evaluation for speech-language pathologists.* San Diego, CA: Plural.

Kummer, A. W. (2014). *Cleft palate and craniofacial anomalies: The effects on speech and resonance* (3rd ed.). Clifton Park, NY: Cengage Learning.

Langmore, S. E., Terpenning, M. S., & Schork, A. (1998). Predictors of aspiration pneumonia: How important is dysphagia? *Dysphagia, 12*, 69-81.

Mayo Clinic, Department of Neurology. (1998). *Clinical examinations in neurology* (7th ed.) St. Louis, MO: Mosby.

Morris, S., & Klein, M. (2000). *Pre-feeding skills: A comprehensive resource for feeding development.* Tucson, AZ: Communication Skill Builders.

Robbins, J. A., & Klee, T. (1987). Clinical assessment of oropharyngeal motor development in young children. *Journal of Speech and Hearing Disorders, 52*, 271-277.

Robertson, S. J. (1982). *Dysarthria profile.* Tucson, AZ: Communication Skill Builders.

Seikel, J. A., Drumright, D. G., & Seikel, P. (2013). *Essentials of anatomy & physiology for communication disorders* (2nd ed.). Clifton Park, NY: Delmar Cengage Learning.

Seikel, J. A., King, D. W., & Drumright, D. G. (2010). *Anatomy & physiology for speech, language and hearing* (4th ed.). Clifton Park, NY: Delmar Cengage Learning.

Sheppard, J. (1995). Clinical evaluation and treatment. In S. R. Rosenthal, J. Sheppard, & M. Lotze (Eds.), *Dysphagia in the child with developmental disabilities, medical, clinical and family interventions.* San Diego, CA: Singular.

Shipley, K. G., & McAfee, J. G. (2009). *Assessment in speech-language pathology: A resource manual* (4th ed.). Clifton Park, NY: Delmar Cengage Learning.

Shipley, K. G., & McAfee, J. G. (2015). *Assessment in speech-language pathology: A resource manual* (5th ed.). Clifton Park, NY: Delmar Cengage Learning.

Swigert, N. (2007). *The source for dysphagia* (3rd ed.). East Moline, IL: LinguiSystems.

Swigert, N. (2010). *The source for dysarthria* (4th ed.). East Moline, IL: LinguiSystems

Webb, W. (2017). *Neurology for the speech-language pathologist.* St. Louis, MO: Mosby/Elsevier.

Wertz, R. (1985). Neuropathologies of speech and language: An introduction to client management. In D. Johns (Ed.), *Clinical management of neurogenic communicative disorders* (2nd ed.; pp. 1-96). Boston, MA: Little, Brown.

Wilson-Pauwels, L., Akesson, E., & Stewart, P. (1988). *Cranial nerves anatomy and clinical comments.* St. Louis, MO: CV Mosby.

Wilson-Pauwels, L., Stewart, P., Akesson, E., & Spacey, S. (2013). *Cranial nerves function and dysfunction* (3rd ed.). Retrieved from https://www.amazon.com/Cranial-Nerves-Function-Dysfunction-3e/dp/1607950316#reader_1607950316

World Health Organization. (2001). International Classification of Functioning, Disability and Health (ICF). Geneva: Author.

Zemlin, W. R. (2000). *Speech and hearing science: Anatomy and physiology* (4th ed.). Englewood, NJ: Prentice Hall.

Additional Recommended Reading

American Speech-Language-Hearing Association. (n.d.). Motor Speech Disorders Evaluation form. Retrieved from https://www.asha.org/uploadedFiles/slp/healthcare/AATMotorSpeech.pdf

Kent, R. D., Kent, J., & Rosenbek, J. (1987). Maximal performance tests of speech production. *Journal of Speech and Hearing Disorders, 52*, 367-387.

McCauley, R. J., & Strand, E. A. (2008). A review of standardized tests of nonverbal oral and speech motor performance in children. *American Journal of Speech Language Pathology, 1*(1), 1-11.

Velleman, S. L. (2002). *Childhood apraxia of speech resource guide*. Clifton Park, NY: Delmar/Thomson/Singular.

Website Resources

American Speech-Language-Hearing Association (ASHA): www.asha.org

ASHA portal: www.asha.org/practice-portal/

Anatomy

The Bartleby.com edition of Gray's *Anatomy of the Human Body*: www.bartleby.com/107

W. R. Zemlin Memorial Website: http://zemlin.shs.uiuc.edu

Netter Atlas of Human Anatomy: https://allmedicalstuff.com/netter-atlas-pdf-buy/

Cranial Nerves

Wright State University, College of Nursing and Health—Physical Assessment Examination Study Guide, Neurologic Examination; General Considerations and Observations: https://nursing.wright.edu/sites/nursing.wright.edu/files/page/attachments/PhysicalAssessmentExamStudyGuidefinaldraft.pdf

Cranial Nerves Illustrated: https://bmc.med.utoronto.ca/cranialnerves

Apraxia

Apraxia Kids: www.apraxia-kids.org

ASHA Portal—Motor Speech Disorders Evaluation Template: www.asha.org/Practice-Portal/Templates

Judith Kuster Website Motor Speech Apraxia: www.mnsu.edu/comdis/kuster2/sptherapy.html#motor

Cleft Palate

Cincinnati Children's Hospital website—Ann Kummer, PhD, has provided handouts on cleft palate, craniofacial anomalies, and velopharyngeal dysfunction: www.cincinnatichildrens.org/service/s/speech/hcp/lecture-notes

Dental Occlusions

Norton, N. (2007). *Netter's head and neck anatomy for dentistry*. Philadelphia, PA: Saunders Elsevier.

Dysphagia

Dysphagia Research Society: www.dysphagiaresearch.org

GI Mortality Online: www.nature.com/gimo/index.html

Medline-Plus Swallowing Disorders: https://medlineplus.gov/swallowingdisorders.html

Infant Reflexes and Development

Lucile Packard Children's Hospital Stanford, Topics, Newborn-Reflexes: www.stanfordchildrens.org/en/topic/default?id=newborn-reflexes-90-P02630

Medical Dictionaries

Mosby's medical dictionary (9th ed.). (2013). St. Louis, MO: Mosby Yearbook. www.online-medical-dictionary.org

Trusted Medline Plus: https://medlineplus.gov/mplusdictionary.html

Oral Motor Assessments

Dworkin-Culatta Oral Mechanism Exam and Treatment System (D-COME-T). California State University East Bay, Department of Communicative Sciences and Disorders. https://www.csueastbay.edu/class/departments/commsci/files/docs/pdf/dworkin-culatta-oral-mech-exam.pdf

Kaufman Speech Praxis Test for Children (KSPT), on Apraxia Kids: www.apraxia-kids.org/library/links-apraxia-assessment-tools

7

Assessment of Speech Sound Disorders

Renee Fabus, PhD, CCC-SLP, TSHH and Felicia Gironda, PhD, CCC-SLP

Key Words

- addition
- alveolar
- alveolarization
- apraxia
- articulation
- articulation disorder
- assimilation
- backing
- cluster reduction
- coarticulation
- depalatalization
- derhotacization
- diadochokinesis
- dialects
- diminutization
- diphthongization
- distinctive features
- distortion
- doubling
- dysarthrias
- epenthesis
- final consonant deletion
- final devoicing
- fricative preference
- fronting
- gliding
- idiopathic
- juncture
- labialization
- linguadental
- liquid simplification
- maximal pairs
- minimal pairs
- morpheme
- morphophenemics
- nasal preference
- neurogenic
- obstruent
- omission
- pattern analysis
- phonetics
- phonological disorder
- phonological processes
- phonology
- phonotactics
- prevocalic voicing
- prosody
- reduplication
- sonorant
- speech sound disorders
- stimulability
- stopping
- stridency deletion
- substitution
- suprasegmentals of speech
- tetism
- unstressed syllable deletion
- velar
- velar fronting
- vocalization
- vowel harmony

Stein-Rubin, C., & Fabus, R. *A Guide to Clinical Assessment and Professional Report Writing in Speech-Language Pathology, Second Edition (pp 131-161).*

The purpose of this chapter is to delineate the various considerations that the student clinician and novice speech language pathologist (SLP) should take into account when planning to evaluate **speech sound disorders** in both children and adults. Speech sound disorders encompass both **articulation** and **phonological disorders**. Because there are numerous etiologies and characteristics underlying these disorders across the life span, this chapter focuses on the assessment of the most typical developmental presentations. For a more exhaustive description of speech sound disorders, the reader is referred to the seminal works of Bauman-Waengler (2012); Bernthal and Bankson (2004); Bernthal, Bankson, and Flipsen (2013); and Peña-Brooks & Hegde (2015).

Let's begin by first defining speech sound disorders. "Speech sound disorders is an umbrella term referring to any combination of difficulties with perception, motor production, and/or the phonological representation of speech sounds and speech segments (including **phonotactic** rules that govern syllable shape, structure, and stress, as well as **prosody**) that impact speech intelligibility" (American Speech-Language-Hearing Association [ASHA], 2016b).

The term **articulation** generally refers to the motor processes involved in the execution of movements for speech production of sounds (Bauman-Waengler, 2012; Bernthal et al., 2013). A client could be diagnosed with an articulation disorder if he or she has difficulty executing these speech movements or difficulty producing speech sounds. In contrast, we could define **phonology** as a description of phonemes and their organization within a language, and a phonological disorder could be defined as an impairment in the organization of these phonemes within a language (Bauman-Waengler, 2012). A client may have both an articulation and phonological disorder, and it may be difficult to distinguish the characteristics of either disorder. Before further differentiating these terms, it is important that the novice clinician understand other important related terms:

- **Phonetics**: The study of speech sounds and their properties. There are different types of phonetics, but they are not discussed in this chapter. Please refer to Bauman-Waengler (2012) and Peña-Brooks & Hegde (2015).
- Phone: A speech sound
- Phonemes: A basic speech segment
- Allophonic variations (phonetic variations): The slight variations in production of a phoneme that do not change the meaning
- Phonotactics: The description of permitted phoneme combinations within a language
- Phonetic inventory: An inventory of different speech sounds, or phones
- Phonemic inventory: An inventory of the smallest segmental unit of sounds used to form meaningful contrasts between utterances
- **Coarticulation**: The influence of one sound by a sound that precedes or follows it
- **Morphophonemics**: The phonological structure of **morphemes**
- **Minimal pairs**: Pairs of words that differ by place, manner, or voicing
- **Maximal pairs**: Pairs of words that differ by multiple contrasts in place, manner and/or voicing (Bauman-Waengler, 2012; Peña-Brooks & Hegde, 2015)

We use the International Phonetic Alphabet (IPA) to describe the different sounds in our client's speech. The IPA is a group of symbols selected to represent the broadest consensus of articulatory characteristics across the world's languages (International Phonetic Association, 2005; Tiffany & Carrell, 1977). There are generally two types of transcription that we could use to transcribe our client's speech: narrow phonetic transcription and broad phonetic transcription (Bauman-Waengler, 2012; Peña-Brooks & Hegde, 2015). Clinicians use broad transcription to indicate the more noticeable phonetic features of an utterance. When we transcribe our client's speech, we place the sounds (phonemes) within brackets, and we may use special symbols or diacritics to further explain the client's speech (narrow phonetic transcription). Diacritics are used in narrow transcription to mark the allophonic variations of a sound (Shriberg & Kent, 2012). They are written on top of the sound, under it, or directly before or after the production of the sound. According to Shriberg and Kent (2012), diacritic marks can be classified into six positions: onglide symbols, stress (nasal and lip) symbols, main symbols (tongue and sound source symbols), offglide symbols, timing symbols, and **juncture** symbols. Onglide symbols are used when there is a brief sound that occurs before the main sound in transcription. Stress symbols indicate where the stress occurs, nasal symbols reveal information about the velopharyngeal closure during that sound production, and lip symbols indicate whether lip rounding has occurred for that production. Tongue symbols describe changes in placement, whereas sound source symbols describe a change in manner

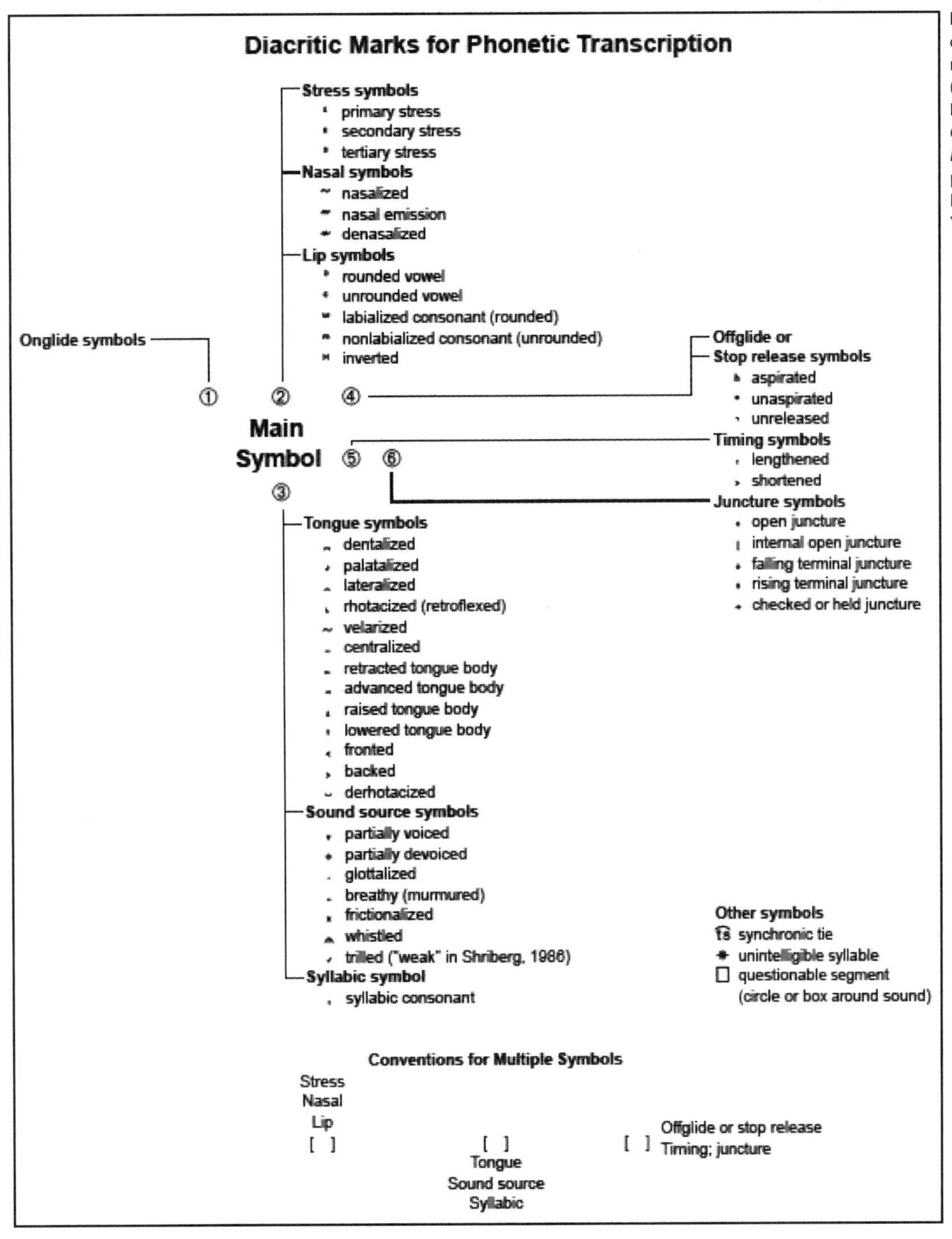

Figure 7-1. List of diacritic marks for phonetic transcription. (Shriberg, Lawrence D.; Kent, Raymond D., *Clinical Phonetics, 4th Ed.*, ©2013. Reprinted by permission of Pearson Education, Inc., New York, New York.)

of production for that sound. Offglide symbols, unlike onglide symbols, indicate the presence of a brief sound after the main sound. Timing and juncture symbols are used to indicate changes in the intonation. See Figure 7-1 for a complete listing of all diacritic marks; see Shriberg and Kent (2012) for a description of all diacritic marks.

Shriberg and Kent (2012) presented the following guidelines for using diacritic marks, which would be helpful for the novice clinician:

- First, choose the phonetic symbol to represent the sound and write it in brackets.
- If the sound is produced with a source modification, write it under the sound.
- If the sound is produced with a place modification, write it.
- If there is any modification of velopharyngeal closure, indicate it.
- If there is any pause, prolongation, or abrupt **stopping** of a sound, indicate it.

Phoneme Classification

Before viewing the IPA table, it is imperative that you understand phoneme classification. Some discussion will take place in this chapter; however, for further discussion, refer to the following references: Bauman-Waengler (2012); Bernthal et al. (2013); Lowe (2009); Peña-Brooks and Hegde (2015); Roach (2004); Shriberg and Kent (2012); and Small (2005). Consonants and vowels are the two main phoneme categories. There are terms used to describe the consonant's position in a word. If the consonant precedes a vowel, the term **prevocalic** is used. If the consonant is after a vowel, it is termed *postvocalic*. When the consonant occurs between two vowels, it is *intervocalic*. Some clinicians prefer to use the terms *initial*, *medial*, and *final position* for where the consonant occurs within a word. Vowels are produced with an open vocal tract, no constriction, and always with vocal fold vibration, whereas consonants are produced with constriction in the oral cavity and may be produced with (voiced) or without (voiceless) vocal fold vibration.

Vowels

Vowels can be classified as either monophthongs (one vowel sound) or diphthongs (**gliding** of two vowel sounds together). Vowels are described according to the following qualities:

- Vowels produced in the front of the oral cavity vs. the back of the oral cavity
- Vowels produced high toward the palate vs. low away from the palate
- The degree of lip rounding for the vowel production
- The amount of tension for vowel production—tense vs. lax vowel production

Refer to the following references for additional information about phoneme classification: Bauman-Waengler (2012), Peña-Brooks and Hegde (2015), Roach (2004), Shriberg and Kent (2012), and Small (2005).

The vowel quadrilateral is illustrated in Figure 7-2 with the vowels produced in the front of the oral cavity on the left side of the chart and those produced in the back of the oral cavity on the right side of the chart. The vowels produced high in the palate are written at the top of the chart, and those produced low away from the palate are at the bottom of the chart (Bauman-Waengler, 2012; Peña-Brooks & Hegde, 2015).

Generally speaking, the other two characteristics of vowel production are described as follows:

1. Tense vowels require greater muscle activity and a longer duration compared to lax vowels.
2. Rounded vowels tend to be produced with the client rounding and protruding his or her lips.

It is imperative to know what sound corresponds with each symbol. Please review Table 7-1 for this information.

Diphthongs

Diphthongs are two vowel sounds combined, meaning there is an onglide and offglide sound. See Table 7-2 for a list of diphthongs and their corresponding sounds in words. For further discussion about diphthongs, please refer to Bauman-Waengler (2012), Peña-Brooks and Hegde (2015), Roach (2004), Shriberg and Kent (2012), and Small (2005).

Consonants

Consonants can be described according to the following characteristics (Bauman-Waengler, 2012; Bernthal & Bankson, 2004; Bernthal et al., 2013; Peña-Brooks & Hegde, 2015; Small, 2005):

- Place of articulation (where along the vocal tract the sound is formed)
- Manner of articulation (the type of airflow constriction to form the sound)
- Voicing (vocal fold vibration or not)
- Organ of articulation (not used often in description; the part of the vocal tract that moves to form the sound)
- When two or more consonants are together, they are called *consonant clusters* (e.g., /str/ in the word street). (We use the terms *prevocalic* [before a vowel], *intervocalic* [between two vowels], and *postvocalic* [after a vowel] to describe where the consonants are placed within the word.)

See the consonant chart in Figure 7-2.

Classification of Consonants and Vowels

IPA Table: Listing of Consonants According to Place, Manner, and Voicing

The IPA table (see Figure 7-2) illustrates groups of speech sound symbols selected to represent the

THE INTERNATIONAL PHONETIC ALPHABET (revised to 2015)

CONSONANTS (PULMONIC)

	Bilabial	Labiodental	Dental	Alveolar	Postalveolar	Retroflex	Palatal	Velar	Uvular	Pharyngeal	Glottal
Plosive	p b			t d		ʈ ɖ	c ɟ	k ɡ	q ɢ		ʔ
Nasal	m	ɱ		n		ɳ	ɲ	ŋ	ɴ		
Trill	ʙ			r					ʀ		
Tap or Flap		ⱱ		ɾ		ɽ					
Fricative	ɸ β	f v	θ ð	s z	ʃ ʒ	ʂ ʐ	ç ʝ	x ɣ	χ ʁ	ħ ʕ	h ɦ
Lateral fricative				ɬ ɮ							
Approximant		ʋ		ɹ		ɻ	j	ɰ			
Lateral approximant				l		ɭ	ʎ	ʟ			

Symbols to the right in a cell are voiced, to the left are voiceless. Shaded areas denote articulations judged impossible.

CONSONANTS (NON-PULMONIC)

Clicks	Voiced implosives	Ejectives
ʘ Bilabial	ɓ Bilabial	ʼ Examples:
ǀ Dental	ɗ Dental/alveolar	pʼ Bilabial
ǃ (Post)alveolar	ʄ Palatal	tʼ Dental/alveolar
ǂ Palatoalveolar	ɠ Velar	kʼ Velar
ǁ Alveolar lateral	ʛ Uvular	sʼ Alveolar fricative

VOWELS

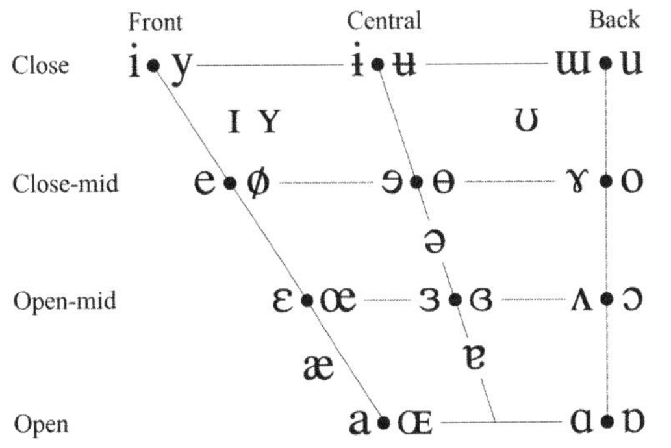

Front Central Back

Close: i • y — ɨ • ʉ — ɯ • u
ɪ ʏ ʊ

Close-mid: e • ø — ɘ • ɵ — ɤ • o
ə

Open-mid: ɛ • œ — ɜ • ɞ — ʌ • ɔ
æ ɐ

Open: a • ɶ — ɑ • ɒ

Where symbols appear in pairs, the one to the right represents a rounded vowel.

OTHER SYMBOLS

- ʍ Voiceless labial-velar fricative
- w Voiced labial-velar approximant
- ɥ Voiced labial-palatal approximant
- ʜ Voiceless epiglottal fricative
- ʢ Voiced epiglottal fricative
- ʡ Epiglottal plosive
- ɕ ʑ Alveolo-palatal fricatives
- ɺ Voiced alveolar lateral flap
- ɧ Simultaneous ʃ and x

Affricates and double articulations can be represented by two symbols joined by a tie bar if necessary. t͡s k͡p

SUPRASEGMENTALS

- ˈ Primary stress ˌfoʊnəˈtɪʃən
- ˌ Secondary stress
- ː Long eː
- ˑ Half-long eˑ
- ˘ Extra-short ĕ
- | Minor (foot) group
- ‖ Major (intonation) group
- . Syllable break ɹi.ækt
- ‿ Linking (absence of a break)

DIACRITICS Some diacritics may be placed above a symbol with a descender, e.g. ŋ̊

̥ Voiceless	n̥ d̥	̤ Breathy voiced	b̤ a̤	̪ Dental	t̪ d̪
̬ Voiced	s̬ t̬	̰ Creaky voiced	b̰ a̰	̺ Apical	t̺ d̺
ʰ Aspirated	tʰ dʰ	̼ Linguolabial	t̼ d̼	̻ Laminal	t̻ d̻
̹ More rounded	ɔ̹	ʷ Labialized	tʷ dʷ	̃ Nasalized	ẽ
̜ Less rounded	ɔ̜	ʲ Palatalized	tʲ dʲ	ⁿ Nasal release	dⁿ
̟ Advanced	u̟	ˠ Velarized	tˠ dˠ	ˡ Lateral release	dˡ
̠ Retracted	e̠	ˤ Pharyngealized	tˤ dˤ	̚ No audible release	d̚
̈ Centralized	ë	~ Velarized or pharyngealized	ɫ		
̽ Mid-centralized	e̽	̝ Raised	e̝ (ɹ̝ = voiced alveolar fricative)		
̩ Syllabic	n̩	̞ Lowered	e̞ (β̞ = voiced bilabial approximant)		
̯ Non-syllabic	e̯	̘ Advanced Tongue Root	e̘		
˞ Rhoticity	ɚ a˞	̙ Retracted Tongue Root	e̙		

TONES AND WORD ACCENTS

LEVEL		CONTOUR	
e̋ or ˥	Extra high	ě or ˩˥	Rising
é ˦	High	ê ˥˩	Falling
ē ˧	Mid	e᷄ ˦˥	High rising
è ˨	Low	e᷅ ˩˨	Low rising
ȅ ˩	Extra low	e᷈ ˧˦˧	Rising-falling
↓	Downstep	↗	Global rise
↑	Upstep	↘	Global fall

Figure 7-2. The IPA. (IPA Chart, http://www.internationalphoneticassociation.org/content/ipa-chart, available under a Creative Commons Attribution-Sharealike 3.0 Unported License. Copyright © 2015 International Phonetic Association.)

Table 7-1. IPA Vowel Symbols and Their Corresponding Sounds in Words

IPA Vowel Symbol	*Example in Word*
ʌ	cup, butter, clutter
ǣ	mat, black, bat
ɛ	set, bed, wet
ə	away, cinema
ɝ	burn, learn, earn
ɪ	hit, bit, sit
i	bee, heat, meat
ɑ	hot, sock, rock
ɔ	call, pour, ball
ʊ	book, could, should
u	blue, food, mood

broadest consensus of articulatory characteristics across the world's languages (International Phonetic Association, 2005; Tiffany & Carrell, 1977). The top horizontal row of the main IPA chart contains the place of articulation/constriction in the vocal tract (oral cavity and laryngopharynx). The column on the far left of the main IPA chart lists the manner of articulation/type of vocal tract closure. Some phonetic symbols are paired in a cell with the voiceless (vocal folds not vibrating) consonant on the left and the voiced (vocal folds are vibrating) consonant on the right. Vowels, pictured below the main IPA chart, are represented by both the front–back and the high–low articulatory position of the tongue. Because each phoneme is represented by one discrete symbol in the consonant and vowel charts, allowances are made to describe the broad scope of variation by the other tables pictured (unusual nonpulmonic consonants, other symbols, diacritics, **suprasegmentals**, and tone and word accents). Shipley and McAfee (2015) provided a listing of consonants by place, manner, and voicing and a listing of vowels by place of articulation and height.

Distinctive Features

Another way to discuss the classification of consonants and vowels is by their **distinctive features**. The distinctive feature system (Chomsky & Halle, 1968) is a binary system in which a phoneme has a unique representation of features that distinguishes it from other phonemes, and we indicate this with a (+) or a (–) feature. Consonants are classified according to 16 binary features and vowels have 7 features. Please see

Table 7-2. Diphthongs and Their Corresponding Sounds in Words

Diphthong in IPA	*Example in Word*
/aɪ/	five, eye, dive
/aʊ/	now, out, cow
/eɪ/	say, eight, day
/əʊ/	go, home, comb
/ɔɪ/	boy, join, coin
/eə/	where, air, hair
/ɪə/	near, here, deer

Table 7-3 for a list of the distinctive features for consonants. The following are some examples of distinctive features by which consonants are classified:

- Vocalic: Like a vowel
- Consonantal: Like a consonant
- High: Body of tongue elevated
- Back: Tongue elevates to velum
- Low: Tongue in lowest position: /h/
- Anterior: Sound made with articulators at **alveolar** ridge (bony ridge behind upper front teeth) or forward
- Coronal: Sound made with tongue blade raised
- Round: Lips rounded
- Tense: Degree of muscle tension
- Strident: Forced airstream creates intense noise quality to sounds
- **Sonorant**: Unimpeded sound through oral cavity
- Interrupted: Completely blocked airflow at some point in production
- Lateral: Air flows along the lateral margins of tongue
- Voice: Vibrating vocal folds

For further discussion about the definition of each feature and the vowel features, refer to Bauman-Waengler (2012), Bernthal & Bankson (2004), Bernthal et al. (2013), Peña-Brooks & Hegde (2015), Roach (2004), Rogers (2000), Shriberg and Kent (2012), Small (2005), and Tiffany and Carrell (1977).

Additional Background Information

The background information presented in Tables 7-1 through 7-3 is essential for a novice clinician

Table 7-3. Distinctive Features of Consonants

	English																							
	p	m	t	b	d	k	n	g	f	v	ʃ	s	z	ʒ	j	h	dʒ	tʃ	ð	θ	l	ʔ	ŋ	ɹ
syllabic	–	–	–	–	–	–	–	–	–	–	–	–	–	–	–	–	–	–	–	–	–	–	–	–
consonantal	+	+	+	+	+	+	+	+	+	+	+	+	+	+	–	+	+	+	+	+	+	+	+	+
continuant acoust.	–	+	–	–	–	–	+	–	+	+	+	+	+	+	+	+	–	–	+	+	+	–	+	+
continuant artic.	–	–	–	–	–	–	–	–	+	+	+	+	+	+	+	+	–	–	+	+	+	–	–	+
sonorant	–	+	–	–	–	–	+	–	–	–	–	–	–	–	+	–	–	–	–	–	+	–	+	+
approximant	–	–	–	–	–	–	–	–	–	–	–	–	–	–	+	–	–	–	–	–	+	–	–	+
nasal	–	+	–	–	–	–	+	–	–	–	–	–	–	–	–	–	–	–	–	–	–	–	+	–
strident	–	–	–	–	–	–	–	–	–	–	+	+	+	+	–	–	+	+	–	–	–	–	–	–
lateral	–	–	–	–	–	–	–	–	–	–	–	–	–	–	–	–	–	–	–	–	+	–	–	–
trill	–	–	–	–	–	–	–	–	–	–	–	–	–	–	–	–	–	–	–	–	–	–	–	–
tap	–	–	–	–	–	–	–	–	–	–	–	–	–	–	–	–	–	–	–	–	–	–	–	–
labial	+	+	–	+	–	–	–	–	+	+	–	–	–	–	–	–	–	–	–	–	–	–	–	–
round	–	–	–	–	–	–	–	–	–	–	–	–	–	–	–	–	–	–	–	–	–	–	–	–
labiodental	–	–	–	–	–	–	–	–	+	+	–	–	–	–	–	–	–	–	–	–	–	–	–	–
coronal	–	–	+	–	+	–	+	–	–	–	+	+	+	+	+	–	+	+	+	+	+	–	–	+
anterior	+	+	+	+	+	–	+	–	+	+	–	+	+	–	–	–	–	–	+	+	+	–	–	+
distributed	–	–	–	–	–	–	–	–	–	–	+	–	–	+	–	–	+	+	+	+	–	–	–	–
dorsal	–	–	–	–	–	+	–	+	–	–	–	–	–	–	+	–	–	–	–	–	–	–	+	–
high	–	–	–	–	–	+	–	+	–	–	–	–	–	–	+	–	–	–	–	–	–	–	+	–
low	–	–	–	–	–	–	–	–	–	–	–	–	–	–	–	–	–	–	–	–	–	–	–	–
back	–	–	–	–	–	+	–	+	–	–	–	–	–	–	–	–	–	–	–	–	–	–	+	–
voice	–	+	–	+	+	–	+	+	–	+	–	–	+	+	+	–	+	–	+	–	+	–	+	+
spread glottis	–	–	–	–	–	–	–	–	–	–	–	–	–	–	–	+	–	–	–	–	–	–	–	–
constricted glottis	–	–	–	–	–	–	–	–	–	–	–	–	–	–	–	–	–	–	–	–	–	+	–	–

Reprinted with permission from Department of Linguistics, University of California, Santa Barbara.

conducting speech sound assessment. The clinician must be comfortable transcribing speech using IPA symbols and diacritics. The two systems of classification discussed (place, manner, and voicing or distinctive features) for consonants and vowels are also crucial to know when the clinician is assessing the client. Clinicians decide, depending on the client and other factors (discussed later in the chapter), which type of assessment approach they will implement with a client.

There is one additional essential topic that must be explained before discussing assessment: syllable structure as a basis for planning and producing speech sounds (Velleman, 2002). Syllable structure should be viewed in terms of the number of syllables, the type of syllable, and syllable stress. This is important information lacking in most norm-referenced measures and therefore must be addressed in an assessment. Phonotactics, which is the analysis of permitted phoneme combinations within a language and within a word, attempts to address this aspect.

Table 7-4. Acquisition of English Vowels: General Age of Mastery of English Vowels

Age of at Least 90% Mastery	*Vowel Sounds*
2:0	/ʌ/
2:0 to 3:0	/i/ /u/ /o/
3:0 to 6:0	/ə/
3:0	/ɛ/ /ɑ/ /aɪ/ /aʊ/ /ɔi/
3:0 to 4:0	/ɪ/
3:0 to 5:0	/æ/ /e/
3:0 to 6:0	/ɝ/ /ɚ/

Adapted from Edwards (2003).

Prevalence and Incidence

ASHA (2016c) discusses that it is difficult to determine the prevalence of speech sound disorders due to inconsistent definitions of speech sound disorders and that the data relied on teacher and parent reports. The likelihood of seeing a client with an articulation problem due to the prevalence of speech sound disorders in various populations is noteworthy for the novice clinician. In 2014, nearly 93% of SLPs in schools indicated that they served individuals with phonological/articulation disorders (ASHA, 2014), and for 80% of children with phonological disorders, the disorders were sufficiently severe to require clinical treatment (Gierut, 1998). In fact, the National Institute on Deafness and Other Communication Disorders (NIDCD, 2010) estimated that the prevalence of speech sound disorders in young children was 8% to 9%. Furthermore, articulation disorders represented more than 75% of all speech disorders in children, and most of them had no identifiable organic, neurological, or physical etiology (Ansel, 1994). In older populations, the prevalence of **neurogenic** (pertaining to the central or peripheral nervous system) communication disorders is high; however, it is difficult to estimate the approximate number of adults in the United States who have motor speech disorders or articulation disorders arising either from nonprogressive brain damage such as cerebrovascular accident or traumatic brain injury or from progressive/degenerative **dysarthrias** such as amyotrophic lateral sclerosis or multiple sclerosis when areas of the brain that control speech musculature are involved (ASHA, 2014; NIDCD, 2010).

Normative Data for Speech Sound Acquisition

One of the primary means of determining whether speech sound production is delayed or disordered is by comparison to developmental norms. As a general developmental rule, vowels emerge and become established before consonants. See Table 7-4 for a list of vowels and the age they emerge and Table 7-5 for the ages of acquisition for consonants. On the ASHA website (n.d.a), there is information about developmental norms for speech and language skills. A number of textbooks cite norms for speech development. The student and novice clinician should review the presentation by Gregory Lof (2004) before reviewing these norms. Lof presented "Confusion About Speech Sound Norms and Their Use" at an online language conference. Shipley and McAfee (2015) included a table indicating the frequency of occurrence of individual consonants.

Although a child's patterns of sound acquisition are fairly predictable when the child's sound inventory corresponds to the age of normal acquisition of phonemes (Khan, 1982), it is important to consider that there is a wide range of individual variability across sound development charts. This variability is due to the how the data in the speech sound acquisition tables are interpreted (Bernthal & Bankson, 2004; Bernthal et al., 2013; Lof, 2004; Sanders, 1972). For example, the data from the Sander's (1972) norms were based on when 50% of the children produced the sound (known as the *age of customary production*), whereas when 90% of the children produced the sound, it was called the *age of mastery production.*

Phonetic development and acquisition data have been customarily derived from initial position, single-word testing; the resulting average age estimates range from the median age of correct articulation to the (older) age level at which 90% of the children tested accurately produced the target (Peña-Brooks & Hegde, 2015). Templin (1957) derived her data from the age levels at which 75% (as well as 90%) of her subjects mastered each sound in the initial, medial, and final positions (Bernthal & Bankson, 2004), whereas Poole (1934) derived data when 100% of the 140 children tested produced the consonant in all three positions. Prather, Hendrick, and Kern (1975) derived data when 75% of the 147 children produced the consonant in the initial and final positions. In addition, Templin (1957)

Table 7-5. Acquisition of English Consonants: Age of Developmental Norms for Sound Acquisition

Consonant	Wellman et al. (1931)	Poole (1934)	Templin (1957)	Prather et al. (1975)	Arlt & Goodban (1976)
m	3	3½	3	2	3
n	3	4½	3	2	3
h	3	3½	3	2	3
p	4	3½	3	2	3
f	3	5½	3	2–4	3
w	3	3½	3	2–8	3
b	3	3½	—	2–8	3
ŋ	—	4½	3	2–8	3
j	4	4½	3½	2–4	—
k	4	4½	4	2–4	3
g	4	4½	4	2–4	3
l	4	6½	6	3–4	4
d	5	4½	4	2–4	3
t	5	4½	6	2–8	3
s	5	7½	4½	3	4
r	5	7½	4	3	5
tʃ	5	4½	—	3–8	4
v	5	6½	6	4	3½
z	5	7½	7	4	4
ʒ	6	6½	7	4	4
θ	—	7½	6	4	5
dʒ	—	7	4	4	—
ʃ	—	6½	4½	3–8	4½
ð	—	6½	7	4	5

identified the ages at which initial and final consonant clusters are accurately produced by 75% of his participants in his study, ranging from 4 to 8 years old:

- At age 4 years:
  - Initial clusters {bl, gl, kl, pl, br, dr, kr, pr, tr, sk, sm, sn, sp, st, kw, and tw}
  - Final clusters {ft, ks, lp, lt, mp, mps, mpt, and pt}
- At age 5 years:
  - Initial clusters {fl, fr, gr, and str}
  - Final clusters {lb, lf, rd, rf, and rn}
- At age 6 years:
  - Initial cluster {skw}
  - Final clusters {lk, lf, nd, nt ,nth, rb, rg, rst, and rth}
- At age 7 years:
  - Initial clusters {shr, skr, sl, spl, spr, sw, and thr}
  - Final clusters {lth, lz, sk, and st}
- At age 8 years:
  - Final clusters {kt and sp}

Speech Sound Disorders

The characteristics of both articulation and phonological disorders will be discussed next.

Articulation Disorders

Articulation disorders are said to occur when the client has difficulty producing the movements associated with the production of a sound (or sound segments; Khan, 1982; Peña-Brooks & Hegde, 2015). A client may have a functional articulation disorder, no known etiology or an organic articulation disorder, or an underlying organic cause, such as a cleft lip or palate. Possible physiological reasons for inaccurate motor productions of sounds or sound segments include structural variations of the lips, teeth, mandible, tongue, and palate; cranial-facial anomalies; hearing loss; and neurological or neuromuscular impairments (Bernthal & Bankson, 2004; Bernthal et al., 2013). Typically, a child with one or two consistent speech sound errors, such as a mild **distortion** of /r/ or an interdental lisp (the **substitution** of /s/ with /θ/), is described as having an articulation disorder (Bernthal et al., 2013; Bleile, 2014; Hodson, 2004).

Classification of Articulatory Errors

ASHA (2016d) describes the following signs and symptoms of speech sound disorders:

- "**Omissions**/deletions: Certain sounds are not produced but omitted or deleted (e.g., "cu" for "cup" and "poon" for "spoon")
- Substitutions: One or more sounds are substituted, which may result in loss of phonemic contrast (e.g., "dood" for "good" and "wabbit" for "rabbit")
- **Additions**: One or more extra sounds are added or inserted into a word (e.g., "buhlack" for "black")
- Distortions: Sounds are altered or changed (e.g., a lateral "s")
- Whole-word/syllable-level errors: Weak syllables are deleted (e.g., "tephone" for "telephone"), a syllable is repeated or deleted (e.g., "dada" for "dad" or "wawa" for "water")
- Prosody errors: Errors occur in stress, intensity, rhythm, and intonation"

Pattern Analysis

Children who produce multiple articulation errors are best served by a **pattern analysis** (an examination and classification of the child's speech sound errors), including the following:

- Place-voicing-manner
- Distinctive feature analysis
- Deep testing, as exemplified in the Deep Test of Articulation (DTA; McDonald, 1964), incorporates the effect of multiple and varying phonetic contexts on the production of sounds to obtain a more realistic sample of the child's sound productions in connected speech (Bernthal & Bankson, 2004; Bernthal et al., 2013).
- Phonotactic analysis (Velleman, 2002) examining the syllable shape of the word:
  - The sounds included in the word
  - The arrangement of those sounds within the word
  - The sequence of its elements

According to Velleman (2002), a child with multiple misarticulation errors may possess an age-appropriate sound inventory yet have difficulty using sounds in the obligatory linguistic shapes such as clusters and polysyllabic words. This is why it is important to examine the context of the errors.

Classification of Phonological Processes

Whereas **phonological processes** are normal systematic changes that can affect a syllable or an entire category of phonemes and that gradually disappear, phonological errors are those attributed to the persistence of these developing patterns from a younger age. Phonological errors can also be caused by the incomplete acquisition of the phonetic/phonemic and phototactic rules of language (Bernthal & Bankson, 2004; Bernthal et al., 2013). Generally, a child who does not eliminate the phonological processes by a certain age may have a phonological delay, whereas children who exhibit unusual or idiosyncratic processes may have a phonological disorder (Hodson, 2004; Khan, 1982). Unusual processes are discussed later in this chapter, but first we discuss normal phonological processes.

Classification of Phonological Processes and Corresponding Normative Data

Phonological processes have been broadly classified as whole word (also referred to as *syllable structure processes*), segment substitution, **assimilation**, and idiosyncratic processes (Lowe, 2009; Table 7-6).

1. Whole-word (syllable structure) processes: Occur when the syllable structure of the target word is altered by a reduction, deletion, or expansion of one or more sounds in the syllable (e.g., /bʊk/ → /bʊ/)
2. Substitution processes: One class of sounds affects another sound class in that the phonemes are altered by changing the place or manner of production (Bernthal & Bankson, 2004; Bernthal et al., 2013; Lowe, 2009; e.g., /sʌn/ → /tʌn/)
3. Assimilation processes: Sounds or sound families that change to become similar to other sounds within the word. These assimilatory processes may be classified as regressive or progressive (or anticipatory) in nature.

Table 7-6. Typical Phonological Processes and Corresponding Normative Data

Process	*Definition*	*Example*	*Approximate Age of Suppression (years)*
Whole Word (Syllable Structure)			
Cluster reduction	Deletion of one or more consonants from a two- or three-consonant cluster	/klin/ → /kin/	4
Diminutization	Addition of an /i/ or a consonant + /i/	/hæt/ → /hæti/	3
Epenthesis	Insertion of a new phoneme, typically the unstressed schwa	/blu/ → /bəlu/	4
Initial consonant deletion	Deletion of the first consonant or consonant cluster in a syllable or word	/kʌp/ → /ʌp/	3
Unstressed syllable deletion	Deletion of an unstressed syllable from a word containing two or more syllables	/bənænə/ → /nænæ/	4
Reduplication (**doubling**)	Repetition of an entire or partial syllable	/ətɚ/ → /wəwə/	3
Substitution			
Alveolarization	Substitution of an alveolar sound for a **lingua-dental** or labial sound	/peən/ → /teən/	6
Deaffrication	An affricate manner changed to a fricative	/ʃu/ → /tʃu/	4
Depalatalization	Substitution of a an alveolar fricative or affricate for a palatal fricative or affricate	/fɪʃ/ → /fɪs/	4
Derhotacization	Omission of the r-coloring for the consonant /r/ and for the central vowels with r-coloring	/zɪpɚ/ → /zɪp/	4
Gliding	Substitution of a glide for a liquid	/rʌn/ → /wʌn/	5 to 7
Labialization	Substitution of a labial sound for an alveolar sound	/dɔg/ → /bɔg/	6
Liquid simplification	Substitution of another sound for a liquid	/leɪk/ → /teɪk/	5
Stopping	Substitution of a stop consonant for a fricative or affricate.	/cætʃ/ → /cæt/	3 to 5
Stridency deletion	Omission or substitution of another sound for a fricative.	/sop/ → /op/	6
Velar fronting	Substitution of sounds in the front of the mouth, usually alveolar sounds, for **velar** or palatal sounds	/keəndi/ → /teəndi/	3
Vocalization	Substitution of a vowel for a final position liquid sound	/pipl/ → /pipo/	7
Assimilation			
Final devoicing	Alteration in voicing affected by a nearby sound	/beɪk/ → /beəg/	3
Prevocalic voicing	Voicing of an initial voiceless consonant in a word	/kʌp/ → /gʌp/	3
Alveolar assimilation	Alveolar sound influences a nearby sound	/jɛlo/ → /lɛlo/	3.5
Labial assimilation	Labial sound influences a nearby sound	/teɪbl/ → /peɪbo/	3.5
Nasal assimilation	Nasal sound influences a nearby sound	/spun/ → /nun/	3.5
Velar assimilation	Velar sound influences a nearby sound	/dɔgi/ → /gɔgi/	3.5

Adapted from Bauman-Waengler (2008), Bernthal & Bankson (2004), Khan (1982), Lowe (2009), and Peña-Brooks & Hegde (2015).

Table 7-7. Idiosyncratic Phonological Processes

Process	*Definition*	*Example*
Apicalization	Labial replaced by a tongue tip consonant	/bou/ → /dou/
Atypical cluster reduction	Deletion of the member that is usually retained	/pleɪ/ → /leɪ/
Backing of stops and fricatives	Substitution of velar stops for consonants that are usually produced further forward in the mouth	/taɪm/ → /kaɪm/
Fricative replacing stops	Substitution of a fricative for a stop	/dɑl/ → /zɑl/
Glottal replacement	Substitution of a glottal stop for another consonant	/pɪk/ → /pɪʔ/
Medial consonant deletion	Deletion of intervocalic consonants	/bitl/ → /bi-o/
Migration	Movement of a sound from one position in a word to another	/sop/ → /ops/
Sound preference substitutions	Replacement of groups of consonants by one or two particular consonants	Usually affricates = stops /ʃɑp/, /tʃɑp/ → /tɑp/
Stops replacing glides	Substitution of a stop for a glide	/jɛs/ → /dɛs/
Vowel Errors, Including Feature Changes in Terms of Tongue Placement		
Backing	Tongue retracted for a front vowel	/kaet/ → /kɪt/
Diphthongization	Splitting apart of the target vowel into two vowel sounds	/kek/ → /ke-ek/
Fronting	Tongue forward for a back vowel	/rak/ → /rek/
Vowel harmony	When vowels are produced like contrastive vowels (elsewhere in a word)	/kuki/ → /ki-ki/

Adapted from Lowe (1994) and Pollack (1991).

- Regressive assimilation occurs as a result of later sounds influencing previous sound production (e.g., /dɔgi/ → /gɔgi/).
- Progressive assimilation results from previous phonemes influencing later occurring sounds in a word or syllable or across words (e.g., /dɔgi/ → /dɔdi/).

In the literature, there are various criteria for determining whether a phonological process exists; however, none of them are clear-cut, and clinicians must use their professional judgment. There are several factors to consider when analyzing the formal and informal testing measures:

- The frequency and percentage of occurrence of the process
- The number of opportunities for the target process to occur
- The number of sounds or sound classes affected

It is not a coincidence that the final suppression of phonological processes occurs simultaneously at the age at which a child becomes intelligible to strangers. When these processes persist beyond the normal age range, the speech pattern is typically considered delayed. It is considered a disorder when the child exhibits unusual or idiosyncratic processes. Idiosyncratic processes are processes that are unique to a child's phonological system (e.g., baby = taty or banana = nini). When the presence of unusual processes or vowel errors is noted, this is a potential hallmark of a child with a disorder rather than a delayed phonological pattern (Khan, 1982). Table 7-7, adapted from the research of Lowe (1994) and Pollack (1991), lists idiosyncratic or unusual processes common in a child with a phonological disorder.

It should also be noted that many speech sound disorders have been found to have no apparent structural or neurological cause and are often referred to as **idiopathic** or functional (i.e., of unknown cause or origin). There are subtle maturational determinates besides those of oromotor musculature and coordination, such as psycholinguistic, speech sound perception, and cognitive-communicative development (Winitz, 1969, cited by Bernthal & Bankson, 2004; Bernthal et al., 2013). For a broader discussion of these aspects, refer to Chapters 5, 6, 8, and 14 in this text.

Nonspeech Oral Motor Exercises

There is controversy about whether performing oral motor exercises facilitates speech production. The student and novice clinician is referred to Kent (2015) Lass and Pannbacker (2008), Lof (2004, 2008), and Lof and Watson (2008).

Specific Parameters for Assessment

According to ASHA (2016b), clinical indications for a speech sound assessment are initiated by referral (from a health or an education professional), the client's medical status, or failing a speech-language screening. There are several published screening measures published, and a list of some could be seen in Bleile (2014) and Shipley and McAfee (2015). Clinicians need not use a published measure but can instead create their own informal measure. It is provided to evaluate both strengths and weaknesses in speech sound discrimination and production, for the objective identification of impairments or speech sound disorders, and to make recommendations and referrals for intervention. To conduct assessment with a younger child, the clinician should have knowledge of the anatomy and physiology mechanism and speech-language development. ASHA (2016a) provided information about the components of a comprehensive speech sound assessment. Generally, the parameters to be assessed by formal and informal means for a child are as follows:

- A case history/intake should be obtained from the child's parent/guardian or client that entails the child's/client's medical history, birth and developmental milestones (including speech-language and motor if a child), language(s) spoken in the home, social and academic history, previous therapy (including speech-language, occupational or physical therapy, psychological services, special education), employment history (if an adult), and presenting complaint.
- The client's oral-peripheral mechanism is examined, including the articulatory **diadochokinetic** rates (see Chapter 6).
- A hearing screening is conducted (see Chapter 5).
- Speech sound assessment is conducted, including single word as well as connected speech; intelligibility in different contexts, **stimulability**, and severity; and conversational speech assessment in different contexts.
- Additional testing measures are performed as necessary (e.g., language, auditory discrimination, phonological awareness).

There are important aspects to consider when designing the assessment protocol for a client. Some of these include the client's cultural and linguistic background and **dialect**; cognitive, social, and physical abilities; interests; family's perceptions of the speech sound delay/disorder; and other possible communication or concomitant disorders.

Special Considerations for Clients Who Speak More Than One Language

The student and novice clinician is referred to the following references for information about clients who speak more than one language: ASHA (2016a, n.d.b), Derr (2003), Fabiano (2007), Hegde and Freed (2013), Hegde and Promoville (2017), Shipley and McAfee (2015).

After administering the norm-referenced measures and obtaining a speech sample, the following information could be obtained about the client (depending on the age of the client):

- A phonetic and/or phonemic inventory, including a list of sounds that the client can produce, organized by either place, manner, and voicing of articulation or distinctive features and discuss the position within the word.
- A vowel inventory.
- A syllable shape inventory (V, CV, VC, CVC, CCV, VCC)—discuss the number of syllables, open vs. closed syllables, and the degree of syllable stress.
- Type, number, and consistency of sound production errors.
- Are there still phonological processes (the child's systematic simplification of adult words)? The type and percent of occurrence of phonological process(es).
- Overall intelligibility (understandability of speech) in isolation, words, connected, and spontaneous utterances, again noting the consistency and frequency of sound production errors.
- Severity is a subjective rating of mild, moderate, or severe based on intelligibility.
- Stimulability is the client's ability to imitate a target sound to correct error sound productions.
- Examination of suprasegmental features by comparing samples of the client's speech in different contexts such as oral reading, automatic speech,

spontaneous speech, and imitating (Shipley & McAfee, 2015).

- Additional testing in the areas of language and auditory discrimination.
- Phonological awareness skills (rhyming, alliteration, phoneme isolation, phoneme manipulation, sound and syllable blending, sound and syllable identification, and sound segmentation) are important to assess. There are norm-referenced measures to assess these skills. Discussion of these areas is beyond the scope of this chapter, but they are no less important than any other aspect discussed here. Children with phonological disorders may exhibit difficulties in phonological awareness skills and then reading (decoding and comprehension).

If you have a young patient with emerging articulation and phonology, you will want to obtain an independent analysis, which only examines the child's productions and does not compare it with norms, because of the limited speech skills of the client. You will be assessing the speech sound inventory and syllable shapes. The severity measure obtained from Paul and Jennings (1992) is based on the average level of complexity of their syllable structures, the number of different consonant phonemes produced, and the percentage of consonants correctly produced in intelligible utterances.

In the protocol for adults with acquired articulation abnormalities secondary to neurological injury, one should consider the following additional testing:

- An extensive examination of the speech mechanism during nonspeech activities (Duffy, 2013; Freed, 2012),
- Nonverbal oral movement control tasks (Darley & Spriestersbach, 1978; Freed, 2012)
- Speech planning and programming tasks (Wertz, LaPointe, & Rosenbek, 1984)
- Use of a dysarthria rating scale (Darley, Aronson, & Brown, 1975; Duffy, 2013)
- A standardized assessment of intelligibility in words, sentences, and conversation

For clients (children and adults) who are speakers of English as a second language or exhibit regional dialects, the following aspects should be considered: vowel and consonant substitution errors that consistently appear in client's connected speech, conversation, oral reading, and speech clarity. Refer to ASHA (2016a) and Shipley and McAfee (2015) for a complete listing of speech and language differences across different dialects. The information for various dialects is placed in table format compared with standard American English.

The assessment process is basically a blending of art and science to include standardized and nonstandardized procedures; an assessment of functional communication abilities; evaluation of intelligibility in a variety of contexts; as well as severity, consistency, stimulability, observations of client and client–parent interactions, the interview information, and a great deal of clinical intuition. The final product is an organized analysis of a collected combination of different pertinent features relating to the client's speech patterns. We begin by gathering the client's background history.

Key Clinical Interview Questions

The clinical interview will likewise be adapted to the age of the client, as developmental concerns differ from the factors considered in acquired or residual cases. Pertinent medical history includes childhood illnesses, particularly ear, tonsil, or adenoid infections; allergies; high fevers; accidents and hospitalizations; dental and orthodontic treatment; and current medications. Determining developmental data such as visual and hearing acuity, hand dominance, and prespeech and speech milestones (e.g., cooing, babbling, first words, and early word combinations) are gathered for younger children. For older children and young adults, their educational, social, and therapeutic experiences are also noted. Adult clients are asked about their occupational background as well as any recent health concerns such as hospitalizations, cancerous conditions, neurological events, or head trauma.

It is essential to ascertain parental concerns and priorities for their children because the parent is the expert on his or her child, as well as self-concerns for older clients because these clients are the experts on their own lives. Therefore, the needs and priorities of parents and clients must be taken into consideration in all decision making. Furthermore, the examiner should make note of inconsistencies in both parental and client reports as well as conflicts between assessment results and interview information. All of these factors will influence the final diagnosis and recommendations.

Key Clinical Interview Questions for Parents

1. What are your concerns regarding your child's speech?
2. When did you first notice any problems?
3. What were your child's first sounds like (babbling, cooing)?
4. Are there times when your child's speech is difficult to understand?
5. Are there times when your child's speech is easier to understand?
6. Do you think your child avoids speaking because of the way he or she talks?
7. Is this your child's first speech-language evaluation? If not, what were the results of previous assessments?
8. Has your child's hearing ever been tested? If so, what were the results?
9. What language is spoken most often at home?
10. What language does your child speak most often?
11. With whom does your child interact, and how (verbally, with gestures)?
12. Is it difficult to understand your child?
13. Does your child add, omit, or substitute sounds at the beginning, middle, or end of words?
14. Is your child aware of his or her speech difficulty?
15. Does your child seem frustrated by his or her speech difficulty?
16. Does your child's speech difficulty affect any of his or her daily play or school activities adversely?
17. Does anyone in your family exhibit any speech problems?

Key Clinical Interview Questions for Teachers

1. What are your concerns regarding your student's speech?
2. When did you first notice any difficulties in your student communicating?
3. Is the student's intelligibility affecting any of his or her daily play or school activities adversely?
4. Does your student avoid interaction and speaking with his or her peers?
5. Does your student avoid participating in the classroom?

Key Clinical Interview Questions for Older Clients

1. What brings you here today?
2. How much education did you have/how many years of schooling did you complete?
3. What is your occupation/where do you work?
4. What are your hobbies/interests/talents?
5. What is your native language?
6. When did you first notice a problem/difference in your speech?
7. What do you think is/are the cause(s) of the change(s) in your speech?
8. Has your speech changed since you first noticed a difference?
9. How well can others understand you when you speak?
10. How do you react to others' difficulty understanding you?
11. Do feel that your speech interferes with any part of your life (school, friends, work, family)?
12. Is it difficult for you to pronounce certain sounds or words?

After gathering relevant background information, the diagnostic section commences with the administration of a selection of formal and informal methods that are appropriate to the client's age and abilities. During administration of informal and formal assessment, the information gathered in the clinical interview is taken into account in synthesizing and analyzing all data.

Formal Assessment Measures

Bleile (2014) suggested that younger children be assessed with mostly nonstandardized procedures supplemented by standardized materials and, conversely, that older children be evaluated primarily with standardized instruments and secondarily with informal activities. They stated that, while nonstandardized assessments are more adaptable to clients with developmental disorders or who are not otherwise "testable," standardized test results are more reliable and are often required by third-party payers and school systems to determine whether a child is eligible for speech-language services. Table 7-8 contains a list of standardized tests of speech sound production for evaluating preschool and school-age children and

Table 7-8. Formal Speech Sound Production Assessment Instruments for Children and Young Adults

Name of Test	*Authors*	*Area Assessed*	*Age Range (Years; Months)*	*Subtests*
Goldman-Fristoe Test of Articulation-3 (GFTA-3)	Goldman & Fristoe (2015)	Articulation	2;0 to 21;11	• Sounds-in-Words subtest • Sounds-in-Sentences subtest • Stimulability • Norm-referenced
Khan–Lewis Phonological Analysis-3 (KLPA-3)	Khan & Lewis (2015)	Phonological processes	2;0 to 21;11	• Phonological processes • Norm-referenced
Clinical Assessment of Articulation and Phonology-2 (CAAP-2)	Secord & Donohue (2013)	Articulation and phonological processes	2;6 to 8;11 2;6 to 11;11	• Articulation inventory • Phonological processes checklist • Norm-referenced
Bankson–Bernthal Test of Phonology (BBTOP)	Bankson & Bernthal (1990)	Articulation and phonological processes	3;0 to 9;0	• Whole-word accuracy • Consonant • Norm-referenced
Photo Articulation Test-3 (PAT-3)	Lippke, Dickey, Selmar, & Soder (1997)	Articulation	3;0 to 8;11	• Articulation omissions, substitutions, and distortions • Norm-referenced
Assessment Link Between Phonology and Articulation—Revised (ALPHA)	Lowe (2000)	Articulation and phonological processes	3;0 to 8;11	• Sound-in-position (I, F) • Phonological processes • Norm-referenced
Diagnostic Evaluation of Articulation and Phonology (DEAP)	Dodd, Hua, Crosbie, Holm, & Ozanne (2006)	Articulation and phonological processes	3;0 to 8;11	• Phonological process use • Single words vs. connected speech • Norm-referenced
Templin–Darley Tests of Articulation-2 (TDTA-2)	Templin & Darley (1969)	Articulation	3;0 to 8;0	• Whole-word accuracy • Consonant and vowel articulation • Norm-referenced
Hodson Assessment of Phonological Patterns-3 (HAPP-3)	Hodson (2004)	Phonological processes	3;0 to 8;0	• Identifies phonological patterns, and deviations and determines severity
DTA	McDonald (1964)	Articulation	3;0 to 12;0	• Contextual tests for individual phonemes
Fisher–Logemann Test of Articulation Competence (F-LTAC)	Fisher & Logemann (1971)	Articulation	3;0 to adult	• Place, manner, and voicing pattern analysis that includes regional dialects

Table 7-9 briefly describes typical intelligibility tests for older children and adults. Note that these tables, although comprehensive, include some of the more typically relied-on instruments and do not encompass all available standardized assessment tools for articulation and phonological disorders. The reader is referred to Bernthal and Bankson (2004), Bleile (2014), Peña-Brooks & Hegde (2015), and Shipley &McAfee (2015) for a more complete inventory. The test selected should be appropriate for the client's age and cognitive and linguistic skills.

Table 7-9. Formal Assessment Instruments for Assessing Intelligibility for Older Children and Adults

Name of Test	*Authors*	*Age Range (Years)*	*Subtests*
Frenchay Dysarthria Assessment-2 (FDA-2)	Enderby & Palmer (2008)	12 to 97	• Eight sections, including intelligibility ratings for words, sentences, and conversation • Norm-referenced
Assessment of Intelligibility in Dysarthric Speakers	Yorkston, Beukelman, & Traynor (1984)	Adolescent to adult (no age range)	• Single-word intelligibility • Sentence intelligibility • Speaking rate • Criterion-referenced
Dysarthria Profile	Robertson (1982)	> 14 to adult (not specified)	• Speech and nonspeech diadochokinesis • Ratings of Normal, Good, Fair, None • Criterion-referenced
Dysarthria Examination Battery	Drummond (1993)	Adolescent to adult (no age range)	• Intelligibility in words and sentences • Norm-referenced

Advantages of Formal Assessment Measures

There are distinct advantages to employing standardized measures when evaluating speech sound production:

- A standardized test is easy to administer and score.
- The standardized measure provides a standard score and percentage compared with norms.

Controlled stimulability testing available in standardized tests is mainly used with children to predict which unit of speech production is optimal to begin intervention with: sounds in isolation; syllables; words; and initial, medial, or final position in words (Berthal & Bankson, 2004; Bernthal et al., 2013). Stimulability reflects a child's ability to correctly imitate a given phoneme when provided with specific instructions or models of the phoneme and, according to Rvachew, Rafaat, and Martin (1999), is therefore a prognostic factor. The clinician can create his or her own stimulability measure based on the client's error sounds.

For clients aged 15 through 90 years, the advantage of formal instruments is that, even though the FDA-2 and the Assessment of Intelligibility in Dysarthric Speakers were originally devised to provide detailed and differential profiles of motor speech disorders, information about the client's articulation can also be discerned. The FDA-2 rates the client's performance on tasks involving eight areas: reflexes, respiration, lips, palate, laryngeal, tongue, intelligibility, and influencing factors. The Assessment of Intelligibility in Dysarthric Speakers contains various stimulus words and sentences designed to yield useful intelligibility and communication efficiency measures (Yorkston et al., 1984, 2010).

Standardized instruments serve to reliably identify the client's speech sound disorders (articulation errors and/or the young client's phonological processes), which are then compared to typical, age-related, normative data. Age and phonological development must be taken into consideration in clinical decision making but should not be the only criteria in diagnosis and intervention (Bernthal & Bankson, 2004; Bleile, 2014).

Disadvantages of Formal Assessment Measures

There are disadvantages to administering only a standardized measure, without considering other options:

- They do not test all sounds in all positions of words.
- Articulation tests alone do not provide information about the child's phonological skills.
- Articulation tests generally tend to test sounds in words, not connected speech.
- Although they offer an inventory of sound production, they offer little in terms of the child's functional communication in everyday life situations. As such, they are low in ecological validity (where they fall in the range or continuum of naturalness).

- They are limited in the inventory of phonemes (especially vowels) assessed as well as in the contexts in which these phonemes are presented.
- Many formal assessment tools do not take into account the effects of coarticulation (the overlapping effects of the articulators during connected speech due to ease or speed of production).
- Most formal assessments do not take phonological processes into account in their inventory.

In line with these drawbacks, formal assessment measures are standardized and their assessment is static, providing merely a snapshot of the client's performance. As such, there is no provision for dynamic assessment (ongoing probing through the use of various prompts to determine the most beneficial cues for the client, which techniques are most helpful, ascertaining the client's learning styles; in short, what will help the client most going forward in therapy).

The end result of formal assessment of articulation does not afford the clinician with a picture of the client as a true communicator in everyday life situations. Therefore, it is essential to take into account informal measures and observations. For example, although a child may score within normal limits on this test, his or her intelligibility may be proportionately poor due to factors not tapped by the norm-referenced measure. Therefore, the resulting "normal" scores may deter the child from possibly obtaining educational services for his or her speech pattern.

To further illustrate this example, several factors that may influence a client's intelligibility are not accounted for on different norm-referenced measures. These include vowel errors, a rapid speech rate, inappropriate prosody (the melody or intonation, timing, and stress patterns of speech), inadequate articulatory excursions, and imprecise articulatory contacts in connected discourse, creating a "mumbled" speech pattern, among others. On the other hand, an 8-year-old child who presents with a distortion of /l/ and /r/ sounds in all positions and contexts may score below his or her age level on a test indicating a more serious problem than his or her actual speech pattern portrays.

In light of these deficiencies, alternative and more informal observations and approaches are essential to fairly and objectively provide an accurate portrayal of the client's speech patterns.

Informal Assessment and Behavioral Measures

Informal measures are more flexible than standardized test procedures and can provide the clinician with a more realistic sample of the client's speech sound production. They are more authentic (true picture of a client as a true communicator in everyday communicative situations) means of assessment; some of the following nonstandardized procedures can be supplemented by standardized materials.

Speech Sample

The importance of obtaining a natural discourse sample from any age client cannot be overemphasized. Speech sound productions generated in spontaneous connected verbal exchange are considered to have the best face validity and are a major factor in deciding the necessity and benefit of treatment (Bauman-Waengler, 2012; Bernthal & Bankson, 2004; Peña-Brooks & Hegde, 2015). According to Kamhi (2005), a useful conversational sample should contain a minimum of 100 different words and should be analyzed for the same elements discussed before testing.

Age-Appropriate Speech Sampling Tasks

- For younger children:
  - Wordless picture books
  - Telling back a story
  - Play activities
  - Autobiographical information
  - Counting 1 to 10; reciting ABCs
  - Describing a favorite birthday party, special fun time, or favorite vacation
  - Describing a contextual picture with lots of action, such as those used in the Comprehensive Assessment of Spoken Language (CASL; Carrow-Woolfolk, 1999; see also Chapter 10 of this text)
  - Shipley and McAfee (2015) as well as the Test of Narrative Language (TNL; Gillam & Pearson, 2004) are also excellent sources for colored contextual pictures to generate spontaneous speech samples.
- For older children:
  - Reading the "Rainbow Passage" (Fairbanks, 1960)

- Conversing about a TV show, school, magazine article, sports, or hobbies
- Discussing favorite parts of school or favorite activities
- Describing how to play a certain sport or make a particular craft
- Shipley and McAfee (2015) and the TNL (Gillam & Pearson, 2004) contain single and sequence pictures of imaginative items such as dragons and aliens that are certain to help elicit spontaneous speech samples from young adults

- For adults:
  - Reading the "Grandfather Passage" aloud (Darley et al., 1975)
  - Reading aloud from a newspaper
  - Discussing current events
  - Describing the plot of a TV show, movie, or book

Intelligibility

Intelligibility can be discerned by subjective description under the following conditions: Could the clinician readily understand the client when the context is known and not known; intelligible with careful listening when context not known; intelligible with careful listening when context is known; and unintelligible with careful listening when context known?

Intelligibility can be derived by dividing the number of words/utterances that can be understood by the total number of words/utterances produced × 100; a word/utterance intelligibility percentage is thus yielded (Peña-Brooks & Hedge, 2015). For example, if the client produced 25 utterances of which 20 could be understood by the clinician, $20 \div 25 \times 100 = 80\%$ of the child's utterances are intelligible.

Factors that influence the intelligibility of an utterance (ASHA, 2016a) include the following:

- Listener's familiarity with the speaker's speech pattern
- Speaker's rate, inflection, stress patterns, pauses, voice quality, loudness, and fluency
- Social environment (e.g., familiar vs. unfamiliar conversational partners, one-on-one vs. group conversation)
- Communication cues for listener (e.g., known vs. unknown context)
- Signal-to-noise ratio (e.g., amount of background noise)
- Listener's skill

As mentioned earlier, factors found to affect subjective appraisals of intelligibility include the client's rate and prosody (stress and intonation pattern), the clinician's familiarity with the client, and the clinician's experience as an astute listener, especially for juncture (the blending of syllables in connected speech). As the rate of speech increases, final consonants simultaneously become initial consonants (Tiffany & Carrell, 1977). Generally, the more errors of frequently made sounds that the client produces, the less intelligible the client will be rated (Bernthal & Bankson, 2004; Bernthal et al., 2013) and the more guarded the prognosis. It has also been observed that abnormal prosody, as a by-product of articulation problems, also decreases intelligibility (Duffy, 2013).

Advantages and Disadvantages of Informal Assessment Measures

Informal methods are more dynamic in their assessment than standardized tests and allow for probing and prompting to determine facilitating techniques and results of assistance, such as repeating or revising instruction or providing an example. Despite their advantages, informal assessment measures are limited in that they are subjective and therefore not as reliable and valid as formal standardized testing. In view of this, the criterion for obtaining speech services and insurance reimbursement cannot be necessarily met by informal assessment alone (Bleile, 2014). Please refer to Chapter 4 for a more in-depth discussion of the rationale for using both formal and informal measures efficiently. One of the many purposes of a speech sound production evaluation is to not only provide an objective identification of impairments or speech sound disorders, but also to make an informed prognosis (ASHA, 2016b).

Prognostic Indicators

- Consistency of errors: The more consistent the error, the less likely the client will be stimulable in therapy or spontaneously remediate his or her error production.
- External error sound discrimination is the ability to differentiate the sound from other sounds when presented auditorily; decreased ability to discriminate a target sound error from other productions is a poor prognostic indicator.

- Internal error sound discrimination is the ability to self-evaluate production of the target sound from incorrect production; decreased internal error sound discrimination is a poor prognostic indicator.
- Stimulability reflects a child's ability to correctly imitate a given phoneme and models of the phoneme when provided with specific instructions. According to Rvachew et al. (1999), stimulability is therefore a significant factor in the success of remediation. There are a variety of ways to correctly articulate a target sound; Shipley and McAfee (2015) provided ample lists of words and phrases to facilitate imitation.
- Idiosyncratic phonological processes (explained earlier in the chapter) are reflective of abnormal phonological development and consist of error patterns such as **backing**, initial and medial consonant deletion, **nasal preference** (substitution of /n/ and /m/ for stops and fricatives), **tetism** (substitution of /t/ for /f/), and **fricative preference** (retention of /s/ in clusters). These unusual patterns are red flags for poorer prognosis (Khan, 1982). Vowel errors (also considered idiosyncratic) may also be indicative of deviant speech development (Pollack, 1991) and include **diphthongization** (the splitting apart of the target vowel into two vowel sounds), **vowel harmony** (when vowels are produced like contrastive vowels elsewhere in a word), and feature changes in terms of tongue placement: backing (tongue retracted for a front vowel; e.g., kite for cat); and **fronting** (tongue forward for a back vowel; e.g., rake for rack). Lastly, there are idiosyncratic phonological processes that are found in children who may have a phonological disorder, childhood **apraxia** of speech, or both diagnoses. The discovery of these bizarre speech patterns can assist the clinician in forming the description of the level of the younger client's severity and the need for and benefits of therapy.
- In addition, the age of the client, type of disorder, severity of the disorder, characteristics of the deviant speech pattern such as idiosyncratic processes or vowel errors, family support and involvement, and client and caregiver motivation are some of the many prognostic indicators clinicians take into consideration.
- Comorbid factors (coexisting conditions) such as hearing loss, ADD, language and learning disorders, intellectual disability, and cerebral palsy must also be considered.
- Parental involvement is essential in determining prognosis.

Another key aspect of careful assessment giving rise to effective intervention is prudently distinguishing between disorders with apparently similar characteristics.

Phonological Awareness

Deficits in phonemic awareness skills are linked to reading disabilities (Shipley & McAfee, 2015). Shipley and McAfee (2015) presented phonemic awareness benchmarks and a list of standardized tests for assessing phonemic awareness. If possible, these skills should be assessed during an evaluation.

Differential Diagnosis

It is important to recognize some typical disorders that may underlie or coexist with articulation and phonological impairment (Bernthal & Bankson, 2004, Bernthal et al., 2013).

- Developmental speech delay may be reflected in the use of phonological processes beyond the typical age.
- Language-learning disabilities by way of the use of phonological processes beyond the typical age is usually associated with difficulty understanding language and the use of simpler, less grammatically formulated utterances.
- With hearing loss, common error patterns include production of voiced sounds instead of voiceless sounds, vowel prolongation, nasality, diphthongs replaced with vowels (e.g., d/t, n/p, w/r).
- Orofacial myofunctional disorders occur when the tongue rests too far forward or may protrude between the teeth during speech and swallowing, although articulation is not always affected. Orofacial myofunctional disorders most often causes misarticulation of fricative, affricate, and alveolar sounds (ASHA, 1991, 2016d).
- Cleft palate speech contains variable errors, with sounds requiring high intraoral pressure most affected (e.g., nasal emission on the following consonants: /p/, /b/, /t/, /d/, /k/ and /g/).
- Dysarthria and apraxia: Neurological lesions of the brain can give rise to both childhood and acquired dysarthrias (speech disorders caused by weakness, incoordination, or paralysis of the

TABLE 7-10. COMPARISON OF DYSARTHRIA, APRAXIA OF SPEECH, AND ARTICULATION AND PHONOLOGICAL DISORDERS

Disorder	*Speech Error Characteristics*
Articulation disorder	• Number of errors: minimal • Predominate types of error: substitutions, omissions, distortions, and additions • Ability to imitate: easy • More complex motorically productions: easy • Diadochokinesis: normal • Effect of increase in rate of speech: neutral • Consistent across productions: yes
Phonological disorder	• Number of errors: moderate • Predominate types of error: substitutions and omissions • Ability to imitate: easy • More complex motorically productions: some difficulty • Diadochokinesis: normal • Effect of increase in rate of speech: neutral • Consistent across productions: yes
Apraxia	• Number of errors: much more • Predominate types of error: substitutions and additions • Ability to imitate: difficult • More complex motorically productions: very difficult • Diadochokinesis: poor • Effect of increase in rate of speech: improves intelligibility • Consistent across productions: no
Dysarthria	• Number of errors: moderate • Predominate types of error: mostly omissions and distortions, fewer substitutions and additions • Ability to imitate: easy • More complex motorically productions: some difficulty • Diadochokinesis: slow • Effect of increase in rate of speech: impairs intelligibility • Consistent across productions: yes

speech musculature that affect respiration, phonation, and resonance, as well as articulation) and apraxia. Apraxia of speech (AOS) is a sound production disorder resulting in difficulty executing the volitional motor plan for speech in the absence of paralysis (Duffy, 2013; Freed, 2012). Speech of the client with dysarthria is characterized mainly by consistently produced sound distortions and omissions due to motor control weakness. In contrast, apraxic speech contains more substitution errors, plus transpositions and prolongations, which are unpredictable; perseverative; and the result of an impaired ability to plan, position, and order the speech musculature to command (Wertz, 1985). In contrast to apraxia of speech, the three hallmarks of developmental verbal dyspraxia have been summarized as difficulty with syllable sequencing, inconsistency in error sound production, and flat or unusual prosody (Velleman, 2003).

- Differentiate further between the cluster of symptoms that define the dysarthrias, apraxia of speech, articulation, and phonological disorders (Table 7-10), keeping in mind that, according to Bernthal and Bankson (2004), the distinction between phonetic/motor and phonemic/linguistic errors is often blurred and challenging to determine.

SUMMARY

At this point in the chapter, we can appreciate the contribution that all of the aspects of a speech sound assessment (e.g., hearing screening, oral peripheral examination, clinical interview, standardized and informal assessment, and clinical observations) lend to a logical synthesis of all of the data gathered to generate a comprehensive written clinical report.

The diagnostic report is an important document illustrating the client's skills, strengths, and weaknesses. It is the means with which we communicate with the client, his or her family, and other professionals including fellow SLPs. This report is the culmination and synthesis of our findings and provides not only a diagnostic label (when necessary) but also a clear description of the client's behavior and his or her speech sound production, in conjunction with his or her strengths and weaknesses, stimulability, severity, intelligibility, prognosis, and recommendations for therapy, if indicated. In addition, further recommendations are explained to outside professionals and agencies when indicated. This document is a clear reflection of ourselves as professionals as well as on the facility where we are employed. It is often a deciding factor in a client securing much needed services that he or her needs and may have been denied, as well as insurance reimbursement for treatment that he or she may not be able to afford. Thus, it is our ethical and professional responsibility that the diagnostic report be clearly and authentically expressed, yet with the utmost sensitivity.

To provide an appropriate report model as well as a vehicle for practice, the following sections include a sample case history, a rationale for instrument selection, a rubric for writing the articulation section of a diagnostic report, an actual model report based on the sample, and a novel case history exercise for reader application.

Case History

M.C., a 4;9-year-old boy, was seen at the speech-language and hearing clinic for a complete speech and language evaluation. He was accompanied by his mother, who was concerned that his speech was very difficult to understand. M had not spoken his first words until he was about 2 years old and did not begin combining words until shortly before his third birthday. Although he was cooperative during play activities, his utterances could not be understood. He produced many inconsistent sound production errors and his speech movements seemed slightly labored and clumsy. M spoke with little expression in his voice, had many phonological processes, and was difficult to understand even with pictures.

Assessment: Tool Selection and Rationale

- The clinical interview helps the clinician ascertain the client's parents' perception of the speech difficulties and possible etiology, discussing background information including birth and developmental history, environmental considerations, medical history, social history, and previous therapy history.
- The audiological screening rules out hearing loss associated with a speech perception/production disorder.
- The oral-peripheral examination helps rule out any possible contributing physical or functional abnormalities (of the articulators).
- Informal tasks:
    - Client's verbal motor planning ability will be assessed by requesting that he imitate words of increasing length (e.g., fun, funnier, funniest).
    - When observing the child's oral motor skills during the production of multisyllabic words and connected speech, ease or degree of effort is noted, particularly during combinations of movements, such as transitional motor activities that are more difficult are indicative of verbal dyspraxia (Velleman, 2003).
    - Client's speech intelligibility will be informally assessed during spontaneous conversational interactions and play activities.
- GFTA-3 and KLPA-3 were selected because the two tests together assess production of sounds categorized by errors of substitution, omission, distortion, and/or addition. Subsequently, a phonological analysis of these error patterns may reveal excessive use of, or persisting, phonological processes (Peña-Brooks & Hegde, 2015). These tests, as well as most standardized testing, also provide a basis for severity rating and screening suprasegmental qualities by including various speech contexts in their subtests. The chief limitation is the absence of a connected speech or conversational speech sample.

Rubric for the Formal Speech Sound Production Section of the Diagnostic Report

❑ Introductory statement to include the complete name of the test (underlined) and in abbreviated form in parentheses (not underlined)

Example: Articulation was formally assessed through the administration of the Goldman-Fristoe Test of Articulation-3 (GFTA-3) and Khan–Lewis Phonological Analysis-3 (KLPA-3). (You may continue to use the abbreviations throughout the report.)

❑ Test construct (what it purports to measure)

Example: The GFTA-3 is a norm-referenced instrument that assesses consonants in various phonetic positions and contexts. The Sounds-in-Words and Sounds-in-Sentences subtests of the GFTA-3 were administered to assess M's articulation on the isolated word and sentence levels, respectively. The KLPA-3 was administered to further clarify the pattern of X's phonological processes.

❑ Elicitation procedures (describe where appropriate)

Example: For the Sounds-in-Words subtest, the GFTA-3 requires the client to name pictured stimuli.

❑ General quantification of results in paragraph form (derived scores from standardized test)

Example: Analysis of error patterns indicated the presence of a combination of typically developmentally lagging and idiosyncratic phonological processes. X obtained a standard score of 85 (mean = 100; standard deviation = 15), placing her at a percentile rank of 20, and at a test age equivalent of 2 to 5 years (Table 1).

Table 1. GFTA-3 Summary of Scores

	Standard Score	*Percentile*	*Test-Age Equivalent*
Sounds-in-Words	85	20th	2 to 5 years

❑ General quantification of results in table form (insert table number and title in bold font, capitalizing each main word)

❑ Discuss error pattern in narrative form, if applicable (note phonological processes in general; refer the reader to the table for specific examples)

Example: Results of the KLPA-3 after administering the GFTA-3 disclosed the presence of several phonological processes to include fronting, stopping, and de-affrication during the testing. Although vowel errors are not targeted by the GFTA-3, it is important to note the presence of several deviations during the testing. These errors were not reflected in X's score but nevertheless affected her intelligibility (Table 2).

Table 2. KLPA-3 Analysis of Phonological Process

Target Word	*Response*	*Phonological Process*	*Examples*

❑ Analyze inventory of errors in table form if applicable (insert table number and title in bold font, capitalizing each main word)

❑ Qualification of findings (additional behavioral and testing observations)

Example: This is an appropriate place to discuss error consistency within and between contexts (e.g., isolated word vs. connected, consistency, and additional behaviors noted during the testing). Include a statement of intelligibility and the factors that influenced diminished intelligibility, if applicable.

❑ Intelligibility

Example: Speech intelligibility was poor with and without context known due to X's multiple phonological processes, vowel alterations, and rapid speech rate. (Note that this is generally included in the informal section)

❑ Consistency between assessments

Example: Make note of the alignment between the formal assessment instruments used as well as between the testing and the client/family interview. In addition, discuss consistency or lack thereof between the formal and informal testing results.

Example: Results of the GFTA-3 and the KLPA-3 were aligned with the connected speech sample. Intelligibility decreased as the utterance length increased.

❑ Interpretation of findings

Example: X presented with a moderate phonological disorder due to the presence of multiple phonological processes, the presence of vowel errors, rapid speech rate, and resulting poor intelligibility.

❑ Stimulability

Example: X was stimulable for production of fricative consonants in the initial position in words.

Sample Report Based on Case History

Patient Information

Client: M.C. **Date of Evaluation:** 09/09/09
Address: *(street)* **Phone number:**
(city, state, zip code)
Date of Birth: 03/05/2005
Diagnosis: Speech disorder

I. Reason for Referral

M.C., a 4;9-year-old boy, was seen at the speech-language and hearing clinic for a complete speech and language evaluation on 09/09/09 due to parental concerns regarding his speech. M was accompanied by his mother, who appeared to be a reliable and concerned informant. It was requested that M return the following week for language testing; however, the client never returned for the second part of the evaluation.

II. Tests Administered/Procedures

- Parent interview
- Audiological screening
- Oral-peripheral mechanism examination
- Goldman-Fristoe Test of Articulation-3 (GFTA-3)
- Khan–Lewis Phonological Analysis-3 (KLPA-3)
- Conversational speech sample

III. Background Information

Birth and Developmental History

M was born following a normal pregnancy, weighing 7 pounds, 6 ounces at birth. According to Mrs. C, M reached all his developmental milestones at the appropriate age, with the exception of speech and language. M produced his first word at 24 months of age and began combining words at 36 months. Presymbolic speech-language development (cooing, babbling, and gesture) was reportedly normal.

Mrs. C explained that she became concerned about her son's speech-language development when he was 2 years old, and he had not yet verbalized his first words.

Medical/Health History

The mother reported that the client's medical history was unremarkable and that there were no hospitalizations or allergies noted.

Family/Social History

The mother indicated that M currently resides at home with his parents and 3-year-old brother. She also indicated that English is the only language spoken in the home. His mother described M as a happy child, who engages in both solitary and cooperative play with other children, such as his cousins and classmates at his preschool. However, Mrs. C stated that she is currently concerned because her son's delayed speech and language skills are interfering with his social skills.

Educational/Therapeutic History

Mrs. C reported that M currently attends P.S. 123 in a mainstream nursery classroom. M initially received a speech and language evaluation in 2008 through the Board of Education and he receives speech and language therapy in his school four times per week. In addition, the mother stated that he receives special education services for 10 hours per week.

IV. Clinical Observations

Behavior

M presented as a sociable child who easily separated from his mother. He displayed an eager attitude both to repeated requests for clarification and to increasing task complexity. Although he was cooperative while engaging in unstructured activities, M often became distracted during more structured tasks such as administration of the GFTA-3. He frequently required redirection on the task.

Audiological Screening

M did not pass a hearing screening at 20 db HL at all test frequencies. Results were considered unreliable due to the client's difficulty comprehending and following test instructions. A complete audiological evaluation was recommended.

Oral-Peripheral Mechanism Examination

An oral-peripheral examination was conducted on 09/09/09. The client exhibited good head and neck support. No facial asymmetry was noted. Facial sensitivity was within normal limits (WNL). Labial and lingual structural integrity was WNL. Labial and lingual functional integrity was reduced. The client exhibited reduced labial retraction and protrusion and lingual protrusion and depression. The jaw was WNL. Dental condition was good. Tonsils present, not enlarged. M exhibited mild limitations in lip rounding and when performing automatic tasks such as to blowing bubbles. He further demonstrated mild difficulty when drinking from a straw. M held the liquid in his mouth for a slightly extended period indicating difficulty in oral transit and propulsion. Dental occlusion, velopharyngeal movement, and diadochokinetic rate for /pʌ, tʌ, kʌ/ could not be assessed due to lack of cooperation. An open mouth posture at rest and mouth breathing were noted.

Speech Sound Production Skills

Formal Assessment

Articulation was formally assessed through the administration of the GFTA-3 and the KLPA-3. The GFTA-3 is a norm-referenced instrument that assesses consonant and consonant blend phonemes in various phonetic positions and contexts. The Sounds-in-Words and Sounds-in-Sentences subtests of the GFTA-3 were administered to assess M's articulation on the isolated word and sentence levels, respectively. Upon administration of the Sounds-in-Sentences subtest, M responded in one-word utterances and in several unintelligible multiple-word sentences. Therefore, target productions could not formally be assessed at the sentence level.

Analysis of error patterns indicated the presence of multiple and inconsistent phonological processes of typically developing children and idiosyncratic phonological productions. M obtained a standard score of 91 (mean = 100; standard deviation = 15), placing him at –.9 standard deviations below the mean and at a percentile rank of 25 and a test age-equivalent of 3;1 years, indicating a moderate delay in speech sound performance. M scored in average range with regard to the phonemes he has in his repertoire; however, due to his multiple phonological processes and vowel errors, M's speech was unintelligible on the isolated word level without contextual support. (Refer to Table 1: Summary of GFTA-3 Scores.)

The KLPA-3 was used to further clarify and analyze the presence and nature of M's speech sound production errors. The results yielded a standard score of 82, placing him in the 13th percentile and at a test age-equivalent of 2;3 years, indicating a moderately severe phonological processing disorder. (See Table 3 for results of the KLPA-3.) M exhibited deletion of final consonants 22.7% out of 44; syllable reduction 8% out of 26; stopping of fricatives and affricatives 16% out of 31; cluster simplification 50% out of 26; liquid simplification 29% out of 31; velar fronting 21% out of 19; initial voicing 15% out of 26; and final devoicing 3% out of 32 items. M's articulation was further characterized by the idiosyncratic process of labialization. The following inconsistent vowel errors were noted in his phonetic inventory: /ɝ/ → /ɔ/, /æ/ → /ɑ/, /ɚ/ → /ə/, /ʌ/ → /ɑ/, and /æ/ → /ɛ/. The presence of so many persisting processes combined with unusual patterns further indicates a moderately severe phonological processing disorder.

Intelligibility

Speech intelligibility was poor with and without context known due to multiple phonological processes and vowel alteration errors. M was stimulable at the single word/syllable level but exhibited difficulty imitating correct productions at the multiple syllable word level.

Summary of Speech Sound Production Abilities

In view of his formal test results, the presence of multiple phonological processes, vowel errors, and poor intelligibility, M presented with a moderately severe phonological disorder. Results of the KPLA-3 were aligned with those derived from the GFTA-3 (Report Tables 2 and 4). Stimulability was good for production of final consonants and simple clusters (e.g., spoon) but poor for multisyllabic words as well as for voicing.

Report Table 1: GFTA-3 Summary of Scores

	Standard Score	*Percentile*	*Test-Age Equivalent*
Sounds-in-Words	91	25th	3;1

Report Table 2 on the next page provides specific error analysis and examples of the various phonological processes identified during testing.

Report Table 3: KLPA-3 Score Summary

Raw Score	*Standard Score*	*Percentile*	*Test-Age Equivalent*
48	82	13	2;3

Report Table 4: Analysis of Vowel Errors

Target Vowel	*Response*	*Vowel Alteration*	*Examples*
/ɝ/	/ɔ/	Vowel retracted	/gɝl/ → /gɔl/
/æ/	/ɑ/	Vowel lowering + retracted	/bənænə/ → /bənɑnə/
/ɚ/	/ə/	Derhotacization	/sɪzɚz/ → /sɪzə/ /zɪpɚ/ → /zɪpə/
/ʌ/	/ɑ/	Vowel lowering	/dʌk/ → /dɑk/
/æ/	/ɛ/	Vowel raising	/læmp/ → /lɛmp/

Report Table 2: GFTA-3 /KPLA-3 Analysis of Phonological Processes				
Target Word	*Response*	*Phonemic Change*	*Phonological Process*	*Examples*
tree	/twi/	/tr/ → [tw]	Cluster reduction	/spun/ → /pun/
monkey	/mʌki/	/ŋk/ → [k]	50% out of 26	
blue	/bju/	/j/ → [bj]		
flowers	/faʊə/	/ɚz/ → [ə]		
blue	/bwu/	/bl/ → [bw]		
clean	/dwin/	/kl/ → [dw]		
crawling	/kwaiɪn/	/kr/ → [kw]		
		/ŋ/ → [n]		
stars	/tɑr/	/st/ → [t]		
		/rz/ → [r]		
chair	/tʃɛ/	/ɛr/ → [ɛ]	Final consonant deletion	/sɪzɚz/ → /sizə/
carrot	/karɛ/	/ɛt/ → [ɛ]	22.7% out of 44	
pencils	/pɛnsəl/	ls (/lz/) → [l]		
flavors	/flavə/	ers (/ɚz/) → [ə]		
balloons	/bəjun/	/l/ → [j]		
		/nz/ → [n]		
stars	/tɑr/	/st/ → [t]		
		/rz/ → [r]		
frog	/frɔk/	/g/ → [k]	Final devoicing	/dɔg/ → /dɔk/
			3% out of 32	
clean	/dwin/	/kl/ → [dw]	Prevocalic voicing	/kʌp/ → /gʌp/
car	/gɑr/	/k/ → [g]	15% out of 26	
telephone	/dɛləfon/	/t/ → [d]		
jello	/wɛlo/	/j/ → [w]	Labialization	/dɔg/ → /bɔg/
blue	/bju/	/j/ → [bj]	Liquid simplification	/kraiɪŋ/ → /kwaiɪn/
glasses	/bwæsɪz/	/gl/ → [bw]	29% out of 31	
tree	/twi/	/tr/ → [tw]		
orange	/ɔwind/	/r/ → [w]		
		/dʒ/ → [d]		
balloons	/bəjun/	/l/ → [j]		
		/nz/ → [n]		
crawling	/kwaiɪn/	/kr/ → [kw]		
		/ŋ/ → [n]		
slide	/swaɪd/	/sl/ → [sw]		
clean	/dwin/	/kl/ → [dw]	Velar fronting	/kar/ → /tar/
glasses	/bwæsɪz/	/gl/ → [bw]	21% out of 19	
vacuum	/vætjum/	/k/ → [t]		

Informal Assessment

M's verbal motor planning ability was assessed by requesting that he imitate words of increasing length (e.g., fun, funnier, funniest). M exhibited marked difficulty imitating words consisting of two or more syllables, even despite repeated trials. M's speech intelligibility was informally assessed during spontaneous conversational interactions and play activities.

Intelligibility was fair upon producing monosyllabic single-word utterances (e.g., no, fish). However, as the length of words or utterances increased beyond this level, M's speech was not intelligible (e.g., *glasses* → /gækses/ and *I want the vacuum* → /ai wand du vatum/) despite contextual support. Factors that contributed to his poor intelligibility included the presence of numerous phonological processes, inconsistent metathetic errors (e.g., *vacuum* → /bækjum/ → /vætum/) vowel alterations and the insertion of a schwa vowel to replace a word (e.g. *One for you* → One /ə/ you.)

Results of the GFTA-3 and KLPA-3 were aligned with the results of informal speech sample analysis.

Voice and Vocal Parameters

Vocal prosody was mildly monotonous in connected discourse. Imitating sentences with rising and falling inflection were assessed during an informal imitation task (e.g., Are you tired↑, No, I am happy↓). M frequently answered the sentences rather than imitating them and required several models when imitating the sentences; however, he was stimulable for varied vocal inflection.

Fluency

Rate and rhythm were judged to be within normal limits.

Language

Not assessed during the day of the evaluation. It was requested that the parent return with the child; however, they never returned for further testing.

V. Clinical Impressions

M, a 4;9-year-old boy, presented with a moderate articulation and phonological delay characterized by numerous errors in articulation and phonological processes (**final consonant deletion**, cluster reduction, velar fronting, and liquid simplification), inconsistent metathetic errors, as well as a restricted prosodic pattern. A mild verbal dyspraxia cannot be ruled out as he exhibited difficulty with verbal sequential motor planning markedly in the production of multisyllabic words. Intelligibility was poor with both context known and not known.

The GFTA-3 results revealed a standard score of 91 and a test age of 3;1 years, and the KLPA-3 was used to further clarify and analyze the presence and nature of M's speech sound production errors on the GFTA-3. The KLPA-3 results yielded a standard score of 82, placing him in the 13th percentile and at a test age-equivalent of 2;3 years, indicating a moderately severe phonological processing disorder. M's articulation was further characterized by the idiosyncratic process of labialization. The following inconsistent vowel errors were noted in his phonetic inventory: /ɝ/ → /ɔ/, /æ/ → /ɑ/, /ɚ/ → /ə/, /ʌ/ → /ɑ/, and /æ/ → /ɛ/. Prognosis is good due to client's age, level of cooperation, additional therapeutic support in the school environment, and parental involvement.

VI. Recommendations

1. Individual therapy is recommended twice per week to address the following goals:
   - To eliminate phonological processes thereby increasing intelligibility, M will suppress the following phonological processes:
     - Final consonant deletion
     - Simple cluster reduction
     - Velar fronting
     - Liquid simplification
   - To correctly produce vowels at the word, phrase, sentence, and conversation level
2. To further assess M for childhood apraxia of speech
3. A complete audiological evaluation is recommended because M failed a hearing screening at 20-db HL at all test frequencies
4. Discuss generalization activities of target skills in the home and classroom environment with M's parents, teachers, and other therapists

____

(Name of clinician or clinical supervisor and credentials)

Speech-Language Pathologist

Sample Case History for a Practice Exercise

Please read the following case history. Then select and list an appropriate battery of formal and informal assessment procedures as well as any other relevant assessment information that might pertain to this specific client. Please include a rationale as to why you selected these specific instruments for this client.

Case History

Y.Z., a 7-year-old boy, was seen at the speech-language and hearing clinic for a complete speech and language evaluation at the request of his father who was concerned about Y's difficulty saying /s/ and /z/. The child did not have any other sound production errors; however, some of his articulatory movements were imprecise, and his speech rate was rapid. The client appeared to have some upper teeth protruding excessively over his lower teeth, and his dentition did not make complete contact when biting down. The client kept his mouth open at all times and his tongue protruded when he swallowed.

Conclusion

When conducting a speech sound production assessment, the clinician must consider all aspects of a client that might have an impact on her articulation and phonology skills: developmental milestones, oral peripheral structures and functions, phonetic inventory, phonological processes, intelligibility, stimulability, cognitive and linguistic maturity, and communication environment. To gather a comprehensive range of clinical information expediently, a logical sequence such as outlined here is strongly suggested by ASHA (2004, 2016b). Appropriate intervention targets can be derived from the results of a well-planned and properly executed articulation and phonology assessment and can determine the direction of effective treatment.

Glossary

Addition: Insertion of an extraneous sound in a target word.

Alveolar: Consonants produced by placing the tongue against the alveolar ridge (the oral area where the gum ridge meets the teeth).

Alveolarization: Substitution of an alveolar sound for a linguadental or labial sound.

Apraxia: An impairment of planning and executing motor movements that could also be classified as developmental verbal dyspraxia in children.

Articulation: The movement of articulators during speech production.

Articulation disorder: Difficulty producing speech sounds or difficulty with the motor production of speech movements.

Assimilation: A phonological process in which one sound changes or is altered by a neighboring sound.

Backing: An unusual process that occurs when a consonant made in the back of the oral cavity is substituted for a consonant made in the front of the mouth (e.g., goggie for doggie).

Cluster reduction: A syllable structure process that occurs with the deletion of one or more consonants from a two- or three-consonant cluster.

Coarticulation: The influence on a sound by a sound that precedes or follows it.

Depalatalization: A substitution phonological process in which an alveolar fricative or affricate for a palatal fricative or affricate.

Derhotacization: Idiosyncratic process that occurs with the omission of the r-coloring for the consonant [r] (and for the central vowels with r-coloring).

Diadochokinesis: Rapid, alternating articulatory movements.

Dialects: Consistent variations of a language spoken by a specific ethnic or sociocultural subgroup.

Diminutization: A syllable structure process in which there is an addition of an /i/ or a consonant + /i/.

Diphthongization: The division of one target vowel into two vowel sounds.

Distinctive features: Chomsky and Halle (1968) described a way to classify consonants and vowels by their distinctive features method of classifying phonemes by place and manner of articulation.

Distortion: A way to describe an articulation error in which there is a mispronunciation of a target sound in a word.

Doubling: A syllable structure phonological process in which there is a repetition of a monosyllabic word.

Dysarthria: A motor speech disorder caused by weakness, incoordination, or paralysis of the speech musculature that affect respiration, phonation, articulation, and resonance.

Epenthesis: A syllable structure process where an insertion of a new phoneme, typically the unstressed schwa occurs.

Final consonant deletion: A syllable structure phonological process in which the final consonant or consonant cluster in a syllable or word is deleted.

Final devoicing (postvocalic devoicing): An assimilation phonological process in which the voiced sound (after the vowel) becomes devoiced.

Fricative preference: An unusual process that occurs when a fricative is used in place of a stop consonant.

Fronting: A substitution phonological process that involves a posterior consonant replaced by a consonant produced anteriorly.

Gliding: A substitution phonological process where liquid consonant is replaced by a glide.

Idiopathic: Having no known cause or etiology.

Juncture: The blending, in connected speech, of the final syllables of words with the initial syllables of subsequent words.

Labialization: A phonological process that occurs when an alveolar sound [t,d] is replaced by a labial sound [p,b].

Linguadental: The place of articulation where the tongue is between the teeth.

Liquid simplification: Substitution of another sound, usually the glide /w/, for a liquid, usually /r/ (e.g., wabbit for rabbit).

Maximal pairs: Pairs of words that differ by multiple contrasts in place, manner, and/or voicing.

Minimal pairs: Pairs of words that differ by only one contrast in place, manner, or voicing.

Morpheme: The smallest unit of meaning within a word where a change in it would constitute a change in meaning.

Morphophenemics: The phonological structure of morphemes.

Nasal preference: The substitution of /n/ and /m/ for stops and fricatives.

Neurogenic: Pertaining to the central or peripheral nervous system.

Obstruent: Sounds produced with constriction in the vocal tract, such as stops and fricatives.

Omission: An articulation error in which there is an absence of the target sound in a word.

Pattern analysis: An examination and classification of the child's speech sound errors.

Phonetics: The science of speech sounds as elements of language.

Phonological disorder: An impairment in the organization of the phonemes within a language.

Phonological processes: The child's systematic simplification of adult words into distinct identifiable categories.

Phonology: The study of cognitive, linguistic, and motor aspects of speech sounds as elements of language.

Phonotactics: The arrangement and sequence of sounds within a word.

Prevocalic voicing: An assimilation phonological process where the voiceless sound before the vowel becomes voiced.

Prosody: Perceived stress and intonation pattern variations that occur during speech.

Reduplication: A syllable structure phonological process where there is a repetition of a partial or entire syllable.

Sonorant: Sounds made with an open vocal tract, such as vowels, nasals, laterals, and glides.

Speech sound disorders: Disorders including both articulation and phonological disorders.

Stimulability: The ability to imitate a target sound when presented with auditory and visual models.

Stopping: A substitution phonological process in which there is a substitution of a stop consonant for a fricative or affricate.

Stridency deletion: The omission or substitution of another sound for a fricative.

Substitution: Replacement of the target sound in a word with an unrelated sound.

Suprasegmentals of speech: Stress, rate of speech, intonation, loudness, pitch, and juncture.

Tetism: The substitution of /t/ for /f/.

Unstressed syllable deletion: A syllable structure phonological process where there is a deletion of an unstressed syllable from a word containing two or more syllables.

Velar: The area in the oral cavity in the area of the velum or soft palate.

Velar fronting: A substitution phonological process in which there is the substitution of sounds in the anterior of the oral cavity, usually alveolar sounds, for velar or palatal sounds.

Vocalization: Substitution of a vowel for a final position liquid sound.

Vowel harmony: This occurs when vowels are produced like contrastive vowels elsewhere in a word.

References

American Speech-Language-Hearing Association. (n.d.a). Developmental norms for speech and language. Retrieved from http://www.asha.org/slp/schools/prof-consult/norms

American Speech-Language-Hearing Association. (n.d.b). Phonemic inventories across languages. Retrieved from http://www.asha.org/practice/multicultural/Phono

American Speech-Language-Hearing Association. (1991). The role of the speech-language pathologist in assessment and management of oral myofunctional disorders. *ASHA, 33*(Suppl. 5), 7.

American Speech-Language-Hearing Association. (2004). Preferred practice patterns for the profession of speech-language pathology: #15, Speech sound assessment. Retrieved from http://staff.washington.edu/jct6/ASHAPreferredPracticePatternsSLP2004.pdf

American Speech-Language-Hearing Association. (2014). 2014 Schools Survey report: SLP caseload characteristics. Retrieved from http://www.asha.org/research/memberdata/schoolssurvey

American Speech-Language-Hearing Association. (2016a). Speech sound disorders-articulation and phonology. Retrieved from http://www.asha.org/PRPSpecificTopic.aspx?folderid=8589935321§ion=Assessment

American Speech-Language-Hearing Association. (2016b). Speech sound disorders-articulation and phonology: Overview. Retrieved from http://www.asha.org/PRPSpecificTopic.aspx?folderid=8589935321§ion=Overview

American Speech-Language-Hearing Association. (2016c). Speech sound disorders-articulation and phonology: Incidence and prevalence. Retrieved from https://www.asha.org/PRPSpecificTopic.aspx?folderid=8589935321§ion=Incidence_and_Prevalence

American Speech-Language-Hearing Association. (2016d). Speech sound disorders-articulation and phonology: Signs and symptoms. Rockville, MD: ASHA. Retrieved from http://www.asha.org/PRPSpecificTopic.aspx?folderid=8589935321§ion=Signs_and_Symptoms

Ansel, B. (1994). Articulation disorders of unknown origin in children (*NIH Guide*, Volume 23, Number 7). Washington, DC: Division of Communication Sciences and Disorders, National Institute on Deafness and Other Communication Disorders.

Bankson, N. W., & Bernthal, J. E. (1990). *Bankson–Bernthal Test of Phonology.* Austin, TX: Pro-Ed.

Bauman-Waengler, J. (2008). *Articulatory and phonological impairments: A Clinical Focus* (3rd ed.). Boston, MA: Allyn & Bacon.

Bauman-Waengler, J. A. (2012). *Articulatory and phonological impairments.* New York, NY: Pearson Higher Education.

Bernthal, J. E., & Bankson, N. W. (2004). *Articulation and phonological disorders: Infancy through adulthood* (5th ed.). Boston, MA: Allyn & Bacon.

Bernthal, J., Bankson, N. W., & Flipsen, P., Jr. (2013). *Articulation and phonological disorders.* New York, NY: Pearson Higher Education.

Bleile, K. (2014). *Manual of speech sound disorders: A book for students and clinicians* (3rd ed.). New York, NY: Cengage.

Carrow-Woolfolk, E. (1999). *Comprehensive Assessment of Spoken Language.* East Moline, IL: LinguiSystems.

Chomsky, N., & Halle, M. (1968). *The sound patterns of English.* New York, NY: Harper & Row.

Darley, F. L., Aronson, A. E., & Brown, J. R. (1975). *Motor speech disorders.* Philadelphia, PA: Saunders.

Darley, F. L., & Spriestersbach, D. (1978). *Differential diagnosis of acquired motor speech disorders* (2nd ed.). New York, NY: Harper & Row.

Derr, A. (2003). Growing diversity in our schools—Roles and responsibilities of speech-language pathologists. *SIG 16: School-Based Issues, 4*, 7-12.

Dodd, B., Hua, Z., Crosbie, S., Holm, A., & Ozanne, A. (2006). *Diagnostic evaluation of articulation and phonology* (DEAP). Bloomington, MN: Pearson Clinical Assessments.

Drummond, S. S. (1993). *Dysarthria examination battery.* Tucson, AZ: Communication Skill Builders.

Duffy, J. R. (2013). *Motor speech disorders: Substrates, differential diagnosis and management* (3rd ed.). St. Louis, MO: Elsevier Mosby.

Edwards, H. T. (2003). *Applied phonetics: The sounds of American English* (3rd ed.). Clifton Park, NY: Delmar Cengage Learning.

Enderby, P., & Palmer, R. (2008). *Frenchay Dysarthria Assessment.* Austin, TX: Pro-Ed.

Fabiano, L. (2007). Evidence-based phonological assessment of bilingual children. *Perspectives on Communication Disorders and Sciences in Culturally and Linguistically Diverse Populations, SIG, 14*, 21-23.

Fairbanks, G. (1960). *Voice and articulation drillbook* (2nd ed.). New York, NY: Harper & Row.

Fisher, H., & Logemann, J. (1971). *The Fisher–Logemann test of articulation competence* (F-LTAC). Boston, MA: Houghton Mifflin.

Freed, D. B. (2012). *Motor speech disorders: Diagnosis and treatment* (2nd ed.). Clifton Park, NY: Delmar Cengage Learning.

Gierut, J. A. (1998). Treatment efficacy: Functional phonological disorders in children. *Journal of Speech, Language, and Hearing Research, 41*, 85-100.

Gillam, R., & Pearson, N. (2004). *TNL: Test of narrative language.* Austin, TX: Pro-Ed.

Goldman, R., & Fristoe, M. (2015). *Goldman–Fristoe test of articulation* (3rd ed.). Bloomington, MN: Pearson Clinical Assessments.

Hegde, M. N., & Freed, D. (2013). *Assessment of communication disorders in adults.* San Diego, CA: Plural.

Hegde, M. N. & Promoville, F. (2017). *Assessment of communication disorders in children.* San Diego, CA: Plural.

Hodson, B. (2004). *Hodson assessment of phonological patterns.* East Moline, IL: LinguiSystems.

International Phonetic Association. (2005). Full IPA chart. Retrieved from https://www.internationalphoneticassociation.org/content/full-ipa-chart

Kamhi, A. G. (2005). Summary, reflections ,and future directions. In A. G. Kamhi & E. E. Pollack (Eds.), *Phonological disorders in children: Clinical decision making in assessment and intervention* (pp. 211-228). Baltimore, MD: Brookes.

Kent (2015). Nonspeech oral movements and oral motor disorders: A narrative review. *American Journal of Speech-Language Pathology, 24*, 763-789.

Khan, L. (1982). A review of 16 major phonological processes. *Language, Speech, & Hearing in Schools, 13*, 77-85.

Khan, L., & Lewis, N. (2015). *Khan-Lewis phonological analysis* (3rd ed.). Bloomington, MN: Pearson Clinical Assessments.

Lass, N. J., & Pannbacker, M. (2008). The application of evidence-based practice to nonspeech oral motor treatments. *Language, Speech, and Hearing Services in Schools, 39*, 408-421.

Lippke, B., Dickey, S., Selmar, J., & Soder, A. (1997). *The photo articulation test* (3rd ed.). East Moline, IL: LinguiSystems.

Lof, G. L. (2004). Confusion about speech sound norms and their use. *On-Line Language Conference 2004.* Thinking Publications. Retrieved from https://myspeechteacher.wikispaces.com/file/view/confusion+about+speech+sound+norms+and+their+use.pdf

Lof, G. L. (2008). Controversies surrounding nonspeech oral motor exercises for childhood speech disorders. *Seminars in Speech and Language, 29*, 253-255.

Lof, G. L., & Watson, M. M. (2008). A nationwide survey of nonspeech oral motor exercise use: Implications for evidence-based practice. *Language, Speech, and Hearing Services in Schools, 39*, 392-407.

Lowe, R. J. (1994). *Assessment and intervention applications in speech pathology.* Baltimore, MD: Williams & Wilkins.

Lowe, R. J. (2000). Assessment Link Between Phonology and Articulation—revised. Mifflinville, PA: ALPHA Speech & Language Resources. Retrieved from http://www.speech-language-therapy.com/alpha.html

Lowe, R. (2009). *Workbook for the identification of phonological processes and distinctive features* (4th ed.). Austin, TX: Pro-Ed.

McDonald, E. T. (1964). *A deep test of articulation*. Pittsburgh, PA: Stanwix House.

National Institute on Deafness and Other Communication Disorders. (2010). Statistics and epidemiology. Voice, speech, and language: Quick statistics. Retrieved from https://www.nidcd.nih.gov/health/statistics/quick-statistics-voice-speech-language

Paul, R., & Jennings, P. (1992). Phonological behavior in toddlers with slow expressive language development. *Journal of Speech and Hearing Research, 35*, 99-107.

Peña-Brooks, A., & Hegde, M. N. (2015). *Assessment and treatment of speech sound disorders in children: A dual-level text* (3rd ed.). Austin, TX: Pro-Ed.

Pollack, K. E. (1991). The identification of vowel errors using traditional articulation or phonological process test stimuli. *LSHS, 22*, 39-50.

Poole, E. (1934). Genetic development of articulation of consonant sounds in speech. *Elementary English Review, 11*, 159-161.

Prather, E., Hedrick, D., & Kern, C. (1975). Articulation development in children aged two to four years. *Journal of Speech and Hearing Disorders, 40*, 179-191.

Roach, P. (2004). *Phonetics*. Oxford, England: Oxford University Press.

Robertson, S. (1982). *Dysarthria profile*. Tucson, AZ: Communication Skill Builders.

Rogers, H. (2000). *The sounds of language: An introduction to phonetics*. Essex, England: Pearson Education.

Rvachew, S., Rafaat, S., & Martin, M. (1999). Stimulabitlity, speech perception skills, and the treatment of phonological disorders. *American Journal of Speech-Language Pathology, 8*, 33-43.

Sanders, E. (1972). When are speech sounds learned? *Journal of Speech and Hearing Disorders, 37*, 55-63.

Secord, W., & Donohue, J. (2013). *Clinical assessment of articulation and phonology* (2nd ed.). Austin, TX: Pro-Ed.

Shipley, K. G., & McAfee, J.G. (2015). *Assessment in speech-language pathology: A resource manual* (5th ed.). Clifton Park, NY: Delmar Cengage Learning.

Shriberg, L. D., & Kent, R. D. (2012). *Clinical phonetics* (4th ed). Boston, MA: Pearson Education.

Small, L. (2005). *Fundamentals of phonetics. A practical guide for students*. Boston, MA: Pearson Education.

Templin, M. C. (1957). Certain language skills in children: Their development and interrelationships. *Institute of Child Welfare, Monograph 26*. Minneapolis, MN: University of Minnesota Press.

Templin, M. C., & Darley, F. L. (1969). *Templin–Darley tests of articulation* (2nd ed.). Iowa City: University of Iowa Press.

Tiffany, W., & Carrel, J. (1977). *Phonetics: Theory and application* (2nd ed.). New York, NY: McGraw-Hill.

Velleman, S. L. (2002). Phonotactic therapy. *Seminars in Speech and Language, 23*, 45-55.

Velleman, S. L. (2003). *Childhood apraxia of speech: Resource guide*. Clifton Park, NY: Delmar Cengage Learning.

Wertz, R. (1985). Neuropathologies of speech and language: An introduction to patient management. In D. Johns (Ed.), *Clinical management of neurogenic communicative disorders* (2nd ed.; pp. 1-96). Boston, MA: Little, Brown.

Wertz, R., LaPointe, L., & Rosenbek, J. C. (1984). *Apraxia of speech: The disorder and its treatment*. New York, NY: Grune & Stratton.

Yorkston, K., Beukelman, D., Strand, E., & Bell, K. (2010). *Management of motor speech disorders in children and adults*. Austin, TX: PRO-ED.

Yorkston, K., Beukelman, D., & Traynor, C. (1984). *Assessment of Intelligibility of Dysarthric Speech*. Austin, TX: Pro-Ed.

Additional Recommended Reading

Hegde, M. N. (2003). *A coursebook on scientific and professional writing for speech-language pathology*. Clifton Park, NY: Thomson Delmar Learning.

Hegde, M.N. (2008). *Pocketguide to treatment in speech-language pathology*. San Diego, CA: Singular.

Hegde, M. N., & Pomaville, F. (2013). *Assessment of communication disorders in children. Resources and protocols*. San Diego, CA: Plural.

Williams, A. L., McLeod, S., & McCauley, R. (2010). *Interventions for speech sound disorders in children*. Baltimore, MD: Brookes.

Website Resources

Also review websites provided in Chapter 6 on oral-peripheral examination.

Academy of Neurological Communication Disorders and Sciences: http://www.ancds.org

American Speech-Language-Hearing Association (ASHA): www.asha.org.

ASHA, Developmental Norms for Speech and Language: www.asha.org/slp/schools/prof-consult/norms

ASHA Portal: www.asha.org/practice-portal

Apraxia Kids: www.apraxia-kids.org

International Phonetic Association: www.internationalphoneticassociation.org/

Judith Maginnis Kuster—Examples of materials that can be adapted for therapy (collection of resources): www.mnsu.edu/comdis/kuster2/welcome.html

Motor Speech Disorders/Childhood Apraxia of Speech: www.mnsu.edu/comdis/kuster2/sptherapy.html#motor

Purdue Online Writing Lab: https://owl.english.purdue.edu

The Articulatory Database Registry: www.cstr.ed.ac.uk/research/projects/artic/.

Type IPA Phonetic Symbols: http://ipa.typeit.org

8

Assessment of Preschool Language Disorders

Diana Almodóvar, PhD, CCC-SLP, TSHH; Liat Seiger-Gardner, PhD, CCC-SLP; and Naomi Shualy, MS, CCC-SLP, TSSLD

Key Words

- autism
- cognitive
- collateral test-taking behaviors
- communicative gestures
- discourse skills
- genetic disorder
- heuristic intentions
- illocutionary stage
- imaginative play
- informative intentions
- intellectual developmental disability
- language delay
- language disorder
- late bloomer
- late talker
- locutionary stage
- obligatory contexts
- phonology
- pragmatics
- prelinguistic skills
- presupposition
- primary language impairment
- sensory
- specific language impairment
- symbolic gestures
- syndrome
- syntax
- visual support
- word retrieval deficit

Introduction: Overview of the Disorder

Signs of a communication disorder can be evident as early as the first few months of life. Typically developing infants demonstrate a number of fundamental **cognitive** processes involving thought, reasoning, and problem solving as well as social behaviors that are critical for the appropriate development of language and communication. When assessing a child who is younger than age 5 years, it is essential to examine not only emerging linguistic behaviors, but also **prelinguistic skills**. Prelinguistic skills include early social knowledge, gestures, and cognitive processes that precede verbal language production but are highly correlated with language development (Adams & Gathercole, 2000; Iverson & Goldin-Meadow, 2005; Mayberry & Nicoladis, 2000; Özçalıskan & Goldin-Meadow, 2005; Tomasello, 1992). This chapter focuses on both early language abilities and prelinguistic skills that must be considered when evaluating preschool children between the ages of 2 and 5 years.

Stein-Rubin, C., & Fabus, R. *A Guide to Clinical Assessment and Professional Report Writing in Speech-Language Pathology, Second Edition (pp 163-188).*

Defining Language Disorder

The American Speech-Language-Hearing Association (ASHA, 1993) defines a **language disorder** as "an impairment in comprehension and/or use of spoken language, written, and/or other symbol system. The disorder may involve (1) the form of language (phonologic, morphologic, and syntactic systems), (2) the content of language (semantic system), and /or (3) the function of language in communication (**pragmatic** system), in any combination" (p. 40). The *Diagnostic and Statistical Manual of Mental Disorders* (5th edition [DSM-5]; American Psychiatric Association [APA], 2013) supports this definition, adding that these deficits can be persistent in nature. However, the terminology used to define young children with a language disorder can vary greatly. It is important to be aware of the differences and implications of the various labels for language-based disorders.

Children with a **language delay** present with protracted development of language; however, they follow the typical course of development. In other words, their profiles more closely match younger, typically developing children rather than chronologically age-matched peers. The use of the term *delay* implies that there is a possibility that the child will eventually "catch up" in development to his or her peers (Leonard, 1998). This is in contrast to children whose difficulties in the areas of receptive and expressive language persist past age 5 years and continue to require intervention and academic assistance.

Late Bloomers Versus Late Talkers

All children who begin producing first words and first word combinations late are often and erroneously referred to as **late talkers**. However, late talkers are specifically defined in the literature as children who demonstrate delays in the early stages of language development and whose deficits persist past age 4 years (Rescorla & Schwartz, 1990). There does appear to be a smaller group of children who demonstrate early language delays, particularly between the ages of 12 to 24 months, and who by age 4 years make substantial gains in their language development. These gains are significant in that they no longer appear to have a delay by age 4 years (Rescorla, 2005). Children who fit this profile are referred to as **late bloomers**. Often, children whose language deficits are the primary deficit but who show persisting language processing difficulties into the school-age years are referred to as children with **specific language impairment** (SLI). This term was originally used to denote the presence of language impairment in the absence of any evidence for gross neurological, emotional, cognitive, or **sensory** (e.g., hearing or visual) deficits (Leonard, 1998; Schwartz, 2009). In more recent literature, school-age children with this profile are described as having a **primary language impairment**. Implied within this preferred term is that, although language deficits represent the primary concern for these children, there may also be underlying weaknesses in working memory, executive functions, attentional processes, and motor coordination (Archibald & Gathercole, 2006; Botting & Conti-Ramsden, 2001; Hill, 2001; Marton, 2008, 2009; Richard, Annette, Robert, & Michael, 2005).

Although there is no definitive way to differentially diagnose late talkers from late bloomers, there are several markers that suggest the likelihood of persisting linguistic deficits. Early receptive language skills, for example, appear to be a strong predictor of later language outcomes. Children who demonstrate appropriate receptive language skills at approximately 13 months of age have been shown to develop stronger expressive language skills in later preschool years compared with children who have early deficits in comprehension (Thal, Reilly, Seibert, Jeffries, & Fenson, 2004; Thal & Tobias, 1992). In addition, **communicative gestures** (such as pointing) and **symbolic gestures** (e.g., panting to indicate a dog) seem to be used more frequently by late bloomers than by late talkers (Thal, Tobias, & Morrison, 1991). In typical language development, children first use gestures (**illocutionary stage**) before actual words (**locutionary stage**) to communicate (Bates, 1976; Capone & McGregor, 2004). The use of early gestures to communicate or symbolize concepts may indicate a better prognosis for a child demonstrating a language delay (Thal et al., 1991). Therefore, it is important for the clinician to assess both nonverbal and verbal communication in toddlers and preschoolers, although the use of gestures and nonverbal communication in a child should not be the sole criterion used to determine the need for services.

Secondary Language Impairments

The terms *late bloomers, late talkers, language delay,* and *SLI* all refer to children whose primary and sole (as understood at this point in time) deficits are in the area of language. However, many children demonstrate language impairment that is secondary to other disorders. Typically, these children are not referred to as having language delays but rather a language impairment secondary to a disorder such as

autism, **intellectual developmental disability** (IDD), or a **genetic disorder**. Autism is a behavioral disorder characterized by significant impairments of communication, socialization, and stereotypical behaviors such as but not limited to no eye contact and self-stimulatory behaviors (e.g., rocking, arm flapping, spinning objects). See Chapter 9 for a more in depth discussion on this topic. IDD refers to individuals with significant deficits in intellectual and adaptive functioning (APA, 2013; Luckasson et al., 2002). Children may also have a language impairment that is one of several features characteristic of a particular **syndrome**. A syndrome is a cluster of anomalies in an individual that are caused by the same source. Children with Down syndrome or fragile X syndrome, for example, demonstrate a variety of deficits that are caused by a single source. For a review of language impairments secondary to specific syndromes, see Paul and Norbury (2012).

Although children with secondary language impairments may demonstrate deficits in any area of language, some aspects of language appear to be more vulnerable than others. In contrast to language delays or SLI, a speech-language pathologist (SLP) typically does not officially diagnose the primary disorders that are associated with language impairment (such as IDD and autism). However, SLPs are integral members of interdisciplinary teams consisting of psychologists, special education instructors, or developmental pediatricians who each contribute to diagnosing these disorders. Therefore, if an SLP suspects that the communication disorder is secondary to an undiagnosed disorder, appropriate referrals should be made to those professionals.

Characteristics of a Language Disorder

As stated in the beginning of this chapter, a language problem can affect a child's receptive and expressive language skills. Deficits in both receptive and expressive language can be found across all areas of language. Early signs of a possible language disorder may include one or more of the following:

- Limited phonetic inventory (number of different sounds produced) within babble (for nonverbal children) or meaningful speech
- Limited nonverbal communication in the form of communicative and symbolic gestures after age 9 months
- Delayed onset of first words after age 12 to 14 months
- Delayed onset of two-word combinations after age 18 to 24 months
- Limited to no eye contact
- Sudden regression in child's development in cognitive, social, and linguistic skill areas
- Slow or limited expansion in the total number of different words produced after age 15 to 18 months
- Limited comprehension of basic vocabulary and simple directives

The severity of a child's delay or impairment will dictate the child's skill level in both receptive and expressive language. Children who demonstrate a mixed expressive-receptive language delay or impairment have a more extensive impairment.

Specific Parameters for Assessment

The main objectives in assessing a toddler or preschool-age child is to identify whether a delay or impairment is present, to accurately diagnose the problem, and to identify the areas that require intervention. Appropriate assessment goes well beyond examining language formally through standardized testing. Informal assessment, consideration of family's concerns, and difficulties in peer interactions are also part of the process. The caregivers and other professionals working with the child (e.g., teachers, therapists, physicians) are a vital part of the assessment.

Evaluation of a child's language and communication skills can be done through the use of standardized or norm-referenced tests, criterion-referenced measures, and informal and dynamic assessment. An evaluation of a young child also includes an examination of language-related areas such as play skills, which are highly correlated with a child's language development.

Parameters for assessment should include the following:

- Consideration of caregivers' concerns and expectations for child
- Consideration of teachers' concerns and expectations of child
- Use of informal and formal testing measures to determine the following:
    - Child's level of communication and socialization with peers and adults
    - Child's interest level and level of attention to toys and objects in the environment

- Appropriate usage of toys and objects in the environment
- Attention span, turn-taking skills, and degree of engagement in activities
- Level of comprehension of directives and questions
- Ability to communicate needs and wants
- Appropriate production of speech sounds
- Expressive and receptive vocabulary skills
- Comprehension and production of grammatical forms
- Ability to imitate new sounds or verbal targets presented
- Amount of support needed to complete activities

Collateral Test-Taking Behaviors

In addition to speech, language, and play skills, **collateral test-taking behaviors** are crucial parameters to highlight and to note within the diagnostic report. These measures typically fall under the heading of "Behavioral Observations" in the written document. In this section, the clinician indicates (1) test-taking strategies the child may be using, (2) behaviors that can influence results of formal testing, (3) support that the child required during the session, (4) patterns the child demonstrates (e.g., consistently selecting to the last option presented), and (5) learning style. Specifically, inattentiveness, the need to redirect a child throughout the evaluation, and a child who requires frequent breaks or reinforcement throughout testing should be documented. In addition, the SLP should take note of the degree of support that the child requires, such as extra time to respond, prompting to take his or her time in responding (impulsivity control), repetition, or visual cues. This information is important in creating a treatment plan for the child.

Key Clinical Interview Questions

The first part of an evaluation process entails an interview with the caregiver to obtain the child's case history. This information is vital as it enables the clinician to determine the diagnosis and severity of the delay or disorder. In addition, the interview allows the clinician to gather information on the child's lifestyle, expectations from family, culture, and degree of interference in daily living. Although many clinicians may have caregiver questionnaire forms readily available to distribute, it is preferable for the clinician to ask the caregivers the questions directly to ensure that a full history is obtained and any necessary follow-up questions are asked.

The case history entails asking questions pertinent to developing an accurate and comprehensive linguistic profile of the child. Information on the mother's pregnancy and delivery are typically obtained (if information is available) to determine whether the child was at risk for a developmental disability while in utero (due to exposure to environmental toxins, alcohol, or drugs) or during and after birth. A full medical history is attained, with relevant medical information included in the diagnostic report. Illnesses or medications that may affect a child's speech and language are delineated as well, such as neurological deficits, seizure activity, recurring episodes of otitis media with effusion (middle ear infections with fluid present), and respiratory problems. Developmental milestones are specified to determine whether there appears to be a pattern of developmental delay based on caregiver report. In addition, a general statement of the current problem is acquired to determine the child's current level of functioning. Caregivers are then asked specifically to elaborate on how they perceive their child's language production, comprehension, play skills, and socialization skills. A list of recommended questions can be found in Table 8-1.

Formal Assessment Measures

Norm-Referenced Measures

Formal testing measures are the most frequently used method for determining a child's eligibility for speech-language services. Standardized tests ensure that the administration and scoring of the tests are uniform across the population. Norm-referenced tests take a child's score and weigh it against the performance of other age-matched peers. This enables a clinician to determine whether there is a presence of language delay or impairment, its severity, and the areas of language affected.

Standardized tests for preschool children vary in their content. The most frequently used tests are more comprehensive in nature, containing a set of subtests that measure various areas of language, in both expressive and receptive language skills (e.g., Preschool Language Scale-5 [PLS-5]). Expressive language subtests typically require a child to formulate a sentence, complete a sentence by filling in a missing word, and label pictures or objects. Receptive language subtests require a child to either point to a specific picture or object, follow directives, and respond appropriately to wh- and yes–no questions. These types

Table 8-1. Most Relevant Interview Questions

Prenatal, Perinatal, and Postnatal Questions	*Clinician's Comments*
Were there any complications during your pregnancy?	
Did you have consistent medical treatment during your pregnancy?	
Were you exposed to any toxins that could have been unhealthy for you or your baby during pregnancy (e.g., lead, mercury)?	
Did you deliver full term or prematurely?	
What type of delivery did you have?	
What was your child's weight at birth?	
Were there any complications at birth?	
How long were you and your child hospitalized after your delivery?	
Medical History	*Clinician's Comments*
Developmental History	
At what age did your child begin to sit up, crawl, walk, and produce words?	
Does your child combine two words? Produce full sentences?	
Does your child have any strong food preferences or aversions?	
Is there a history of feeding difficulties?	
Language History	
What languages other than English are spoken at home?	
Does your child have exposure to another language at school or day care?	
Did your child babble during infancy?	
Does your child seem to understand you? Do you have to repeat yourself frequently and point and gesture to be understood?	
Is it difficult to understand your child's speech?	
Does your child play with a variety of toys? Does your child play appropriately or demonstrate limited interest in toys?	
Social and Family History	
Is there a history of speech-language-learning problems in the family?	
Does you child enjoy being with others or prefer to be alone?	
Does your child attend a nursery school or preschool? What do the teachers report about his or her behavior?	

of tests are used most frequently to determine the presence of a delay or disorder because they provide a broader overview of a child's language functioning, with each subtest being relatively quick to administer. Other tests are devoted to examining a specific area of language in finer detail (e.g., Expressive One-Word Picture Vocabulary Test-4 [EOWPVT-4], Preschool Language Assessment Instrument-2 [PLAI-2]).

Typically, norm-referenced tests provide standard scores or quotients, composite scores, percentile ranks, and age-equivalent scores. The most frequently used scores for determining the presence of a delay or impairment are the quotients or standard scores.

Criterion-Referenced Measures

Criterion-referenced measures enable a clinician to explore a specific area of a child's development in depth. These measures differ from norm-referenced tests in that their scores are not compared with age-matched peers. Often, scoring on criterion-referenced tests relies on a pass–fail score or a percentage correct. Of greater importance, however, is the nature of the errors in criterion-referenced tests because this provides the clinician with a better understanding of a child's weaknesses. This provides valuable baseline information on a child's performance in a given area before intervention as well.

Table 8-2. Most Frequently Used Formal Tests

Test Name (Author)	*Age Range (Years)*	*Areas Assessed*
Boehm 3—Preschool (Boehm, 2001)	3 to 5;11	Receptive language concepts
Clinical Evaluation of Language Fundamentals-2 (CELF-2; Wiig, Secord, & Semel, 2004)	3 to 6	Receptive language concepts, auditory processing, expressive vocabulary, expressive morphology
Detroit Test of Learning Aptitude Primary-3 (DTLA-P-3; Hammil & Bryant, 2005)	3 to 9;11	Expressive language narrative and discourse following directions word opposites, memory visual skills
EOWPVT-4 (Brownell, 2011a)	2 to 18	Expressive vocabulary
PLAI-2 (Blank, Rose, & Berlin, 2003)	3 to 6	Assesses the ability to understand and use language at increasing levels of abstract reasoning
PLS-5 (Zimmerman, Steiner, & Pond, 2011)	Birth to 6;11	Assesses receptive and expressive language, auditory comprehension semantics, syntax/morphology
Receptive One-Word Picture Vocabulary Test-4 (ROWPVT-4; Brownell, 2011b)	2;11 to 12	Receptive identification of single words
Test of Auditory Comprehension of Language-4 (TACL-4; Carrow-Woolfolk, 2014)	3 to 9;11	A test of receptive language; includes concepts, grammatical morphemes, syntax, and elaborated sentences
Test of Early Language Development-3 (TELD-3; Hresko, Redi, & Hammill, 1999)	2:7 to 11	Receptive and expressive semantics, syntax/morphology
Test of Language Development-4 (TOLD-4; Newcomer & Hammil, 2008)	4 to 8;11	Receptive and expressive semantics, syntax/morphology, expressive language formulation
Test of Auditory Perceptual Skills-3 (TAPS-3; Martin & Brownell, 2005)	4 to 18	Assesses auditory processing at the phoneme word and sentence level

Table 8-3. Selective Tests for Infants Birth to 3 Years of Age

Test Name (Author)	*Age Range*	*Areas Assessed*
Birth to Three Checklist of Language and Learning Behaviors (BTC-3; Bangs & Ammer, 1999)	Birth to 3 years	Assesses receptive and expressive language and cognitive and play skills
Rossetti Infant-Toddler Language Scale (Rossetti, 1990)	Birth to 3 years	Assesses receptive and expressive language, play, and early pragmatic skills
Communication and Symbolic Behavior Scales (CSBS; Wetherby & Prizant, 2003)	6 to 24 months	Assesses communication, gestures, symbolic play, and social language skills

There is an extensive array of standardized tests available to clinicians. Table 8-2 lists some of the most frequently used tests to date.

Additional Instruments

When evaluating a child, criterion-referenced tools such as checklists and questionnaires provide a detailed representation of a child's level of functioning (Table 8-3).

Advantages and Disadvantages of Formal Assessment Measures

Standardized testing tends to be viewed as one of the most critical components of an evaluation. The standardization ensures that tests are as unbiased and consistent as possible in administration and scoring so that children's scores can be accurately compared with one another. Because this is viewed as one of the more "objective" measures in an evaluation, external funding for services through the board of education and early-intervention agencies rely predominantly on these scores to determine whether a child qualifies for services. However, it is important to keep in mind that standardized tests are not without limitations.

Although many tests purport to provide a general overview of a child's level of linguistic functioning, not all areas of communication and language are always tested. The scope of these tests, although broad, rarely covers all areas of language, nor does it sufficiently target each specific area in depth. For example, a subtest that uses a sentence completion task to examine production of grammatical morphemes may provide one or two opportunities only for a child to produce an particular morpheme (e.g., the plural -s). Children with language impairment who have morphosyntactic deficits may inconsistently produce a particular grammatical morpheme. However, given that the formal testing allowed them only one opportunity to produce that morpheme, a chance exists that they either produce it correctly or that it results in an incorrect production, but in spontaneous speech, they produce the morpheme with 80% to 90% accuracy. Therefore, children could potentially run the risk of being over- or underidentified. In addition, although questions tapping into language form and content are usually well represented, language use, the area of pragmatic language skills, and play skills are frequently overlooked in these tests. To compensate for these limitations, it is imperative that the clinician also include informal assessment in the evaluation process.

Informal Assessment Measures

The interpretation of formal testing scores should comprise not only the quantitative results of standardized testing, but also additional information on the child's performance within more naturalistic contexts. This information provides the clinician with a more accurate picture of a child's receptive and expressive language skills in everyday life. Two of the best ways to informally assess a child aged 5 years or younger is through both play and language sampling.

Play Skills

Play skills are highly correlated with language ability and provide information on how children interpret the world around them. At about 12 to 18 months of age, symbolic play skills—the ability to use one object to represent another (e.g., pretending a tissue is a blanket for a doll; using a banana as a phone)—emerges (Patterson & Westby, 1998). Symbolic play is significant in that it is analogous to the use of a word to symbolize a concept, idea, or object. Informal assessment of toddlers and preschoolers should include play-based observations. The use of play during the evaluation process not only sheds light on a child's understanding of the functions of objects and symbolism, but it also serves as a means of establishing rapport with the child in a very naturalistic way. Through the use of play, language samples can be obtained and information on social interaction skills and problem solving can be readily observed.

Children's play progresses through stages (Table 8-4). Initially, infant play involves reaching for objects, banging the objects, placing objects in the child's own mouth to explore them, and resisting removal when another person attempts to take the toy away. Toddler play progresses to actual object use, such as placing a block in a hole or pushing a car and imitation of actions performed by others. Imitation can be immediate or delayed. At this point, symbolic play begins to emerge. According to Westby (2000), symbolic play also progresses through stages.

Table 8-4 lists of the stages of play development that can be used to determine a child's level of functioning in play.

When conducting a play assessment, the clinician should have a variety of age-appropriate toys available. However, the environment should not be "overloaded" with toys to avoid overstimulation and to ensure to which toys the child is attending. Ideally, provide the child with a choice of two or three toys. Keeping a few toys within a child's visual field but out of reach provides opportunities to assess how a child requests—if he or she points, vocalizes, verbally requests, or becomes agitated. The use of toys can also facilitate the elicitation of a language sample.

Language Sampling

Language sampling is one of the most common methods of assessing language form (**phonology**, **syntax**, morphology), content (semantics), and use (pragmatics). A language sample can be obtained in a less structured context for a more verbal child, where the child's spontaneous speech is recorded during the evaluation. For children who are less verbal or less inclined to initiate conversation, more structured activities might be set up through the use of story retelling, scripts, and props. The language sample is then transcribed and analyzed by the clinician, and developmental norms (such as Brown's stages of morphological development) are used to determine the presence of a delay. It is important to keep in mind that the main purpose of obtaining a language sample is to obtain a sample that is representative of a child in everyday life. A good representative sample should contain between 50 to 100 utterances. When eliciting the sample, it is important for the clinician to avoid having the child label objects in his or her environment or asking predominantly yes–no questions.

Table 8-4. Westby's Play Scale

Stage	*Play Behaviors*
Presymbolic Level I; age 9 to 12 months	The child is developing means–end and will pull a string to obtain the object at the other end. Object permanence is also developing as the child understands that an object remains even after it is hidden from view. The child will search for a ball that rolls under a couch and is out of view. The child is also developing new schema for toys and will not immediately mouth or bang the toy. Functional play emerges, consisting of repetitive actions and movements carried out with or without objects, such as rolling a toy vehicle back and forth repeatedly or squeezing Play-Doh without attempting to construct with it.
Presymbolic Level II; age 13 to 17 months	The child explores toys and attempts to discover how each toy operates. Cause-and-effect actions are more readily observable as the child will push a large button to activate a noise or song. The child is also becoming more aware of how adults can assist in play and will hand the toy to an adult when he or she has difficulty activating it.
Symbolic Level I; age 17 to 19 months	Representational skills emerge. Autosymbolic play is evident as the child will perform an action on him- or herself, such as drinking from an empty cup.
Symbolic Level II; age 19 to 22 months	Play is extended beyond the child to include others in the environment. The child may feed a doll, brush the doll's hair, or brush his or her mother's hair.
Symbolic Level III; age 24 months	Pretend play develops. The child can represent his or her own experiences in play. The child can pretend to be another child or the mother or father. The beginning of sequences emerge such as two actions together (e.g., placing pretend food in a pot and stirring it on a pretend stove). Constructive play emerges. Play activities involve various materials, including blocks or Play-Doh. You can find children in the sensorimotor stage playing with construction type materials but in a more functional/practicing way, such as banging blocks together; lining up, stacking, and knocking over blocks; and putting blocks in containers.
Symbolic Level IV; age 30 months	The child begins to represent experiences that are less frequent in his or her life, such as going to a doctor. Props continue to be realistic, and roles may shift such that at one moment the child is the mommy and the next moment he or she is the child.
Symbolic Level V; age 3 years	Sequences become longer and more complex. The child can produce a play schema involving assembling the items to bake a cake, pouring the ingredients into a mixing bowl and placing the cake in the oven.
Symbolic Level VI; age 3 to 3.5 years	The child begins to use less realistic toys and props such as dollhouse characters. Blocks may be used to build fences and gates. The child will also be observed using one object to represent another (e.g., a stick to comb a dolls hair).
Symbolic Level VII; age 3.5 to 4 years	Language is now used to invent props and set the scene. The child is now able to hypothesize "what would happen if?" in a play schema.
Symbolic Level VIII; age 5 years	Children now set the scene and assign roles to others. Play is highly imaginative and may include events the child has never actually experienced.

Adapted from Westby (2000).

When collecting a language sample, there are several issues to take into account:

- Duration of recordings: It is always better to record a little more than a little less. You can always delete extra data you have recorded, but it is difficult to go back and get more data. If a child does not produce adequate spontaneous speech in the first 15 to 30 minutes of observation, it is probably better to switch contexts. For a very talkative child, a full 1-hour session may be too long. In general, you should attempt to record a minimum of 30 minutes.
- The context of observation: Ideally, when assessing a child's language and communication development, a child should be observed in a number of situations (at school, at home, with different people). However, when only one direct observation is possible, it is important to arrange a setting that will allow for the largest and most representative sample possible. The interactions should be as

relaxed and natural as possible and should not be designed to test the child or to elicit specific words or linguistic structures. Less structured conversational settings elicit more language and more complex language structures.

- Open-ended questions: When questions are used, they should be open-ended and not yes–no questions, which tend to elicit single-word responses. Questions (even yes–no questions) followed with a request of "tell me about it" are helpful in eliciting stories of personal experience.
- The site of the recording session: Young children are usually more likely to talk freely and use more grammatically complex linguistic constructions when they are in a familiar environment. The area should be quiet to ensure that all data are obtained.
- Participants in the recording session: When recording young children, it is usually best to have the caregiver in the room. Other participants, as siblings or friends, may be problematic; their speech may mask the speech of the target child, which will pose some difficulties on the examiner later in the analysis.
- Interactive situations: Some of the richest interactive and linguistic situations may be embedded in a range of daily activities including bathing, cooking, eating, and playing outdoors. Noise factors, such as running water, TV, washing machine, or cooking noises in the background may mask the child's speech and make it difficult for the examiner to later analyze the data. The interactive situation should be in a quieter room in the house with quieter activities. One could begin by presenting one or two toys that may be of interest to the child but keeping it at a distance to create a situation in which the child has to request the toy or initiate interaction with the clinician. If the child does not initiate interaction, simple questions with choices (e.g., "Which would you like to play with first?" or "Do you want to play with the ball or the car?") can be presented.
- Props: If the child is not talkative, you may want to prepare some toys or props in advance that will help you elicit the speech sample. You may want to consult with the caregiver regarding the child's interests.
- Different types of equipment: Speech samples can be collected using an audio recorder or video camera. Some of the benefits in using videotaping over audio recording are the ability to capture the interactive situation (the props, location, stimulation in the environment), observe the interactive roles the child and caregiver are taking (initiating or following), and observe nonlinguistic aspects (body language, gestures, and facial expression), which are particularly important when assessing a prelinguistic child. For example, a child may point to something in the room with or without vocalizations (but without using a specific word), showing developmental abilities for joint reference, request for action, or labeling. This would be difficult if not impossible to capture using audio recording.

  Clinicians should consider supplementing the videotaping with audiotaping to ensure a high-quality sample for later analysis. In addition, ensure that the caregiver has provided permission to record the child.

General Recommendations

- Limit questions significantly. Commenting often yields longer responses from the child. A comment such as, "There are so many trains" may result in more language than, "What is that?"
- Make sure you do not talk over the child and that no conversation between you and the caregiver are taking place during recordings. Any questions to the caregiver should be addressed before or after recordings take place.
- If the child is irritated or tired, do not insist on recording; try another day. You may not get a representative speech and language sample in these situations. If another session is not possible, make sure that you note the child's behaviors in your write-up.
- The child may show interest in or be distracted initially with the recording device. You can show the child the camera and allow him or her to act in front of it for a short time. In fact, the audio or video recorder motivates some children to talk when used as a radio or TV show. Slowly try to take the child's attention from the camera by introducing new props.
- A child in the first-word or two-word stage may sometimes be unintelligible when referring to something or may use portions of the words to refer to items (e.g., *da da* for *daddy* or *ba ba* for *bottle*). If you understand from the context what is the referent the child refers to or if the child

points, holds, or reaches the referent, you can repeat the child's utterance or name the referent out loud so you will have this information later for the analysis. For example, after the child says "ba ba" (requesting the bottle on the shelf), you can expand and clarify, "Bottle? You want the bottle?" which will signal you later in the analysis to the referent and the child's intention.

Once the language sample is obtained, it is necessary to transcribe the sample in a manner that will facilitate analysis.

Transcribing the Language Sample

This section is adapted from Bloom and Lahey (1978), Retherford (2000), and Shipley and McAfee (2009).

- Transcribe any and all speech produced by the child in standard English. Include single words, partial words, word approximations, phrases, and sentences. Transcribe all of the utterances produced by the examiner or other adult present in a separate column. Indicate the play context for each utterance or group of utterances in another column. A chart, such as the one that follows, may be used for this purpose.
- Number each of the child's utterances consecutively as they are produced in the sample.
- Transcribe words produced as a single unit as one word (*gimme* for *give me* should be one word).
- Transcribe unclear words, partial words, or word approximations using the International Phonetic Alphabet.
- A slash (/) mark is generally used to mark the end of an utterance.
- A question mark should be used to indicate a question by either the adult or the child. When a child uses a rising intonation to indicate a question, use an upward arrow (↑).
- Use a dot to indicate a short pause within an utterance.
- Use a line (_) to indicate when the child stops in the middle of an utterance either due to his or her own interruption or another speaker's interruption.
- Use three Xs (XXX) to indicate an unintelligible utterance. Transcribe using the International Phonetic Alphabet or provide a description or context for the utterance.

Sample Transcription Chart

In the first column, transcribe the utterance number, which will be beneficial to have readily available when determining mean length of utterance (MLU), discussed in greater detail later. In the second column, the child's utterance is transcribed. Ideally, it is best to transcribe both phonetically and orthographically to perform the phonological and morphosyntactic analyses with greater ease. Including a column that describes the context is advantageous in that it aids in analyzing the referents against the objects in the environment. Providing information on the adult utterance adds to the context of the child's utterances and can help measure pragmatic language skills, such as how often the child initiates conversation, how relevant his or her responses are to the adult, as well as the child's overall receptive language skills.

SAMPLE TRANSCRIPTION CHART

Number	*Child's Utterance*	*Play Situation/ Context*	*Adult Utterance*

Analysis of Spontaneous Language Samples

Once the sample has been transcribed, the sample is analyzed according to semantics (language content), morphology, syntax, and phonology (language form) and pragmatics (language use).

Semantic Analysis

Semantics is defined as a specific rule system that governs the meaning or the content of words and word combinations. First words typically emerge at approximately 12 months of age, with word combinations being produced between 18 to 24 months of age. These word combinations create new meanings through the relationship between the words. Therefore, if the context supports this, an utterance from a child, such as "Mommy shoe" indicates possession. There are a number of methods of analyzing and interpreting the child's mastery of words and word combinations.

Word combinations can be analyzed according to the types of semantic relations represented in the language sample. Table 8-5 provides a list of the most common types of word combinations produced by children at approximately 18 months and older, followed by definitions of the semantic categories.

By 36 months of age, the child is also coding conjoined sentences that include the semantic categories

Table 8-5. Examples of Two-Word Utterances Using Brown's Prevalent Semantic Relations

Rule	*Utterance*
Recurrent + X*	More cup
Action + Object	Find mitten, cook pizza
Agent + Action	Car crash
X + Locative	Look here
X + Dative	Give mommy
Negative + X	No juice
Possessor + Possession	Daddy shoe
Attributive + Entity	Big ball
Semantic Categories	
Action	Movement or activity some agent is doing
Agent	The person or noun performing the action
Locative	The place where an object is located or moved
Object	The thing that receives the action
Demonstrative	Use of pronouns or adjectives to draw attention or point out (this, that, there, look, and see)
Recurrence	Requesting "more" or an event to reoccur
Possessor	The person to which the object belongs
Quantifier	The amount or number of an item
Recipient	The person who receives the object
Dative	The person or object to whom something is given
Entity	A label for a person or object without the action involved
Negation	Any negative meaning including objects not present or not wanting an object or action to occur

*X is typically a noun or a verb.

Adapted from Brown (1973).

of additive, temporal, and causal relationships. In addition to examining the relationship between words, it is important to examine the diversity of words produced. Children with language impairment often present with a limited vocabulary, with particular difficulty with verbs, adjectives, and abstract words (e.g., words that describe emotional states). Often, nondescript words such as *thing* and *stuff* may be substituted for nouns, and general all-purpose verbs (GAP verbs) such as "He's doing the cake" instead of "He's baking the cake" are substituted for specific verbs.

After age 3 years, some children may not only show difficulty in vocabulary knowledge (deficits in both comprehension and production of words), but also in word retrieval. This is a transient inability to retrieve already known words from the lexicon. The characteristics of **word retrieval deficits** include repetitions (the, the, the), substitutions (nurse for doctor), pauses, the use of nonspecific words such as thing (Faust, Dimitrovsky, & Davidi, 1997), expressing the function or description of the word (cutting thing for scissors) and circuitous responses.

Morphosyntactic Analysis

One important analysis in this area is that of MLU. The MLU is the average length of the child's utterance as calculated by the number of morphemes.

The following *Guidelines for Determining MLU From a Spontaneous Speech Sample* are adapted from Paul and Norbury (2011):

1. Transcribe the child's entire sample using a new line for each utterance.
2. Use the first 50 consecutive utterances. Delete any utterance that is unintelligible. Only count utterances that are produced the first time. A repetition is counted only one time, unless the word is repeated for emphasis (i.e., "no, no, not that one"—five morphemes).
3. Count each free morpheme (single words) as one. Count each bound morpheme (plural s, ed, ing...) as one. Compound words (bedroom), proper nouns (Cookie Monster), and reduplicated words (bye-bye) are counted as one. Fillers and interjections (um, uh) are not counted but words like yeah and uh-oh are counted as one morpheme.
4. Count irregular past tense verbs (gave, came) as one morpheme. However, the immature use of the regular -ed ending as in goed is counted as two morphemes, but the incorrect addition of -ed to the irregular form (roded) is only counted as one.
5. Auxiliary verbs are counted as one morpheme (is, are, was, have, can, should, etc.) unless they are contracted (*he's* is counted as two), except for *can't* and *don't*, which each count as one.
6. Words with diminutive endings (doggie) count as one morpheme.
7. Finally, add up the total number of morphemes in the sample and divide by the total number of

Table 8-6. Brown's Stages

Stage	Age (Months)	Mean Length of Utterance
I	12 to 26	1.0 to 2.0
II	27 to 30	2.0 to 2.5
III	31 to 34	2.5 to 3.0
IV	35 to 40	3.0 to 3.75
V	41 to 46+	3.75 to 4.5

utterances (usually 50 or 100). The resultant number is the MLU. For example, a child who produces 256 morphemes across 100 utterances has an MLU of 2.56.

$$\frac{\text{Total number morphemes}}{\text{Total number of utterances}} \quad \frac{256}{100} = 2.56$$

Note that MLU should never be used as the sole diagnostic instrument to assess language impairment. Rather, it is an integral part of the child's expressive language (Paul, 2007).

Brown (1973) created a list of developmental stages that correspond to a child's MLU at various ages (Table 8-6).

Once the MLU has been calculated, the next step is to analyze the morphosyntactic productions of the child. Children with morphosyntactic deficits will inconsistently produce grammatical morphemes, more frequently omitting them in **obligatory contexts** (contexts in which a specific word or grammatical form should occur). Table 8-7 presents a list of Brown's 14 morphemes and the ages of acquisition for each (Brown, 1973). MLU is less reliable after age 3 years (Owens, 2008).

Morphological analysis would include a detailed review of the language sample assessing the obligatory contexts (when a particular grammatical morpheme is expected to be used; Table 8-8). For example, the irregular past tense (went, sat) appearing in a young child's language at 25 to 46 months not be given credit for the obligatory context "went" because the child used the overgeneralized regular past -ed instead. A simple chart may be created that lists the preceding morphemes in one column, the obligatory contexts (note the utterance number where a grammatical morpheme should have been produced) in the next column, its actual use in the third column, and the percentage of correct productions in the fourth column. This enables the clinician to calculate the percentage of authentic production for each grammatical morpheme (see Table 8-8).

Table 8-7. Brown's Fourteen Morphemes and Ages of Acquisition

Order of Appearance	Morpheme	Example	Age of Mastery (Months)
1	Present progressive *ing*	Baby *crying*	19 to 28
2 and 3	Prepositions (in, on)	*in* car, *on* table	27 to 30
4	Regular plural	toys	24 to 33
5	Irregular past	went, sat	25 to 46
6	Possessive	Mommy's car	26 to 40
7	Uncontractible copula	Mommy got angry	27 to 39
8	Articles	*a, the*	28 to 46
9	Regular past -ed	*jumped, poured*	26 to 48
10	Regular third person s	Daddy walks	26 to 46
11	Irregular third person	*does, has*	28 to 50
12	Uncontractible auxiliary	He *was* cooking	29 to 48
13	Contractible copula	*He's* happy	29 to 49
14	Contractible auxiliary	I'm going	30 to 50

Adapted from Brown (1973).

Table 8-8. Morphological Analysis

Grammatical Morpheme	Obligatory Context	Child's Production	% Correct

Syntax

Syntax is defined as the rules that govern word, phrase, and clause order in a sentence. It includes sentence organization and the relationship between words as well as which word combinations are acceptable and which are not.

When analyzing the syntax of a child, it is important to look at both the variety and complexity of the sentences produced. According to Miller (1981), there are five key aspects to this sentence structure analysis.

Table 8-9. Development of Communicative Intentions

Age (Months)	*Intention*
8	Preverbal language to communicate the following intentions: attention-seeking, requesting, greeting, protesting, informing
12	Emergence of first true words
12 to 24	Begin to infer the intentions of others and may begin to take turns in a verbal interaction (Pence & Justice, 2008)
24 to 36	Heuristic (using language top explore and categorize), imaginative (using language during play), and informative (using language to share knowledge with others) communicative intents emerge (Halliday, 1975), as well as the ability to change a topic, clarify, and request clarification

1. Increased progression of noun phrases from a single noun phrase standing alone to a complex noun phrase that includes articles, demonstratives, and pronouns
2. Increased progression of verb phrases to include auxiliary verbs, copulas, past tense, and subject–verb agreement
3. Use of negative sentences
4. Ability to produce yes–no questions
5. Use of complex sentences

Children with language impairment tend to produce shorter utterances, incomplete and disorganized sentences, a higher percentage of noun phrases compared with verb or adjective phrases, restricted sentence types, and limited use of morphological markers and correct pronouns. Verbal children on the autism spectrum have a great deal of difficulty with syntax, particularly with proper use of pronouns (e.g., he, she, it) and negatives (e.g., not, no).

Phonology

Phonology is defined as the sound system of the language and the rules that govern how those sounds may be combined to form meaningful units. The language sample can provide information on a child's phonetic inventory (total number of sounds produced), syllable shape structure, and error patterns. The error patterns can be analyzed to determine the presence of a phonological or articulation disorder. Children at 2 years of age who demonstrate limited verbal output with few varying sound productions require a full evaluation to determine the source of the difficulty. Difficulties in phonetic or phonological productions impact not only intelligibility of speech, but also have a trickle down effect on vocabulary output, and later, reading development. See Chapter 7 for a full review.

Pragmatic Language Skills

Pragmatic language skills are defined as the rules that govern the use of language in context such that meaning is created from the combination of the utterance and the social setting in which it occurs (Pence & Justice, 2008). Pragmatics also includes the study of speaker and listener interactions, and it covers the rules of conversation, narrative, discourse, and repair. Preschool-age children are only just beginning to learn the complex rules of conversation. These skills develop more fully as the child progresses through the school-age years.

Pragmatic skills develop as young children mature and as their language grows. Early infant pragmatic skills are nonlinguistic in nature and include eye gaze and becoming familiar with caregivers. By 8 months of age, the child may use preverbal language skills to communicate the following intents: attention-seeking, requesting, greeting, protesting, and informing. The first true words emerge at approximately 12 months of age and are often accompanied by gestures that assist in communicating these intents. From 12 to 24 months, toddlers begin to infer the intentions of others and may begin to take turns in a verbal interaction (Pence & Justice, 2008). This can be seen when a caregiver and child sing a song together. The caregiver may begin a song and then stop as the child produces a phrase from the song. From 24 to 36 months, the **heuristic** (using language top explore and categorize), **imaginative** (using language during play), and **informative** (using language to share knowledge with others) communicative intents emerge (Halliday, 1975), as well as the ability to change a topic, clarify, and request clarification. See Table 8-9 for a summary of the development of communicative intentions.

As language skills progress, preschoolers begin to gain knowledge of **discourse skills**. Discourse skills involve the use of language in larger units than a

Table 8-10. Primitive Speech Acts

Speech Act	*Description*	*Example*
Labeling	A word or a prosodic pattern that function as a label and is produced while attending to an object	The child picks up a toy horse and says, "horsey."
Repeating	A word or prosodic pattern that repeats part of the adult utterance	The caregiver stands up and says, "Let's have some cookies." The child in response says, "kiki" (for cookies).
Answering	A word used to respond to an adult question	The caregiver asks the child, "Do you want some cookies?" and the child answers "Ya."
Requesting action	A word or a prosodic pattern that functions as a request for an action	The child stretches his or her arms up to the caregiver and says "uppi."
Requesting an answer	A word that functions as a request for an answer	The child holds up a toy, looks at the caregiver, and says "dog?" asking the caregiver for conformation of the label.
Calling	A word used to obtain another's attention	The child is in bed and calls for his mother, "ma."
Greeting	A word used to mark arrival or leaving	The child is being put to bed by his mom and says, "ni, ni" (for night-night).
Protesting	A word or a prosodic pattern used to express disapproval of or dislike for an object or action	The child protests his mother's attempt to wipe his face by saying, "no."

Adapted from Owens (2016).

sentence. For young children, the components of discourse are conversations and narratives. As preschoolers (36 to 60 months) begin to learn the rules of conversation, they gain an understanding of the knowledge that a listener might implicitly have, their feelings in reference to the topic, and their role in the conversation. This skill includes **presupposition**, in which the speaker assumes or takes into account the background knowledge of a given topic of the listener. For example, if the speaker says, "Do you want to play again?" the presupposition is that the child has already played the game at least one time. By age 3 years, children learn to take more than two turns in a conversation, and they begin to produce utterances that are contingent on the conversational partners responses. They also begin to recognize and verbally repair a breakdown in conversation and learn how to adjust their utterances in length, complexity, and intonation to the listener.

Children with language impairment often have difficulty initiating, maintaining, and appropriately ending conversations and social interactions. They initiate interactions less frequently, have difficulty repairing conversational breakdowns, interject at inappropriate times, and change topics abruptly. Use and comprehension of changes of vocal tone, body posture, and facial expressions to convey meaning or emotions are of great difficulty as well. Each of these areas should be included in an evaluation.

Assessment of pragmatic skills in the prelinguistic stage are as follows:

- Maintenance of eye contact; following of eye gaze
- Turn-taking skills
- Joint attention and joint action
- Initiation of play
- The use of gestures—pointing, reaching, yes–no, bye-bye
- The use of facial expressions to reflect intent
- The use of pragmatic functions such as protesting
    - Three categories of pragmatic functions develop during the first year of life:
        1. Behavioral regulation: Controlling another's behavior to get him or her to perform an action (giving a bottle, manipulating a toy)
        2. Social interaction: Getting another's attention for social purposes (playing peek-a-boo, showing off)
        3. Joint attention: Directing another's attention to establish a shared focus on an activity, object, or person

Assessment of pragmatic skills in the first-word stage includes the assessment of Primitive Speech Acts (PSA; Table 8-10), which are single words or single prosodic patterns that function to convey the child's intentions before he acquires sentences (Owens, 2016).

Table 8-11. Conversational Acts

Conversational Act	*Description*	*Example*
Requests	Utterances used to request information, action, or acknowledgment, including yes–no questions, wh- questions, clarification questions, action requests, permission requests, and rhetorical questions that seek acknowledgment from the listener	The child reaches his or her hand and says, "Want cup."
Responses to requests	Utterances following requests and respond directly to the request, including yes–no answers, wh- answers, clarifications that supply relevant repetition, compliance that verbally express acceptance, denial, or acknowledgment for prior request	The mother is looking for the child's shoes and asks, "Where are the shoes?" The child answers, "No shoes."
Descriptions and statements	Utterances used to describe events, actions, properties, traits or conditions, rules, attitudes, feelings, and beliefs; expressions of locations or directions and reports of time	Mother and child are building a tower with blocks and the child says, "These are the ones we need."
Acknowledgment	Utterances used to indicate recognition of responses and non-requests: approvals/disapproval, agreement/disagreements not in response for requests	The mother says to the child, "I'm going to put the toy in the closet," and the child answers, "OK" (the child's utterance indicates acceptance of the mother's action).
Organizational devices	Utterances that regulate conversation, including boundary markers that indicate openings, closing, and other significant points in the conversation; speaker selection that explicitly indicates the speaker of the next turn; politeness markers and soliciting attention	The child sees his or her mother in the morning and says, "Good morning" (this greeting regulates the conversation).
Performatives	Utterances that are accomplished by being said, including protests against the listener's behavior, jokes, warnings, and teases	The mother attempts to wipe the child's face and the child says, "Don't do it."

Adapted from Owens (2016).

Assessment of pragmatic skills in the multiword stage includes the assessment of conversational acts (Table 8-11), which consist of the conceptual information (what the utterance means), the grammatical structure, and the speaker's intention regarding how the utterance is perceived by the listener (Owens, 2016).

Narratives

Narratives or stories are extended monologues about a particular topic. They include retelling a familiar story, attempting to describe a movie or television show or relating a personal experience or event. Between the ages of 2 and 3 years, children begin to tell short narratives that are linked to a central event. However, they generally do not consider the listener such that there is no introduction or setting the scene, no specific description of the characters involved, and no clear ending. By age 4 years, preschoolers have developed a general method of sequencing the events in a narrative. As they reach their fifth birthday, there is evidence of greater complexity in the narrative.

A sample of a narrative is a useful addition to the informal assessment as it provides information on a child's ability to organize information, his or her attention to relevant details, and his or her morphological and syntactic abilities (Scott & Windsor, 2000). Narratives can be obtained from children using sequencing cards and wordless books or having children describe routine events and personal experiences. They may be elicited one of two ways: through story generation and story retelling. In story generation, a child is provided with a book or picture cards and is asked to independently generate a story. In story retelling, the child is read a story by the clinician. The child is then asked to retell the story. In either case, the story topics selected must be age and culturally appropriate for the child (Miller et al., 2005).

Westby (2005) discussed two approaches for assessing a child's narrative ability (1) comprehension-based measures and (2) production-based measures. The authors state that the tasks selected for narrative production tap into different processes. In the case

Table 8-12. Story Grammar Analysis

Story Grammar Element	*Description*
Setting	Reference to time and place, usually including the introduction of one or more characters
Initiating event or problem	Complication sets the event of the story in motion including a problem that requires a solution
Internal response	How the character feels in response to the initiating event; usually contains an emotion word
Internal plan	A statement of an idea that might fix the problem
Attempt	Some action taken by the main character that is meant to solve the problem; there may be several attempts without a statement of consequence before the end of the story
Consequence	Event(s) following the attempt and causally linked to it; there may be several consequences of an attempt
Resolution or reaction	The final state or situation triggered by the initiating event; it does not cause or lead to other actions or states
Ending	A statement or phrase that clearly states the story is over

of comprehension-based measures, which examine a child's ability to comprehend a story's schema, a child may be required to look at a wordless picture book and asked to "tell the story." However, this task automatically provides the child with the structure and organization required to produce the story. Therefore, the child does not have to generate this on his or her own.

Another example of a comprehension-based task would involve eliciting the narrative through specific questions and prompts such as, "Why do you think the girl is crying?" or "Tell me what's happening in this picture." The main information gained from such tasks is a child's understanding of main characters and events in a story and how they relate to one another. Inferencing abilities, predictions, and understanding of causal events can also be assessed through such tasks. Similar to other receptive/expressive language tasks, however, children often may perform better with these types of narrative measures. Therefore, it is important to also elicit a narrative in a less structured context to get a true representation of their production.

Narrative production can be more accurately assessed through tasks that provide less context to a child. Rather than providing a full wordless picture book, which depicts all main events for a child, using more "open-ended" tools, such a few toys, a single picture, or a verbal story prompt ("tell me about your favorite sport"), more accurately taps into a child's true narrative production ability. This allows the clinician to examine a child's ability to sequence events and include all relevant story elements and grammar in his or her narrative. The child's narrative production can be evaluated on the basis of macrostructure, the cohesion of the narrative (which is detailed later in the chapter), and microstructure, which is the examination of individual linguistic units (such as morphological analyses discussed earlier in the chapter). For a more detailed explanation, see Chapter 10.

There are several methods of story grammar analysis available; however, two of the most commonly employed analyses include story grammar analysis (Jones & Lodholz, 1999; Stein & Glenn, 1979) and Applebee's six levels of narrative development (Applebee, 1978). The story grammar analysis allows the clinician to identify elements that must be present for a complete story (Table 8-12).

Under the story grammar model, the narrative is scored as *proficient* (proficient use of all elements was demonstrated), *emerging* (emerging use requiring prompts or inconsistent use of elements), or *immature/minimal* (immature use where the child leaves out elements).

An alternative approach for narrative analysis is Applebee's (1978) six levels of narrative development (Table 8-13).

Summary of narrative assessment:

- Comprehension of story schema and story knowledge can be obtained though the following methods:
  - Use of wordless picture books, sequencing cards
  - Asking wh- questions and providing prompts for additionally information
  - Children may sometimes perform well on these tasks but will have difficulties in providing narratives in less structured contexts, which more directly tap into their production

Table 8-13. Applebee's Six Levels of Narrative Development

Level	*Age of Emergence (Years)*	*Description*
Heaps	2	• Few links form one sentence to another • Primarily labels and descriptions of events and actions • No central theme • No organization • Sentences are usually simple declaratives
Sequences	2 to 3	• Labeling and descriptions around a central theme or character • There is no plot to the story • The events in the story do not necessarily follow a temporal or causal sequence
Primitive narratives	3 to 4	• There is a central event, theme, or character • Contain three of the story grammar elements: an initiating event, an attempt or action, and some consequence around the central theme. • There is no real resolution or ending and little evidence of what motivates the characters
Unfocused chains	4 to 4.5	• There is evidence of cause-and-effect and temporal relationships • The ending does not really follow logically from the events, and may be very abrupt • Contains four story grammar elements: initiating event, attempt or action, some consequences around a central theme, and some notion of a plan or character motivation
Focused chains	5	• The center is a main character who experiences a series of events, but nothing abstract to indicate a true concept
True narratives	5 to 7	• There is a central theme, character, and plot • Includes the motivations behind the characters' actions as well as logical and temporally ordered sequences of events • Contains at least five story grammar elements: initiating event, an attempt or action, consequence, and an ending with a resolution to the problem

- Assessment of production of narratives can be determined by the following:
    - Using single pictures or toys as prompts and asking the child to create a story based on those props
    - Providing the child with a topic for a story

Informal Assessment of Receptive Language

Assessment of receptive language skills requires the clinician to determine whether the child comprehends language independently or requires **visual support**.

Assessment of comprehension skills entails determining whether the child understands receptive vocabulary, has knowledge of receptive language concepts, understands syntax and morphology, and processes language:

- Receptive vocabulary: Understanding of single words. Can the child point to an object when it is named, choose an object from of field of three (discrimination), point to a picture when it is named, and discriminate among three or four pictures?
- Understanding of receptive language concepts: Concepts are broader than single words; they generally encompass an idea that combines several elements from different sources into a single notion (e.g., size: big, little, tall, short; attributes (descriptions): colors, shapes; spatial relations (prepositions): in, on, under, next to; negatives: no, not, none; quantity: one, all, some, many, few). However, children must learn the vocabulary associated with each concept.

- Understanding the syntax of a sentence and the grammar, including morphology: Syntax is the order ("The boy ran home" does not mean the same thing as "The home ran boy." Morphology is the grammatical markers that change meaning, such as -s, -ed, and -ing. A section on grammar in terms of expressive language is discussed later. For now, we are talking about understanding the difference when word order changes and understanding how different morphological markers change meaning.
- Auditory processing: The ability to understand what we hear, to act on the message, and what we do with what we hear. This includes following directions that may have concepts embedded ("Get the green ball under the table"); understanding questions and the difference between questions ("Who is laughing?" does not mean "Why is he laughing?"); and following the flow of conversation, understanding the words, phrases, and sentences so other skills such as forming a response can operate.

A battery of formal tests may be used to assess each individual area; however, informal assessments and informal observations of test behaviors provide the examiner with the ability to ascertain whether the child is processing language. Informal measures that are not always presented on formal tests for young children might include differentiating how the child responds with and without visual cues. Tasks should begin with no visual support. If the child does not respond, varying levels of support may be provided, although it is imperative that the examiner make note of the varying levels of cues. Some of these cues include stimulus repetition, providing additional processing time, or even pointing at visual images. Following directions with both objects and using crayon and paper activities that are not visually self-explanatory may allow for the discovery of this information. For example, if you give a child a ball and ask him or her to throw it, that is visually self-explanatory. If you ask the child to roll the ball under a chair, that is not visually self-explanatory and requires some measure of language comprehension. It is also necessary to determine whether the child's comprehension difficulties are a result of issues working with memory.

Hierarchy for Receptive Language

The following task hierarchy is in a following directions format, written as instructional objectives, and is for language ages of 9 months to 5 years. The hierarchy can be used to assess receptive vocabulary knowledge, understanding of receptive language concepts, and understanding or processing of "larger chunks" of language.

1. Child will identify three objects from a set of five by pointing.
2. Child will follow "give me" command using familiar play materials.
3. Child will follow simple one-step direction using action words (e.g., "kick the ball," "push the car").
4. Child will follow one-step + attribute direction (color, size, shape).
5. Child will follow one-step + spatial direction.
6. Child will follow one-step + object function direction (category/description).
7. Child will follow one-step + negative direction (although often does not stand alone).
8. Child will follow one-step + quantity direction.
9. Child will follow one-step + attribute + spatial direction.
10. Child will follow one-step + attribute + spatial + object function

May start two-step directions here; base this on individual child.

11. Child will follow one-step + attribute + spatial + object function + negative.
12. Child will follow one-step + attribute + spatial + object function + negative + quantity direction
13. Child will follow two-step + object + action directions ("Push the car and bring it back").
14. Child will follow two-step + (follow the previous pattern until child will follow two-step + attribute + spatial + object function + negative + quantity direction).

Child must be able to follow a variety of these combinations in play, then in a structured context with crayons and pictures.

Example: two-step + attribute + spatial = "Put a green circle around the car and a red X under the airplane."

Example: two-step + attribute + spatial + negative + object function = "Put a yellow X under the vehicle but not the car, and a green square around the food but not the hamburger."

By age 5 years, children are able to follow these directions with embedded concepts such as time (before and after) and sequence/order (first in line, last in line).

Understanding Questions

In addition to following directions, the child's ability to answer questions is also critical. This information can be obtained from play context ("What are you cooking?"; "Who are you giving the sandwich to?") and a shared book reading with questions posed following each segment of reading. Questions follow a hierarchy as well and include Yes/No, Who, simple What (what + noun phrase), Where, more complex What ("What else can we do?"; "What will happen if…?"), Why, and then How ("How do you know?").

Sample Report Case History

John is a 3-year-old boy who was evaluated for speech and language deficits. He is an only child. His parents' primary concerns are regarding the intelligibility of his speech and his inability to express himself effectively. John has received home-based speech-language services for approximately 9 months through Early Intervention. He is attending a preschool; however, his teachers have voiced concerns about his language development in terms of production and comprehension.

Assessment Procedures and Rationale

The following assessment measures were selected for John's case history. A corresponding rationale is provided for each assessment selection.

- Audiological screening
  - To rule out the influence of hearing loss on language development
  - This examination should be conducted on all clients regardless of disorder
- Oral-peripheral speech mechanism examination
  - To assess the structural and functional integrity of the speech mechanism
  - This examination should be conducted on all clients regardless of disorder
- Parent interview
  - To obtain full case history/developmental history for child
  - Determine parent concerns and perception of problem
  - Determine parental involvement attitude and motivation
- The PLS-5
  - To formally assess the child's auditory comprehension and expressive language skills
- A language sample was elicited through play
  - A naturalistic language sample analysis is an essential component of a speech-language evaluation for a preschool-age child (Paul, 2007)
- Play analysis
  - Play is a natural window into a child's development (Almodòvar & Levey, 2017; Owens, 2016).
  - Play provides an opportunity to compare cognitive level to language level. This provides important information with respect to diagnosis and therapy (Owens, 2016).
  - Play is a nonthreatening, low-pressure, child-friendly assessment medium (Owens, 2016).
- Developmental norms were used to analyze the language and play samples.

Instructional Writing Rubric for Formal Language Section of the Diagnostic Report

Writing Rubric for Formal Language Section of the Diagnostic Report

☐ Introductory statement to include name of test in full (underlined) and in abbreviated form in parentheses (not underlined)

Example: Language was formally assessed through the administration of the Preschool Language Scale-5 (PLS-5).

☐ Test construct (What it purports to measure)

Example: The PLS-5 is a norm-referenced instrument that measures receptive (auditory comprehension) and expressive language skills in children from 0 to 6;0 years.

☐ Elicitation procedures (Describe where appropriate)

Example: The Auditory Comprehension subtest requires the child to demonstrate vocabulary comprehension by pointing to pictures and follow simple and complex directives, using familiar objects and toys. The Expressive Communication subtest has the child label pictures and objects and assesses his or her production while responding to simple questions and in spontaneous speech.

☐ General quantification of results in paragraph form (derived scores from standardized test)

Example: John scored a standard score of 21 on the Auditory Comprehension subtest, yielding a standard score of 71 and percentile rank of 3. This score is two standard deviations (SDs) below the mean, indicating a significant receptive language delay. On the Expressive Communication subtest, he scored a raw score of 14, yielding a standard score of 55, and percentile rank of 1. This score is three SDs below the mean, indicating a significant expressive language delay.

☐ General quantification of results in table form

Table 1. PLS-5 Summary of Scores

Subtest	*Standard Score*	*Percentile Rank*
Auditory comprehension	71	3
Expressive communication	55	1

☐ Qualification in narrative form

Example: Results of the Auditory Comprehension and Expressive Communication subtests of the PLS-5 indicate a significant, mixed expressive–receptive language delay. This was characterized by John's difficulties in identifying and producing words that referred to animals, common household objects, and body parts. His productions were predominantly single words, with rare two-word combinations. John demonstrated difficulty in following simple, two- and three-step directives.

Sample Report

John Doe **D.O.E.**: 5/29/06 **Age**: 3;0 years old
123 Main Street **D.O.B.**: 5/15/03
New York, NY 10016
Language: English

I. Reason for Referral

John Doe, a 3-year-old boy, was seen at the Speech & Language Center for a complete speech-language evaluation. John was referred and accompanied to the center by his mother, Heather Doe. Mrs. Doe expressed concerns over the intelligibility of John's speech, his difficulties expressing himself, and following directions at his nursery school and at home. Mrs. Doe served as the informant and appeared to be concerned and reliable.

II. Tests Administered/Procedures

- Parent Interview
- Audiological Screening
- Oral-Peripheral Speech Mechanism Evaluation
- Preschool Language Scale-5 (PLS-5)
- Informal measures and clinical observations performed in the home setting
- Play Analysis
- Language Sample Analysis

III. Background Information

Birth and Developmental History

Mrs. Doe's pregnancy with John was unremarkable until approximately the 30th week, at which point she experienced contractions and was placed on bed rest. John was born full-term via cesarean delivery because the umbilical cord wrapped around his neck during labor. His postnatal medical history is unremarkable, and he is reportedly in good health.

Developmental milestones were achieved within a typical range: crawled at 10 months, sat at 5 months, walked at 10 to 13 months, and his first word ("dada") was uttered at 11 months. He does not have a history of feeding difficulties.

Health History

John has seasonal allergies. He has no history of recurring ear infections. An audiological evaluation performed in August 2005 reported his hearing as within normal limits.

Family/Social History

John currently lives with his parents, Carl Doe and Heather Doe. He is cared for during the daytime by his mother, who served as the reliable informant. The only language John is exposed to is English. Mrs. Doe reports that in English, John is producing short sentences to request (e.g., "I want orange juice please."), to protest ("You stop now!"), and to request ("I need shoes."). Mrs. Doe states that John's speech continues to be difficult to understand. In addition, on the basis of the final progress report through early intervention, John continued to demonstrate delayed use and comprehension of language.

Educational History

John is currently attending a nursery school three afternoons per week. His teachers have reported concerns regarding John's willingness to engage and participate during group activities. He reportedly becomes "nervous" or shy when he is required to perform in front of others after a directive. His observed verbal output at school is reduced in comparison to observed verbalizations within his home.

Therapeutic History

John has received home-based speech-language services for approximately 9 months through Early Intervention.

IV. Clinical Observations

Behavior

John is a happy, sweet, engaging child. He initiates and maintains appropriate eye contact. Although he does not consistently actively participate in activities, John observes actions and play routines with minimal prompting. When directed to carry through directives, he often shook his head "no" and responded, "You do it."

Because of John's reluctance to follow through directives, he was not responsive to many of the probe questions. Midway through the session, he sought out his mother. He did not initiate play, but with mild to moderate prompting, he observed the examiner's actions and passively participated in play, with frequent activity changes.

Audiological Screening

John received an audiological evaluation in August 2005. Hearing was determined to be within normal limits. He has no reported history of recurring ear infections. John responds appropriately to speech delivered at a typical conversational level.

Oral-Peripheral Speech Mechanism Examination

A full oral-peripheral examination could not be performed. Informal assessment determined appropriate extension, elevation, and depression of tongue. Facial features appear to be symmetrical and functional for speech.

Articulation

Intelligibility of John's speech was judged to be fair. John demonstrated the following phonological processes during spontaneous speech: Final consonant deletion (cah for cat, no for nose) and weak syllable deletion (ephant for elephant). These are whole-word processes that should be extinguished by age 3. It is recommended that these processes be monitored and targeted within the upcoming months because their presence affects John's intelligibility.

Language Skills

The PLS-5, a norm-referenced instrument for children 0 to 6;11 years of age, was administered to assess receptive and expressive language skills. Following are the standard scores, based on a mean of 100, and SD of 15.

Table 1. PLS-5 Summary of Scores

Subtest **Mean = 100; SD = 15**	*Standard Score*	*Percentile Rank*
Auditory comprehension	70	2
Expressive communication	68	2
Total language	73	4

Auditory Comprehension

On the Auditory Comprehension subtest of the PLS-5, John received a standard score of 70, placing him at a percentile rank of 2 (mean = 100; SD = 25), and at 2.0 SDs below the mean. His scores indicated deficits in auditory comprehension of spoken information.

John had difficulty following one- and two-step directives, particularly during formal testing. When asked to point to a picture, he either did not respond or shook his head while saying, "No, no, you do it." During identification of pictures, where John was required to point to a picture that matched the provided label (i.e., "Show me cookie"), John was largely unresponsive. Of six possible pictures, he identified one by pointing (ball). This probe is reported to be a skill containing vocabulary that is typically acquired from 18 to 23 months of age. While this could be indicative of limited comprehension of basic vocabulary, John at other times pointed independently and labeled some of the objects, demonstrating comprehension of these concepts. His resistance to performing actions following directives has been reported in school as well.

John demonstrated comprehension of basic body parts and inhibitory words (i.e., stop, wait). He did not respond to directives that required him to carry out actions (e.g., "The bear is hungry. Give him something to eat."). John's comprehension of nouns is stronger than his comprehension of action words. He demonstrated some difficulty in comprehending descriptive concepts (such as big, small, wet).

Formal and informal assessment demonstrates that John presents with a receptive language delay. It is important to note that John's performance on auditory comprehension tasks varies a great deal and appears to be largely influenced by his willingness to carry through directives at that particular moment. Therefore, the formal test scores need to be viewed with caution.

Expressive Communication

On the Expressive Communication subtest of the PLS-5, John received a standard score of 68, placing him in a percentile rank of 2 (mean = 100; SD = 15), placing him at least 2.0 SDs below the mean, indicating significant expressive language deficits.

John's vocalizations during the evaluation consisted mainly of imitations of the evaluator's statements. He imitated words without prompting. John was more inclined to vocalize, when he was not explicitly told to imitate or produce a word or sound. For example, imitations of words were provided mainly when he spontaneously imitated them, rather than when explicitly asked, "John, can you say *tiger*?"

Similar performance was observed during formal expressive language testing, as on the auditory comprehension portion of the PLS-5. John independently labeled "banana" when presented with a page filled with six pictures. For the remaining five, when asked to label the pictures, he did not respond, asked, "What's that?" or stated, "You do." His expressive vocabulary skills are limited for his age, particularly in his ability to describe actions. He produces mainly nouns to convey messages and produces related words to describe actions (i.e., "night-night" for sleeping).

John spontaneously produced short sentences to request and protest when speaking to his mother. He requested "orange juice" while pointing to the refrigerator. When told that he had to drink water instead, he protested "no water." His mother reported observing longer sentence production (up to four words). John predominantly produced two-word utterances, but he has reportedly produced up to four word sentences, although none were noted during the evaluation. A 50-utterance language sample obtained from John, yielded a MLU of 2.36, corresponding to Brown's Stage II. In addition, John uses visual cues to expand utterances. Formal and informal assessment demonstrates that John presents with an expressive language delay.

Social Communication and Play Skills

Pragmatically, John prefers to perform activities with someone else, in parallel play style, or independently on his own rather than performing through turn-taking. Within the classroom, he reportedly becomes nervous with the anticipation of his turn and refuses to perform during his turn. Similar behaviors were noted the evaluation when a new activity was introduced. Functional use of toys was noted. John used toys as a means of initiating communication or engaging the therapist during the evaluation. A limited amount of exploration of toys was noted.

Fluency

Rate and rhythm were judged to be within normal limits.

Voice

Vocal parameters were subjectively assessed as appropriate.

V. Clinical Impressions

John Doe is a 3-year-old boy who was evaluated for speech and language. The results of today's evaluation supported the linguistic and speech behaviors reported by his mother as well as by school report. John presents with a significant expressive and receptive language delay. It is recommended that speech-language services be continued.

In addition, John's reluctance to perform and follow through directives should be explored further. Although some of this is supported by his language delay, a portion of it could be attributable to nervousness or anxiety. This may affect him academically in the future. Consultation with his school and his SLP determined that his true abilities are not well represented in an academic setting.

VI. Recommendations

It is strongly recommended that John continue to receive speech-language services to address the aforementioned issues with special emphasis on the following:

1. Increasing ability to carry through multistep directives
2. Increasing expressive and receptive vocabulary skills
3. Increasing mean length of utterances

I certify that I personally evaluated the above-mentioned child, employing age-appropriate instruments and procedures as well as informed clinical opinion. I further certify that the findings contained in this report are an accurate representation of the child's level of functioning at the time of my assessment.

____

(Name of clinician or clinical supervisor and credentials)

Speech-Language Pathologist

Practice Exercises

The following practice exercises provide an opportunity to integrate what you have learned in this chapter. The instructional writing rubric and sample report should serve as guides when completing your exercises. These are especially relevant for Practice Exercise 3.

Practice Exercise 1

Read the following summary of a 4;6-year-old boy recently evaluated. Discuss the formal and informal testing measures this clinician used to observe these behaviors. What additional measures could you use to add more information to the linguistic profile outlined in this summary?

Peter is a 4;6-year-old preschooler who exhibits a mild to moderate expressive language impairment. His language was characterized by minimal inclusion of age-expected grammatical elements. The following grammatical morphemes were used inconsistently: present progressive (-ing), plural (s), possessive ('s), contractible and uncontractible copula and auxiliaries (is, are, was, were), prepositions (in, on), regular and irregular past tense verbs (e.g., walked and ate, respectively), and third-person singular(s). He also presented with a limited expressive and receptive vocabulary. He often used nonspecific words and phrases, such as this, that, and over there, to describe objects and locations, and GAP verbs (e.g., go, make, do) to mark actions. Peter's pragmatic skills were typical for his age. He demonstrated eye contact, turn-taking, joint attention, and joint action, and enjoyed playing and interacting with the SLP.

Practice Exercise 2

The following sample is provided for the student to practice preparing for a diagnostic testing session.

Shannon is a 4;8-year-old girl who is enrolled in the local public school preschool program. Mrs. P, Shannon's mother had been concerned about her daughter's slow language growth at age 2;6 years. Shannon struggled to use new words, and her utterance length was not expanding as much as other children her age. The summer before Shannon turned 3, Mrs. P brought her to the local public school district for a complete set of evaluations. Shannon was 2;10 years old when those evaluations took place. The school district evaluated Shannon and concurred with Mrs. P. Shannon was mandated for speech and language therapy twice weekly and additional special education itinerant services in her local mainstream preschool classroom. Shannon made a great deal of progress during the 18 months that she was provided with therapy, and although her mother still felt that she continued to need services, she was unclear about where to place her for kindergarten in the fall. It is now March, and Mrs. P has two choices. Her first choice is the local Catholic parochial school, which has an SLP who provides services at the school 3 days per week. However, there are no other services provided except for extra reading help for second graders 2 days per week. Shannon's brother and sister attend the Catholic school, and Mrs. P is extremely pleased with the education they are receiving. However, she questions whether this is the correct choice for Shannon. Her other choice for Shannon is the local public school, which would provide the option of an integrated program for Shannon, continued itinerant special education services if Shannon still needed it, and the speech therapy that Mrs. P wanted to continue. Mrs. P sought the current evaluation from a private independent agency to (a) assess her daughters current language skills and (b) help her decide whether Shannon would "make it" in a regular classroom with only the speech therapy as her related service.

1. On the basis of this child's age and background, determine which formal test instruments would provide the most information.
2. Which informal assessment measures would you choose?
3. Provide a rationale for each of the instruments and informal measures chosen.

Practice Exercise 3

A father brings his 2;5-year-old child to your office due to concerns about the child's ability to communicate. He states that the child does not seem to understand what he and his mother say to him. He produces about five or six real words and some babble. He is concerned that the child's "delay" in development is due to a history of language problems in the family.

1. List all pertinent questions you need to ask when obtaining the case history, with a brief explanation as to the relevance to this case.
2. Describe your methods of assessment for this child. What standardized test will you use? What supplemental testing methods will you employ?

Practice Exercise 4

A 3;5-year-old girl was recently administered the PLS-5. She scored a raw score of 31 on the Auditory Comprehension subtest and a raw score of 20 on the Expressive Communication subtest.

1. Using the PLS-5 manual, look up the standard scores and percentile ranks for this child.
2. What is the SD from the mean for these scores?
3. On the basis of these results, does this child demonstrate a language delay?
4. Is the delay expressive, receptive, or mixed?
5. Present your answer by creating a table for the scores,
6. Write a short narrative, reporting test scores and type of language delay.

Glossary

Autism: A disorder characterized by significant impairments in the areas of communication and socialization, with the presence of stereotypical behaviors.

Cognitive: Pertaining to thought processes such as memory, problem-solving, and reasoning skills.

Collateral test-taking behaviors: Test-taking behaviors that can add to the scope of an evaluation; these behaviors provide information on a child's test-taking strategies, attention, turn-taking behaviors, and support needed.

Communicative gestures: Gestures use to communicate an idea (e.g., pointing, raising arms, to indicate "up").

Discourse skills: Skills that involve the use of language in larger units than a sentence.

Genetic disorder: A disorder that is acquired genetically.

Heuristic intentions: Using language to explore and categorize.

Illocutionary stage: Prelinguistic stage of development in which child communicates primarily through gestures.

Imaginative play: Using language during play.

Informative intentions: Using language to share knowledge with others.

Intellectual developmental disability: Significantly low intellectual and adaptive functioning, which is present early on in a child's development.

Language delay: Early language skills are late developing; however, the term implies that there is a potential for the child to "catch up" to peers. Typically used for children age 4 years and under.

Language disorder: Impairment of comprehension and production in the modalities of oral, written, or sign system; can affect any of the five areas of language—syntax, semantics, phonology, morphology, pragmatics.

Late bloomer: A child who appears delayed before age 3 years, but after this age makes sufficient developmental gains linguistically so that he or she demonstrates appropriate skills by age 4 years.

Late talker: A child who appears delayed before age 3 years, and by age 4 years demonstrates a more persistent impairment.

Locutionary stage: Follows illocutionary stage of development; child communicates using words and gestures.

Obligatory contexts: Contexts in which a specific word or grammatical form should occur.

Phonology: Study of the rules of the sequencing and distribution of sounds in a language.

Pragmatics: Language use.

Prelinguistic skills: Skills acquired before verbal language development; entails skills such as play and attention.

Presupposition: Where the speaker assumes or takes into account the background knowledge of a given topic of the listener.

Primary language impairment: Language is the primary area of deficit; language impairment is not secondary to another developmental disorder such as a syndrome or autism.

Sensory: Regarding the senses, such as vision/sight or hearing.

Specific language impairment (SLI): Language is impaired in the absence of any gross cognitive, behavioral, sensory, or emotional deficits.

Symbolic gestures: The use of a gesture to symbolize an object or idea.

Syndrome: A cluster of anomalies in an individual that are caused by the same source.

Syntax: The rules that govern word, phrase, and clause order in a sentence.

Visual support: Additional visual cues, such as pointing, gesturing, or the use of pictures to aid an individual in a task.

Word retrieval deficit: A deficit in which an individual has difficulty retrieving a word, despite having comprehension of the word.

References

Adams, A.-M., & Gathercole, S. E. (2000). Limitations in working memory: Implications for language development. International *Journal of Language & Communication Disorders, 35*, 95-116.

Almodòvar, D. & Levey, S. K. (2017). Preschool language development. In S. K. Levey, ed., *Introduction to language development* (2nd ed., pp. 119-147). New York, NY: Plural Publishing.

American Psychiatric Association. (2013). *Diagnostic and statistical manual of mental disorders* (5th ed.). Washington, DC: American Psychiatric Association.

American Speech-Language-Hearing Association. (1993). *Definitions of communication disorders and variations.* Rockville, MD: Author.

Archibald, L. M. D., & Gathercole, S. E. (2006). Short-term and working memory in specific language impairment. *International Journal of Language & Communication Disorders, 41*, 675–693.

Applebee, A. (1978). *The child's concept of story.* Chicago, IL: University of Chicago Press.

Bangs, T. E., & Ammer, J. (1999). *Birth to three checklist of language and learning behaviors* (BTC-3). Austin, TX: Pro- Ed.

Bates, E. (1976). *Language and context: The acquisition of pragmatics.* New York, NY: Academic Press.

Blank, M., Rose, S., & Berlin, L. (2003). *Preschool language assessment instrument* (PLAI-2). Austin, TX: Pro- Ed.

Bloom, L., & Lahey, M. (1978). *Language development and language disorders.* New York, NY: Wiley.

Boehm, A. E. (2001). *Boehm 3—preschool assessment.* San Antonio, TX: Harcourt.

Botting, N., & Conti-Ramsden, G. (2001). Non-word repetition and language development in children with specific language impairment (SLI). *International Journal of Language & Communication Disorders, 36*, 421-432.

Brown, R. (1973). *A first language, the early stages.* Cambridge, MA: Harvard University Press.

Brownell, R. (2011a). *Expressive one-word picture vocabulary test* (4th ed.). Novato, CA: Academic Therapy.

Brownell, R. (2011b). *Receptive one-word picture vocabulary test* (4th ed.). Novato, CA: Academic Therapy.

Capone, N., & McGregor, K. (2004). Gesture development a review for clinical and research practices. *Journal of Speech, Language, and Hearing Research, 47*, 173-186.

Carrow-Woolfolk, E. (2014). *Test of auditory comprehension of language.* Austin, TX: Pro-Ed.

Faust, M., Dimitrovsky, L., & Davidi, S. (1997). Naming difficulties in language-disabled children: Preliminary findings with the application of the tip-of-the-tongue paradigm. *Journal of Speech, Language, and Hearing Research, 40*, 1037-1047.

Halliday, M. A. K. (1975). *Learning how to mean.* London, England: Edward Arnold

Hammil, D. D., & Bryant, B. R. (2005). *Detroit test of learning aptitude primary.* Austin TX: Pro-Ed.

Hill, E. L. (2001). Non-specific nature of specific language impairment: A review of the literature with regard to concomitant motor impairments. *International Journal of Language & Communication Disorders, 36*, 149-171.

Hresko, W. P., Redi, K., & Hammill, D. D. (1999). *Test of early language development.* Austin, TX: Pro-Ed.

Iverson, J. M., & Goldin-Meadow, S. (2005). Gesture paves the way for language development. *Psychological Science, 16*, 367-371.

Jones, M. A., & Lodholz, C. (1999). *Rubric for completing a story grammar analysis.* Madison, WI: Madison Metropolitan School District.

Leonard, L. (1998). *Children with specific language impairment.* Cambridge, MA: MIT Press.

Luckasson, R., Borthwick-Duffy, S., Buntinx, W., Coulter, D. L., Craig, E. M., Reeve, A., . . . Tasse, M. (2002). *Mental retardation. Definition, classification and systems of supports* (10th ed.). Washington, DC: American Association on Mental Retardation.

Martin, N., & Brownell, R. (2005). *Test of auditory perceptual skills.* Novato, CA: Academic Therapy.

Marton, K. (2008). Visuo-spatial processing and executive functions in children with specific language impairment. *International Journal of Language & Communication Disorders, 43*, 181-200.

Marton, K. (2009). Imitation of body postures and hand movements in children with specific language impairment. *Journal of Experimental Child Psychology, 102*(1), 1-13.

Mayberry, R. I., & Nicoladis, E. (2000). Gesture reflects language development. *Current Directions in Psychological Science, 9*, 192-196.

Miller, J. (1981). *Assessing language production in children.* Baltimore, MD: University Park Press.

Miller, J. F., Long, S., McKinley, N., Thorman, S., Jones, M. A., & Nockerts, A. (2005). *Language sample analysis II: The Wisconsin guide.* Madison: Wisconsin Department of Public Instruction.

Newcomer, P. L., & Hammil, D. D. (2008). *Test of language development.* Austin, TX: Pro-Ed.

Owens, R. (2008). *Language development: An introduction* (7th ed.). Boston, MA: Allyn & Bacon.

Owens, R. E. (2016). *Language development: An introduction* (9th ed.). Boston, MA: Pearson.

Özçalİskan, S., & Goldin-Meadow, S. (2005). Gesture is at the cutting edge of early language development. *Cognition, 96*, B101-B113.

Patterson, J., & Westby, C. (1998). The development of play. In B. Shulman & W. O. Haynes (Eds.), *Communication development* (2nd ed.; pp. 135-164). Englewood Cliffs, NJ: Prentice Hall.

Paul, R. (2007). *Language disorders from infancy through adolescence: Assessment and intervention* (3rd ed.). St. Louis, MO: Mosby.

Paul, R., & Norbury, C. (2012). *Language disorders from infancy through adolescence: Listening, speaking, reading, writing, and communicating* (4th ed.). St. Louis: Elsevier Mosby.

Pence, K., & Justice. L. (2008). *Language development from theory to practice.* Upper Saddle River, NJ: Pearson Education.

Rescorla, L. (2005). Age 13 language and reading outcomes in late-talking toddlers. *Journal of Speech, Language, and Hearing Research, 48*, 459-472.

Rescorla, L., & Schwartz, E. (1990). Outcome of toddlers with expressive language delay. *Applied Psycholinguistics, 11*, 393-407.

Retherford, K. S. (2000). *Guide to analysis of language transcripts* (3rd ed.). Greenville, SC; Thinking Publications.

Richard, I. W., Annette, M., Robert, W. P., & Michael, I. S. (2005). Motor function at school age in children with a preschool diagnosis of developmental language impairment. *The Journal of Pediatrics, 146*(1), 80-85.

Rossetti, L. (1990). *Rossetti infant toddler language scale.* Austin, TX: LinguiSystems.

Schwartz, R. G. (2009). *The handbook of child language disorders.* New York, NY: Psychology Press.

Scott, C. M., & Windsor, J. (2000). General language performance measures in spoken and written narrative and expository discourse of school-age children with language learning disabilities. *Journal of Speech, Language, and Hearing Research, 43*, 324-339.

Shipley, K., & McAfee, J. (2009). *Assessment in speech-language pathology: A resource mannual.* Clifton Park, NY: Cengage Learning.

Stein, N. L., & Glenn, C. G. (1979). An analysis of story comprehension in elementary school children. In R. O. Freedle (Ed.), *New directions in discourse processing* (pp. 53-120). Norwood, NJ: Ablex.

Thal, D. J., Reilly, J., Seibert, L., Jeffries, R., & Fenson, J. (2004). Language development in children at risk for language impairment: Cross-population comparisons. *Brain & Language, 88*, 167-179.

Thal, B., & Tobias, S. (1992). Communicative gestures in children with delayed onset of oral expressive vocabulary. *Journal of Speech and Hearing Research, 35*, 1281-1289.

Thal, D., Tobias, S., & Morrison, D. (1991). Language and gesture in late talkers: A 1-year follow-up. *Journal of Speech and Hearing Research, 34*, 604-612.

Tomasello, M. (1992). The social bases of language acquisition. *Social Development, 1*(1), 67-87.

Wetherby, A. M., & Prizant, B. M. (2003). *Communication and symbolic behavior scales.* Baltimore, MD: Brookes.

Westby, C. (2000). A scale for assessing development of children's play. In K. Gitlin-Weiner, A. Sandgrund, & C. Schaefer (Eds.), *Play diagnosis and assessment* (2nd ed., pp. 15-57). New York, NY: Wiley.

Westby, C. (2005). Assessing and remediating text comprehension problems. In H. Catts & A. Kamhi (Eds.), *Language and reading disabilities* (2nd ed., pp. 157-232). Boston, MA: Allyn & Bacon.

Wiig, E. H., Secord, W., & Semel, E. (2004). *Clinical evaluation of language fundamentals.* San Antonio, TX: Harcourt Assessment.

Zimmerman, I. L., Steiner, V., & Pond, R. (2011). *Preschool language scale—5th edition.* San Antonio, TX: Harcourt Assessment.

9

Assessment of Speech, Language, and Communication in Autism Spectrum Disorders

Susan Longtin, PhD, CCC-SLP, TSHH

KEY WORDS

- Asperger disorder
- autism
- autism spectrum disorders
- childhood disintegrative disorder
- contact gestures
- deixis
- delayed echolalia
- distal gestures
- hyperlexia
- immediate echolalia
- joint attention
- pervasive developmental disorder
- pervasive developmental disorder—not otherwise specified
- presuppositional skills
- Rett disorder
- scripted language
- splinter skills
- theory of mind

INTRODUCTION

Autism spectrum disorder (ASD) refers to a neurodevelopmental condition currently defined by two core areas: (1) impairments in social communication and social interaction (SCSI) and (2) the presence of restricted, repetitive patterns of behaviors, interests, and activities (American Psychiatric Association [APA], 2013). Deficits in both of these areas must be present for an individual to be diagnosed as having ASD. In addition, the onset of the condition must occur in the early developmental period, usually before age 3 years, although the symptoms might not manifest until somewhat later when the demands of social communication exceed the child's capacities. Diagnosis of this condition is based on behavioral rather than physiological characteristics. If comorbid conditions such as language impairment and intellectual disability accompany the condition, the clinician must specify this information because these are not defining features of ASD.

The behavioral manifestations of ASD within an individual child change over time (National Research Council, 2001). A 1-year-old who does not engage in back-and-forth reciprocal interactions during a peek-a-boo game with a caregiver and a 4-year-old who does not show interest in engaging with peers both demonstrate challenges in the first core characteristic, social interaction and social communication. Similarly, a 2-year-old who lines up his trains in the same way every time he plays with them and a 6-year-old who talks only about trains to the exclusion of other topics of conversation both demonstrate restrictive, repetitive behaviors and interests.

Stein-Rubin, C., & Fabus, R. *A Guide to Clinical Assessment and Professional Report Writing in Speech-Language Pathology, Second Edition (pp 189-222).*

Ideally, a multidisciplinary team of varied professionals makes the diagnosis because ASD is a complex neurodevelopmental disability, which requires the expertise and input of different disciplines (Volkmar, Reichow, Westphal, & Mandell, 2014). The interprofessional evaluation team could include a developmental pediatrician, pediatric neurologist, psychologist, psychiatrist, social worker, special educator, speech-language pathologist (SLP), occupational therapist, and physical therapist. SLPs play a critical role in multidisciplinary team assessment for this population because their clinical expertise lies in social interaction and social communication, one of the core characteristics of ASD. If not part of an multidisciplinary team, SLPs are frequently the first professional that parents approach because their initial concerns often center around their child's difficulties in social interaction and communication as well as limited speech and language development. Whether as part of a multidisciplinary team or an individual practitioner in an educational or clinical setting, SLPs have both the foundational knowledge and clinical skills to evaluate these core deficits (American Speech-Language-Hearing Association [ASHA], 2006).

Classification

Currently, the most commonly used classification system for categorizing ASD in the United States is the *Diagnostic and Statistical Manual, Fifth Edition* (DSM-5; APA, 2013), which replaced the *Diagnostic and Statistical Manual, Fourth Edition* (DSM-IV; APA, 1994) and its revision (DSM-IV-TR; APA, 2000) in May 2013. The *International Classification of Diseases, Tenth Revision* (ICD-10; World Health Organization, 1993), which is currently in the process of revision, was closely aligned with the former DSM-IV (APA, 1994). Both the DSM-IV and ICD-10 recognize five categories of ASD with impairment in three core areas: (1) social reciprocity, (2) communication (including language), and (3) restricted, repetitive behaviors and interests. The convergence of social interaction and communication into a single core area rather than two separate ones was a major change from the DSM-IV to the DSM-5 (Volkmar, Reichow, et al., 2014). With social interaction and communication merged into one core area, language was removed from the mix. Consequently, the clinician now needs to specify if ASD occurs with or without language impairment (DSM-5; APA, 2013). Another notable change was the substitution of the overall categorical term *ASD* for the previously used **pervasive developmental disorder** (PDD), which suggested challenges across several different developmental domains. Another revision was the introduction degrees of severity of social communication impairment and restricted, repetitive behaviors and interests (DSM-5; APA, 2013). This topic of the diagnostic criteria for ASD in the DSM-5 is revisited in the Differential Diagnosis section at the end of this chapter before the case history and sample report. In addition, the reader is referred to Volkmar, Reichow, et al. (2014) and the DSM-5 itself (APA, 2013).

The five ASDs recognized in the former DSM-IV that mapped onto the five diagnostic categories delineated in the ICD-10 are autistic disorder, **Asperger disorder**, **childhood disintegrative disorder** (CDD; also known as *Heller syndrome*), **Rett disorder**, and **pervasive developmental disorder—not otherwise specified** (NOS), called *atypical autism* in the ICD-10 system. Although these separate categories are no longer used in the DSM-5, it is helpful for clinicians to be familiar with these terms because they might appear in reports of the individual being evaluated. Of note, children classified as having autistic disorder, Asperger disorder, and PDD NOS in the DSM-IV are considered to have ASD in the current DSM-5, whereas children diagnosed with CDD and Rett disorder are not. See Volkmar, Reichow, et al. (2014) for further discussion of this complex issue. The five PDDs in the former classification system are briefly described next.

Autistic disorder, sometimes called *classic autism* as originally described by Leo Kanner (1943) was more common in males than in females. However, recent evidence suggests that a greater number of females may have ASD than previously realized because females are more skillful than males at compensating for their social challenges (Kothari, Skuse, Wakefield, & Micali, 2013). The onset of autistic disorder occurred before age 3 years and was characterized by impairments across the three core areas. Classic autism was often associated with delays in other developmental domains such as cognition. The level of intellectual functioning in classic autism, as in the case of ASD in the current DSM-5 framework, ranges from severe intellectual disability to the normal range and above. Individuals with autistic disorder who have normal intelligence were considered to have high-functioning autism (HFA; Volkmar & Klin, 2005).

Asperger syndrome (AS), first described by Hans Asperger in 1944, was traditionally thought of as more common in males than females. Identification of AS was often made after age 3 years because this syndrome was characterized by normal intelligence, with concomitant satisfactory language in morphosyntax and vocabulary, but impaired social skills with associated pragmatic language difficulties. Individuals with AS were noted to have circumscribed interests, which could interfere with their social functioning, especially in adolescence and adulthood (Klin, McPartland, & Volkmar, 2005). Additional characteristics of individuals with AS included possible motor delays, sensory issues, and emotional liability. The literature sometimes distinguished between individuals with HFA and AS. Currently, individuals with both HFA and those with AS are considered to have ASD. Following the introduction of AS into the DSM-IV, interest in AS increased tremendously by both professionals and the general public (Volkmar, Reichow, et al., 2014).

Unlike the other ASDs, which occur in both males and females but predominantly in males, Rett disorder occurs only in females. The girls with this disorder begin a normal developmental trajectory, but their development is arrested after age 5 months. This progressively degenerative condition is caused by a mutation of the MECP2 gene. Characteristics of Rett disorder include deceleration of head growth, severe or profound intellectual disability, loss of intentional hand movements, regression in motor skills and social interaction, and severely impaired language. Although loss of social engagement occurs early in the course of the disorder, interest in social interaction often develops later in childhood or early adolescence. Individuals with Rett syndrome are prone to seizures, respiratory problems, and feeding difficulties (Van Acker, Loncola, & Van Acker, 2005). According to Volkmar, Reichow, et al. (2014), Rett disorder could be listed as a comorbid condition of ASD in the current DSM-5 if an ASD diagnosis is justified. However, given its known genetic etiology, Rett disorder is no longer listed as a separate disorder in the DSM-5.

Initially described more than 100 years ago by Theodore Heller (1908), CDD is marked by severe developmental regression. The onset of this rare condition is usually between 3 and 4 years, but it can begin anytime between 2 and 10 years. In these cases of later regression, CDD is not subsumed under the broader AS because, to be considered an ASD, the onset must occur during the early developmental period (DSM-5; APA, 2013), before 3 years. In the former DSM-IV (APA, 1994), diagnosis was made on the basis of deficits in any two of the three core areas that defined the ASDs. In CDD, regression is reported in at least two of the following areas: receptive or expressive language, social skills, bowel or bladder control, motor skill, or play. Individuals with this rare disorder have lower IQs and poorer prognosis than those with classic autism (Volkmar, Koenig, & State, 2005). CDD is no longer classified as a separate disorder in the current DSM-5 system. However, it can be subsumed under the broader autism spectrum if the onset occurs before age 3 years. In addition, the child must demonstrate the two core features of significant challenges in social interaction and social communication and the presence of restricted, repetitive behaviors and interests (Volkmar, Reichow, et al., 2014).

The last category, PDD-NOS, was used in the former DSM-IV (APA, 1994) when the diagnostic criteria for the other four ASD categories were not met. This milder form of ASD was considered primarily a disorder of reciprocal social interaction with associated impairments in verbal or nonverbal communication and the presence of repetitive behaviors and/or restricted interests. Expressions of the core characteristics in PDD-NOS were not as pronounced as in classic autism or Asperger disorder. Prognosis for individuals with PDD-NOS was considered better than for those with classic autism (Towbin, 2005). Children who met the former criteria for PDD-NOS may not meet the criteria for ASD under the DSM-5. Volkmar, Reichow, et al. (2014) noted that some children previously classified as PDD-NOS may lose their ASD diagnosis and instead receive the new DSM-5 social (pragmatic) communication disorder classification.

Speech-Language-Communication Characteristics of Children on the Spectrum and Parameters for Assessment

In terms of speech, language, and communication, the clinician needs to keep in mind that variability is the rule rather than the exception. Despite poor performance and areas of significant challenge, children with ASD may have **splinter skills** such as **hyperlexia**, precocious decoding skills for reading in the absence of reading comprehension, which can give the impression of a higher level of functioning and misrepresent the child's more typical abilities (Kim, Paul, Tager-Flusberg, & Lord, 2014; National Research Council, 2001). Furthermore, no single characteristic of children on the spectrum is unique to this heterogeneous group to distinguish this disorder from other developmental disabilities. Some individuals on the spectrum remain nonverbal for their entire lives, whereas others achieve high levels of linguistic skills with difficulties only in the pragmatic domain. The speech, language, and communication challenges vary with the child's developmental level, the individual's profile, and environmental factors. Any description of the speech, language, and communication characteristics of individuals with ASD must take these factors into account. Where applicable, the possible speech, language, and communication characteristics of individuals with ASD are described with respect to language developmental stages (e.g., Gerber & Prizant, 2000; Tager-Flusberg et al., 2009), the language domains, and their interactions (Lahey, 1988). In evaluating children with ASD a developmental perspective is critical because of the high comorbidity of intellectual disability in ASD (National Research Council, 2001) and the strong association of intellectual impairment and language impairment. The specific parameters for assessment of a child with ASD will depend on the individual's profile and developmental level. The areas delineated in the following section are ones the clinician will wish to evaluate in any particular child on the spectrum.

A comprehensive speech-language assessment for children on the spectrum who are functioning at the preintentional stage (the period before purposeful communication) should include an examination of the cognitive-social precursors to language (reciprocal interaction, affective engagement, **joint attention**, intentionality, and imitation).

Social-Cognitive Precursors to Communication and Language

The following abilities are the social and cognitive underpinnings for oral communication as well as for literacy.

Reciprocal Interaction and Affective Engagement

During the first 6 to 8 months of life, the child demonstrates a variety of behaviors such as gazing, crying, touching, and smiling. The child does not intend to communicate with these behaviors, but the adult often responds to them as if they were intentional (Gerber & Prizant, 2000). At this earliest preintentional stage, children on the spectrum have difficulties engaging in the joyful reciprocal interactions so characteristic of infancy. Reciprocal interaction at the preverbal level is foundational to the social skill development of the child. The following aspects of reciprocal interactions typically characterize young children on the spectrum:

- Flat affect and gaze aversion
- Preference to be left alone
- Difficulty with engagement
- Responsiveness to linguistic input (Some evidence suggests that very young children on the spectrum do not orient to their mother's voice [Klin, 1991] or their own names [Osterling & Dawson, 1994], missing much of the speech directed to them.)

These characteristics compromise the ability of children on the spectrum to engage in the social world (Carpenter & Tomasello, 2000), a precursor to the use of language (Lahey, 1988). The quality and frequency of these social behaviors are best assessed through direct observation of the child interacting with a significant other.

Joint Attention

During the second half of the first year, the typically developing child communicates intentionally using a combination of gestures, vocalizations, and gaze. A key communication challenge of children on the spectrum that emerges during this prelinguistic intentional stage is the ability to engage in joint attention. Joint attention requires orienting and attending to a social partner, then drawing that person's attention to objects or events of interest at the moment in order to share experience (Carpenter & Tomasello, 2000; Jones & Carr, 2004). Engaging in joint attention requires coordinating attention between objects and people and sharing affect or emotional states with others. The proto-declarative acts of indicating and showing objects to others for the purpose of social interaction are pragmatic functions associated with initiating joint attention.

The clinician should note whether the child:

- Initiates joint attention with another (e.g., shows an object to the parent or clinician)
- Responds to another's bids for joint attention (e.g., follows the clinician's point to an object across the room)
- Uses social referencing in which the child might "check" the adult's facial expressions to influence his or her own behavior

Intentionality

The intention to communicate with others emerges toward the end of the first year at around 7 to 8 months of age in typically developing children.

Children with ASD are compromised in their ability to read the intentions of others and to express their own intentions. (See the section on the Pragmatic Use of Language on the next page for a discussion of intentionality.)

Imitation

Children with autism generally show impaired performance on traditional imitation tasks such as clapping hands. Role reversal imitation, in which the action imitated requires a change in orientation or perspective such as waving hands while facing another, poses particular difficulty for children on the spectrum. Children with ASD may not reverse the position of their hand toward the social partner who modeled the gesture. Instead, they may wave with the palm of their hand facing themselves (Carpenter & Tomasello, 2000). Both traditional imitation tasks such as clapping hands and role reversal imitation such as waving to someone should be evaluated. Impairments in imitation including oral-motor imitation among those with ASD have been observed across the life span and intellectual abilities (Rogers, Cook, & Meryl, 2005; Vivanti & Hamilton, 2014).

Social Interaction Across Development

As noted in the introduction to this chapter, the domain of social interaction is now considered a core area of deficit in ASD. Expected behaviors in the social interaction domain vary significantly with development. For example, affect, gaze, body orientation, and synchronous vocalizations are behaviors that suggest attunement to another during infancy (Stern, 1985). The child at the preschool level should be interested in social interaction with peers and be able to engage with them in imaginative, cooperative play. During the school-age years, forming friendships and pleasing others are considered appropriate social behaviors. During adulthood, one is expected to get along with coworkers and employers and to maintain a socially appropriate distance between self and others. Thus, social interaction demands, as in other domains, vary developmentally so that challenges in this core area have different manifestations within the same individual over time (Davis & Carter, 2014). Consequently, the particular social interaction skills evaluated must be appropriate for the developmental level of the individual. Across the lifespan from earlier to later levels of social sophistication, this could include the following areas:

- Affective attunement to and engagement with others
- Interaction with peers
- Forming friendships
- Getting along with coworkers and employers
- Dating
- Other interpersonal relationships

A form–content–use (Bloom & Lahey, 1978; Lahey, 1988) paradigm can be useful to capture the relative strengths and weakness of verbal children on the spectrum who have achieved intentional communication. Language *form* refers to the structural components of language and includes phonology (units of sound), morphology (units of meaning that are words or inflections), and syntax (the way the units of meaning are put together through rules of word order). Linguistic form is the code of language, which interacts with content and use. *Content* refers to the ideas that are expressed through language, and *use* includes the functions and context language (Bloom & Lahey, 1978; Lahey, 1988).

A comprehensive speech-language assessment for children on the spectrum who are verbal should include an evaluation of these different aspects of language, especially pragmatics (the use of language in real communicative contexts), aspects of phonology (in particular, suprasegmental phonology or prosody) and articulation (see Chapter 7), unusual uses of linguistic forms (e.g., pronoun reversals and echolalia), the more tradition aspects of language form/content (semantic relations and grammatical morphology), conversational and narrative discourse, language comprehension, and play (see Chapter 8). Although the SLP's primary focus is on the child's speech, language, and communication, allied professionals can provide valuable information on related areas such as social problems, motor impairment, sensory issues, hearing status, cognitive abilities, and medical problems such as seizures.

Patterns of Lexical Development and Parameters of Language Content

Typically developing children begin to understand and use their first words within the context of their daily life and develop symbolic communication (Gerber & Prizant, 2000). First words or lexical development is one aspect of language content, the meanings or notions that are represented through language. The lexical development of children on the spectrum may be characterized by the following:

- Unusual patterns of development including delayed onset of first words, arrested growth, or regression after initial acquisition

- Similar types of words as typically developing children at the earlier stages of lexical development
- Exclusion of words that code mental states such as *know* or *think* (Tager-Flusberg, 1992) and words that express emotions in later lexicons

In addition to noting the preceding areas of lexical development, the clinician will want to assess the range and variety of semantic notions (e.g., possession) the child expresses and coordinates with other categories (e.g., possession + existence).

Language Content–Form Interactions

The utterances of verbal children with ASD are often grammatically correct, with linguistic structure considered a relative strength. The language of children on the spectrum, as with all children, should be assessed for the following aspects of morphosyntax:

- The types of structures spontaneously used and the variety of words used to express them (e.g., "I threw the ball," "he ate a cookie," and "she drove my car" are different sentences that have the same underlying subject–verb–complement construction)
- The child's use of grammatical morphemes in obligatory contexts
- For all aspects of language content and form, the clinician should determine what is missing, emerging, and productive. For developmentally expected items for which there is no evidence, the clinician should note these as areas in need of further assessment (Lahey, 1988).

These parameters of language are best assessed through natural language samples (see Chapter 8 for a detailed discussion of language assessment).

Pragmatic Use of Language

The current DSM-5 recognizes a new category of social (pragmatic) language disorder as separate from ASD. For individuals with autism and language impairment, problems in the pragmatic use of language are usually the most salient (Paul & Norbury, 2012) across developmental levels. The pragmatic challenges of individuals with ASD vary in severity and scope. For verbal children with ASD and language impairment, challenges in both conversational and narrative discourse compromise the individual's achievement of communicative competence. Challenges in the pragmatic use of language are reflected in various areas, as described next.

Theory of Mind

A deficit in **theory of mind** (ToM), sometimes called *mindblindness* (Baron-Cohen, 1995), is a social cognitive impairment that has been used to explain communicative-linguistic problems in individuals on the spectrum. The following are characteristics ToM development:

- ToM development begins in infancy with the ability to comprehend the intentions and emotional states of others.
- ToM continues to develop with perspective taking (the ability to take another's viewpoint) and related **presuppositional skills** (information that is shared by speaker and listener).
- ToM development culminates with understanding the truth and falsity of others' beliefs and knowledge during the early school years. Most children with ASD show problems in all aspects of ToM understanding (Baron-Cohen et al., 2005; Bauminger-Zviely, 2014).

Communicative Intentions

The clinician should delineate the frequency and range of the child's communicative intentions (labels, comments, requests, protests) and the means (or form) used to express them (e.g., vocalizations, gestures, echolalia, or spontaneous speech). The following are characteristic of communicative intent in children on the spectrum:

- Limited range of communicative intentions
- Less frequent initiation of communication
- More frequent initiation of communication for the proto-imperative acts of requesting or regulating the behavior of others
- Compromised ability to read the intentions of others
- Difficulty responding to adults' bids for joint attention
- Less frequent social referencing; use of the adult's facial expressions to influence their own behavior (Carpenter & Tomasello, 2000)
- Difficulties using nonverbal means of communication such as eye contact and gestures
- Use of fewer **distal gestures** such as pointing, but more frequent use of **contact gestures** such as hand leading, which occurs infrequently in typical development

When assessing communicative intent, the clinician should note (1) the types of gestures the child uses and whether the gestures are conventional (e.g., pointing) or unconventional (e.g., hand leading), and (2) the range and variety of communicative functions (e.g., commenting) expressed through vocalizations, gestures, words, or an alternative means (e.g., signs or picture symbols).

The Use of Linguistic Forms in Unusual Ways

Several of the language characteristics of children on the spectrum reflect problems in the interaction of linguistic form and use. Echolalia, idiosyncratic language, and pronoun reversals are problems that reflect difficulties in using linguistic forms appropriately.

Echolalia

Children with autism who have limited verbal skills may use echolalia, one of the most salient features of deviant language in autism (Kim et al., 2014). Echolalia, the repetition of a prior utterance, can be immediate or delayed.

- **Immediate echolalia** occurs directly after the prior utterance and usually shares both its linguistic and paralinguistic features (e.g., you say, "Hi Jenny" and Jenny replies, "Hi Jenny").
- **Delayed echolalia** refers to repetitions that are removed from the time and place in which they were initially heard (e.g., the child says "Don't touch that," a phrase that the child has heard his or her parents say on a previous occasion when the child was about to touch something that he or she is not supposed to). Sometimes delayed echolalia originates in **scripted** forms of **language** such as television commercials, YouTube videos, or movies.
- Both immediate (Prizant & Duchan, 1981) and delayed echolalia (Prizant, 1983) can serve communicative functions.

Idiosyncratic Language

Instances of delayed echolalia can have private or idiosyncratic meanings that do not make sense to the listener unless the context of the original utterance is known.

- An example of an idiosyncratic or form–use interaction was provided in Kanner's (1943) seminal report. He noted that a child said, "Don't throw the dog off the balcony" in many contexts where there was neither a dog nor a balcony present. In asking the boy's mother about the origin of this utterance, she explained that it was first used to prevent the boy from throwing his toy dog off of a balcony when the family was staying in a hotel. The child subsequently used this utterance in varied contexts to regulate his own behavior when he was about to do something prohibited, resulting in idiosyncratic use of the command. Consequently, the unconventional form–use interaction (Lahey, 1988) lacked meaning except to those familiar with the original connection. For this child, the utterance appears to have served a self-regulatory function (discussed subsequently).
- Idiosyncratic forms of language can serve communicative functions for children with ASD with impaired expressive language. They may be used at moments of limited comprehension, to fill a conversational turn, or to serve a pragmatic function (Kim et al., 2014).

Pronoun Reversals

The use of second-person for first-person pronouns, called pronoun reversals, in children with ASD may be rooted in echolalia (Kanner, 1943). For example, the child who says "pick you up" after the adult's query, "Do you want me to pick you up?" uses the latter part of the adult's utterance for his or her own. This atypical language behavior may reflect the child's difficulties with **deixis**, the aspect of language that codes the shifting discourse relationship between speaker and listener (Kim et al., 2014). In the preceding example, the child did not make the deictic shift from person spoken to—the second person—in which the pronoun "you" is appropriate to the speaker role—the first person—in which the pronoun "me" is correct. Characteristics of pronoun reversal errors include the following:

- The child mistakenly used these pronouns as if they were static forms with stable referents rather than as dynamic forms, which shift with speaker–listener discourse role. The shifting reference is particularly difficult for children on the spectrum because of their difficulty with abstraction and lack of flexibility (Paul & Norbury, 2012).
- These errors do not occur in all children on the spectrum but are more common in individuals with autism than in other clinical populations (Kim et al., 2014).

Assessment Parameters Related to Discourse

Engaging in conversation and producing narratives requires the child's understanding of speaker–listener roles (Gerber & Prizant, 2000). The following section includes considerations for the assessment of conversational and narrative discourse skills in verbal children with ASD who are capable of engaging in discourse.

Conversational Skills

Engaging in conversation requires a wide range of pragmatic language behaviors that one can observe in varied settings during everyday communicative interactions. When conversing with others, individuals on the spectrum may have difficulty with one or more of the following areas:

- Producing alternative forms of a message that are adapted to the needs of the listener. Simply stated, verbal individuals with ASD may have difficulty knowing when to say what to whom. One explanation for these pragmatic language difficulties is that individuals with autism do not take the listener's perspective (the listener's point of view) into account because of deficits in ToM, an aspect of social cognition mentioned earlier.
- Excessive talk about a circumscribed, narrow range of topics such as dinosaurs. Grice's (1975) conversational maxims of quantity, quality, relation, and manner provide a useful framework for clinicians in describing the conversational challenges of individuals with HFA/AS. For example, the principle of manner suggests that the speaker be clear, concise, and coherent.
- Initiating, maintaining, and terminating topics; making topic-relevant contributions to a conversation; and engaging in the back and forth flow of two-way discourse

When assessing the conversational skills of a child with ASD and more advanced language skills, the clinician should note whether the individual:

- Adapts the message for varied listeners (e.g., contains politeness markers with an unfamiliar adult or simplifies language addressed to a younger child)
- Talks about a range of topics removed in time and place
- Engages in a number of back and forth turns
- Extends own talk within a turn
- Converses about a topic generated by another (in addition to topics chosen by the child)
- Repairs or clarifies the message (a discourse function that indicates responsiveness to the needs of the listener) when communication breakdown occurs
- Uses presupposition (shared background information) in formulating the message, a skill based on the child's ability to understand which information is shared with the listener and which is not (Gerber & Prizant, 2000)
- Requests clarification of the listener and responds to the listener's clarification requests, functions of language that are used when communication breakdown occurs between the speaker and listener during conversation

Narrative Discourse

The ability to produce narratives, a type of extended discourse or social monologue, emerges during the preschool years and develops during the school-age years. By the early school-age years, individuals should have developed an internalized story grammar (Stein & Glenn, 1979), which consists of several components such as the setting, characters, problems, and consequences. In addition to their structural properties, narratives have pragmatic aspects such as how well the narrator adapts to the needs of the listener in terms of shared prior knowledge and includes evaluative comments about how the narrator feels about the events of the story (Lahey, 1988). Narrative discourse draws on the social-emotional, cognitive, and linguistic domains—all areas that can challenge individuals in this population. Research on the narratives of verbal school-age children with ASD indicates that they:

- Narrate less frequently in conversational contexts
- Rely on prompting from the listener to clarify information
- Lack complexity, coherence, and reference to the mental states of the characters
- Contain more frequent off topic, irrelevant comments (Losh & Capps, 2003)

To assess narrative skills from individuals on the spectrum who are able to spontaneously engage in extended discourse, the clinician must obtain narrative language samples. Guidelines for obtaining narrative samples from children on the spectrum include the following:

- Obtaining different types of narratives such as:
    - A narrative of personal experience in which the background information is not shared with the clinician. For example, the child can be asked to tell the funniest or scariest thing that ever happened to him or her. The clinician can note whether the child provided sufficient background information to take the listener's needs into account.

- Telling or retelling a story from a wordless picture book such as *Frog, Where are You?* (Mayer, 1969) or an almost wordless picture book such as *Tuesday* (Weisner, 1997), which provide shared nonlinguistic contexts. The clinician can note whether the child appropriately specifies the presupposed referents, which are available to the clinician from the shared context of the pictures.
- Retelling a familiar story that is known by both child and clinician or one that is unknown to the child but modeled by the clinician with various degrees of nonlinguistic contextual support.
- For all narrative contexts with children on the spectrum, the clinician can determine if the child referred to the mental states, feelings, and intentions of the characters and provided evaluative comments about them.

See Chapter 10 for a more detailed discussion of narrative skills.

Literacy Skills

Literacy skills in ASD are usually commensurate with overall developmental level. Reading comprehension for some children on the spectrum may typically be weak relative to word recognition. A subset of these individuals on the spectrum, considered hyperlexic, demonstrate decoding abilities that are advanced relative to their cognitive, social, and other linguistic skills. Characteristics of hyperlexia include the following:

- Advanced word recognition
- A compulsive preoccupation with reading, letters, or writing
- A significant gap between strong decoding skills, word recognition, and spelling in comparison to weak reading comprehension (Kim et al., 2014)
- Early interest in letters
- Learning to read without direct instruction

See Chapter 10 for a more detailed discussion of literacy.

Phonology and Articulation

Phonology refers to the sound system of language and includes the rules for speech sound segment (consonants and vowels) combinations. Articulation refers to the vocal tract movements for speech sound production involving placement of the articulators and the modifications in the size and shape of the resonating cavities. Like other aspects of linguistic form, segmental phonology and articulation are usually areas of relative strength in children with ASD who follow the same sequence of development that occurs in typically developing children (Kim et al., 2014). However, Needleman, Ritvo, and Freedman (1981) identified "imprecise articulation" in a large proportion of children with autism. More recently, in a study of males aged 10 to 50 years, Shriberg et al. (2001) found significantly more articulation errors in individuals with HFA and AS than in a comparison groups without ASD. Thus, in articulation and phonology, as in other aspects of speech and language, variation is the rule in this heterogeneous population. At the earliest stages, the clinician can note the child's phonetic inventory and syllabic structures and the presence of phonological processes and misarticulations for those at the preschool level and beyond (see Chapter 7 for a detailed discussion).

Prosody

Whereas segmental phonology and articulation can be relative strengths in children on the spectrum, the suprasegmental aspects of phonology, or prosody, is often impaired. These suprasegmental aspects of speech, also referred to as *paralinguistic features*, include intonation, stress, and volume. Kanner's (1943) original description of autism included disordered prosody, one of the immediately recognizable signs of the disorder. Problems with prosody among individuals on the spectrum vary widely and can include the following:

- An exaggerated, high-pitched "sing-song" intonation to a flat, monotonous tone of voice
- Misplaced stress in adolescents and adults (Shriberg et al., 2001)
- Problems with volume including poor control, unexplained fluctuations, and excessive loudness (Shriberg et al., 2001)
- Whispering among children with echolalia (Kim et al., 2014)
- Pedantic speech reflects a qualitative difference in word use and speech style in some individuals with ASD
- Difficulty interpreting the meaning of vocal tone, such as whether a message conveys sarcasm vs. sincerity (Alpern & Zager, 2007)

For all verbal individuals on the spectrum, the suprasegmental or paralinguistic features of intonation, stress, volume, and tone of voice should be assessed because children on the spectrum are known to have problems in this area. The clinician should note any unusual speech patterns such as a pedantic speech style. Prosody is best evaluated through a spontaneous speech sample.

Nonverbal Oral Apraxia

Nonverbal oral apraxia refers to difficulty imitating or sequencing volitional oral movements not related to speech, such as puckering and licking the lips. Children with ASD often have impaired imitation skills (Vivanti & Hamilton, 2014). Some clinicians believe that apraxia, a motor planning disorder, is a major factor that accounts for the failure of many children with ASD to develop speech, but this explanation is controversial (Paul & Sutherland, 2005). Apraxia refers to impairments in the ability to plan and execute movements in the absence of other motor symptoms (Ayers, 2000). This disorder is associated with difficulty sequencing speech sounds, groping and reduced intelligibility, nasality, silent posturing, inconsistent errors, and abnormal prosody (ASHA, 2007; see Chapters 6 and 7 for a discussion of childhood apraxia.)

Language Comprehension

In addition to expressive language impairments, difficulties in receptive language can accompany ASD. The following language comprehension challenges may contribute to the individual's limited understanding of linguistic input and communicative intent:

- Lack of response to the speech of others (e.g., a child's failure to respond to his or her name is a good discriminator of ASD; Paul & Fahim, 2014)
- Following simple directions
- Difficulty interpreting and integrating nonverbal cues such as gestures and facial expressions and paralinguistic cues such as tone of voice

Problems with the comprehension of language continue at later language levels. In fact, comprehension can be more impaired than production among verbal children with autism (Kim et al., 2014; Tager-Flusberg, 1981), which is atypical of other populations of children with language impairment. Comprehension of nonliteral language including idioms, jokes, similes, and metaphors can be particularly challenging because they are characterized by less transparent, form-meaning relationships. Children with ASD have difficulty accepting that individual words or entire utterances can have multiple meanings or interpretations.

Gerber and Prizant (2000) provided guidelines for assessing the language comprehension of children from the prelinguistic through later language levels. The following is an inventory of those guidelines.

- For children at the earliest stages, the clinician can note the child's use of nonlinguistic response strategies such as attending to the object mentioned and following simple directions such as "show me ____."
- At later levels, the child should understand simple wh- questions and word combinations.
- With further language development, the child should understand utterances based less on nonlinguistic response strategies and more on morphsyntactic rules.
- At all linguistic stages, the clinician should assess receptive vocabulary.
- Across development, the clinician should assess the ability to interpret and integrate nonverbal cues such as gestures and facial expressions and paralinguistic cues such as tone of voice.

The following areas for assessment are relevant to the comprehension of individuals with more advanced language skills:

- Understanding nonliteral language including idioms, jokes, similes, and metaphors as well as words with multiple meanings (Paul & Norbury, 2012).
- Understanding what is inferred in addition to what is explicitly stated.
- Understanding the false beliefs of others to probe ToM.

Play

Children on the spectrum have impairments in the quantity, quality, and duration of play, a reflection of their limited capacity for symbol use. Lack of varied, spontaneous make-believe or social imitative play appropriate to developmental level is a hallmark of autism. Their play is characterized by the following:

- More repetition (Kasari & Chang, 2014)
- Less novelty
- Less diversity of schemas (Rogers et al., 2005)
- More solitary, constructive play of a repetitive nature (Kasari & Chang, 2014)

- Less parallel, cooperative, or symbolic play of a dynamic, creative nature
- Restricted, stereotypic patterns of play such as rolling a car back and forth instead of richly nuanced imaginative play, which is characteristic of the play of typically developing children (Rogers et al., 2005)
- Unusual sensory interests in play materials
- Deficiency in the self-other dimension of symbolic play related to impaired ToM (see previous discussion on ToM) because children on the spectrum are unlikely to attribute feelings and desires to their play partners, whether dolls, toy animals or people (Westby, 2000)

See Chapter 8 for information about the assessment of play.

Concomitant Problems and Related Areas

In addition to problems in the core area of social interaction and communication and the possibility of comorbid language impairment, individuals with ASD present with additional challenges. These possible additional areas of challenge are discussed in the following subsections.

Motor Skills

For some children on the spectrum, motor abilities, at least in the first 2 years of life, may be an area of relative strength. However, with the passage of time, some children with an ASD develop challenges in both gross and fine motor skills (National Research Council, 2001) as well as in the related area of praxis—the ability to conceptualize, plan, and execute voluntary, goal-directed actions (Baranek, Parham, & Bodfish, 2005). Bodison and Mostofsky (2014) preferred the term *developmental dyspraxia* to *apraxia* for challenges in this area because the latter implies acquired adult loss of skills and the former early childhood onset. The following information is relevant to the motor skills of individuals with autism:

- The range of motor problems in autism is considerably broad (Rogers et al., 2005) and occurs in multiple domains (Bodison & Mostofsky, 2014).
- Some individuals with autism demonstrate stereotypical motor movements such as rocking or hand flapping, which can be a manifestation of the core repetitive behaviors characteristic of the disorder.
- Despite the prevalence of motor challenges in some children on the spectrum, others have relative strength in:
    - Gross motor skills that are encountered in everyday life such as stair climbing
    - Visuomotor skills such as completing form boards and puzzles (Baranek et al., 2005)

To date, motor problems that are unique to ASD have not been identified.

- Nonverbal oral apraxia, mentioned earlier, is a type of motor imitation deficit seen in autism.
- The SLP can judge the degree of severity of the motor problem in the individual with ASD. If the child is receiving a multidisciplinary team assessment, the occupational and physical therapists will conduct in-depth evaluations of the individual's motor skills. If the SLP is not evaluating the child as part of a multidisciplinary team, the clinician can note gross motor skills such as climbing stairs, fine motor skills such as cutting, and visuomotor skills such as completing puzzles or writing, as well as praxis or motor planning such as imitating body movements. If concerns arise, then referral should be made to an occupational or physical therapist, or both.
- Finally, the clinician can observe the presence of repetitive motor behaviors such as rocking.

Sensory Processing

Sensory processing is a comprehensive term that refers to the way in which the nervous system manages sensory information, which includes the registration, modulation, integration, and organization of sensory input. Sensory processing problems are relatively common in individuals on the spectrum with about 42% to 88% of individuals having some challenges in this area. In contrast to the previous DSM-IV (APA, 1994, 2000) the current DSM-5 (APA, 2013) includes sensory sensitivities under the core characteristic of restrictive repetitive behaviors and interests (Volkmar, Reichow, et al., 2014). Sensory-seeking behaviors may be intense and repetitive. Baranek, Little, Parham, Ausderau, and Sabatos-DeVito (2014) suggested that the same unknown mechanism might underlie both sensory features and restrictive, repetitive behaviors. The following sensory challenges are typical in this population:

- Motor-planning difficulties, mentioned earlier, which often have a sensory base (Gal, Cermack, & Ben-Sasson, 2007)

- Under- or over-responsiveness to sensory stimuli
- Hypo- and hypersensitivities
- Preoccupations with sensory features of the environment
- Paradoxical responses to sensory stimuli

Although these problems are manifested across all sensory modalities including the visual, auditory, gustatory, olfactory, tactile, proprioceptive, and vestibular systems, auditory sensitivities have been the most commonly reported among those with ASD (Baranek et al., 2014). Temple Grandin (2005), a well-known advocate with ASD, has written about her hypersensitivities to sound and touch. Information about a child's sensory processing, which is included in the scope of practice of occupational therapists, is gained through caregiver report, clinical observations, and direct assessment through standardized measures.

The SLP may consult with an occupational therapist to clarify the nature and extent of the child's sensory processing issues (Baranek et al., 2014). Gal et al. (2007) provided clinicians with a helpful overview of this area. In addition, the Sensory Processing Disorder Network website (www.sinetwork.org) offers current information and resources on this disorder that could be helpful for the SLP to more fully understand this area. The assessment of sensory processing should include information about the individual's:

- Hyposensitivities (under-responsiveness) or hypersensitivities (over-responsiveness) to sensory stimuli
- Preoccupations with sensory features of the environment
- Paradoxical responses to sensory stimuli
- Sensory regulation
- Behavioral organization

Intellectual Abilities

Historically, estimates of children with autism also diagnosed with intellectual disability have been in the 70% to 80% range. However, given the broadening of the spectrum since the late 1990s to include higher functioning populations, the figures are now considerably lower. For example, a 2010 study found that approximately 40% to 50% of school-age children with ASD have intellectual impairments (Charman et al., 2010). Furthermore, given the difficulty children with ASD have in participating in formal, standardized tests, these results can be questionable. In terms of the level of intellectual functioning, IQs in this population vary from severe or profound intellectual disability to the gifted range (National Research Council, 2001).

Epilepsy

When a child experiences two or more unprovoked seizures, the condition is considered epilepsy, a neurologically based medical condition that occurs in approximately 11% to 39% of the ASD population (Howlin, 2014), a figure far above chance. Children on the spectrum are at risk for developing seizure disorders throughout the developmental period (National Research Council, 2001) with one peak chance of onset before 5 years and another after 10 years (Volkmar, Rowberry, et al., 2014). By adulthood, one-third of individuals with ASD will have developed epilepsy (Volkmar, Rowberry, et al., 2014). Epilepsy in autism is associated with lower IQ, sex (with higher risk among females), greater behavioral challenges, and more impaired language skills (Howlin, 2014).

Oral Motor and Feeding Skills

For a detailed discussion, see Chapters 6 and 14.

Audiological Status

For a detailed discussion, see Chapter 5.

Augmentative Alternative Communication

Augmentative alternative communication (AAC) may be a necessary component of a comprehensive speech-language assessment, especially for older nonverbal children with ASD (Paul & Fahim, 2014). Evaluation in this area is likely to be conducted as a follow-up assessment after an initial intake has been conducted. The purpose of an AAC assessment is to identify differences between an individual's communication needs and capabilities and to determine what type of AAC techniques or systems would most likely enhance his or her ability to communicate (Mirenda, 2014). These clients may be candidates for visual graphic AAC systems such as picture boards, picture schedules, computers, or tablets (e.g., iPad [Apple]). For older nonverbal children with ASD, a form of AAC could provide them with a means of expressing their wants and needs (Paul & Fahim, 2014). The growth of relatively affordable handheld devices over the past few years has made AAC technology both more accessible and acceptable. Shane and colleagues (2012) suggested that this has caused a paradigm shift in the use of AAC as a tool for communication.

During an AAC assessment, the clinician gathers information from a wide range of sources to gain an understanding of an individual's current means of communicating as well as his or her patterns and opportunities to communicate (Beukelman

& Mirenda, 2013). The clinician would also need to determine the individual's motor skills, symbolic capacities, language comprehension abilities, literacy skills, and sensory-motor functioning (Mirenda, 2014). An AAC assessment for an individual with ASD should be both family- and person-centered, taking into consideration the needs and preferences of both. For comprehensive information about AAC assessment, the reader is referred to Beukelman and Mirenda (2013).

Areas of Strength and Splinter Skills

The developmental trajectories of children on the spectrum often diverge from that of their neurotypical peers. In addition to challenges, some individuals with ASD have areas of significant strength, including rote memory, visual spatial processing, and attention to detail. Many individuals with higher-level intellectual abilities have splinter skills in areas such as music (Paul & Norbury, 2012), art, computers, mathematics, and mechanics (Grandin, 2005). Hyperlexia, described earlier, can be considered a splinter skill for some children on the spectrum.

Key Clinical Interview Questions

The clinical interview process provides the clinician with an opportunity to obtain information from the parents or other primary caregivers and to determine their priorities and concerns. In evaluating speech, language, and communication in individuals with ASD, parental input is crucial as parents know their child best. Furthermore, the social interactive nature of the evaluation process involving language sampling and play is perhaps a greater challenge to individuals with ASD than for those with other types of disorders. The questions asked during a clinical interview will depend on the developmental level of the individual being evaluated. The questions that follow are organized according to individual's level of functioning or domain of communication-language that they address.

Prelinguistic Intentionality

- Does your child try to communicate with others? If so, how?
- Does your child bring objects to you just to show them to you?
- Does your child point or make sounds to get you to look at something?
- If you point to something in the distance, does your child look at it?
- Does your child physically lead you to what he or she wants?
- Does your child use parts of your body as tools (e.g., putting your hand on a doorknob that he or she wants turned)?

Early Language Comprehension

- Does your child respond to his or her name?
- Does your child understand words outside of the usual situation in which he or she hears them?
- Does your child follow simple directions without gestural cues?
- Does your child follow complex directions such as, "Get your car and put it on the table"?

Early Language Production

- Does your child use any meaningful words (consistently for a specific purpose in an appropriate context) or word approximations spontaneously (not in imitation or on request)?
- Does your child repeat words that he or she does not understand?

Social Referencing

- Does your child ever look at your face to check your reaction to an unfamiliar person or situation?

Social Interaction and Play

- Does your child enjoy playing games such as peek-a-boo or hide and seek?
- Does your child ever pretend while he or she is playing?
- Does your child play with you or other children?
- Does your child take turns in play with you or other children?
- Does your child have friends?
- How does your child get along with other children at home or in school?
- Does your child have any deep interests that he or she talks about a lot?

Social Skills for an Adolescent or Adult With HFA/AS

- How comfortable are you in social situations?
- How easily do you make friends?
- How do you get along with others at home, in school, or on the job?

Table 9-1. ASD-Specific Screening Tools

Screening Tool and Source	*Ages*	*Domains Assessed*	*Format*
Checklist for Autism in Toddlers (CHAT; Baron-Cohen, Allen, & Gillberg, 1992)	18 months	Symbolic play, taking interest in other children, gestures, and gaze monitoring	Interview questions asked of parents and observation by clinician
Infant–Toddler Checklist of Communication and Symbolic Behavior Scales Developmental Profile (Wetherby & Prizant, 2003)	6 to 24 months	Emotions and eye gaze, communication, gestures, sounds, words, understanding, and object use	Checklist items completed by primary caretaker; norm-referenced
Modified Checklist for Autism in Toddlers (M-CHAT; Robins, Fein, Barton, & Green, 2001)	18 months	Symbolic play, social relatedness, communication, sensory and motor skills	Checklist completed by parent at pediatric visit
Screening Tool for Autism in Two-Year-Olds (STAT; Stone, Coonrod, & Ousley, 2000)	24 to 35 months	Symbolic and social interactive play, motor imitation, and nonverbal expression of communicative intents	20-minute play interaction with child
Social Communication Questionnaire (Rutter, Bailey, & Lord, 2003)	>4 years	Social interaction; communication/language; repetitive, stereotyped behaviors	Parent questionnaire with 40 yes/no questions
Systematic Observation of Red Flags for Autism Spectrum Disorders in Young Children (SORF; Wetherby & Woods, 2002)	12 to 36 months	Reciprocal interaction, unconventional gestures, unconventional sounds or words, repetitive behaviors, restricted interests, and emotional regulation	Review of caregiver–child videotaped interactions

Behaviors

- Does your child engage in any repetitive behavior (such as flipping through magazine pages, rocking)?
- How does your child react to changes in routine?
- Does your child demonstrate any usual hand or finger mannerism or movements?
- Does your child overreact or underreact to certain sensations such a sights, sounds, smells, or touch? If so, explain.

Medical

- Does your child have a history of any physical problems such as seizures?

Formal Assessment Measures

Children on the spectrum present significant challenges to clinicians who wish to use formal standardized tests as part of their assessment tools (McCauley, 2001). Any assessment for children on the spectrum should rely on multiple sources of information. These ideally include natural language samples, parent reports, and direct standardized assessment (Tager-Flusberg et al., 2009). Given the child's core deficits in the area of social interaction and the fact that an assessment is an opportunity for social interaction, parent questionnaires and behavioral checklists are important clinical tools to assist in screening and diagnosis. Table 9-1 lists screening measures used in the identification of individuals with ASD. Most were developed with the goal of early identification so that they target the infant, toddler, and preschool ages. In terms of format, the majority of these assessments use rating scales, checklists, interviews, and questionnaires completed by those most familiar with the individual (i.e., a parent or other primary caregiver).

Individuals who may have been identified as at risk for having an ASD may be administered an autism-specific diagnostic assessment. Like the screening measures, many of these begin at 18 months; however, unlike the screening tools, they can be used through adulthood. In terms of format, the diagnostic tools use direct observation in addition to checklists, rating scales, and other parent report procedures that are also used for screening. Lord, Corsello, and Grzadzinski (2014) discussed diagnostic instruments in ASD. Table 9-2 lists ASD-specific diagnostic tools.

Considerations in Standardized Language Assessment

More traditional, standardized assessments can be a helpful component for the assessment of some children on the spectrum, especially those who are verbal

Table 9-2. ASD-Specific Diagnostic Tools

Assessment Tool and Source	*Ages*	*Domains Assessed*	*Criterion- or Norm-Referenced*	*Test Construct, Format, Elicitation Techniques*
Autism Diagnostic Interview-Revised (ADI-R; Le Couteur, Lord, & Rutter, 2003)	18 months to adult	Reciprocal social interaction, communication, language, and repetitive behaviors and interests	Criterion	Semistructured, standardized parent interview and response coding; uses a diagnostic algorithm for classification
Autism Diagnostic Observation Scale-2 (ADOS-2 Toddler Module; Lord, Luyster, Gotham, & Guthrie, 2012)	12 to 30 months	Communication, social interaction, and play	Criterion	Semistructured, standardized observations for toddlers who do not consistently use "phrase speech"; uses a diagnostic algorithm for classification
Autism Diagnostic Observation Scale-2 (ADOS-2; Lord, Rutter, et al., 2012)	2 years to adult	Communication, social interaction, and play	Criterion	Semistructured, standardized observations using one of four modules based on expressive language level and age; uses a diagnostic algorithm for classification
Childhood Autism Rating Scale-2 (CARS-2; Schopler, Van Bourgondien, Wellman, & Love, 2010)	2 years to adult	Social-emotional, imitation, body movements, object use, adaptation to change, sensory peculiarities, communication, activity, intellectual functioning	Criterion	Structured interview and observation; behaviors in 15 areas are rated on scale of 1 to 4; includes two versions, each designed for different populations of children with ASDs—those younger than age 6 years or below average estimated IQs, and those older than age 6 years, higher functioning, and with IQs estimated above 80; parent/caregiver questionnaire also available
Gilliam Autism Rating Scale-3 (GARS-3; Gilliam, 2013; Western Psychological Services, 2013)	3 to 22 years	Stereotyped behaviors, social interaction, and communication	Norm	Parent interview and checklist used by for parents, teachers, or clinicians to identify autism and indicate severity level; behaviors consistent with DSM-5, rated on scale of 1 to 4

(McCauley, 2001). However, the clinician may need to make accommodations to standardized assessment procedures to administer a formal test to a child with ASD. Such accommodations could include providing reinforcement, changing the order of presentation items to keep the child's interest, repeating items or instructions, and providing additional demonstrations if the child fails or does not understand the task (Paul & Fahim, 2014). As usual, these departures from standard administration procedures must be noted in reporting the test results (Paul & Norbury, 2012).

These tests could be included as part of a comprehensive communication-language evaluation for individuals with ASD whether they have received a formal diagnosis or not. These measures, which are mostly norm-referenced, cover the age range from infancy through late adolescence. Several tests, which are listed in Table 9-3, were selected because they either include a pragmatic component in addition to the more traditional aspects of form and content tapped by standardized tests such as understanding or producing grammatical morphemes (e.g., Comprehensive Assessment of Spoken Language-2 [CASL-2; Carrow-Woolfolk, 2016]) or they claim to focus exclusively on the pragmatic domain (e.g., Test of Pragmatic Language-2 [TOPL-2; Phelps-Terasaki & Phelps-Gunn, 2007]). However, a major drawback of using standardized tests to assess pragmatics in individuals with ASD is that their language is often learned by rote, is scripted, and may not vary with the context and interactant. Furthermore, standardized assessments by their very nature are static and not responsive to the dynamic, nuanced, and variable nature of language use in everyday contexts, the essence of pragmatics. Table 9-3 lists assessment tools that address the pragmatic component of language.

Table 9-3. Standardized Assessments That Address Aspects of Pragmatic Language

Assessment Tool and Source	*Ages*	*Domains Assessed*	*Criterion- or Norm-Referenced*	*Test Construct, Format, Elicitation Techniques Relevance for ASDs*
Children's Communication Checklist-2 (CCC-2; Bishop, 2006)	4 to 17 years	Language: speech, syntax, semantics, coherence Pragmatics: initiation, scripted language context, nonverbal communication, social relations, and interests	Norm	Parent or caregiver rating scale of 70 items to identify children with pragmatic language impairment including those who would benefit from further assessment for ASD
Clinical Evaluation of Language Fundamentals-5 (CELF-5; Wiig, Semel, & Secord, 2013)	5 to 21 years	Semantics, syntax, memory, receptive and expressive language, and pragmatics profile	Norm	Includes 16 subtests including a pragmatics profile, which is relevant to the verbal children with ASD
Communication and Symbolic Behavior Scales-Developmental Profile (CBSC-DP; Wetherby & Prizant, 2003)	6 to 24 months	Emotion and eye gaze, communication, gestures, sounds, expressive language, receptive language, object use/play	Norm	Caregiver questionnaire and 30-minute behavior sample using communicative temptations, book sharing, symbolic and constructive play contexts, and comprehension probes
CASL-2 (Carrow-Woolfolk, 2016)	3 to 21 years	Lexical/semantic skills, syntactic skills, supralinguistic skills, pragmatic skills; paragraph comprehension and pragmatic judgment subtests are most relevant to ASDs	Norm	Six clinician administered subtests for age 3 to 6 years; 14 subtests for age 7 to 21 years; most relevant subtests for ASDs are paragraph comprehension, idiomatic language, nonliteral language, inference, and pragmatic judgment
Diagnostic Evaluation of Language Variation-2 (DELV-2; Seymour, Roeper, & de Villiers, 2005)	4 to 9 years	Syntax, phonology, semantics, and pragmatics which includes communicative role taking, short narratives, and question asking	Norm	Clinician administered subtests; the short narrative items of the pragmatics subtest includes some questions related to ToM
Evaluating Acquired Language Skills in Communication-3 (EASIC-3; Marcott, 2009)	3 months to 6 years	Prelanguage, semantics, syntax, morphology, and pragmatics	Criterion	A five-level inventory that yields developmental profiles that focus on communication
MacArthur-Bates Communicative Development Inventories-2 (CDI-2; Fenson et al., 2006)	8 to 30 months	Comprehension and production of gestures, vocabulary, morphology, and phrases/sentences	Norm	Checklist completed by parent or caregiver reports current and emergent behaviors including early gestures, words and phrases; two forms available: "words and gestures" and "words and sentences"

(continued)

Table 9-3. Standardized Assessments That Address Aspects of Pragmatic Language (continued)

Assessment Tool and Source	*Ages*	*Domains Assessed*	*Criterion- or Norm-Referenced*	*Test Construct, Format, Elicitation Techniques Relevance for ASDs*
Pragmatic Language Skills Inventory (PLSI; Gilliam & Miller, 2006)	5;0 to 12;11 years	Personal interaction skills, social interaction skills, classroom interaction skills	Norm	Rating scale consisting of 45 items to be completed by parent, caregiver and/or classroom teacher that can serve as part of an assessment battery or screening measure.
Rossetti Infant-Toddler Language Scale (Rossetti, 2006)	Birth to 3 years	Interaction-attachment, pragmatics, gesture, play, language comprehension and expression	Criterion	Parent or caregiver questionnaire and checklist used by clinicians to develop a profile of behaviors that are observed, elicited, or reported by caregiver
Social Language Development Test—Elementary (Bowers, Huisingh, & LoGiudice, 2008)	6 to 11;11 years	Making inferences, interpersonal negotiations, multiple interpretations, supporting peers	Norm	Students respond to orally presented situations of peer situations accompanied by colored photographs requiring inferences of what another is thinking or feeling; relevant to ToM
Test of Linguistic Competence—Expanded Edition (Wiig & Secord, 1989)	5 to 9 years Level 1 10 to 18 years Level 2	Ambiguous sentences, listening comprehension, making inferences, oral expression, recreating speeches, figurative language	Norm	Measures higher level metalinguistic language functions
TOPL-2 (Phelps-Terasaki & Phelps-Gunn, 2007)	6 to 18 years	Pragmatic evaluation: judge the effectiveness of a response to a social problem situation	Norm	Individual monitors and responds to social situations represented by pictures
Test of Problem Solving 2—Adolescent (Huisingh, Bowers, & LoGiudice, 2007)	12 to 17;11 years	Inferential thinking, determining solutions, problem solving, interpreting perspectives, and transferring insights	Norm	Students listen to passages presented orally then answer questions that require a range of critical thinking skills
Test of Problem Solving 3—Elementary (Bowers, Huisingh, & LoGiudice, 2005)	6 to 12;11 years	Inferential thinking, sequencing, predicting, problem solving, and determining causality	Norm	Students respond to orally presented situations accompanied by pictorial representations that they must respond to with a range of critical thinking skills

Table 9-4. Measures of the Social-Emotional Domain

Assessment Tool and Source	*Ages*	*Domains Assessed*	*Criterion- or Norm-Referenced*	*Test Construct, Format, Elicitation Techniques, Relevance for ASDs*
Ages and Stages Questionnaire—Social Emotional Screener-2 (ASQ-SE-2; Squires, Bricker, & Twombly, 2015)	1 to 72 months	Self-regulation, compliance, communication, adaptive behaviors, autonomy, affect, and social interaction	Norm	Parent-completed 30-item questionnaires
FEAS (Greenspan, DeGangi, & Wiede, 2001)	7 to 48 months	Child's functional social-emotional core capacities and related sensory, motor, cognitive, and linguistic capacities including self-regulation, reciprocal interactions, and play; caregiver's ability to support their child in each area	Criterion	Videotaped observations of unstructured parent–child interactions; requires specialized training to administer
Social Responsiveness Scale-2 (SRS-2; Constantino, 2012)	2;5 to 18 years	Social awareness, social cognition, social communication, social motivation, and autistic mannerisms	Norm	Parent or teacher completed rating scale measures severity of social impairment in ASD
Vineland Adaptive Behaviors Scales-2 (Sparrow, Cicchetti, & Balla, 2005)	0 to adult	Communication, daily living, socialization, and motor skills	Norm	Parent or caregiver rates child on 3-point scale in each domain

Social-Emotional Functioning

The clinician may want to include an assessment of an individual's social-emotional functioning, a core deficit in ASD that influences the use of communication and language. Some measures evaluate only the social-emotional domain (e.g., Functional Emotional Assessment Scale [FEAS; Greenspan, DeGangi, & Wieder, 2001]), whereas others were developed to assess various domains including the social (e.g., Vineland Adaptive Behaviors Scale-2 [Sparrow, Cicchetti, & Balla, 2005]). Table 9-4 lists some measures that can be used for this purpose. In terms of format, all but the FEAS (Greenspan et al., 2001) uses parental ratings of social impairment.

Informal Assessment Measures

Given that pragmatics is the use of language in context (Bates, 1976), it is difficult to see how standardized assessment measures can effectively capture the dynamic act of using language in an actual communicative situation. This complex act depends on aspects of the linguistic context, including what was said before, the relationship between the interactants that determine what can be said to whom, and a host of other linguistic and nonlinguistic variables. Given the complexity of an actual communicative event, clinicians who evaluate children with ASD include nonstandardized, informal measures such as behavioral observations, communication-language sampling and analysis, play sampling and analysis, and elicitations such as communicative temptations as core components of a comprehensive clinical assessment.

Behavioral Observations

The clinician will note the presence of any unusual behaviors or difficulties the child has in the two core areas: social interaction and social-communication-language, and repetitive, restricted behaviors, actions, or interests. These behavioral observations will occur throughout the entire evaluation, especially during informal receptive language assessment and expressive communication-language sampling.

Receptive Language

The clinician will note whether the child responds to the clinician's attempt to direct the child's interest to something he or she turns toward and points to. In addition, the clinician can note whether the child responds to his or her name when spoken by the parent or clinician. The clinician can also assess the child's ability to identify names for objects, actions, and attributes through object or picture identification. The child can be asked to carry out identifications by following directions in a low-structured context (e.g., "Give me a cookie" while having a snack) or in a more structured situation where the child is asked to identify items by pointing in a field of two, three, or four. The child can also be asked to identify body parts in the context of a play routine or in more structured activities. Information about receptive language can also be obtained from the standardized assessments listed in Table 9-4 as well as in information derived from Chapters 8 and 10 on the assessment of preschool-age and school-age language, respectively.

Receptive language assessment for school-age children with ASD who have more developed verbal skills can include many of the same higher-level receptive language tasks that one might use with other populations of language-impaired children, such as the ability to understand nonliteral language and make inferences. In addition, the clinician can assess these children's ToM by giving them false-belief tasks, which evaluate their ability to predict the thoughts, feelings, and mental states of others. In a classic ToM task described in the literature (Baron-Cohen, Leslie, & Frith, 1985), a girl hides a small object in one of two containers while another girl watches. When the girl who is watching leaves, the other girl switches the hiding place. The question for the child being evaluated is whether the girl who left the room will know where the object is after she returns. Most children with ASD who performed this task falsely predicted that the girl who left would know that the object was moved to a new location, failing to take the girl's perspective into account. The creative clinician who wishes to probe this area can construct vignettes based on this paradigm.

Communication-Language Sample

The core of a comprehensive language assessment for children with ASD is the communication-language sample. Although considered primarily a means of assessing expressive language, the clinician can glean information about comprehension as well as production by noting the child's responsiveness to language throughout the sample. In addition to communication and language, this naturalistic observational procedure can serve as an excellent opportunity for the clinician to observe the presence of the two core deficits in autism: social interaction and social communication, and restricted, repetitive behaviors, interests, and activities (RRBIA). Finally, the sample can serve as the basis for a play analysis.

Considerations for Obtaining the Communication-Language Sample

- The samples should be video-recorded to capture the nonlinguistic context and aspects of the child's nonverbal expression including affect, body orientation, gestures, and vocalizations.
- The clinician should interact with the child for part of the sample; more importantly, the sample should include parent–child interaction for younger children.
- The sample should incorporate child–child interaction with a peer if possible for a school-age child. In the event that a peer is not available, a sibling could serve as an interactant to ensure that the sample includes multiple conversational partners.
- The clinician will want to note how the child interacts with these varied communicative partners, including any modifications in linguistic form that the child makes with different listeners.
- Depending on the purpose of the assessment as well as practical logistical considerations, the sample could be obtained in different settings such as home, clinic, or school.
- The time needed to obtain the sample will vary but typically lasts about 30 minutes.
- The clinician should obtain the sample in a variety of low-structure contexts such free play, shared book reading, or having a snack. The particular contexts the clinician chooses will depend on the age, developmental level, and interests of the child.

Considerations for Transcribing and Coding the Sample

- Transcribing the sample is a lengthy but worthwhile endeavor because it can provide a wealth of information about the child's linguistic and nonlinguistic behavior.
- The level of transcription such as phonetic or lexical, and the inclusion of adult language input will depend on the purpose of the assessment

(Tager-Flusberg et al., 2009), such as describing regularities in the child's performance or intervention planning (Lahey, 1988).

- Finally, the clinician must select a means of coding the transcribed data, including manual coding or using computer-based software such as Systematic Analysis of Language Transcripts (Miller, Andriacci, & Nockerts, 2015) or Child Language Data Exchange System (MacWhinney, 2000), among others.
- In choosing a computer-based system over manual coding, the clinician needs to ensure that important aspects of the child's behavior such as shared attention, affective engagement, reciprocity, and shared intentions (Interdisciplinary Council on Development and Learning Disorders, 2005), which are so challenging for children on the spectrum, are not lost to the convenience of computer transcription and coding.
- When coding the data, whether by hand or computer, the clinician should also note whether the child's prelinguistic and linguistic forms were imitative, prompted, or spontaneous.

The areas selected for coding will depend on the communicative-linguistic and developmental level of the child. For the preintentional child, responsiveness to linguistic input and the ability to ability to engage in the social world through affect, gaze, body orientation can be noted through direct observation of the child interacting with a significant other. The clinician can comment on the child's affective engagement, reciprocity, and shared meanings (Interdisciplinary Council, 2005). For children who have achieved intentionality, the range of the child's communicative intentions and the forms through which they are expressed can be noted. For example, the clinician will note if the child points, vocalizes, or uses language for a range of intentions such as to direct the clinician's attention to something of interest. The clinician can also wave to the child to elicit an imitation, noting whether the child can role reverse his or her waving response to orient the greeting gesture toward the clinician.

Consideration for Analyzing the Sample

- The sample should be analyzed for the frequency, diversity, and types of forms produced; range of semantic relations expressed; and diversity of forms to express semantic content categories.
- The clinician should note the presence of any remarkable form–use interactions such as nonconventional, idiosyncratic use of words; examples of immediate and delayed echolalia; and pronoun reversals.
- The clinician may use a form–function checklist to chart the child's range of communicative intentions and the forms through which they were expressed. See Paul and Fahim (2014) for an example.

Conversational Sample Analysis

For children who engage in extended discourse, the sample can be analyzed for the variety of conversational skills described previously. If the clinician does not obtain evidence about these conversational skills through a natural language sample, the clinician can use contexts such as referential communication tasks to assess these skills. For further information on the elicitation and analysis of perspective-taking at the preschool, early school, and later school, the reader is referred to Geller (1989). For further information about the broader topic of language sampling analysis procedures, the reader is referred to Lahey (1988) and Retherford (2000).

Narrative Sample Analysis

Narrative language samples can be used to evaluate the following parameters:

- Pragmatic aspects such as adapting to the needs of the listener in terms of shared content
- Macrostructure (overall level of structural sophistication) using a system such as one of the following:
  - Applebee's (1978) levels that describe young children's narrative sophistication, such as the primitive narratives of 3- to 4-year-olds and the true narratives of 6- to 7-year-olds
  - Stein and Glenn's (1979) story grammar elements, which is suited to the fictionalized stories typical of the early school years
- Microstructure (smaller units within the narrative) elements, such as the types of clauses that are used to make it coherent and the types of linguistic devices that make it cohesive (In analyzing for cohesion, the clinician can note whether the child uses forms such as personal pronouns and definite articles to link his or her present utterance to what was said before.)

For guidelines for the collection and analysis of narrative samples, the clinician is referred to Lahey (1988) and Hughes, McGillivrey, and Schmidek (1997) and Chapter 10 on the assessment of school-age language and literacy disorders.

Communicative Temptations

If the child does not spontaneously communicate during the sampling procedure, the clinician can attempt to elicit intentions from the child through the use of communicative temptations (Wetherby & Prizant, 1989). These contexts were designed to entice the young child to engage in communicative interactions. These situations work best with children functioning between the prelinguistic through early language stage. Because communicative temptations may be presented nonverbally, they can be used with children with limited comprehension. For example, the clinician can blow up a balloon, then slowly deflate it, and wait for the child's response. Of note, this particular context appears on two standardized measures mentioned earlier: the ADOS-2 (Lord, Luyster, et al., 2012; Lord, Rutter, et al., 2012) and the CSBS (Wetherby & Prizant, 2003). In adapting this context for informal use, the clinician can note whether the temptation elicited a communicative function and, if so, the form of the child's response such as a vocalization, gesture, or word. For a description of several communicative temptations that can easily be used as part of a clinical assessment, the reader is referred to Wetherby and Prizant (1989) and Wetherby and Prutting (1984).

Play Sample and Analysis

The clinician who evaluates a child from about 8 months to 5 years of age will want to evaluate the child's play. The data obtained from direct observations of the child's play can complement the information gleaned through the interview, checklists, or standardized instruments the clinician selected to administer such as the CSBS (Wetherby & Prizant, 2003) or Rossetti Infant-Toddler Language Scale (Rossetti, 2006). The play analysis should be based on a representative sample of the child's play behaviors using a varied set of toys. Roth and Worthington (2016) provide suggestions for developmentally appropriate toys for use with children from birth through 5 years. The play sample should be about 30-minutes long and, depending on the child and contexts, the clinician can use parts of the language sample for the play analysis. Like language behaviors, the child's play can be coded as imitative, prompted, or spontaneous. In addition to levels, the child's play is analyzed in terms of four dimensions: decontextualization, thematic content, organization, and self–other relationships (Westby, 2000; see Chapter 8).

The clinician must use a variety of nonstandardized, informal measures in order to conduct a comprehensive communication-language assessment for an individual with ASD. These include behavioral observations of the core challenges that define the disorder as well as the related areas that have been described. At the heart of the assessment will be communication-language sampling and analysis with a variety of interactants and contexts, play sampling and analysis, and elicitations such as communicative temptations. The importance of evaluating comprehension through informal means and tasks has also been emphasized.

Differential Diagnosis

As noted in the introduction, ASD is a neurodevelopmental disability that represents a broad spectrum of disorders with challenges in two core areas: SCSI and the presence of RRBIA. According to the current DSM-5 criteria (APA, 2013), for children to be diagnosed with ASD, they must demonstrate deficits in these three areas of SCSI:

1. Social-emotional reciprocity such as reduced shared interests, affect, and emotions
2. Nonverbal communication such as impaired understanding or use of gestures
3. Developing, maintaining, and understanding, relationships such as difficulty forming friendships or engaging with peers

In terms of the second core area, RRBIA, the individual must demonstrate two of the following four criteria to receive an ASD diagnosis:

1. Stereotyped, repetitive speech, motor movements, or object use, such as repeatedly lining up toys
2. Insistence on sameness, inflexible routines, ritualized patterns of speech or behavior, such as the need to eat the same food daily
3. Highly restricted, intense, fixated interests such as only talking about or playing with trains
4. Hyper- or hyporeactivity to sensory input or unusual sensory responses to the environment, such as excessive smelling of objects

For each of these two domains, the clinician needs to specify the severity of the individual's symptoms based on the level of support required for that person to be able to function. The symptoms must cause the individual with ASD clinically significant challenges and be present in the early developmental period or by 3 years of age. In terms of differential diagnosis, the challenges that the individual experiences in the two core domains cannot be better explained by another disorder such as intellectual disability or global developmental delays. When an individual demonstrates challenges in SCSI but not RRBIA, the individual is diagnosed with social (pragmatic) language disorder rather than ASD (APA, 2013). This new diagnostic category is particularly important to SLPs.

In addition to intellectual disability and language impairment, other comorbid conditions that must be specified, including medical problems such as epilepsy, genetic disorders such as Rett syndrome, or associated neurological disorders such as ADHD. The reader is referred to Volkmar, Reichow, et al. (2014) for further discussion of comorbidity and other issues related to the differential diagnosis of ASD.

Case History for Sample Report

Following is the background information on a preschool-age child with an ASD. This case history will form the basis for the following sections, which list the formal and informal procedures the clinician selected for this child's speech and language evaluation.

J.B. is a 2;5-year-old boy who resides with his parents and older brother. His birth and medical history is unremarkable. His parents describe him as a quiet baby who was often happiest when left alone. At first, they thought he was deaf because he often did not respond when they called his name, but his hearing was found to be within normal limits. His responses to his name and other language input are still inconsistent. J's affect is described as relatively flat, and he does not engage in the back-and-forth games of infancy, such as peek-a-boo. In addition, he would peer at objects held close to the corner of his eyes, and when he was about 1 year old, he began to repeatedly flick his fingers. J acquired a few single words, which he used to communicate his wants and needs, between 12 and 15 months, but he stopped using them by the time he was 20 months. J's pediatrician referred the family to a neurodevelopmental specialty clinic, where J was diagnosed with ASD based on an assessment, which included the Toddler Module of the ADOS-2 at 24 months.

J has since been enrolled in a behaviorally oriented center-based early intervention program 3 half-days weekly. In addition, he receives home-based speech-language therapy for two individual 30-minute sessions weekly, which is also behaviorally oriented. Although the parents have noticed some gains, they feel their son is not progressing adequately and do not feel comfortable following up on the therapist's behaviorally oriented suggestions at home. They would like to supplement their son's therapy with another approach and have just begun to explore alternatives. In addition, the parents would like some suggestions on how to further develop their son's communication and language skills at home.

Formal and Informal Measures Selected With Provided Rationales for the Choices

- CARS-2, Standard Version: This scale allows the clinician to assign an overall severity rating of J's autism symptoms as well as ratings in the specific areas of social-emotional functioning, imitation, body movements, object use, adaptation to change, sensory peculiarities, communication, activity level, and intellectual functioning based on parental input. The standard version of the test was selected because J's chronological age was less than 6 years.
- Rossetti Infant-Toddler Language Scale: This scale allows the clinician to assign a developmental level to J's behaviors in the areas of interaction-attachment, pragmatics, gesture, play, language comprehension, and expression.
- Communication-Language Sample Analysis (Lahey, 1988): This informal assessment allows the clinician to analyze parent–child interaction patterns and all aspects of communication-language, determine J's level of language development, and develop goals for intervention.
- Communicative Temptations: This informal procedure adapted from the CSBS allows the clinician to elicit J's pragmatic functions and the forms through which they were expressed. The procedure is used informally because the CSBS was normed on children up to 24 months, which is below J's chronological age of 2;5 years.
- Informal Comprehension Assessment: J's responses to language were noted while he responded to requests to identify objects, people, actions, and body parts and to follow directions with and without gestural cues.
- Westby Play Scale: This informal assessment allowed the clinician to evaluate the level of J's

play in a naturalistic context. Play assessment was important because children on the spectrum usually are impaired in symbolic play.

Rubric Outline for Writing Observations, Communication-Language Assessment Section of Diagnostic Report

1. Label the first section "Formal Assessment."
2. Provide an introductory statement about how severity of autism was assessed using the CARS-2 (Schopler et al., 2010) and how these finding relate to the findings of the Toddler Module of the ADOS-2 (Lord, Luyster, et al., 2012), which was administered to the child prior to this assessment as part of a neuropsychological workup. State which behaviors were rated on the CARS-2, the child's overall severity rating, and an example of his behaviors for each area.
3. Provide an introductory statement about the Rossetti Infant-Toddler Language Scale (Rossetti, 2006) and the domains that it assesses. List the child's age ranges on the various domains. Place information in a table.
4. Label the next section "Informal Assessment."
5. Provide an introductory statement of how the communication language sample served as an informal measure. Describe how the sample was obtained, recorded and transcribed. Describe the instructions given to the parent/interactant. List the toys and objects that were available. Describe child's communication-language and other relevant behaviors (e.g., play) that occurred during the sample. Provide examples.
6. Provide an introductory statement about the communicative temptations as an informal assessment adapted from the CSBS (Wetherby & Prizant, 2002). Describe the contexts and the child's responses. Summarize the child's forms and functions from this elicitation in a table.
7. Label the next section "Receptive Language."
8. Provide an introductory statement about the challenges of assessing comprehension deficits in this child. In the next paragraph, provide examples of evidence of the child's comprehension problems from the informal assessment. Compare the results of the informal assessment to the comprehension results on the formal assessment with the Rossetti Infant-Toddler Language Scale (2006).
9. Label the next section "Expressive Communication Language."
10. Provide an introductory statement how behaviors from both the spontaneous language sample and the communicative temptations section will be used together to assess this child's communication-language. Describe the child's overall stage of expressive language development, the content categories that were expected, and those that were observed. Provide examples from the data.
11. Write an introductory statement about the child's pragmatic use of language including his communicative functions and his reliance on linguistic or contextual support. Compare the findings on pragmatics from the informal assessment to the pragmatic level based on the Rossetti Infant-Toddler Language Scale. Summarize the child's linguistic form, content, and use in a table with examples from the data.
12. Label the next section "Play."
13. Provide an introductory statement about the selection of the Westby (2000) Play Scale as an informal measure of play. Provide examples that support your description of the child's level of play and the relevant dimension of play. Provide a statement of the consistency of the findings based on the Westby Play Scale and the Rossetti Infant-Toddler Language Scale.

Sample Report

Speech and Language Evaluation

Client: JB **DOE**: *(mm/dd/yr)*
Address: **DOB**: *(mm/dd/yr)*
Phone number(s):
Parents' Names: SB and VB
Diagnosis: Autism spectrum disorder

I. Reason for Referral

J.B., a 2;5-year-old boy, attends a half-day center-based early intervention program for children with autism spectrum disorder (ASD) at XYZ. In addition, he receives two half-hour sessions weekly of speech-language therapy. He was seen at the Speech-Language-Hearing Center for a speech and language evaluation over two sessions on mm/dd/yr and mm/dd/yr. The director of the speech-language services at XYZ referred J's family to the clinic upon their request for additional services.

II. Tests Administered/Procedures

- Parent Interview
- Childhood Autism Rating Scale-2 (CARS-2)
- Rossetti Infant-Toddler Language Scale
- Language Sample Analysis (Lahey, 1988)
- Communicative Temptations adapted from Communication and Symbolic Behavior Scales (CSBS)
- Westby Play Scale
- Oral-Peripheral Examination
- Feeding Observation

III. Background Information

Birth and Developmental History

J.B. was the result of a full-term pregnancy and normal delivery. Birth weight was 7 lbs, 2 oz. His birth history was unremarkable. His parents described him as a "good" baby who was often happiest when left alone. At first, they thought he was deaf because he rarely made sounds and often did not respond when they called his name. A formal audiological assessment done at that time revealed hearing sensitivity to be in the normal range bilaterally. His responses to his name and other language input are still inconsistent. When asked about other early concerns, the parents recalled that, as an infant, J would peer at objects held close to the corner of his eyes, and at about 1 year, he began to flick his fingers repeatedly. In addition, they were concerned about J's flat affect and lack of interest the back-and-forth games of infancy such as peek-a-boo. They further reported that if J wanted something, he would take one of them by the hand to lead them to what he wanted. In addition, they noted that he did not point to objects just to show them and rarely made sounds except for high-pitched squeals.

In terms of feeding, J was breastfed until about 6 months and did not experience any difficulties transitioning to the bottle, but seemed to dislike solid foods with a mushy texture. His parents reported that he is now able to tolerate foods of a greater variety of tastes and textures, although they still considered him a picky eater.

J's motor developmental milestones were achieved at the upper limits of the normal range with sitting unassisted at age 6 months and walking unassisted at age 18 months. J has not yet shown any interest in becoming toilet trained.

A few single words, which were used to communicate wants and needs, emerged between 12 and 15 months, which is the typical time frame. At 18 months, he began to talk less, and by the time he was 20 months, he stopped using words at all. The only sounds J made were high-pitched squeals when he was angry or frustrated. These sounds were often accompanied by behaviors such as jumping up and down. J currently communicates through vocalizations, picture symbols, manual signs, and some words. He now has a vocabulary of about 20 words.

Medical/Health History

J was characterized as a healthy baby who has never had any serious illnesses or hospitalizations. J's inconsistent response to his name, lack of interest in social routines, tendency to peer at objects out of the corners of his eyes, emergence of finger flicking, and loss of his early words led the family to seek a neurodevelopmental assessment at age 24 months. J's pediatrician referred the family to a neurodevelopmental pediatric clinic affiliated with a university hospital, where J received a comprehensive assessment at 24 months that included administration of the Toddler Module of the ADOS-2. As a result of this multidisciplinary evaluation, J was diagnosed with ASD with language impairment. Mr. and Mrs. B were devastated upon learning of J's diagnosis but tried to learn as much as possible about their son's problems.

Family/Social History

J resides with his mother, S, his father, V, and 5-year-old brother, E, who is in a general education kindergarten class. Mrs. B works part-time as a school crossing guard, and Mr. B edits television commercials. J's maternal grandmother also lives with the family and assists with child care until Mrs. B returns from work. Mrs. B reported that E tries to play with J but that J does not seem to know how to play with his older brother. The only games they enjoy together are physical games such as "chase" and cars, but J only plays with E in a limited way. For example, if E tries to play "garage," J takes the cars and lines them up in a particular order. When E suggests making the cars go somewhere, J does not respond. Outside of the home, at family gatherings where other children are present, J often appears overwhelmed and does not usually play with them. On these occasions, he either remains close to his parents or plays alone. Family history was negative for speech, language, or hearing problems. English is the only language spoken in the home.

Educational/Therapeutic History

After J's diagnosis, the family obtained services through early intervention. He was enrolled in a center-based behaviorally oriented program for children with autism at 25 months. He currently attends that program 3 half-days weekly and receives individual speech-language therapy at home 2 afternoons weekly. The parents reported that the therapist uses similar behavioral techniques. The educational program has focused on J's responses to commands such as "look at me" and the use of picture symbols to communicate. Although the family has seen some progress, they do not feel that this is the best approach for their son and would like him to make more rapid gains. Mr. and Mrs. B, who have done extensive reading on ASD interventions over the past few months, indicated that they would like to explore more developmental relationship-based approaches, which they have recently heard about. In addition, they would like their son to receive occupational therapy to address his sensory-regulatory issues, which was not funded through early intervention. They are currently looking into different program options for their son when he transitions from early intervention into the Committee on Preschool Education (CPSE) system when he turns 3 years old.

IV. Clinical Observations

J presented as a handsome, ambulatory little boy who reticently entered the evaluation room with his parents. He initially remained in close physical proximity to them but slowly explored his surroundings, picking up various toys then putting them down. He did not show the toys to his parents or attempt to share his focus of attention with them. He remained aloof of the clinical staff for most of the evaluation and was difficult to engage. The parents remained in the room throughout the evaluation. There was no attempt to have J separate from them during the session. When the clinician showed J a fire engine that made noise, he jumped up and down as if excited, then covered his ears as if hypersensitive to this sound.

Audiological Screening

An audiological screening was not attempted, but a complete audiological examination with thorough play audiometry is recommended as a follow-up.

Oral Motor and Feeding Skills

J exhibited normal muscle tone in the oral-facial region. He generally maintained a closed mouth posture at rest. His oral-peripheral structures appeared symmetrical. An oral-peripheral examination was attempted, but J did not follow all of the directions to complete this activity even when a model was provided. For example, he did not imitate the clinician's oral motor lingual movements of tongue tip protrusion, elevation, lateralization, and elevation. He was able to imitate the labial movements of protrusion and retraction following a model.

The clinician assessed J's feeding skills by observing him eat a snack of goldfish crackers. Instead of placing a cracker in his mouth, J held it in the front of his mouth in the space between his lips and front teeth until the cracker softened. Then J sucked it into his oral cavity. J consumed all of the crackers in this way. This behavior appeared to be sensory seeking. J did not demonstrate tongue lateralization or rotary chewing at any time during the snack. He drank single sips of liquid from an open cup without spillage.

Formal Assessment

The CARS-2, a criterion-referenced measure, was administered to determine severity ratings of J's autistic symptoms on a 4-point scale in the areas of social-emotional functioning, imitation, body movements, object use, adaptation to change, sensory peculiarities, communication, activity level, and intellectual functioning based on parental input and clinician observations. His ratings ranged from 2.5 to 4.0, with the mean of his ratings at 3.5, falling in the moderately to severely impaired range. Table 1 indicates J's ratings on 15 categories of the CARS-2.

The Rossetti Infant-Toddler Language Scale, a criterion-referenced measure, was used to identify J's age performance in the domains of interaction-attachment, pragmatics, gesture, play, language comprehension, and expression based on behaviors that were observed, elicited, or reported. He demonstrated scatter in performance across these domains with significant delays in all areas. His age performance levels

Table 1. Severity Ratings of J's Behaviors on the CARS-2

Categories	*Ratings* **1 = Age appropriate** **2 = Mildly abnormal** **3 = Moderately abnormal** **4 = Severely abnormal**	*Examples*
Relating to people	3	J was not attentive to adults in the room at times; the clinician needed to persist to obtain his attention.
Imitation	3.5	J did not imitate the clinician's symbolic play behaviors.
Emotional response	3	J responded with laughter when he was reprimanded.
Body use	3.5	J jumped up and down and flapped his hands.
Object use	3	J shows limited interest in toys; he rarely used toys symbolically.
Adaptation to change	2.5	J had difficulty transitioning from the wind-up toy to the balloon activity.
Visual response	4	J held a block near the corner of his eye, peering at it for a prolonged period.
Listening response	4	J covered his ears when the toy fire engine alarm sounded. He inconsistently responded to his name.
Taste, smell, and touch response	2.5	Reportedly, J is a picky eater. He was observed to lick pretzels before he ate them.
Fear or nervousness	3	Reportedly, J has an unexplainable fear of swings.
Verbal communication	4	J demonstrated limited use meaningful speech; he produced nonlinguistic squeals.
Nonverbal communication	3	J demonstrated limited affective engagement and gestures; he has difficulty reading the nonverbal signals of others.
Activity level	2	J roamed around the room but was able to sit to attend when directed.
Level and consistency of intellectual response	3.5	Child did not exhibit superior intellectual functioning in any one specific domain.
General impressions	3.5	Child shows limited shared attention, affective engagement, reciprocity, shared intentions, symbolic play, inconsistent responses, unusual sensory responses, repetitive behaviors and impaired receptive and expressive language.
Total ratings	44	J's ratings placed him in the severe autism range.

ranged from 9 to 12 months through 18 to 21 months. Table 2 indicates J's age performance levels on the six domains assessed with examples of his behaviors.

Informal Assessment

Communication Language and Play Sample

A spontaneous communication-language sample analysis was obtained while J interacted with his mother for a 30-minute period. The sample was video recorded for later transcription and analysis. Mrs. B was instructed to play with J as if she had some free time to spend with him. A variety of toys were available for them to choose from. These included a pop-up toy, jack-in-the-box, baby doll, stuffed Elmo toy, blanket, pretend food, toy pot, spoon, cup, two cars, several blocks, airplane, box, picture book, and garage. During the sample, J demonstrated intermittent shared positive affect, reciprocity, and shared attention while playing with the toys. Of note, he favored the pop-up toy but became self-absorbed while playing with it. When his mother suggested playing with something else, he said "no, no, no," shook his head, and flapped his hands. When his mother successfully coaxed him to play with something else, he turned the handle of

Table 2. Age Performance Levels on the Rossetti Infant-Toddler Language Scale in Six Domains

Domain	*Age Performance Level*	*Examples*
Interaction/ attachment	15 to 18 months	J stayed in close proximity to his parents when the clinician greeted him.
Pragmatics	9 to 12 months	J indicated a desire to change activities by pushing away an object.
Gesture	12 to 15 months	J shook his head "no."
Play	18 to 21 months	J used two toys together in pretend play when he held a bottle to a doll's mouth.
Language comprehension	12 to 15 months	J responded to a "give me" command when he gave the clinician a balloon.
Language expression	12 to 15 months	Reportedly, J uses 8 to 10 words spontaneously.

Table 3. J's Communicative Forms and Functions During Four Communicative Temptations

Communicative Temptation	*Function/Intention*	*Form Nonlinguistic Linguistic*
Wind-up toy	Request for action	Gesture: gives toy to clinician Word: *more*
Balloon	Request for action Label Comment	Gesture: gives balloon to clinician Word: *blow* *balloon* *up*
Bubbles	Request for action Label Comments	Gesture: gives bubbles to clinician Word: *more* *bubble* *pop; all gone*
Jar	Request for action	Gesture: gives jar to clinician Word: *open*

the jack-in-the-box but became fearful and covered his ears when the toy popped up and made a sound. Again, he said, "no, no, no," flapped his hands, and pushed it away. He peered at the cars out of the corners of his eyes, and then repeatedly rolled them back and forth. When his mother attempted to engage him with the airplane, J shifted his gaze from the airplane to his mother and said "up." While looking at the book together, J produced the words bear and boy to label pictures. He did not spontaneously play with any of the representational toys but imitated his mother's action of holding the spoon to Elmo's mouth. When she covered the Elmo doll with the blanket to hide it, J pulled the blanket off, looked at his mother, and smiled.

Communicative Temptations

Four communicative temptations from the CSBS were administered by the clinician and used informally to provide additional sampling opportunities in which to observe J's communication and language. These contexts—a wind-up toy, balloon, bubbles, and jar—were designed to elicit communicative intentions. During the first temptation, the clinician activated a wind-up toy, let it deactivate, and then handed it to J. During the next context, the clinician blew up a balloon, held it up, and then slowly deflated it. Next, the clinician blew some bubbles, then closed the jar tightly, and then gave it to J. Finally, the clinician shook an opaque jar containing a small object to make a noise and then gave J the jar. During these contexts J demonstrated a variety of communicative intentions that were expressed through gestures and words. In addition, he occasionally shifted his gaze from the clinician to the object of interest, indicating some initiations of joint attention. Table 3 lists J's form–function interactions that were elicited through these contexts.

Table 4. Results of J's Level 2 Form: Content–Use Analysis

Content	*Form*		*Use*
	Item	**Frequency**	**Function**
Existence	balloon	1	Request
	bubble	1	Label
	bear	1	Label
	boy	1	Label
Nonexistence	bubble	1	Label
Recurrence	more	2	Request
Rejection	no	2	Protest
Action	blow	1	Request
	pop	1	Comment
	open	1	Request
Locative action	up	2	Comment

Receptive Language

Given J's communication profile, it is difficult to capture his strengths and weaknesses through a receptive language age range. J's difficulties strongly suggest significant difficulties in comprehending spoken language and possible auditory processing challenges. His inconsistent responses to auditory input suggest that his comprehension may be somewhat greater than he was able to demonstrate.

J inconsistently responded to his name. He identified several common objects by pointing to them when they were named. These included the spoon, car, and airplane during play and crackers, juice, and a cup during a snack. He did not identify eyes, ears, nose, or mouth by pointing. He identified his mother and father by looking at each of them in response to the clinician's questions, "Where's mommy?" and "Where's daddy?" He did not pick up the Elmo doll when asked, although his mother indicated that he was familiar with that character. He followed one-step commands such as "sit down" and "give me the book" when gestural cues were provided. His significantly impaired performance during the informal comprehension assessment corroborate with parental report and the results of the Rossetti Infant-Toddler Language Scale.

Expressive Communication-Language

On the basis of both the spontaneous language sample and the communicative temptations, J's expressive language and communication development is at the single-word stage. On the basis of a Level 2 analysis (Lahey, 1988), J coded six of the nine phase 1 content categories, including existence (bear; balloon), nonexistence/disappearance (e.g., all gone), recurrence (e.g., more), rejection (no), action (e.g., blow; pop), and locative action (up). Although coding the semantic notions of possession and attribution was not observed, Mrs. B reported that J has expressed them with words such as mine and hot. Reportedly, he has not coded denial.

In terms of early pragmatic intentions, J used language to label, comment, regulate, and protest. He also communicated with gestures sometimes coordinated with gaze. All of J's utterances were in the "here and now," requiring the perceptual support of the nonlinguistic context. Given these observations and parental report, J's expressive language, which is significantly impaired, approximates the 15-month level. These findings corroborate with the results of the Rossetti Infant-Toddler Language Scale. J's expressive language performance during the evaluation is described in Table 4.

Play

J's play was analyzed according to the Westby Play Scale, an informal measure that allowed the clinician to evaluate the level and dimensions of J's play in a naturalistic context while he interacted with his mother. J's play was considered presymbolic because his play was predominantly sensorimotor rather than symbolic. He demonstrated the dimensions of sensorimotor, presymbolic play along the dimensions of object permanence (e.g., pulling the blanket off of Elmo when he was hidden), means–end problem solving (pushing a button to activate the pop-up toy), and object use (e.g., rolling a car). Only one imitative symbolic play scheme was observed when J copied his mother's action of holding the spoon to Elmo's mouth. His level of play in the 13- to 17-month range on the Westby Play Scale was lower than his level the Rossetti Infant-Toddler Language Scale (18 to 24 months), but both represent significant delays.

Speech, Articulation, and Prosody

J's speech, articulation, and prosody were assessed through the communication-language sample. He demonstrated a limited repertoire of speech sounds and syllabic structures. Most of the sounds in his phonemic inventory such as /p/, /b/, and /m/ are produced in the front of the mouth. The syllabic structure of most of his word productions consisted of CV or CVCV sequences. J sometimes spoke in a high-pitched voice as when he uttered "no, no, no" to protest. Several of his words were produced with a terminal rising intonation contour, which gave his speech an unusual prosodic pattern.

Fluency

On the basis of informal assessment, the fluency of J's speech was rated within normal limits.

V. Clinical Impressions

J.B. is a 2;5-year-old boy who presents with behaviors consistent with ASD and language impairment. He has difficulties with the foundational communication domains of shared attention, affective engagement, and reciprocity although a few episodes of joint attention were observed over the session. J has recently begun to use words after a history of language regression and is currently at the single-word stage of language development, where he has begun to share meanings through gestures and words with others. His language challenges are in both comprehension and production in the domains the form, content, and use. In addition, his speech is characterized by an unusual prosodic pattern and he demonstrates some oral motor difficulties. J also has challenges in symbolic play and demonstrates some sensory regulatory issues.

VI. Recommendations

A. J would benefit from developmentally based communication-language therapy on a twice-weekly basis for individual 45-minute sessions to supplement the services that J currently receives through early intervention. The clinician should establish a collaborative partnership with J's teacher and the SLP in his educational setting. Therapy should incorporate a parent education component that emphasizes J's communication challenges and allows members of his family to work closely with the clinician to facilitate J's development in the areas in which he is challenged. This supplemental therapy could also incorporate J's older brother as a typically developing peer.

B. J would benefit from continued attendance at his center-based early intervention program and then transition into a preschool program that will address his communication challenges in the areas of shared attention, affective engagement, and reciprocity. The parents could use this time before J ages out of early intervention to visit a variety of preschool programs representing different intervention approaches so that they can become more informed about available treatment options. They could benefit from exploring the range of treatments options available for children with ASD, including both behavioral and developmental social pragmatic approaches.

C. J should receive an occupational therapy evaluation by a clinician who is knowledgeable about sensory regulatory issues.

D. J should receive an audiological evaluation to determine his current hearing status.

E. The following Long-Term Goals and Short-Term Goals related to the Long-Term Goals were established for J's intervention:

1. Long-Term Goal: J will demonstrate a range of communicative intentions with a variety of single words expected at Phase 1 (Lahey, 1988).
   - Short-Term Goal: J will produce 5 to 10 novel words to comment on activities and events in the immediate context during a 30-minute play interaction with a familiar adult.
   - Short-Term Goal: J will request objects or actions of others with 5 to 10 novel words during a 30-minute play interaction with a familiar adult.
2. Long-Term Goal: J will coordinate his nonverbal communication with his verbal communication.
   - Short-Term Goal: J will coordinate gesture + word three to five times during joint action routines with a familiar adult.
   - Short-Term Goal: J will coordinate gaze + word three to five times during joint action routines with a familiar adult.
3. Long-Term Goal: J will comprehend a variety of familiar words and phrases during familiar routines.
   - Short-Term Goal: J will look at a familiar adult in response to his name five times during a 15-minute play routine.
   - Short-Term Goal: J will give or show objects when named by a familiar adult five times during a 15-minute play routine.
   - Short Term Goal: J will perform an action on an object when named by a familiar adult five times during a 15-minute play routine.

____

(Name of clinician or clinical supervisor and credentials)

Speech-Language Pathologist

Case History for a Practice Exercise

In this section, a novel case history is presented. The reader's task is to develop a speech-language evaluation protocol for the child described. Outline the formal and informal procedures that would be included in a comprehensive speech and language evaluation. Be sure to include the specific measures you would select and your rationales for choosing them. In addition, list concomitant areas for which the clinician should obtain further information.

M.G. is a 4;11-year-old boy who is enrolled in a regular pre-kindergarten class. He talks in complete sentences that are grammatically correct. On the basis of the results of previous psychological testing, M has intelligence in the normal range. Development milestones were achieved at the normal times, but M was characterized as "clumsy." His parents were seeking a speech and language evaluation because of concerns regarding their son's difficulty sustaining conversations at home and at school. Both parents reported that M often resorts to scripted speech that he has heard others use in previous conversations. The parents noted that they are able to understand M's speech, but that sometimes he speaks in a "sing-song" voice that is too loud for the situation. They also reported that M is a picky eater who avoids foods with mushy textures such as pudding.

During a recent parent–teacher conference, M's teacher told the parents about their son's difficulties in making friends at school. The teacher reported that, although M is interested in his classmates, he does not know how to interact or play with them. Specifically, the teacher reported that when M approaches other children, he does not take turns with them in play or conversation. The teacher noted that sometimes M monopolizes the conversation and will talk only about topics that interest him such as trains. At other times, M remains quiet and needs to be brought into the conversation by the teacher or another adult. The teacher further reported that MG sometimes tells jokes that do not make sense and will laugh. Furthermore, he does not seem to know when others are joking. In terms of comprehension, the teacher felt that M's answers to questions were sometimes off target. The teacher further reported that M is beginning to decode written material, but it is not clear whether he understands what he is reading.

Summary

In this chapter, we have seen that the comprehensive evaluation of individuals with ASD is a complex process with numerous areas that need to be addressed. This heterogeneous population has core challenges in two domains—SCSI and RRBIA—that often co-occur with cognitive and linguistic impairment. As a first step, the clinician should determine the developmental level of the individual, which will direct the rest of the assessment. Furthermore, it is crucial that the clinician gather as much background information from the parents or other primary caregivers who should be key players in all aspects of the assessment process. This will help the clinician become attuned to the concerns of the family. In addition, the clinician should obtain information from allied professionals who might provide an understanding of the child's associated challenges. This will enable the clinician to think outside of the box of speech-language pathology and embrace a broad, interprofessional perspective. This chapter also included information on formal, standardized and informal, nonstandardized procedures. In terms of standardized procedures, despite the myriad formal assessments presented in this chapter, the clinician needs to remember the important role of both clinical judgment and informal observations in evaluating individuals on the spectrum. Finally, the clinician should remember that the social interactive nature of the evaluation process is particularly challenging to these individuals.

Glossary

Asperger disorder: One of five ASDs in the DSM-IV characterized by normal cognitive abilities, impaired social interaction skills, and retracted, repetitive patterns of behavior; language difficulties are often restricted to the pragmatic domain; similar to high-functioning autism.

Autism: Sometimes called *classic autism* in the diagnostic literature that preceded the DSM-5; represents a wide range of functioning in two core areas of deficit: SCSI and the presence of RRBIA.

Autism spectrum disorders: An umbrella term for a disability in which individuals share two core areas of deficit: SCSI and the presence of RRBIA. The term *spectrum* represents a broad range of challenges in the two core areas.

Childhood disintegrative disorder: One of five ASDs in the former DSM-IV that was characterized by regression between the ages of 2 and 10 years in the following areas: communication-language, social interaction, motor skills, bowel or bladder control, or play; also called *Heller syndrome*. CDD is no longer classified as a separate disorder in the current DSM-5 system but rather subsumed under the broader term autism if the onset occurs before age 3 years, the early developmental period.

Contact gestures: A form of nonverbal communication in which the individual makes physical contact with an object or person to request objects or actions (e.g., putting an adult's hand on a door knob to request going outside).

Deixis: A linguistic device that anchors an utterance to the communicative context in which it occurs; person deixis indicates who the speaker and listener are (e.g., I/you); place deixis indicates where the speaker and listener are at the time of the utterance (e.g., here/there); time deixis indicates when an utterance is taking place (e.g., now/later).

Delayed echolalia: The repetition of an original utterance at some later time; may contain scripted language; may appear idiosyncratic to listeners who do not know the context of the original utterance; can serve communicative functions for children on the autistic spectrum.

Distal gestures: Pointing to objects and events at a distance; one means to initiate joint attention when coordinated with gaze and vocalizations or words; an ability that is often a challenge for children with ASDs.

Hyperlexia: Exceptionally well-developed reading skills relative to IQ or mental age; a splinter skill found in some high-functioning children with ASD; phonological decoding skills are significantly advanced relative to semantic comprehension.

Immediate echolalia: The instant repetition of an original utterance; often occurs in contexts of limited comprehension; may serve communicative function such as turn-taking for children on the spectrum.

Joint attention: The ability to use gesture, body language, facial expression, vocalization, or language to direct another's attention to or share interest in an object or an event. Children with ASD are often impaired in their ability to both initiate joint attention and to respond to other's bids for joint attention.

Pervasive developmental disorders: An umbrella term used in the former DSM-IV that had often been used synonymously with ASDs. The term reflected the varied domains that affected in these individuals—namely, the cognitive, social, and linguistic.

Pervasive developmental disorder—not otherwise specified: One of five ASDs in the former DSM-IV characterized by milder symptoms than classic autism; characteristics included impaired social interaction and impaired communication-language or repetitive, restricted behaviors. Individuals with this disability might not qualify for ASD under the current DSM-5 system.

Presuppositional skills: The aspects of pragmatics related to background information that is not contained in the utterance but must be known and understood if that utterance is to make sense. Presuppositional knowledge includes how speakers differentiate new information from old information and the linguistic devices that mark this distinction such as articles, ellipsis, and topic introductory devices.

Rett disorder: One of five ASDs in the former DSM-IV with a known genetic cause that affects only females; characterized by regression after 5 months in purposeful hand movements, social engagement, and language, cognitive, and gross motor development. Rett disorder is no longer considered an ASD, but is to co-occur with ASD.

Scripted language: An utterance or utterances that can originate in a story, commercial or some other memorized whole. Some delayed echolalia of children with ASDs contains such gestalt, unanalyzed language that differs from spontaneous, generative language.

Splinter skills: Areas of extraordinary talent in some people with autism such as music, art, or hyperlexia; reflect strengths of individuals on the spectrum who often have an uneven profile of abilities.

Theory of mind: The ability to perceive the predictable thoughts, complex emotions, or mental states of another; deficits in the normal process of empathizing with another; sometimes called mindblindness.

References

Alpern, C. S., & Zager, D. (2007). Addressing communication needs of young adults with autism in a college-based inclusion program. *Education and Training in Developmental Disabilities, 42*, 428-436.

American Psychiatric Association. (1994). *Diagnostic and statistical manual of mental disorders* (4th ed.). Washington, DC: Author.

American Psychiatric Association. (2000). *Diagnostic and statistical manual of mental disorders* (4th ed., text revision). Washington, DC: Author.

American Psychiatric Association. (2013). *Diagnostic and statistical manual of mental disorders* (5th ed.). Washington, DC: Author.

American Speech-Language-Hearing Association. (2006). Knowledge and skills needed by speech-language pathologists for diagnosis, assessment, and treatment for autism spectrum disorders across the lifespan. Retrieved from www.asha.org/members

American Speech-Language-Hearing Association. (2007). Childhood apraxia of speech [technical report]. Retrieved from http://www.asha.org/policy/tr2007-00278.htm

Applebee, N. (1978). *The child's concept of story.* Chicago, IL: University of Chicago Press.

Asperger, H. (1944). Die "Autistischen Psychopathen" im Kindesalter. *Arcive fur Psychatrie und Nervenkrankheiten, 117*, 76-136.

Ayers, A. J. (2000). *Developmental dyspraxia and adult onset apraxia.* Torrance, CA: Sensory Integration International.

Baranek, G. T., Little, L. M, Parham, D., Ausderau, K. K., & Sabatos-DeVito, M. G. (2014). Sensory features in autism spectrum Disorders. In F. R. Volkmar, S. J. Rogers, R. Paul, & K. A. Pelfrey (Eds.) *Handbook on autism and pervasive developmental disorders: Vol. 1. Diagnosis, development, and brain mechanisms* (4th ed., pp. 378-407). New York, NY: Wiley.

Baranek, G. T., Parham, D., & Bodfish, J. W. (2005). Sensory and motor features in autism: Assessment and intervention. In F. R. Volkmar, R. Paul, A. Klin, & D. Cohen (Eds.), (2005). *Handbook on autism and pervasive developmental disorders: Vol. 2. Assessment, interventions, and policy* (pp. 831-857) New York, NY: Wiley.

Baron-Cohen, S. (1995). *Mindblindness: An essay on autism and theory of mind.* Boston, MA: MIT Press/Bradford Books.

Baron-Cohen, S., Allen, J., & Gillberg, C. (1992). Can autism be detected at 18 months? The needle, the haystack and the (CHAT). *British Journal of Psychiatry, 161*, 839-843.

Baron-Cohen, S., Leslie, A., & Frith, U. (1985). Does the autistic child have a "theory of mind"? *Cognition, 21*, 37-46.

Baron-Cohen, S., Wheelwright, S., Lawson, J., Griffin, R., Ashwin, C., Billington J., & Chakrabarti, B. (2005). In F. R. Volkmar, R. Paul, A. Klin, & D. Cohen (Eds.), *Handbook on autism and pervasive developmental disorders: Vol. 2. Assessment, interventions, and policy* (3rd ed., pp. 628-639) New York, NY: Wiley.

Bauminger-Zviely, N. (2014). School-age children with ASD. In F. R. Volkmar, S. J. Rogers, R. Paul, & K. A. Pelfrey (Eds.), *Handbook on autism and pervasive developmental disorders: Vol. 1. Diagnosis, development, and brain mechanisms* (4th ed., pp. 148-175). New York, NY: Wiley.

Bates, E. (1976). *Language and context: The acquisition of pragmatics.* New York, NY: Academic Press.

Beukelman, D. R., & Mirenda, P. (2013). *Augmentative alternative communication: Supporting children and adults with complex communication needs.* Baltimore, MD: Brookes.

Bishop, D. (2006). *Children's communication checklist—2.* San Antonio, TX: Pearson Assess.

Bloom, L., & Lahey, M. (1978). *Language development and language disorders.* New York, NY: Wiley.

Bodison, S., & Mostofsky, S. (2014). Motor control and motor learning processes in autism spectrum disorders. In F. R. Volkmar, S. J. Rogers, R. Paul, & K. A. Pelfrey (Eds.), *Handbook on autism and pervasive developmental disorders: Vol. 1. Diagnosis, development, and brain mechanisms* (pp. 354-377). New York, NY: Wiley.

Bowers, L., Huisingh, R., & LoGiudice, C. (2005). *Test of problem solving 3—Elementary.* East Moline, IL: LinguiSystems.

Bowers, L., Huisingh, R., & LoGiudice, C. (2008). *Social language development test—Elementary.* East Moline, IL: LinguiSystems.

Carpenter, M., & Tomasello, M. (2000). Joint attention, cultural learning, and language acquisition. In A. M. Wetherby & B. M. Prizant (Eds.), *Autism spectrum disorders: A transactional developmental perspective* (pp. 31-54). Baltimore, MD: Brookes.

Carrow-Woolfolk, E. (2016). *Comprehensive assessment of spoken language—Second edition.* Los Angeles, LA: Western Psychological Services.

Charman, T., Pickles, A., Simonoff, E., Chandler, S., Loucas, T., & Baird, G. (2010). IQ in children with autism spectrum disorders: Data from the special needs and autism project (SNAP). *Psychological Medicine, 41*, 619-627.

Constantino, J. (2012). *Social responsiveness scale, second edition.* Los Angeles, CA: Western Psychological Corporation.

Davis, N. O., & Carter, A. S. (2014). Social development in autism. In F. R. Volkmar, S. J. Rogers, R. Paul, & K. A. Pelfrey (Eds.) *Handbook on autism and pervasive developmental disorders: Vol. 1. Diagnosis, development, neurobiology, and behavior* (4th ed., pp. 212-229). New York, NY: Wiley.

Fenson, L., Marchman, V., Thal, D., Dale, P., Reznick, J. S. & Bates, E. (2006). *MacArthur-Bates communicative development inventories, second edition.* Baltimore. MD: Brookes.

Gal, E., Cermak, S. A., & Ben-Sasson, A. (2007). Sensory processing disorders in children with autism: Nature, assessment, and intervention. In R. L. Gabriels & D. E. Hill (Eds.), *Growing up with autism* (pp. 95-123). New York, NY: Guilford Press.

Geller, E. (1989). The assessment of perspective taking skills. *Seminars in Speech and Language, 10*, 28-41.

Gerber, S., & Prizant, B. F. (2000). Speech, language, and communication assessment and intervention for children. In *Clinical practice guidelines: Redefining the standards of care for infants, children, and families with special needs* (pp. 85-122). Bethesda, MD: ICDL Press.

Gilliam, J. E. (2013). *Gilliam Autism rating scale—2.* Los Angeles, LA: Western Psychological Services.

Gilliam, J. E., & Miller, L. (2006). *Pragmatic language skills inventory.* Austin, TX: PRO-ED.

Grandin, T. (2005). A personal perspective of autism. In F. R. Volkmar, R. Paul, A. Klin, & D. Cohen (Eds.), *Handbook on autism and pervasive developmental disorders: Vol. 2. Assessment, interventions, and policy* (pp. 1276-1286) New York, NY: Wiley.

Greenspan, S., DeGangi, G., & Wieder, S. (2001). *Functional emotional assessment scale.* Bethesda, MD: Interdisciplinary Council on Development and Learning Disorders Press.

Grice, H. P. (1975). Logic and conversation: In P. Cole & J. Morgan (Eds.) *Speech acts: Syntax and semantics* (Vol. 3, pp. 41-58). New York, NY: Academic Press.

Heller, T. (1908). Dementia infantilis. *Zeitschrift fur die Enforschung und Behandlung des Jugenlichen Schwachsinns, 2*, 141-165.

Howlin, P. (2014). Outcomes of adults with autism spectrum disorders. In F. R. Volkmar, S. J. Rogers, R. Paul, & K. A. Pelfrey (Eds.), *Handbook on autism and pervasive developmental disorders: Vol. 1. Diagnosis, development, and brain mechanisms* (4th ed., pp. 97-116). New York, NY: Wiley.

Hughes, D., McGillivrey, L., & Schmidek, M. (1997). *Guide to narrative language: Procedures for assessment.* Eau Claire, WI: Thinking Publications.

Huisingh, R., Bowers, L., & LoGiudice, C. (2007). *Test of problem solving 2—Adolescent.* East Moline, IL: LinguiSystems.

Interdisciplinary Council on Development and Learning Disorders. (2005). *Diagnostic manual for infancy and early childhood.* Bethesda, MD: Author.

Jones, E. A., & Carr, E. G. (2004). Joint attention in children with autism: Theory and intervention. *Focus on Autism and Other Developmental Disabilities, 19*, 13-26.

Kanner, L. (1943). Autistic disturbances of affective contact. *The Nervous Child, 23*, 217-250.

Kasari, C., & Chang, Y. (2014). Play development in children with autism spectrum disorders: Skills, object play, and interventions. In F. R. Volkmar, S. J. Rogers, R. Paul, & K. A. Pelfrey (Eds.), *Handbook on autism and pervasive developmental disorders: Vol. 1. Diagnosis, development, and brain mechanisms* (4th ed., pp. 263-277). New York, NY: Wiley.

Kim, S. H., Paul, R., Tager-Flusberg, H., & Lord, C. (2014). Language and communication in autism. In F. R. Volkmar, S. J. Rogers, R. Paul, & K. A. Pelfrey (Eds.), *Handbook on autism and pervasive developmental disorders: Vol. 1. Diagnosis, development, and brain mechanisms* (4th ed., pp. 230-262). New York, NY: Wiley.

Klin, A. (1991). Young autistic children's listening preferences in regard to speech: A possible characterization of social withdrawal. *Journal of Autism and Developmental Disorders, 21*, 29-42.

Klin, A., McPartland, J., & Volkmar, F.R. (2005). Asperger syndrome. In F. R. Volkmar, R. Paul, A. Klin, & D. Cohen (Eds.), *Handbook on autism and pervasive developmental disorders: Vol. 1. Assessment, interventions, and policy* (3rd ed.; pp. 88-125). New York, NY: Wiley.

Kothari, R., Skuse, D., Wakefield, J., & Micali, N. (2013). Gender differences in the relationship between social communication and emotion recognition. *Journal of the American Academy of Child and Adolescent Psychiatry, 52*, 1148-1157.

Lahey, M. (1988). *Language disorders and language development.* New York, NY: Macmillan.

Le Couteur, A., Lord, C., & Rutter, M. (2003). *Autism diagnostic interview—Revised.* Los Angeles, CA: Western Psychological Services.

Lord, C., Corsello, C., & Grzadzinski, R. (2014). Diagnostic instruments in autistic spectrum disorders. In F. R. Volkmar, S. J. Rogers, R. Paul, & K. A. Pelfrey (Eds.), *Handbook on autism and pervasive developmental disorders: Vol. 2. Diagnosis, development, and brain mechanisms* (pp. 609-660). New York, NY: Wiley.

Lord, C., Luyster, R. J., Gotham, K., & Guthrie, W. (2012). *Autism diagnostic observation scale, second edition manual (part II): Toddler module.* Torrance, CA: Western Psychological Services.

Lord, C., Rutter, M., DiLavore, P. C., Risi, S., Gotham, & Bishop, S. L. (2012). *Autism diagnostic observation scale—Second edition manual part I: Modules 1-4.* Torrance, CA: Western Psychological Services.

Losh, M., & Capps, L. (2003). Narrative ability in high-functioning children with autism or Asperger's syndrome. *Journal of Autism and Developmental Disorders, 33*, 239-251.

MacWhinney, B. (2000). *The CHILDES Project: Tools or analyzing child talk* (3rd ed.). Mahwah, NJ: Erlbaun.

Marcott, A. (2009). *Evaluating acquired language skills in communication.* San Antonio, TX: Pearson Assess.

Mayer, M. (1969). *Frog, where are you?* New York, NY: Dial Press.

McCauley, R. J. (2001). *Assessment of language disorders in children.* Mahwah, NJ: Erlbaum.

Miller, J., Andriacci, K., & Nockerts, A. (2015). *Assessing language production using SALT software: A clinician's guide to language sample analysis.* Middleton, WI: SALT Software.

Mirenda, P. (2014). Augmentative and alternative communication. In F. R. Volkmar, S. J. Rogers, R. Paul, & K. A. Pelfrey (Eds.), *Handbook on autism and pervasive developmental disorders: Vol. 2. Assessment, interventions, and policy* (4th ed., pp. 813-825). New York, NY: Wiley.

National Research Council. (2001). *Educating children with autism* (Committee on Educational Interventions for Children with Autism, Commission on Behavioral and Social Sciences and Education; C. Lord & J. P. McGee, Eds.). Washington DC: National Academy Press.

Needleman, R., Ritvo, E. R., & Freedman, B. J. (1981). Objectively defined linguistic parameters in children with autism and other developmental disabilities. *Journal of Autism and Developmental Disorders, 10*, 389-398.

Osterling, J., & Dawson, G. (1994). Early recognition of children with autism: A study of first birthday home videotapes. *Journal of Autism and Developmental Disorders, 24*, 247-257.

Paul, R., & Fahim, D. (2014). Assessing communication in autism spectrum disorders. In F. R. Volkmar, S. J. Rogers, R. Paul, & K. A. Pelfrey (Eds.), *Handbook on autism and pervasive developmental disorders: Vol. 2. Assessment, interventions, and policy* (4th ed., pp. 673-694). New York, NY: Wiley.

Paul, R., & Norbury, C. F. (2012). *Language disorders from infancy through adolescence: Listening, speaking, reading, writing and communicating, fourth edition.* St. Louis, MO: Elsevier Mosby.

Paul, R., & Sutherland, D. (2005). Enhancing early language in children with autism spectrum disorders. In F. R. Volkmar, R. Paul, A. Klin, & D. Cohen (Eds.), *Handbook on autism and pervasive developmental disorders: Vol. 2: Assessment, interventions, and policy* (3rd ed., pp. 946-976). New York, NY: Wiley.

Phelps-Terasaki , D., & Phelps-Gunn, T. (2007). *Test of pragmatic languge—2.* East Moline, IL: LinguiSystems.

Prizant, B. M. (1983). Language acquisition and communicative behavior in autism: Toward an understanding the "whole" of it. *Journal of Speech and Hearing Disorders, 48*, 296-308.

Prizant, B. M., & Duchan, J. (1981). The functions of immediate echolalia in autistic children. *Journal of Speech and Hearing Disorders, 46*, 241-250.

Retherford, K. S. (2000). *Guide to the analysis of language transcripts* (3rd ed.). Eau Claire, WI: Thinking Publications.

Robins, D. L., Fein, D., Barton, M. L., & Green, J. A. (2001). The Modified Checklist for Autism in Toddlers: An initial study investigating the early detection of autism and pervasive developmental disorders. *Journal of Autism and Developmental Disorders, 31*, 131-144.

Rogers, S. J., Cook, I., & Meryl, A. (2005). Imitation and play in autism. In F. R. Volkmar, R. Paul, A. Klin, & D. Cohen (Eds.), *Handbook on autism and pervasive developmental disorders: Vol. 1. Assessment, interventions, and policy* (3rd ed., pp. 382-405). New York, NY: Wiley.

Rossetti, L. (2006). *Rossetti infant-toddler language scale.* East Moline, IL: LinguiSystems.

Roth, F. P., & Worthington, C. K. (2016). *Treatment resource manual for speech-language pathology* (4th ed.). Clifton Park, NY: Cengage Learning.

Rutter, M., Bailey, A., & Lord, C. (2003). *Social communication questionnaire.* Los Angeles, CA: Western Psychological Services.

Schopler, E., Van Bourgondien, M. E., Wellman, G. J., & Love, S. R. (2010). *Childhood autism rating scale—Second edition.* Los Angeles, CA: Western Psychological Services.

Seymour, H., Roeper, T., & de Villiers, J. (2005). *Diagnostic evaluation of language variation—2.* San Antonio, TX: Pearson Assess.

Shane, H., Laubscher, E., Schlossser, R., Flynn, S., Sorce, J., & Abramson. J. (2012). Applying technology to visually support language and communication in individuals with autism spectrum disorders. *Journal of Autism and Developmental Disorders, 42*, 1128-1235.

Shriberg, L. D., Paul, R., McSweeny, J. L. Klin, A., Cohen, D. J., & Volkmar, F. R. (2001). Speech and prosody characteristics of adolescents and adults with high-functioning autism and Asperger syndrome. *Journal of Speech, Language and Hearing Research, 44*, 1097-1115.

Sparrow, S., Cicchetti, D., & Balla, D. (2005). *Vineland adaptive behaviors scales, second edition.* San Antonio, TX: Pearson Assess.

Squires, J., Bricker, D., & Twombly, E. (2015). *Ages and stages questionnaire—Social emotional screen, second edition* (ASQ-SE-2). Baltimore, MD: Brookes.

Stein, N., & Glenn, C. (1979). An analysis of story comprehension in elementary school children. In R. Freedle (Ed.), *New directions in discourse processing* (pp. 53-120). Norwood, NJ: Ablex.

Stern, D. N. (1985). *The interpersonal world of the infant.* New York, NY: Basic Books.

Stone, W. L., Coonrod, E. E., & Ousley, O. Y. (2000). Brief report: Screening Tool for Autism in Two-Year-Olds (STAT): Development and preliminary data. *Journal of Autism and Developmental Disorders, 30*, 607-612.

Tager-Flusberg, H. (1981). Sentence comprehension in autistic children. *Applied Psycholinguistics, 2*, 5-24.

Tager-Flusberg, H. (1992). Autistic children's talk about psychological states: Deficits in the early acquisition of a theory of mind. *Child Development, 63*, 161-172.

Tager-Flusberg, H., Rogers, S., Cooper, J., Landa, R., Lord, C., Paul, R., Rice, M. ... Yoder, P. (2009). Defining spoken language benchmarks and selecting measures of expressive language for young children with autism spectrum disorders. *Journal of Speech, Language, and Hearing Research, 52*, 643-652.

Towbin, K. E. (2005). Pervasive developmental disorder not otherwise specified. In F. R. Volkmar, R. Paul, A. Klin, & D. Cohen. (Eds.), *Handbook on autism and pervasive developmental disorders: Vol. 1. Assessment, interventions, and policy* (3rd ed., pp.165-200). New York, NY: Wiley.

Van Acker, R., Loncola, J. A., & Van Acker, E. Y. (2005). Rett syndrome: A pervasive developmental disorder. In F. R. Volkmar, R. Paul, A. Klin, & D. Cohen (Eds.), *Handbook on autism and pervasive developmental disorders: Vol. 1. Assessment, interventions, and policy* (3rd ed., pp. 126-164). New York, NY: Wiley.

Vivanti, G., & Hamilton, A. (2014). Imitation in autism spectrum Disorders. In F. R. Volkmar, S. J. Rogers, R. Paul, & K. A. Pelfrey (Eds.), *Handbook on autism and pervasive developmental disorders: Vol. 1. Diagnosis, development, and brain mechanisms* (4th ed., pp. 278-301). New York, NY: Wiley.

Volkmar, F. R., & Klin, A. (2005). Issues in the classification of autism and related conditions. In Volkmar, F. R., Paul, R., Klin, A., & Cohen, D. (Eds.) *Handbook on autism and pervasive developmental disorders, third edition, vol.1: Assessment, interventions, and policy* (pp.5-41). New York, NY: Wiley.

Volkmar, F. R., Koenig, K., & State, M. (2005). Childhood disintegrative disorder. In Volkmar, F. R., Paul, R., Klin, A., & Cohen, D. (Eds.) *Handbook on autism and pervasive developmental disorders, third edition, vol.1: Assessment, interventions, and policy* (pp.70-87). New York, NY: Wiley.

Volkmar, F. R., Reichow, B., Westphal, A., & Mandell, D. S. (2014). Autism and the autism spectrum: Diagnostic concepts. In F. R. Volkmar, S. J. Rogers, R. Paul, & K. A. Pelfrey (Eds.), *Handbook on autism and pervasive developmental disorders: Diagnosis, development, and brain mechanisms* (4th ed., Vol. 1; pp. 3-27). New York: Wiley.

Volkmar, F.R., Rowberry, J., DeVinck-Baroody, O., Gupta, A.R., Leung, J., Meyers, J., . . . Wiesner, L. A. (2014). Medical care in autism and related conditions. In F. R. Volkmar, S. J. Rogers, R. Paul, & K. A. Pelfrey (Eds.), *Handbook on autism and pervasive developmental disorders: Vol. 1: Diagnosis, development, and brain mechanisms* (pp. 532-555). New York, NY: Wiley.

Weisner, D. (1997). *Tuesday.* New York, NY: Clarion Books.

Westby, C. E. (2000). A scale for assessing development of children's play. In K. Gilllin-Weiner, A. Sandgrund, & C. Schaefer (Eds.), *Play diagnosis and assessment* (2nd ed., pp. 15-57). New York, NY: Wiley.

Wetherby, A. M., & Prizant, B. M. (1989). The expression of communicative intent: Assessment guidelines. *Seminars in Speech and Language, 10*, 77-91.

Wetherby, A. M., & Prizant, B. M. (2003). *Communication and symbolic behavior scales.* Baltimore, MD: Brookes.

Wetherby, A. M., & Prutting, C. (1984). Profiles of communicative and cognitive-social abilities in autistic children. *Journal of Speech and Hearing Research, 27*, 364-377.

Wetherby, A. M. & Woods, J. (2002). *Systematic observation of red flags for Autism spectrum disorders in young children* (SORF). Unpublished manual. Tallahassee: Florida State University.

Wiig, E., & Secord, W. (1989). *Test of language competence—Expanded edition.* San Antonio, TX: Pearson Assess.

Wiig, E., Semel, E., & Secord, W. (2013). *Clinical evaluation of language fundamentals—5.* San Antonio, TX: Pearson Assess.

World Health Organization. (1993). *The ICD-10 classification of mental and behavioral disorders.* Geneva, Switzerland: Author.

Website Resources

American Speech-Language-Hearing Association: Autism. www.asha.org/PRPSpecificTopic.aspx?folderid=8589935303§ion=Assessment

Centers for Disease Control and Prevention: Autism spectrum disorders. www.cdc.gov/ncbddd/autism/screening.html

Autism Research Institute: Assessment and diagnosis. www.autism.com/knowthesigns

National Institute of Neurological Disorders and Stroke: Autism Spectrum Disorder fact sheet. www.ninds.nih.gov/Disorders/Patient-Caregiver-Education/Fact-Sheets/Autism-Spectrum-Disorder-Fact-Sheet

10

Assessment of School-Age Language and Literacy Disorders

Gail B. Gurland, PhD, CCC-SLP, TSHH and Klara Marton, PhD

KEY WORDS

- attention-deficit/hyperactivity disorder (ADHD)
- attention
- collateral measures
- developmental dyslexia
- differential diagnosis
- discourse
- executive functions
- expository discourse
- formal assessment
- informal assessment
- lexical diversity
- macrostructure
- metalinguistic knowledge/skills
- narrative discourse
- phonotactic rules
- sequential bilingualism
- specific language impairment
- type/token ratio
- working memory

The focus in this chapter is on children who have primary language impairment that is not part of another recognized syndrome or the consequence of intellectual disability, hearing impairment, neurological deficit, emotional disturbance, or environmental deprivation. The terminology in the literature is not uniform; some authors refer to this population as children with expressive or receptive language impairment; researchers prefer the term **specific language impairment** (SLI) or *primary language impairment*, and there are references to this population by the term *developmental language disorders*, particularly in the neuropsychology literature. The prevalence of the impairment is approximately 6% to 8% in kindergarten children. It is more frequent in male students than in females, and approximately 80% of the children with this diagnosis show both expressive and receptive problems (Tomblin, Records, Buckwalter, Zhang, & Smith, 1997). The percentage of children identified with language impairment varies across studies because it is influenced by the age of the sample, cut-off point for diagnosis, and definition used (Gilger & Wise, 2004).

Providing a "pure" diagnosis is further complicated by the fact that childhood language impairment is not a unitary disorder. Although all children with this diagnosis show significant language difficulties, there are differences in these children's cognitive-linguistic profiles and in their motivation to learn. The cognitive-linguistic system is a dynamic system that shows continuous development with age and with intervention (Botting & Conti-Ramsden, 2004).

Stein-Rubin, C., & Fabus, R. *A Guide to Clinical Assessment and Professional Report Writing in Speech-Language Pathology, Second Edition (pp 223-244).*

There are variations in the severity and pervasiveness of the language impairment that these children exhibit. They differ in the range of the language areas that are problematic (phonology, morphology, syntax, vocabulary, etc.) and in the language modality that is most severely affected (i.e., expressive language, receptive language, or both). Given the complexity of the cognitive-linguistic system, the definition of *primary language impairment* is based on a diagnostic threshold and on some exclusionary criteria. These criteria serve to distinguish children with language impairment from children with other developmental disorders. The determination of the diagnostic threshold is based on the presence of significant language difficulties. Typically, it is either defined relative to the child's age or to his or her nonverbal intelligence (Peterson & McGrath, 2009).

Traditional definitions of childhood language impairment were based on a discrepancy between the child's nonverbal cognitive performance and his or her language abilities. There are a number of children, however, who show severe problems in everyday communication and would clearly benefit from language intervention but do not fit the definition of significant discrepancy between expected language level based on age or nonverbal intelligence and actual language performance. There is no consensus regarding the size of the discrepancy and the threshold for the diagnosis. There are different views about the minimum amount of standard deviation below the mean to diagnose the language impairment (1 or 1.25 or 1.5, etc.). Another common way of defining language impairment is to compare language age to chronological age based on the results of comprehensive language tests. In this case, language impairment is diagnosed if the child's language age is at least 12 months lower than the chronological age. The main problem with this criterion is that a 1-year discrepancy between the language age and the chronological age at 3 to 4 years of age signals a larger difference than at 12 years of age. A further issue is related to the poor psychometric properties of age equivalents. A third option for defining child language impairment is based on language measures expressed in percentile. Percentile scores show what percentage of same-age children would obtain an equivalent or lower score than the client. In overall language score, the cutoff point between 1.25 and 1.5 standard deviations corresponds to the 10th percentile.

A related question is how many components of language must be impaired to meet the criteria for the diagnosis of language impairment (Tager-Flusberg, 2005). Typically, childhood language impairment is diagnosed if the child shows difficulties in at least two components of language (e.g., semantics, morphology, syntax, etc.). The problems may occur with different severity in different modalities (expressive and receptive language; oral and written form). As an alternative, Tomblin (2008) suggested a different approach—the use of socially valued outcomes for justifying clinical services. The focus within this perspective is on communication function and competence. This viewpoint is embedded in a framework that integrates development and cultural values. The author argues that children who enter school with poor language performance show lower competence as adolescents, regardless of their nonverbal IQ. Thus, even if there is no significant discrepancy between their language scores and their nonverbal IQ at the time they enter school, they clearly need services to improve their social and academic competence.

Assessment

Specific Parameters for Assessment

The assessment of language disorders in school-age children (5 to 6 years to 13 to 14 years) requires the examination of the levels of the linguistic rule system, individually, interactively, and within context. Thus, formal standardized test administration and informal, dynamic, and curriculum-based assessment must include measurements of semantic, syntactic, morphological, pragmatic, and phonological levels of the linguistic system. Each of these levels of the rule system influences not only spoken language (i.e., listening and speaking), but written language (i.e., reading and writing) as well. Furthermore, rather than constrain evaluation by dichotomizing spoken and written language, the assessment process would be better served by reframing its parameters to consider the demands oral and literate language place on listening and speaking, as well as on reading and writing in addressing the needs of the school-age child and adolescent.

Thus, the parameters of the assessment process would include the areas of reading, writing, and spelling, along with oral **discourse** to obtain a thorough evaluation of the individual. Additionally, various cognitive-linguistic interactions would have to be examined to understand the influence of attentional control, **working memory**, and other **executive functions** on language performance. As a result, the assessment process would also involve an examination of **metalinguistic knowledge/skills**, working memory, and executive functions. Depending on the developmental age of the child, metalinguistic knowledge would include phonemic awareness for reading, conscious knowledge of definitions, synonyms and antonyms, analogies, grammaticality judgments, and the ability to distinguish between literal and figurative meanings. Working memory would include storage and manipulation of information needed to carry out a task. Working memory skills are closely related to executive functions, an umbrella term that refers to a range of cognitive skills, such as **attention** switching, monitoring behavior, maintaining goals, inhibiting irrelevant information, and avoiding distraction.

Collateral measures allow the clinician to assess the child's communication skills in more depth and to look behind the easily observable behaviors by taking a multiperspective approach. Collateral test-taking behaviors may reveal a wide range of linguistic and communicative skills such as turn-taking, initiation, requests for clarification, and the ability to follow and integrate verbal directions. They may also indicate whether the child uses strategies to cope with the challenges of increased language processing demands and the extent to which these strategies are or are not helpful for the child. Is the child aware of what he or she does and does not understand? Does the child repeat and rehearse verbal information before responding, and does this strategy facilitate or impede performance? Does the child examine response choices, and does this increase the likelihood of a correct response? Whether during formal standardized testing or the administration of informal discourse and curriculum-based tasks, does the child demonstrate sustained and controlled attention, persist at tasks even when they are challenging, switch easily from one task to another, and maintain goals in active memory?

Moving beyond traditional correct/incorrect (+/–) scoring to consider error patterns may also reveal deficiencies not otherwise easily measured. How does the availability of visual referents affect the accuracy and consistency of the child's comprehension of spoken or written text? How does the demand to hold in memory and manage more than one piece of information at a time influence response accuracy? Are there instances when the child does not respond at all, indicates that he or she does not know, or guesses randomly or impulsively? Are the child's errors somewhat related to the correct responses or are they completely irrelevant? Does the child monitor and self-correct his or her responses?

The resulting assessment framework provides for the examination of the comprehension, retention, organization, retrieval, and formulation of single words, phrase and sentence structures, and extended discourse, heard and read, spoken and written. These measures may be obtained during formal standardized testing and informal discourse and curriculum-based tasks. Furthermore, it requires that this information be obtained and analyzed within the context of the background information provided by parents, caregivers, and teachers about the child's birth, health, and developmental histories, language learning history, social-communicative interactions, educational achievements and challenges, and prior assessments and treatment, where applicable.

The essential components of such a framework are summarized as follows.

- Comprehension and Production of the Linguistic Rule System
  - Semantic
  - Syntactic
  - Morphological
  - Pragmatic
  - Phonological
- Cognitive-Linguistic Interactions
  - Metalinguistic knowledge
  - Working memory
  - Executive functions
- Language-Related Skills
  - Reading
  - Writing
  - Spelling
  - Text comprehension and reformulation across subject areas
- Collateral Test-Taking Behavior
  - Linguistic and communicative behaviors
  - Sustained and controlled attention
  - Strategies for managing and coping with challenging tasks
  - Effectiveness of management and coping strategies
- Analysis of Error Patterns
  - Influence of modality of input (auditory, visual, tactile)
  - Relationship of error response to correct response
  - Self-monitoring and self-correction

- Background Information
    - Pregnancy, birth, health, developmental histories
    - Language learning history
    - Social-communicative interactions
    - Educational achievements and challenges

Essential Clinical Interview Questions

The clinical interview provides the examiner with much of the background information needed to assess the nature, severity, and functional impact of the school-age child's language difficulties. Additional information may be obtained with parent/guardian permission through the review of prior diagnostic and therapy reports, and through the use of parent and teacher questionnaires. Although these other sources are important, face-to-face contact with the parent/guardian and child is a critical component of the assessment process. In fact, the clinical interview might be best viewed as consisting of two interviews: one with the parent/guardian and one with the child. Clearly, the information provided by the parent/guardian will provide the context for understanding the child's difficulties as well as offer further direction in the selection of specific assessment procedures. However, the child is a valuable resource, not to be overlooked in developing the most complete assessment possible.

It is always best to begin the clinical interview with the parent/guardian by posing open-ended questions, keeping in mind that parents may have considerable knowledge and familiarity with language learning or very little background about language apart from the most obvious awareness of whether the child understands and can be understood. Thus, it is important to explain your use of terminology and not take anything for granted. Some possible introductory questions might include the following:

- Why did you decide to have your child evaluated? Could you describe your concerns?
- Has your child previously been evaluated or received services related to your present concerns?
- How would you describe your child's early development? Were there any aspects of his or her early development that were particularly noteworthy?
- How would you describe your child's speech and language development? Do you recall any instances when she had difficulty understanding you or other family and friends? Do you recall any instances when he or she had difficulty expressing him- or herself with words and sentences?
- How would you describe your child's overall health? Are there any specific health issues either past or present that are noteworthy?
- How is your child doing in school? Have teachers brought any specific concerns to your attention? Does he or she favor or dislike any particular subjects?

The answers to these questions will direct the examiner accordingly and suggest a number of specific and perhaps somewhat more close-ended questions to obtain the necessary background information relative to the presenting problem. For example, if the examiner learns that the child's native language is not English or that he or she has been exposed to more than one language, it is essential to determine the age and extent of experience with other languages, the relative balance of current language use, and whether difficulties are apparent in all languages. If difficulties are described with the child's overall speech and language development, then more specific questions might be raised with respect to his or her following directions, interest in having stories read aloud, ability to discuss and answer questions about books that have been read to him or her, compensatory strategies he or she may have used to communicate if he or she was not readily understood, and whether anyone else in the family has had similar difficulties. If health issues are raised, then questions might be presented regarding the nature and duration of any illness, treatments administered, and influence on the child's communication or performance in school. If concerns are described with respect to school, then questions might be focused on the child's interest in recreational reading as compared to reading for school, the nature of the curriculum, specific subject difficulties, and the child's persistence and/or frustration in view of academic challenges.

The child's contribution as an informant is of equal importance to that of the parent/guardian. Again the usefulness of open-ended questions cannot be overstated. Caution is advised with terminology and, of course, the nature of the questions will vary considerably depending upon the child's age and level of maturity. Some possible introductory questions might include the following:

- Why do you think your mom/dad brought you here today?
- Tell me about your family and some of the things you do when you spend time together.
- What kinds of things do you like to do with your friends?

- Tell me something about school. Do you have any favorite subjects or subjects that you dislike? What is it that you do or do not like about that subject?
- What kinds of books do you like to read for fun when you're not in school?
- What kinds of things do you like to do when you're not in school or busy with homework?

The answers obtained from the child will indicate the need for more specific follow-up questions. If the child has no apparent awareness of the nature of his or her difficulties, then the examiner needs to learn more about his or her routines both in and out of school. If the child is aware of any problems, then the examiner will need to provide the opportunity for the child to discuss his or her feelings and coping strategies in dealing with family, friends, and teachers. If the child identifies a particularly troublesome teacher or subject, then questions need to be directed toward learning as much as possible about the nature of the child's frustration. It is essential to keep in mind that even the most insightful child is likely to become somewhat defensive about his or her problems and find blame with others rather than assume responsibility him- or herself. This, too, is a critical piece of information that will contribute to a deeper understanding and a more complete assessment of the problem.

Formal Assessment Measures

The selection of **formal assessment** measures will depend on the age and estimated developmental level of the child as well as the aspect of language, cognitive-linguistic interaction, and language-related skill under consideration. The list of available formal assessment tools for the school-age child is long and growing. A list of the most widely used and well-regarded procedures is provided in Table 10-1 according to specific area(s) of consideration. Comprehensive test batteries are those that examine a range of language and related skills at varying levels of the linguistic rule system. These are likely to assess both receptive and expressive skills and may include tasks to measure spoken and/or written language. Some of these also may measure underlying cognitive-linguistic interactions.

Several formal assessment tools are available for more in-depth examination of semantic, syntactic and/or morphological knowledge and performance (Table 10-2). They may specifically examine receptive and/or expressive skills; word retrieval; or metalinguistic knowledge of lexical, semantic, or grammatical aspects of language.

A number of assessment tools are designed to examine metalinguistic skills at the phonological level of the rule system or phonological and phonemic awareness, a set of language related skills that has been determined to be critical to the attainment of early decoding and literacy (Table 10-3).

Although formal tests of pragmatic language skills are more likely measuring metalinguistic or metapragmatic skills where the child is asked to reflect on how to use language within a particular social context rather than providing opportunities to actually observe the child engage in these communicative exchanges, there are specific procedures that could be helpful in the assessment process (Table 10-4).

Finally, there are several formal assessment tools to be considered in examining the school-age child's narrative skills, reading, writing, spelling, and even mathematics to better understand the impact that language difficulties may have on academic achievement (Table 10-5).

The advantages of formal assessment are numerous when tests are selected carefully with respect to their validity and reliability, are administered and analyzed according to guidelines detailed in specific test manuals, and results are considered within the context of the child's overall social and academic functioning. They provide the opportunity to examine a range of knowledge and skills efficiently and to compare the child's performance to established norms and criteria to determine strengths and weaknesses. They offer the examiner a window onto a selection of representative behaviors whose measurement can explain and potentially direct remediation of the challenges the child faces.

However, these tests are only as good as the clinician who administers them and interprets their findings. They often measure skills independent of the contexts in which they occur in the home, playground, or classroom. Furthermore, they isolate skills in a somewhat artificial way so that the examiner does not always see them engaged interactively. Certainly, the results of a specific expressive vocabulary measure are useful, but only to the extent that the clinician considers how the child incorporates vocabulary when asked to produce increasingly complex syntactic and morphological structures. Similarly, measures of the child's comprehension as he or she hears individual phrases and sentence structures are important, but only to the extent that he or she might understand those phrases and sentences when they are linked together into longer extended units of spoken or written instructional

Table 10-1. Comprehensive Assessment Batteries

Test, Author	*Age Range (year;month)*	*Description*
Clinical Evaluation of Language Fundamentals-5 (CELF-5; Wiig, Semel, & Secord, 2013)	5;0 to 21;11	Overall core language; receptive and expressive language; language content; language structure; and language memory indices; various levels of the linguistic rule system; metalinguistic skills; reading comprehension; structured writing; social communication skills
Comprehensive Assessment of Spoken Language-2 (CASL-2; Carrow-Woolfolk, 2017)	3;0 to 21;11	Lexical, semantic, morphosyntactic, and pragmatic knowledge; literal and nonliteral comprehension
Detroit Test of Learning Aptitude-4 (DTLA-4; Hammil, 1998)	6;0 to 17;0	Receptive and expressive language and related memory and motor tasks; verbal and nonverbal linguistic; attention-enhanced and attention-reduced; and motor- enhanced and motor-reduced composite domains
Illinois Test of Psycholinguistic Abilities-3 (ITPA-3; Hammil, Mather, & Roberts, 2001)	5.0 to 12;11	Semantics, morphosyntax, and phonological awareness; oral language, reading, writing, and spelling
Test of Adolescent and Adult Language-4 (TOAL-4; Hammil, Brown, Larsen & Wiederholt, 2007)	12;0 to 24;11	Comprehension and production of lexical, semantic, morphosyntactic structures, spoken and written language
CELF-5 Metalinguistics (Wiig, Semel, & Secord, 2014)	9;0 to 21;11	Higher level language; metalinguistic skills and figurative language
Test of Language Development: Intermediate-4 (TOLD: I-4; Hammil & Newcomer, 2008a)	8;0 to 17;11	Comprehension and production of lexical, semantic, morphosyntactic structures; multiple meanings
Test of Language Development: Primary-4 (TOLD: P-4; Hammil & Newcomer, 2008b)	4;0 to 8;11	Comprehension and production of lexical, semantic, morphosyntactic, and phonological structures
Test of Integrated Language and Literacy Skills (TILLS; Nelson, Plante, & Helm-Estabrooks, 2015)	6;0 to 18;11	Listening, speaking, reading, and writing
Receptive, Expressive, and Social Communication Assessment-Elementary (RESCA-E; Hamaguchi & Ross-Swain, 2015)	5;0 to 1;11	Receptive and expressive vocabulary, syntax/morphology, narrative, and social communication

discourse which he or she is likely to encounter in the classroom.

Traditional language tests measure end products and not the underlying processes; therefore, these tasks are often not sensitive to the changes that occur with development and intervention in the cognitive-linguistic system. Traditional measures are also more biased than processing measures in culturally diverse populations. Thus, traditional formal language measures must be supplemented with informal language and information processing tasks that are less biased. These tasks appear to be valuable in distinguishing populations that on the surface show similar language problems (e.g., children with language impairment, children with reading disorders, **sequential bilingual** children, English language learners [ELL]).

It is precisely because of these limitations of formal testing that informal measures must be included in the assessment process. Whereas formal assessment tools allow for the identification of specific strengths and weaknesses, **informal assessment** provides an examination of the interaction of a range of skills within a more dynamic and, perhaps, natural context. For example, it is possible to determine how vocabulary usage might be influenced by sentence complexity, how sentence formulation is affected by whether output is spoken or written, and how comprehension of text is determined by familiarity of the material presented.

TABLE 10-2. ASSESSMENT OF SEMANTIC, SYNTACTIC, AND MORPHOLOGICAL SKILLS

Test, Author	*Age Range (year, month)*	*Description*
Boehm Test of Basic Concepts-3 (Boehm, 2001)	Kindergarten to second grade	Vocabulary related to basic conceptual knowledge used in the classroom
Comprehensive Receptive Expressive Vocabulary Test-3 (CREVT-3; Wallace & Hammil, 2013)	5;0 to adult	Receptive and expressive vocabulary
Expressive One-Word Picture Vocabulary Test-4 (EOWPVT-4; Brownell, 2011a; Spanish-Bilingual edition, 2012)	2;0 to 18;11	Expressive vocabulary
Peabody Picture Vocabulary Test, Fourth Edition (PPVT-4; Dunn & Dunn, 2007)	2;0 to adult	Receptive vocabulary
Preschool Language Assessment Instrument-2 (PLAI-2; Blank, Rose, & Berlin, 2003)	3;0 to 5;11	Discourse abilities related to typical early educational exchanges
Receptive One Word Picture Vocabulary Test-4 (ROWPVT-4; Brownell, 2011b; Spanish-Bilingual edition, 2012)	2;0 to 18;11	Receptive vocabulary
Test of Auditory Comprehension of Language-3 (TACL-3; Carrow-Woolfolk, 1999)	3;0 to 9;11	Comprehension of vocabulary, grammatical morphemes, and elaborated phrases and sentences
Test of Word Finding-2 (TWF-2; German, 2015)	4;0 to 12;11	Word-finding ability based on accuracy and speed
The Word Test 3—Elementary and Adolescent (Bowers, Huisingh, LoGiudice, & Orman, 2014)	6;0 to 11;11; 12;0 to 17;11	Lexical and semantic knowledge; metalinguistic skills
Token Test for Children-2 (TTFC-2; McGhee, Ehrler, & DiSimoni, 2007)	3;0 to 12;11	Semantic-syntactic structures related to following spoken directions

TABLE 10-3. ASSESSMENT OF METALINGUISTIC SKILLS

Test, Author	*Age Range (year, month)*	*Description*
Comprehensive Test of Phonological Processes-2 (CTOPP-2; Wagner, Torgesen, Raschotte, & Pearson, 2013)	4;0 to 24;11	Phonological awareness, phonological memory, rapid naming
Lindamood Auditory Conceptualization Test-3 (LAC-3; Lindamood & Lindamood, 2004)	5;0 to 18;11	Perception and conceptualization of speech sounds related to phonological awareness
Test of Auditory Processing-3 (TAPS-3; Martin & Brownell, 2005)	4;0 to 18;11	Word discrimination, phonological awareness, word and sentence memory
Test of Phonological Awareness-2 (TOPA-2; Torgesen & Bryant, 2004)	5;0 to 8;11	Phonological awareness related to early decoding and spelling
The Phonological Awareness Test-2 (Robertson & Salter, 2017)	5;0 to 9;0	Phonological awareness related to early decoding and spelling

TABLE 10-4. ASSESSMENT OF PRAGMATIC LANGUAGE SKILLS

Test, Author	*Age Range (year, month)*	*Description*
Test of Pragmatic Language-2 (TOPL-2; Phelps-Terasaki & Phelps-Gunn, 2007)	5;0 to 13;11	Social communication in context
Test of Problem Solving 3—Elementary (Bowers, Huisingh, & LoGiudice, 2005)	6;0 to 11;0	Analysis, reasoning, inferencing, prediction related to various communicative contexts

Table 10-5. Assessment of Narrative and Academic Literacy Skills

Test, Author	*Age Range (year;month)*	*Description*
Assessment of Literacy and Language (ALL; Lombardino, Lieberman, Jaumeiko, & Brown, 2005)	Preschool to first grade	Receptive vocabulary, basic conceptual knowledge, listening comprehension, alphabet knowledge and print awareness, phonological awareness
Gray Oral Reading Tests-5 (GORT-5; Weiderholt & Bryant, 2012)	6;0 to 23;11	Reading rate, accuracy, fluency, and comprehension
Gray Diagnostic Reading Tests-2 (GDRT-2; Bryant, Wiederholt, & Bryant, 2004)	6;0 to 13;11	Oral reading, letter/word identification, phonetic analysis, reading vocabulary, meaningful reading
Gray Silent Reading Tests (GSRT; Wiederholt & Blalock, 2000)	7;0 to 25;11	Silent reading comprehension
Peabody Individual Achievement Test (PIAT; Markwardt, 1997)	5;0 to 22;11	General information, reading recognition, reading comprehension, spelling, math, and written expression
Kaufman Test of Educational Achievement-3 (KTEA-3; Kaufman & Kaufman, 2014)	4;0 to 25;11	Phonological processing, math concepts and applications, letter and word recognition, math computation, nonword decoding, silent reading comprehension, written expression, spelling, reading vocabulary, listening comprehension, oral expression
Key Math—3 Diagnostic Assessment (Connolly, 2007)	4;6 to 21;0	Basic concepts, numerical operation, applications, and mathematical problem-solving
Test of Narrative Language-2 (TNL-2; Gillam & Pearson, 2017)	5;0 to 11;11	Story comprehension, retelling and original narrative formulation
Test of Reading Comprehension-4 (TORC-4; Brown, Wiederholt, & Hammil, 2009)	7;0 to 17;11	Silent reading comprehension of vocabulary, sentence structures, and paragraphs
Test of Written Language-4 (TOWL-4; Hammil & Larsen, 2009)	9;0 to 17;11	Semantic, morphosyntactic, and discourse aspects of writing; writing conventions
Test of Written Spelling-5 (TWS-5; Larsen, Hammil, & Moats, 2013)	First to 12th grade	Written spelling based on oral dictation
Written Language Assessment (WLA; Grill & Kirwin, 1989)	8;0 to 18;0	Narrative and expository written expression
Woodcock Reading Mastery Tests-III (WRMT-III; Woodcock, 2011)	4;6 to 79;11	Phonological awareness, listening comprehension, letter and word identification, rapid automatic naming, oral reading fluency, word attack, word recognition, word and passage comprehension

Informal Assessment Measures

The selection of informal assessment measures will also depend upon the age and estimated developmental level of the child as well as the aspect of language, cognitive-linguistic interaction, and language related skill under consideration. It is important that the nature of the task itself not artificially constrain the complexity of the child's linguistic output (Ebert & Scott, 2014). Generally speaking, they may be categorized into discourse and curriculum-based tasks. They may also involve dynamic and portfolio assessment) i.e., organized collections of a child's work such as reading logs, writing samples, and various school related projects; Lipson & Wixson, 2009). They may include listening and speaking as well as reading and writing activities. They may require the use of checklists and coded observations completed one-on-one within the clinical suite or as part of the group within the classroom. Although several formal tests have been developed to examine discourse skills, it is essential that the assessment process includes the collection and analysis of one or more natural discourse or curriculum-based samples. The clinician may choose to include both oral and written samples incorporating various discourse genres, depending on the age and developmental level of the child.

Tasks to be included involve having the child make up a story about a picture, tell a personal experience story, retell a previously heard or read story, explain how to perform an activity or accomplish a goal, and answer open-ended questions based on previously presented text, either spoken or written. These activities provide the opportunity to examine a range of different strengths and weaknesses, such as appropriateness and diversity of vocabulary; syntactic, morphological, and phonological structure; text cohesion and referencing; overall hierarchical organization or **macrostructure** and its relationship to individual detail and linguistic structure or microstructure; spelling; and application of writing conventions. Discourse genres include conversation, question/answer, narrative, and expository. Within the **narrative discourse** genre, the examiner may sample recounts (verbalization of past experiences in the presence of those who shared those experiences), eventcasts (verbalization of ongoing events), accounts (verbalization of experiences not shared with the listener), and stories (fictional narratives; Heath, 1986). Within the expository genre, the examiner may sample descriptive/enumerative, persuasive, compare–contrast, procedural, problem–solution, and cause–effect discourse (Ukrainetz, 2006).

It is neither practical nor desirable to collect samples of all of these discourse genres. Rather, the clinician needs to obtain a representative selection of discourse types that offer a view of the communicative exchanges relevant to the child's social-interactive and academic experiences. These exchanges may be more oral (i.e., structurally informal) or literate (i.e., structurally formal) depending on the demands of the task and the child's ability to adapt to those demands. Once the discourse tasks are administered, the clinician must select appropriate indices, coding systems, or rubrics with which to analyze the samples. The analysis of vocabulary usage may be accomplished using **type/token ratio** (TTR; Templin, 1957), which is the ratio of different words to total words in the sample. Although the validity and reliability of the TTR may vary depending on sample size and context as well as age of the child, it has been a useful clinical tool for measuring vocabulary diversity (Hess, Sefton, & Landry, 1986). TTR is computed by counting and dividing the number of total words (NTWs) in the sample into the total number of different words (NDWs) in the sample. If a 100-utterance sample consisted of a total of 500 words, of which there were 200 different words or tokens, the TTR would be 0.4 (40%). The higher the ratio, the greater **lexical diversity** observed within the sample. Alternately, a measure of lexical diversity may be obtained by simply counting the NDWs in the sample. Paul (2007) provides data on normal ranges of NDWs and NTWs for children between 5 and 11 years of age. For example, the normal range of NDWs is 156 to 206 for 5-year-olds; 173 to 212 for 7-year-olds; 183 to 235 for 9-year-olds; and 191 to 267 for 11-year-olds.

Analysis of syntax and morphology for the school-age child must reach beyond the calculation of mean length of utterance or the simple declarative sentence. Specific measures have been shown to vary with respect to their accuracy in differentiating language impairment in school-age children (Guo & Schneider, 2016). Furthermore, different units of analysis have been proposed depending on whether the discourse sample is oral or written. The communication unit (CU) consisting of an independent clause and its modifiers (Loban, 1976) is primarily used for oral discourse, whereas the terminable unit (T-unit) consisting of a main clause and all subordinate or dependent clauses attached to it, developed by Hunt (1965), is used for written samples. Analysis may be done by measuring average number of words per CU or T-unit. For written discourse, the clause length (average number of words per clause), and subordination index (average number of clauses, both main and subordinate, per T-unit) may be used to measure more complex sentence forms (Scott, 1988; Scott & Stokes, 1995). In these analyses, clauses are critical linguistic units that vary in length and in density. A clause is a group of words that consists of a subject and a predicate. Hughes, McGillivray, and Schmidek (1997) presented data on mean number of words per CU and per T-unit, mean number of dependent clauses per CU, and subordination indices for either spoken or written samples for children across the grades. Justice et al. (2006) provided a framework for the analysis of internal linguistic structure in the Index of Narrative Microstructure (INMIS) in which measures may be obtained of both productivity and complexity by calculating total number of words (TNW), total NDW, total number of T-units (LENGTH), mean length of T-units in words (MLT-W), mean length of T-units in morphemes (MLT-M), total number of complex T-units (COMPLEX), total number of coordinating conjunctions (COORD), total number of subordinating conjunctions (SUBORD), proportion of complex T-units (PROPCOMPLEX).

Hierarchical organization and cohesion or macrostructure of narratives may be evaluated using various rubrics such as Applebee's (1978) stages of narrative development, consisting of heaps (labeling or describing events without a central theme), sequences (labeling or describing events about a central theme), focused chains (describing a sequence of events related to a each other and a central theme), unfocused chains (labeling a sequence of events without a clear relationship to a central theme), primitive narratives (describing a sequence of connected events and actions related to a central theme without an ending related to the initiating event), and true narratives (describing a sequence of connected events and actions with a central theme in which the ending or resolution is related to the initiating event), or Stein and Glenn's (1979) story grammar, consisting of setting or orientation, initiating event or complicating action, internal response, consequence or outcome, resolution, and ending or coda. Paul, Hernandez, Taylor, and Johnson (1996) provide a rubric for the analysis of narrative macrostructure that combines elements of both Applebee's (1978) and Stein and Glenn's (1979) frameworks in which they use the categories heap, sequence, primitive narrative, chain, and true narrative.

Expository discourse analysis typically involves measurements of various aspects of lexical variation and syntactic usage previously described for narrative structures. Nippold, Mansfield, and Billow (2008) focus on sentence length using mean length of T-units, subordinate clause production, and clausal density (average number of clauses per T-unit) to examine syntactic complexity in expository discourse of adolescents. Scott and Windsor (2000) include NWD as a measure of lexical diversity and percent of T-units with mazes (revision of an utterance) as a measure of discourse fluency. When considering written expository text, the clinician may also apply more traditional curriculum-based rubrics for the analysis of paragraph and essay structure (i.e., topic, supporting, and concluding sentences; introductory paragraph, body, and conclusion). Lexical diversity may be measured using TTR or NDW; grammatical complexity may be measured using sentence length, subordinate clause production, and clausal density.

Informal assessment is also useful in supplementing the information obtained from formal reading tests. Word recognition and oral reading fluency may be assessed by having the child read aloud from samples of literature and curriculum-based materials. The clinician can do a miscue analysis to determine the nature and pattern of the child's deviations from the printed text, measure the number of words read correctly per minute to judge overall fluency, and evaluate comprehension through story retelling and responses to factual and inferential questions about the text (Lipson & Wixson, 2009).

It is important for the clinician to consider that different tasks target different skills and therefore yield different pictures of children's reading/language comprehension. The following are examples to demonstrate how various tasks may be used to examine the child's cognitive-linguistic strengths and weaknesses in relation to reading comprehension. Multiple-choice questions and cloze tasks are widely used methods for testing reading comprehension. Cloze tasks contain sentences with omitted words. It is the child's task to fill in the blank. Multiple-choice questions are useful if the clinician wants to see how the student understands main ideas vs. details, but performance on these tasks will not reveal how the student constructs mental representations of the text while reading. Multiple-choice questions and cloze tests are not appropriate to assess understanding and recall of ideas, but cloze tests will indicate the child's sensitivity to grammatical and semantic constraints. If the clinician wants to see a more complex picture of the child's reading comprehension skills, then story retelling might be the appropriate task. When using free recall, the clinician may observe how the student organizes and remembers information from the text and whether he or she uses higher-level metacognitive abilities efficiently. This method, however, is highly demanding on expressive language. If the clinician wants to assess reading comprehension without tapping expressive language abilities, then a picture organization task or sentence verification test may be administered. This latter task consists of text and a series of sentences; some are related, some are unrelated to the text. The child is asked to indicate whether the information in the sentences was presented in the original text. The sentence verification test is a sensitive measure of memory for text and of understanding text structures. The limitation of the picture selection task is that it is not appropriate for assessing abstract ideas or relations among ideas.

Finally, coded observations and checklists can be used to provide an understanding of the child's pragmatic abilities within a conversational or classroom context. Damico's (1991) Clinical Discourse Analysis is an example of a checklist in which calculations are made of the sufficiency, accuracy, and situational appropriateness of the child's message; specificity of vocabulary; ability to maintain topic; and overall turn-taking. Craighead and Tattershall's (1991) checklist of

Communicative Skills Required in School examines the child's knowledge of communicative routines, use of strategies to facilitate comprehension, ability to follow and give oral and written directions, and use of figurative/nonliteral language within the classroom setting. Whether the clinician adapts one of these checklists or creates his or her own, the importance of considering these pragmatic language skills within the assessment process cannot be overemphasized as they provide a view of the child as communicator within a dynamic and naturalistic context.

In addition to the examination of various language skills, informal assessment involves the evaluation of numerous underlying cognitive skills such as working memory and executive functions. There are several working memory tasks that speech-language pathologists (SLPs) may administer. These informal measures include nonsense word repetition and complex listening and reading span tasks. In the former task, children repeat strings of phonemes that follow the **phonotactic rules** of the given language; however, the syllables do not carry meaning. These nonsense words may differ in length (2-3-4-5 syllables). This task provides the clinician with information about the child's phonological processing and storage skills. In complex listening and reading span tasks, children are required to process the content and structure of sentences and to repeat the sentence final words. The sentences may vary in syntactic complexity and length. The results reveal how much the child's working memory performance is affected by the length and the complexity of the linguistic material. This information is useful for diagnostic purposes as well as for intervention planning.

The assessment of executive functions during speech-language evaluation may include the examination of sustained and controlled attention, development and maintenance of goals in active memory, allocation of processing resources, active maintenance of information, and comprehension monitoring. Although many of these parameters may be readily measured by formal standardized tests, others require the administration of informal procedures or the observation of collateral behaviors and analysis of error patterns during formal and informal assessment. Depending on the instructions and task administration procedures, informal assessment may provide the clinician with further knowledge about the processes and the strategies that the child used during task performance.

Differential Diagnosis

To establish a **differential diagnosis**, the clinician needs to weigh all the evidence, including parent and teacher reports, family history, behavioral observations of the child and formal testing. Each specific diagnosis is supported by a converging pattern of performance and by diverging results for rivaling diagnoses (Pennington, 2009). As noted in the Introduction, children with language impairment demonstrate varied cognitive-linguistic profiles that reflect significant individual differences and show the dynamic nature of the cognitive-linguistic system. Although most children with language impairment evidence extraordinary difficulty with morphosyntax including grammatical morphemes, function words, and syntactic structures during the preschool years (Leonard, 2007), as these children age, their strengths and weaknesses change and many of them show shifts in their performance patterns. As a result of therapy and maturation, children with language impairment may evidence improvement in vocabulary acquisition or in morphosyntax. On the other hand, with changing academic and social demands, these children may demonstrate difficulties in new areas, such as written language, narrative production, or social language.

Although some clinical markers for language impairment have been identified over the years, standardized tests for these constructs are not available for each age group. Performance on nonword repetition is one of the hallmarks of child language impairment (Tager-Flusberg & Cooper, 1999). Nonword repetition is an effective tool in distinguishing child language impairment from language difference, such as low language proficiency level related to second language acquisition. These two groups (children with language impairment and ELL) may perform similarly in traditional language tests though for very different reasons (Kohnert, Windsor, & Ebert, 2009). The lack of distinguishing power in traditional language tests leads to numerous misidentifications of bilingual children as language impaired. Traditional language screening tasks incorrectly identified 50% to 65% of ELL students as language impaired (Peña & Bedore, 2011). Nonword repetition is one task that typically signals a difference between these two populations. One task, however, is never sufficient for differential diagnosis.

According to the neuroconstructivist approach, there has been a shift in focus from dissociations to cross-syndrome associations over the years in the study of atypical development. The parameters of neurodevelopmental disorders (e.g., SLI, attention deficit disorders, autism, etc.) may vary little at the beginning of life; the more pronounced differences will emerge with maturation (Karmiloff-Smith, 1998). Thus, depending on the severity of the disorder, age of the child, and secondary problems, children with distinct diagnoses may show many overlapping symptoms. Given that the developmental disorders reflect the interplay across genes-brain-environment–behavior, it is not surprising that, on one hand, we see a large number of individual variations within a disorder, and on the other hand, we experience many similarities at the behavioral level across disorders. This explains at least in part why it is so difficult to establish a differential diagnosis of primary language impairment in children. Despite these difficulties, there are a number of tasks and procedures that can be efficiently used when differentiating among developmental disorders. In the following part of this chapter, we present examples of these methods.

Children with a history of language impairment during the preschool years are at high risk for reading disorder, but not all children with reading disorder have difficulties in oral language, and some language-impaired children have no reading problems during the first years of elementary school. Bishop and Snowling (2004) suggested using a two-dimensional model for differentiating among children with SLI, **developmental dyslexia**, and poor reading comprehension. Their model is based on phonological skills and on other nonphonological language abilities. Children with primary or SLI may evidence difficulty in both phonological and nonphonological skills. These children show a weakness in phonological awareness (segmenting and manipulating syllables and phonemes in words) and in other language areas, such as morphosyntax and semantics. Their reading problems are usually complex and they may evidence difficulties in decoding, using contextual cues (semantic and syntactic bootstrapping), and analyzing structural information; differentiating between the main ideas and supporting details; and extracting meaning from the text.

Oral language skills appear to have a strong relationship with both decoding and reading comprehension. A number of studies demonstrated that a high percentage of children with SLI have both decoding and reading comprehension deficits (e.g., Catts, Fey, Tomblin, & Zhang, 2002; Conti-Ramsden, Botting, Simkin, & Knox, 2001). In contrast to these problems, children with dyslexia primarily show a weakness in phonology. These children demonstrate poor performance on phonological tasks, particularly in tests of phonological awareness, but have either age-appropriate morphosyntactic skills and vocabulary or they exhibit oral language problems that are neither severe nor persistent. These children's main weakness is in decoding.

The third group of children with reading problems consists of children with good phonological skills but poor reading comprehension. These children may read fluently but do not process the meaning of the text adequately. Children with poor reading comprehension may demonstrate success in learning to read, but not in reading to learn. Thus, despite their relatively good decoding skills, these children are not able to use reading as a tool for learning and information processing. A large number of children with reading comprehension problems have difficulty in listening comprehension as well. Further, reading comprehension deficits often co-occur with **attention-deficit/hyperactivity disorder** (ADHD; Cutting, Koth, Mahone, & Denckla, 2003). These two disorders co-occur at a greater rate than would be expected by chance; however, the nature of this association is not well understood (Purvis & Tannock, 2000). A deficit in executive functions is in part responsible for some of the overlapping symptoms (Berninger, Abbott, Cook, & Nagy, 2016).

Table 10-6 provides a summary of the distinguishing and overlapping characteristics in children with language impairment, dyslexia, reading comprehension difficulties, and ADHD. It should be noted that many children show mixed profiles and that the categorization involves generalization.

Summary

This chapter illustrated the challenges of diagnosing and describing primary language impairment in school-age children and adolescents. A central theme of the chapter was the critical relationship across different components within the linguistic rule system and among the linguistic, social, and cognitive systems. In assessing children's cognitive-linguistic functions, it is essential that SLPs understand the complexity of these systems as well as their interaction with external factors (e.g., task complexity and type) that influence children's speech-language performance. These functions may be measured by formal standardized tests and with informal procedures. In addition

Table 10-6. Comparison of Cognitive-Linguistic Skills Across Populations

	Children With Language Impairment	*Children With Dyslexia*	*Children With Reading Comprehension Deficit*	*Children With ADHD*
Phonological Skills	Weakness in phonological processing, poor phonological awareness	Weakness in phonological processing, poor phonological awareness	Average phonological processing skills	Average phonological processing skills
Morphosyntactic Skills	Deficit in morphosyntactic processing	Good morphosyntactic skills	Weakness in morphosyntax, difficulty with syntactic cues	Average morphosyntax
Vocabulary	Limited lexical knowledge	Good vocabulary	Limited lexical knowledge	Average lexical knowledge
Executive Functions	Weakness in executive functions, particularly in inhibition and attention switching	Average executive functions	Weakness in planning and monitoring own behavior, but relatively good inhibition	Poor inhibition control and behavioral organization
Working Memory	Working memory impairment across domains	Poor phonological working memory	Weakness in verbal working memory	Working memory impairment, particularly in spatial WM
Attention Control	Weakness in attention control	Average attention control	Average attention control	Deficit in attention control
Speed of Processing	Deficit in speed of processing	Average speed of processing	Deficit in speed of processing	Deficit in speed of processing
Social Communication Skills	A weakness in social communication, particularly in peer relationships	Good social communication skills	Good social communication skills	A weakness in social communication, particularly in peer relationships

to norm-referenced scores, the qualitative analyses of the child's cognitive-linguistic profile, error patterns, and strategy use reveal important information for the clinician. These data provide support for the clinician in establishing a differential diagnosis and in intervention planning. While formal test results offer a reliable reference in evaluating the child's social-cognitive-linguistic performance, informal assessment provides an examination of the child's competency across these areas within a more dynamic context. In contrast to measures of end products of formal tests, informal assessment procedures reveal information about the underlying processes and their interactions with internal and external factors (e.g., the impact of various conversational partners on discourse performance, the effect of text complexity on reading fluency). Both formal and informal assessment procedures are tools to assist the SLP in accomplishing his or her task to support the child's social-cognitive-linguistic development within an optimal learning environment.

Writing Rubric for Formal and Informal Language Assessment Sections of the Diagnostic Report

Identification of the section, followed by the full name of each test administered and its abbreviated form, followed by a brief introductory statement of the purpose of each test and what it purports to measure.

Formal Language Assessment

Clinical Evaluation of Language Fundamentals-5 (CELF-5)

Administration of the CELF-5 was designed to examine and compare receptive and expressive language and related abilities.

☐ Report of overall and domain scores

Example: Sam obtained a Core Language Score of 90, which is at the 25th percentile, a Receptive Language Index of 92, which is at the 30th percentile, an Expressive Language Index of 90, which is at the 25th percentile, a Language Content Index of 98, which is at the 45th percentile, and a Language Structure Index of 90, which is at the 25th percentile.

☐ Report of specific subtest scores, using a table format

Example: Specific subtest standard and percentile rank scores were as follows:

Table 1. Subtest Scores

Subtest	*Standard Score*	*Percentile Rank*
Sentence comprehension	9	37th
Linguistic concepts	9	37th
Word structure	8	25th
Word classes	11	63rd
Following directions	9	37th
Formulated sentences	11	63rd
Recalling sentences	6	9th
Understanding spoken paragraphs	11	63rd
Pragmatics profile	11	63rd

☐ Interpretation of findings of each test

Example: Findings indicate that overall composite language abilities are in the low average range. It is important to note that Sam exhibits performance scatter with subtest scores ranging from below average to high average. Specific weaknesses are apparent in tasks that require short-term recall and retrieval of information he has not fully processed, such as in the Sentence Recall task.

The other areas in which Sam exhibits low average performance involve expression of specific vocabulary and grammatical forms where he demonstrates inconsistent retrieval of specific lexical forms and weak generalization of morphemic structures.

By contrast, when Sam processes and comprehends information adequately, he retains and responds much more consistently, as evidenced in tasks where he has to identify and describe the relationship between words and respond to questions about a story that has been read to him.

Overall, it appears that Sam's language difficulties are related to deficits in immediate short-term rote recall, word retrieval, and incomplete rule generalization. Although it may seem as if his receptive skills are stronger than his expressive language skills, expressive difficulties occur when Sam does not fully process spoken input or is asked to retrieve information based on rote recall. The more meaningful and contextualized the language input is for him, the more successful he is at storing, retrieving, and expressing information.

☐ Comparison of findings of each test to other procedures administered that may measure similar skills sets

Example: These findings confirm those previously described on the Test of Language Development: Primary-4 (TOLD: P-4), and confirm deficits in short-term recall and word retrieval.

Informal Language Assessment

☐ Analysis of Oral Discourse and Listening Skills

Description of specific tasks administered to examine and compare informal conversational social interactions with more structured narrative and expository oral discourse. Include relevant collateral behaviors and strategies as well as specific measures of vocabulary and grammatical complexity if available.

Example: Sam interacted easily with the examiner during informal conversational and question/answer exchange. He was responsive to questions and comments about familiar topics, such as his family and school. He initiated, took his turn, and demonstrated a full range of communicative intentions. These findings are consistent with those previously reported on the Pragmatics Profile of the CELF-5.

Although he generally maintained topic about familiar subjects, when he seemed uncertain about a subject or did not understand a question, Sam shifted to another topic and continued without necessarily responding to his listener. He often interrupted to make comments that were only marginally related to the topic at hand. Because Sam is a very engaging and social child, these interruptions and continuous talking seemed to be a strategy he used to keep the exchange going when he either did not comprehend a question or did not know an answer.

Overall, range of vocabulary and sentence structures was appropriate to the conversational context. Speech sound production was within expected levels.

Analysis of more formal discourse was based on having Sam (a) retell stories that were told or read aloud to him and (b) make up original stories based on pictures. He seemed quite engaged by the stories that were told or read to him and listened attentively as he followed along with the pictures. During story retelling, he provided a logical sequence of actions related to a main idea, and responded accurately to most factual questions about the narratives. He had greater difficulty making up his own story. Rather than provide a cohesive narrative, he described specific objects and actions in the picture but did not readily connect them to a main idea or theme. He presented a sequence of actions but did not offer a clear beginning or end to his story.

Range of vocabulary and sentence structures was appropriate to the content of the narratives. However, Sam was unlikely to incorporate any new vocabulary into his story retelling, and exhibited occasional word retrieval difficulties even after repeated presentation of previously unfamiliar words.

Overall, Sam's oral discourse skills are within expected levels for informal social-interactive exchange with respect to initiation, turn-taking, range of communicative intentions, and lexical and grammatical usage. Topic maintenance and responsiveness to questions are variable and appear related to inconsistencies in attention, processing, and comprehension rather than to lack of awareness of social-pragmatic conventions. Clearly, when Sam perceives something as too difficult, he seeks to change the subject and return to safer ground.

With respect to more formal oral discourse, Sam enjoys hearing stories and being read to. His listening, retention, and reformulation are facilitated by the availability of pictorial referents, modeling, and question prompts to guide his story retelling. He appears to require repeated exposure and time to incorporate novel vocabulary and unfamiliar or more abstract concepts, but he is responsive to the teaching with supportive modeling and reinforcement.

- ☐ Clinical Impression

  Comparison of findings from formal and informal assessment procedures to identify consistencies and/or inconsistencies in observed patterns of findings.

  Example: Sam is a 5;6-year-old child who presents with receptive and expressive language deficits related to weaknesses in short-term rote memory, word retrieval, processing and formulation of more abstract concepts, and phonological awareness.

  Although it may seem as if his receptive skills are stronger than his expressive language skills, expressive difficulties are most likely to occur when Sam does not fully process spoken input and is asked to retrieve information based on rote recall. Findings from both formal and informal assessment procedures indicate that the more meaningful and contextualized the language input is for him, the more successful Sam is at storing, retrieving, and expressing information.

Case History for the Sample Report

David is an 11;8-year-old boy, who is one of triplets. He has been evaluated as having learning difficulties related to possible attention deficit and is in a special education self-contained class. His mother indicates that, while David has received special education services, persistent problems are evident with listening and reading comprehension, as well as oral and written expression which she suspects may be related to language processing weaknesses that were not previously identified.

Selection of Assessment Procedures for the Sample Report

The CELF-5 was selected as an age-appropriate formal standardized test to provide an overview of receptive and expressive language abilities. Selected subtests from the DTLA-4 were chosen as age-appropriate formal standardized measures to clarify discrepancies in language processing observed among specific subtests from the CELF-5. The GORT-5 was administered to examine and compare decoding and comprehension for oral paragraph reading given parental concerns about text comprehension. The WLA was selected as a formal standardized procedure to measure and compare written language expression for different discourse genres.

Informal assessment procedures were selected to provide a measure of the youngster's oral expression in conversation and during question/answer exchange. Additionally he was asked to retell previously read stories to examine narrative and expository discourse.

Sample Report

David Benjamin	D.O.E. 12/14/15; 12/21/15
201 James Street	D.O.B. 4/18/04
Brooklyn, NY 11210	Age: 11 years, 8 months

I. Reason for Referral

Mrs. Benjamin requested a speech and language evaluation for her son because of persistent difficulties observed in his language processing and reading.

David has been diagnosed previously as having a learning disability. He attends P.S. 20, where he is in a self-contained class.

II. Tests Administered/Procedures

- Parent Interview
- Clinical Evaluation of Language Fundamentals-5 (CELF-5)
- Selected subtests from the Detroit Test of Learning Aptitude-4 (DTLA-4)
- Gray Oral Reading Tests-5 (GORT-5)
- Written Language Assessment (WLA)
- Informal Assessment of Oral Discourse and Listening Skills

III. Background Information

David is one of triplets; his two brothers, Ethan and Timothy, have also been diagnosed with learning disabilities. All three boys attend the same self-contained class with a 12:1:1 ratio at P.S. 20, in Brooklyn. Whereas his brothers have received speech and language services as part of their special education program, David previously had not received a formal speech and language evaluation.

The triplets were delivered by cesarean section at 33 weeks following maternal gestational diabetes and toxemia. David was on a ventilator in the neonatal intensive care unit because of respiratory distress. Cardiac problems were identified during the first few months.

David received occupational and physical therapy, as well as the services of a special education itinerant teacher as part of his early intervention and preschool special education programs.

A pediatric neurodevelopmental evaluation, administered in November 2010 and January 2011 confirmed the presence of a learning disability and possible attention deficit. A psychological and educational evaluation administered in June 2011 revealed performance to be in the low average range, with the recommendation for continued placement in a self-contained classroom.

Unlike his two brothers, Mrs. Benjamin reports that David's self-esteem has been significantly affected by his placement in a special education setting. Her sense is that, given some of his strengths, his potential may be limited by the current educational program. Furthermore, as a trained speech-language pathologist, she has observed inconsistencies in his processing abilities that belie his apparently strong vocabulary knowledge, and she questions whether there may be other underlying issues that have not been fully addressed.

IV. Clinical Observations

David was cooperative and participated willingly in all assessment activities. He interacted easily with the examiner and did not exhibit any particular test anxiety. He appeared motivated to do his best and requested assistance appropriately. He demonstrated sustained attention and focus, worked carefully, and persisted at tasks to completion. He exhibited a thoughtful and reflective response style, and considered his choices before selecting an answer. At times, he returned to a previously answered test item and self-corrected his initial response. Although he demonstrated reasonably good frustration tolerance, he was observed to have some difficulty with more complex spoken input that required sustained listening, analysis of more abstract information, and higher-level critical thinking.

Language Skills

Formal Assessment

Clinical Evaluation of Language Fundamentals-5 (CELF-5)

Administration of the CELF-5 was designed to examine and compare receptive and expressive language and related abilities. Results revealed a Core Language Index of 81, which is at the 10th percentile, a Receptive Language Index of 78, which is at the 7th percentile, an Expressive Language Index of 89, which is at the 23rd percentile, a Language Content Index of 104, which is at the 61st percentile, and a Language Memory Index of 91, which is at the 27th percentile.

Specific subtest standard and percentile rank scores were as follows:

Table 1.

Subtest	*Standard Score*	*Percentile Rank*
Word classes	8	25th
Following directions	9	37th
Formulated sentences	9	37th
Recalling sentences	8	25th
Understanding spoken paragraphs	11	63rd
Word definitions	13	84th
Sentence assembly	8	25th
Semantic relationships	2	2nd
Pragmatics profile	11	63rd

Findings indicate that overall language abilities are below average, with relative performance strength observed in expressive compared with receptive language. Considerable performance scatter is observed with specific subtest scores ranging from below average to above average. Most notable is David's knowledge of specific vocabulary as evidenced by his performance on the Word Definitions task. Despite this considerable area of strength, he demonstrates noteworthy weakness in language processing and retrieval, as evidenced in his performance on the Semantic Relationships task. It appears that, although David has a strong vocabulary, he has difficulty processing, storing, reorganizing, and reformulating longer, more complex segments of spoken input.

Furthermore, the rather significant discrepancy observed between his performance on the Semantic Relationships and Understanding Spoken Paragraphs tasks suggests that David makes good use of world knowledge and contextualized information to process language input. His apparent struggle with discrete and decontextualized information is indicative of specific interactions between language processing and working memory deficits.

Detroit Tests of Learning Aptitude-4 (DTLA-4, selected subtests)

Administration of selected subtests from the DTLA-4 was designed to clarify some of the performance discrepancies previously described on the CELF-5. Results revealed a Linguistic-Verbal Domain composite score of 78, which is at the 7th percentile. Specific subtest standard and percentile rank scores were as follows:

Table 2.

Subtest	*Standard Score*	*Percentile Rank*
Word opposites	7	16th
Sentence imitation	6	9th
Reversed letters	6	9th
Story construction	9	37th
Basic information	6	9th
Word sequences	6	9th
Story sequences	13	84th

Findings indicate that performance in the linguistic-verbal domain is below average, with significant weaknesses apparent in language processing, storage, and retrieval as length and complexity of spoken input increases. As previously described on the CELF-5, David has difficulty holding on to and organizing increasingly complex linguistic information in working memory for later use.

Again, although there is notable scatter in his performance on various tasks, it is quite apparent that these discrepancies are attributable to the extent to which David is asked to process discrete, often decontextualized segments of input without pictorial referents, compared with formulating contextualized narrative sequences with pictorial referents.

These findings confirm those previously described on the CELF-5 and suggest significant interactions between language processing and working memory deficits.

Gray Oral Reading Tests-5

Administration of the GORT-5 was designed to examine and compare decoding and comprehension for oral paragraph reading. Results revealed an Oral Reading Quotient of 85, which is at the 16th percentile. Specific subtest standard and percentile rank scores were as follows:

Table 3.

Subtest	*Standard Score*	*Percentile Rank*
Reading rate	7	16th
Reading accuracy	7	16th
Reading fluency	6	9th
Reading comprehension	9	37th

Findings indicate that overall oral reading skills are below average, with weaknesses in decoding and reading fluency appearing to interfere with text comprehension. As observed with listening comprehension previously, David makes good use of his world knowledge and contextualized information to derive meaning from text. However, he is a slow and inefficient reader. He makes frequent errors as length and linguistic complexity of text increase, still seemingly sounding out words that he would be expected to recognize as whole linguistic units within the structure of a sentence.

With decoding still demanding significant processing resources, it is difficult for David to fully attend to and integrate meanings of sentences within the overall flow of the text. Although David exhibits strong vocabulary knowledge for spoken language, he does not always apply this knowledge to decode and interpret written text. These difficulties become more apparent as length and grammatical complexity of sentence structures increase within the text.

Written Language Assessment (WLA)

Administration of the WLA was designed to examine and compare written expression for narrative and expository text. Results revealed a Written Language Quotient of 79, which is at the 8th percentile.

Findings indicate that David provides a clearly stated main idea and related sequence of ideas in both his narrative and expository writing. However, lexical and grammatical usage is surprisingly limited, given his previously described strong vocabulary knowledge. Sentence forms are generally simple and conjoined structures; range of vocabulary is limited; there is little elaboration of ideas, particularly for original expository writing. David does follow rules for writing conventions, including capitalization and punctuation; spelling errors are predominantly phonetic. Overall, written language expression is below expected levels and surprisingly limited, given apparent strengths in oral discourse.

Informal Assessment

Analysis of Oral Discourse and Listening Skills

David interacted easily with the examiner during conversational and question–answer exchange. He was responsive to questions and comments about familiar topics, such as his family and school. He maintained and extended topics, demonstrated a full range of communicative intentions, and exhibited a range of vocabulary and sentence structures that was appropriate to the conversational context. Speech sound production was well within expected levels. These findings are consistent with those previously reported on the Pragmatics Profile of the CELF-5.

Analysis of more formal oral discourse was based on having David retell previously read stories that were well within his reading level. He did somewhat better with narrative compared with expository discourse, in that his narrative was more logically organized, while his expository discourse was somewhat fragmented. In both instances, however, David provided a sequence of facts related to a main idea. Although he offered many details, he needed to be prompted to elaborate on the information presented. Overall, range and variety of vocabulary and sentence structures were within expected levels and clearly more developed than that previously described for written discourse.

Overall, oral discourse skills are within expected levels for both social interactive exchange and more formal narrative and expository structures. Oral discourse is clearly a strength for David compared with written discourse and, as a strength, may mask some of his more subtle weaknesses in language processing, storage, retrieval, and reformulation of less familiar and decontextualized material.

V. Clinical Impressions

David Benjamin is an 11-year, 8-month-old boy who presents with specific language processing deficits that contribute to his learning disability. The presence of relatively strong oral communication skills, particularly for social-interactive exchange, appear to have masked more subtle, but nonetheless significant, weaknesses in processing, storage, retrieval, and reformulation of both spoken and written language as length and complexity of text increase and as text becomes less familiar and decontextualized.

Significant performance inconsistency is evident in the scatter observed across language-based tasks. Although David makes good use of his world knowledge and contextualized information to process language input, his struggle with discrete and decontextualized information is indicative of specific interactions between language processing and working memory deficits.

Furthermore, persistent weaknesses in reading fluency interfere with text comprehension. He remains a slow and inefficient reader, particularly as grammatical complexity and length of text increase, again despite reasonably strong vocabulary skills.

Finally, discrepancies observed between David's oral and written discourse skills may become clearer when the simultaneous, competing demands of processing, retrieval, formulation, and motor execution are considered.

The overall impression is that David's academic potential is indeed greater than he is currently demonstrating. This impression is largely the result of (a) observations of considerable performance scatter and (b) successful attempts to prompt David's self-monitoring, self-correction, revision, and elaboration of his responses.

VI. Recommendations

It is recommended that David be placed in a collaborative educational setting where he may have the opportunity to work alongside typical learners and be exposed more consistently to higher-level processing, increasingly abstract reasoning, and critical thinking activities. This will be fruitful only if he has adequate support services including language therapy on an individual basis, minimally twice per week.

Language therapy should address listening comprehension, reading fluency, reading comprehension, and written expression. Treatment goals should include (a) processing, retention, and reformulation of increasingly complex segments of spoken information, using visualization and paraphrase, at first with and then eventually without pictorial cues; (b) formulation of original narrative and expository text based at first on pictures and then on previously heard and read text, in which David is required to incorporate novel vocabulary and increasingly complex grammatical forms; (c) alternately listening to and reading increasingly higher levels of text aloud to enhance word recognition and overall reading fluency; and (d) writing increasingly complex sentence forms and paragraph structures to describe, explain, and provide information based on information David has heard or read, using Hochman's (1995) *Basic Writing Skills* program to facilitate the use of varying sentence types and expanded sentence structures.

Finally, it is suggested that the family provide David with more consistent exposure to literacy experiences. If he is not particularly motivated at this time to engage in recreational reading, then some consideration should be given to providing him with books on tape, read aloud experiences, and opportunities for discussion, analysis, and prediction about texts.

____

(Name of clinician or clinical supervisor and credentials)

Speech-Language Pathologist

Practice Exercises

Given the following concluding paragraphs from the reports of an assessment conducted with Kate, a 7;4-year-old child; Anthony, a 9;5-year-old child; and Beth, a 13;8-year-old adolescent, identify and describe specific formal and informal assessment procedures and analyses that could have led to the diagnostic conclusions regarding these children's deficits. Explain how each of these procedures might have contributed to and clarified the stated findings.

Case 1

Kate is a 7;4-year-old child who presents a specific language deficit, characterized by weaknesses in processing, storage, and retrieval of spoken and written language. Although overall language skills are within expected levels, significant discrepancies are observed between receptive and expressive abilities. Kate has difficulty following directions, comprehending stories, learning and retrieving precise vocabulary, and listening to and reading extended text, particularly if pictorial referents are limited. Listening and reading comprehension deficits are interacting with difficulties in sustained attention and working memory, and place her at risk for academic achievement as language processing demands of the curriculum increase.

Case 2

Anthony is a 9;5-year-old child who presents specific language deficits, characterized by weaknesses in processing, storing, retrieving, and reformulating input as length and linguistic complexity and abstractness increase. Although expressive language skills are stronger than receptive skills, inconsistencies are apparent in vocabulary formulation and retrieval, as well as in the specificity with which he presents and elaborates on his ideas. Interactions are evident between language processing and working memory which affect both listening and reading comprehension, as well as more formal oral discourse. Written expression does not appear to be affected to the same extent as oral expression, possibly because writing is slower and allows him more time to organize, plan, and formulate his ideas. Nevertheless, even in writing, the range of vocabulary usage and sentence structures is somewhat concrete and below expected levels.

Case 3

Beth is a 13;8-year-old adolescent who presents with language processing, storage, and retrieval weaknesses that become evident as length and complexity of text increase and as information is decontextualized and less familiar. Additionally, she presents weaknesses in vocabulary knowledge and usage, which are as likely the result of limited reading as they are the cause of decoding and reading fluency problems. Despite overall decoding accuracy, Beth approaches previously unfamiliar words and even familiar words without sufficient regard for context, attempting to read words by sounding them out rather than by recognizing them as whole units. With decoding still demanding significant processing resources, it is difficult for Beth to attend to and integrate meanings of sentences within the overall flow of the text, particularly when the information presented is unfamiliar. These difficulties become more apparent as length and grammatical complexity of sentence structures increase within the text.

Glossary

Attention-deficit/hyperactivity disorder (ADHD): A neurobehavioral developmental disorder characterized by a deficit in attention control (inattention, impulsiveness, hyperactivity).

Attention: A complex term that refers to the process of focusing on certain features of the environment while excluding others. There are various types of attention, such as sustained attention, selective attention, and divided attention.

Collateral measures: The clinician's observations of communication skills and other observable behaviors during assessment. These behaviors may not be accounted for by the standardized assessment instrument, but allow for a more in depth analysis of the child's skills.

Developmental dyslexia: A neurocognitive developmental disorder; a specific reading impairment characterized by a weakness in decoding words via phoneme-grapheme correspondence rules despite adequate environmental input and intellectual abilities.

Differential diagnosis: The process of evaluating the probability of different disorders and selecting the most likely diagnosis based on the well-known symptoms.

Discourse: A spoken or written unit that is greater than a sentence. There are various types of discourse including narratives, conversations, quizzes, and self talk.

Executive functions: A set of cognitive abilities that play an important role in inhibition, planning, monitoring, and regulating goal-directed behavior.

Expository discourse: The use of language to describe a topic or provide an explanation organized around a certain theme.

Formal assessment: A data-driven process that involves measurements and documentation of knowledge, skills, and abilities by using tests as standardized measures.

Informal assessment: A performance-driven and process-oriented method including observations, recordings of behavior in natural settings, checklists, and inventories.

Lexical diversity: Richness and variety of vocabulary in an individual's repertoire.

Macrostructure: The framework or story grammar elements that comprise the episodic structure of a narrative.

Metalinguistic knowledge/skills: The ability to think about language and to manipulate linguistic units, such as phonemes, morphemes, and sentences.

Narrative discourse: Account of shared experiences; sequential retell of a past event; telling of a fictional story.

Phonotactic rules: Typically expected sound sequences and patterns and their placement within the segments of language.

Sequential bilingualism: The process of acquiring two languages successively. Exposure to the second language typically occurs after age of 3 years.

Specific language impairment: A developmental language disorder that is not the consequence of intellectual disability, hearing impairment, neurological deficit, emotional disturbances, or environmental deprivation. Children with SLI may show weaknesses in both expressive and receptive language.

Type/token ration (TTR): Clinical tool for measuring lexical diversity, calculated by determining the ratio of different words to total words in a child's language sample.

Working memory: A short-term memory system for storing and simultaneously manipulating information.

References

Applebee, A. (1978). *The child's concept of story.* Chicago, IL: University of Chicago Press.

Berninger, V., Abbott, R., Cook, C. R., & Nagy, W. (2016). Relationships of attention and executive functions to oral language, reading, and writing skills and systems in middle childhood and early adolescence. *Journal of Learning Disabilities, 50*, 434-449.

Bishop, D. V. M., & Snowling, M. J. (2004). Developmental dyslexia and specific language impairment: Same or different? *Psychological Bulletin, 130*, 858-886.

Blank, M., Rose, S. A., & Berlin, L. J. (2003). *Preschool Language Assessment Instrument (PLAI-2).* Austin, TX: Pro-Ed.

Boehm, A. E. (2001). *Boehm Test of Basic Concepts-3.* San Antonio, TX: Pearson.

Botting, N., & Conti-Ramsden, G. (2004). Characteristics of children with specific language impairment. In L. Verhoeven & H. van Balkom (Eds.), *Classification of developmental language disorders* (pp. 23-38). Mahwah, NJ: Erlbaum.

Bowers, L., Huisingh, R., & LoGuidice, C. (2005). *Test of Problem Solving (TOPS-3).* Austin, TX: Pro-Ed.

Bowers, L. Huisingh, R., LoGuidice, C., & Orman, J. (2014). *The Word Test-3.* Austin, TX: Pro-Ed.

Brown, V. L., Wiederholt, J. L., & Hammil, D. D. (2009). *Test of Reading Comprehension (TORC-4).* Austin, TX: Pro-Ed.

Brownell, R., & Martin, N. A. (2011a). *Expressive One Word Picture Vocabulary Test (EOWPVT-4).* Austin, TX: Pro-Ed.

Brownell, R., & Martin, N. A. (2011b). *Receptive One Word Picture Vocabulary Test (ROWPVT-4).* Austin, TX: Pro-Ed.

Bryant, B. R., Weiderholt, J. L., & Bryant, D. P. (2004). *Gray Diagnostic Reading Tests (GDRT-2).* Austin, TX: Pro-Ed.

Carrow-Woolfolk, E. (2017). *Comprehensive Assessment of Spoken Language (CASL-2).* Austin, TX: Pro-Ed.

Carrow-Woolfolk, E. (1999). *Test of Auditory Comprehension of Language (TACL-3).* Austin, TX: Pro-Ed.

Catts, H. W., Fey, M. E., Tomblin, J. B., & Zhang, X. (2002). A longitudinal investigation of reading outcomes in children with language impairments. *Journal of Speech, Language, and Hearing Research, 45*, 1142-1157.

Connolly, A. J. (2007). *Key Math-3 Diagnostic Assessment.* San Antonio, TX: Pearson.

Conti-Ramsden, G., Botting, N., Simkin, Z., & Knox, E. (2001). Follow-up of children attending infant language units: Outcomes at 11 years of age. *International Journal of Language and Communication Disorders, 36*, 207-219.

Craighead, N. A., & Tattershall, S. S. (1991). Observation and assessment of classroom pragmatic skills. In C. S. Simon (Ed.), *Communication skills and classroom success: Assessment and therapy methodologies for language and learning disabled students* (pp. 106-124). Eau Claire, WI: Thinking Publications.

Cutting, L. E., Koth, C. W. Mahone, E. M., & Denckla, M. B. (2003). Evidence for unexpected weaknesses in learning in children with attention-deficit/hyperactivity disorder without Reading Disabilities. *Journal of Learning Disabilities, 36*, 259-269.

Damico, J. S. (1991). Clinical discourse analysis: A functional language assessment technique. In C. S. Simon (Ed.), *Communication skills and classroom success: Assessment and therapy methodologies for language and learning disabled students* (pp. 125-150). Eau Claire, WI: Thinking Publications.

Dunn, L. M, & Dunn, D. M. (2007). *Peabody Picture Vocabulary Test (PPVT-4).* San Antonio, TX: Pearson.

Ebert, K. D., & Scott, C. M. (2014). Relationships between narrative language samples and norm-referenced test scores in language assessments of school-age children. *Language, Speech, and Hearing Services in Schools, 45*, 337-350.

German, D. J. (2015). *Test of Word Finding (TWF-2).* Austin, TX: Pro-Ed.

Gilger, J. W., & Wise, S. E. (2004). Genetic correlates of language and literacy impairments. In C. A. Stone, E. R. Silliman, B. J. Ehren, & K. Apel (Eds.), *Handbook of language and literacy: Development and disorders* (pp. 25-48). New York, NY: Guilford Press.

Gillam, R., & Pearson, N. A. (2017). *Test of Narrative Language (TNL-2).* Austin, TX: Pro-Ed.

Grill, J. J., & Kirwin, M. M. (1989). *Written Language Assessment.* Novato, CA: Academic Therapy Publ.

Guo, L., & Schneider, P. (2016) Differentiating school-aged children with and without language impairment using tense and grammaticality measures from a narrative task. *Journal of Speech, Language, and Hearing Research, 59*, 317-329.

Hamaguchi, P., & Ross-Swain, D. (2015). *Receptive, Expressive, and Social Communication Assessment-Elementary (RESCA-E).* Novato, CA: Academic Therapy Publications.

Hammil, D. D. (1998). *Detroit Test of Learning Aptitude (DTLA-4).* Austin, TX: Pro-Ed.

Hammil, D. D., Brown, V. L., Larsen, S. C., & Wiederholt, J. L. (2007). *Test of Adolescent and Adult Language (TOAL-4).* Austin, TX: Pro-Ed.

Hammil, D. D., & Larsen, S. C. (2009). *Test of Written Language (TOWL-4).* Austin, TX: Pro-Ed.

Hammill, D. D, Mather, N., & Roberts, R. (2001). *The Illinois Test of Psycholinguistic Abilities (ITPA-3).* Austin, TX: Pro-Ed.

Hammil, D. D., & Newcomer, P. L. (2008a). *Test of Language Development-Intermediate (TOLD: I-4).* Austin, TX: Pro-Ed.

Hammil, D. D., & Newcomer, P. L. (2008b). *Test of Language Development-Primary (TOLD: P-4).* Austin, TX: Pro-Ed.

Heath, S. B. (1986). Taking a cross cultural look at narratives. *Topics in Language Disorders, 7*, 84-94.

Hess, C. W., Sefton, K. M., & Landry, R. G. (1986). Sample size and type-token ratios for oral language of preschool children. *Journal of Speech and Hearing Research, 29*, 129-134.

Hochman, J. (1995). *Basic writing skills.* Harrison, NY: CSL.

Hughes, D., McGillivray, L., & Schmidek, M. (1997). *Guide to narrative language: Procedures for assessment.* Eau Claire, WI: Thinking Publications.

Hunt, K. (1965). *Grammatical structures written at three grade levels* (Research Report No. 3). Urbana, IL: National Council of Teachers of English.

Justice, L. M., Bowles, R. P., Kaderavek, J. N., Ukrainetz, T. A., Eisenberg, S. L., & Gillam, R. B. (2006). The index of narrative microstructure: A clinical tool for analyzing school-age children's narrative performance. *American Journal of Speech Language Pathology, 15*, 177-191.

Karmiloff-Smith, A. (1998). Development itself is the key to understanding developmental disorders. *Trends in Cognitive Sciences, 2,* 389-398.

Kaufman, A. S., & Kaufman, N. L. (2014). *Kaufman Test of Educational Achievement (KTEA-3).* San Antonio, TX: Pearson.

Kohnert, K., Windsor, J., & Ebert, K. D. (2009). Primary or "specific" language impairment and children learning a second language. *Brain & Language, 109,* 101-111.

Larsen, S. C., Hammil, D. D., & Moats, L. (2013). *Test of Written Spelling (TWS-5).* Austin, TX: Pro-Ed.

Leonard, L. B. (2007). Processing limitations and the grammatical profile of children with specific language impairment. In R. V. Kail (Ed.), *Advances in child development and behavior* (pp. 139-172). Academic Press Elsevier.

Lindamood, P. C., & Lindamood, P. (2004). *Lindamood Auditory Conceptualization Test (LAC-3).* Austin, TX: Pro-Ed.

Lipson, M. Y., & Wixson, K. K. (2009). *Assessment and instruction of reading and writing difficulty.* Boston, MA: Pearson.

Loban, W. (1976). *Language development: Kindergarten through grade twelve.* Urbana, IL: National Council of Teachers of English.

Lombardino, L. J., Lieberman, R. J., & Brown, J. C. (2005). *Assessment of Literacy and Language (ALL).* San Antonio, TX: Pearson.

Markwardt, F. C. (1997). *Peabody Individual Achievement Test (PIAT-R/NU).* San Antonio, TX: Pearson.

Martin, N. A., & Brownell, R. (2005). *Test of Auditory Processing (TAPS-3).* Austin, TX: Pro-Ed.

McGhee, R. L., Ehrler, D. J., & DiSimoni, F. (2007). *Token Test for Children (TTFC-2).* Austin, TX: Pro-Ed.

Nelson, N., Plante, E., & Helm-Estabrooks, N. (2015). *Test of Integrated Language and Literacy Skills (TILLS).* Baltimore, MD: Brookes Publ. Co.

Nippold, M. A., Mansfield, T. C., & Billow, J. L. (2008). Expository discourse in adolescents with language impairments: Examining syntactic development. *American Journal of Speech Language Pathology, 17,* 356-366.

Paul, R. (2007). *Language disorders from infancy through adolescence.* St. Louis, MO: Mosby.

Paul, R., Hernandez, R., Taylor, L., & Johnson, K. (1996). Narrative development in late talkers: Early school age. *Journal of Speech and Hearing Research, 39,* 1295-1303.

Peña, E. D., & Bedore, L. M. (2011). It takes two: Improving assessment accuracy in bilingual children. *The ASHA Leader, 16,* 20-22.

Pennington, B. F. (2009). *Diagnosing learning disorders: A neuropsychological framework* (2nd ed.). New York, NY: Guilford Press.

Peterson, R. L., & McGrath, L. M. (2009). Speech and language disorders. In B. F. Pennington (Ed.), *Diagnosing learning disorders: A neuropsychological framework* (pp. 83-107). New York, NY: Guilford Press.

Phelps-Terasaki, D., & Phelps-Gunn, T. (2007). *Test of Pragmatic Language (TOPL-2).* Austin, TX: Pro-Ed.

Purvis, K. L., & Tannock, R. (2000). Phonological processing, not inhibitory control, differentiates ADHD and reading disability. *Journal of the American Academy of Child and Adolescent Psychiatry, 39,* 48-494.

Robertson, C., & Salter, W. (2017). *Phonological Awareness Test (PAT-2:NU).* Austin, TX: Pro-Ed.

Scott, C. (1988). Spoken and written syntax. In M. Nippold (Ed.), *Later language development.* San Diego, CA: College-Hill Press.

Scott, C. M., & Stokes, S. L. (1995). Measures of syntax in school-age children and adolescents. *Language, Speech, and Hearing Services in Schools, 26,* 309-319.

Scott, C., & Windsor, J. (2000). General language performance measures in spoken and written narrative and expository discourse of school-age children with language learning disabilities. *Journal of Speech Language and Hearing Research, 43,* 324-339.

Stein, N. L., & Glenn, C. G. (1979). An analysis of story comprehension in elementary school children. In R. O. Freedle (Ed.), *New directions in discourse processing* (pp. 53-120). Norwood, NJ: Ablex.

Tager-Flusberg, H. (2005). Designing studies to investigate the relationships between genes, environments, and developmental language disorders. *Applied Psycholinguistics, 26,* 29-39.

Tager-Flusberg, H., & Cooper, J. (1999). Present and future possibilities for defining a phenotype for specific language impairment. *Journal of Speech, Language, and Hearing Research, 42,* 1275-1278.

Templin, M. (1957). *Certain language skills in children: Their development and inter-relationships.* Minneapolis: University of Minnesota Press.

Tomblin, J. B. (2008). Validating diagnostic standards for specific language impairment using adolescent outcomes. In C. F. Norbury, J. B. Tomblin, & D. V. M. Bishop (Eds.), *Understanding developmental language disorders: From theory to practice* (pp. 93-114). New York, NY: Psychology Press.

Tomblin, J. B., Records, N. L., Buckwalter, P., Zhang, X., & Smith, E. (1997). Prevalence of specific language impairment in kindergarten children. *Journal of Speech, Language, and Hearing Research, 40,* 1245-1260.

Torgesen, J. K., & Bryant, B. R. (2004). *Test of Phonological Awareness (TOPA-2).* Austin, TX: Pro-Ed.

Ukrainetz, T. A. (2006). The many ways of exposition: A focus on discourse structure. In T. A. Ukrainetz (Ed.), *Contextualized language intervention* (pp. 247-288). Eau Claire, WI: Thinking Publications.

Wagner, R. K., Torgesen, J. K., Raschotte, C. A., & Pearson, N. A. (2013). *Comprehensive Test of Phonological Processes (CTOPP-2).* Austin, TX: Pro-Ed.

Wallace, G., & Hammil, D. D. (2013). *Comprehensive Receptive Expressive Vocabulary Test (CREVT—3).* Austin, TX: Pro-Ed

Wiederholt, J. L., & Blalock, G. (2000). *Gray Silent Reading Test (GSRT).* Austin, TX: Pro-Ed.

Wiederholt, J. L., & Bryant, D. P. (2012). *Gray Oral Reading Test (GORT-5).* Austin, TX: Pro-Ed.

Wiig, E. H., Semel, E., & Secord, W. A.(2013). *Clinical Evaluation of Language Fundamentals (CELF-5).* San Antonio, TX: Pearson.

Wiig, E. H., Semel, E., & Secord, W. A. (2014). *Clinical Evaluation of Language Fundamentals, Metalinguistics (CELF-5, Metalinguistics).* San Antonio, TX: Pearson.

Woodcock, R. W. (2011). *Woodcock Reading Mastery Tests-III (WRMT-III).* San Antonio, TX: Pearson.

11

Assessment of Aphasia

Elizabeth E. Galletta, PhD, CCC-SLP and Amy Vogel-Eyny, MPhil

Key Words

- agnosia
- agrammatism
- agraphia
- alexia
- aneurysm
- anomia
- aphasia
- apraxia
- arterial-venous malformation
- cerebrovascular accident
- cognition
- concomitant
- dysarthria
- embolic stroke (embolism)
- fluent aphasia
- hemianopsia
- hemiplegia
- hemorrhagic stroke
- infarct
- ischemic stroke
- neglect
- neologistic paraphasic error
- nonfluent aphasia
- paraphasic error
- random paraphasic error
- speech fluency
- spontaneous recovery
- stroke
- thrombotic stroke
- word-retrieval difficulty

Introduction (Overview of the Disorder)

Aphasia is often defined as an acquired cognitive-linguistic disorder, typically secondary to left hemisphere **stroke**. Aphasia involves the processes underlying receptive and expressive language modalities caused by damage to areas of the brain responsible for language function (Ferrand & Bloom, 1997). Descriptions of aphasia often include two components: a definition of language and an explanation of the underlying neuroanatomical correlates of language. When assessing aphasia, it is important to evaluate receptive and expressive language as well as the cognitive processes involved in communication. This chapter will focus on the language and cognitive skills that need to be formally and informally assessed in adults who have sustained a left hemisphere stroke.

Stein-Rubin, C., & Fabus, R. *A Guide to Clinical Assessment and Professional Report Writing in Speech-Language Pathology, Second Edition (pp 245-264).*

Defining the Disorder

The World Health Organization (WHO; 2001) *International Classification of Functioning Disability and Health* (ICF) views a disorder with respect to the terms *impairment, disability*, and *handicap*. This model classifies an individual's functioning as it relates to his or her participation in life events. Aphasia can be considered within the WHO framework in relation to the preceding terms: *impairment* refers to the disordered language; *disability* refers to the functional consequences of the impairment (i.e., the measureable communication deficits due to the language impairment); and *handicap* refers to the social consequences of the disability. The latter includes how aphasia affects an individual's peer relationships, employment and/or education. Specific to each individual, activities and participation as well as the environment interface with these domains within the WHO framework.

Cognitive and Language Perspectives

Aphasia is often described as a language disorder involving processes underlying communication. When considering these underlying processes, the pure language definition for aphasia broadens to include **cognition** (or thought processes) in addition to the core components of language, which include semantics, syntax, morphology, phonology, and pragmatics.

Aphasiologists consider cognition and all of the following components of language when defining aphasia:

1. Semantics refers to individual word meaning and the meaning of sentences.
2. Syntax is the grammar of the language; complex syntactic structures can have an effect on both language comprehension and language production.
3. Morphology is the study of word formation, with a morpheme defined as the smallest unit of meaning.
4. Phonology is a rule-governed component through which sounds combine to form words.
5. Pragmatics refers to "an interaction between language behavior and the specific contexts in which language occurs" (Strauss & Pierce, 1986, p. 246).

The term *aphasia* as described in this chapter includes language and cognitive processes. When we think, our thoughts are in words, and cognitive processes—including attention, memory, reasoning, concentration, problem-solving, processing speed, and sequencing—are intertwined with our thoughts (the basis for the cognitive perspective of aphasia). Cognitive processes in individuals with aphasia remain relatively intact following stroke. However, depending on the site of the lesion, such as in frontal lobe damage, some of these cognitive abilities may be negatively affected. Similarly to language impairments, cognitive functioning can be more or less severe depending on the location and extent of the lesion. Therefore, aphasia is described in this chapter to include language and cognitive processes. Assessments of cognitive-linguistic skills are listed in Appendix 11-A.

Typically, it is a left hemisphere stroke that causes aphasia because language is represented in the left hemisphere for the majority of people. A right hemisphere stroke, however, can also occur and cause aphasia in rare cases. For the purposes of this chapter, we consider aphasia as an acquired language disorder secondary to left hemisphere brain damage, usually related to a left hemisphere **cerebrovascular accident** (CVA) or stroke.

Aphasia is most frequently caused by focal lesions in the language specialized areas of the brain. A stroke or CVA is one of the most common causes of aphasia and can cause an **infarct** (death of tissue). A CVA is caused by an interruption of the blood supply to the brain because of a blood vessel occlusion (**ischemic stroke**) or to bleeding in the brain (**hemorrhagic stroke**). Ischemic strokes can be **thrombotic** (cerebral thrombosis), where an artery is occluded by material that accumulates at a given place in the artery, or **embolic** (embolism), in which case an artery is suddenly occluded by traveling material (e.g., a piece of a broken clot). Another type of stroke is a hemorrhagic stroke, secondary to a rupture in the blood vessels, causing blood to accumulate in the brain. This type of stroke can occur secondary to a weakened blood vessel wall, an **arterial-venous malformation** (AVM), or an **aneurysm** (an out-pouching of the vessel). Whether the CVA is ischemic or hemorrhagic, it will result in a disruption of blood supply to certain brain areas and subsequently in death of brain tissue (infarct) and loss of connections in this particular region; this disruption makes it difficult for those areas affected to perform their language functions. Additionally, aphasia may occur as a result of other disorders such as brain tumors, head trauma, dementia, hydrocephalus, brain infections, toxins, and nutritional and metabolic disorders (Brookshire, 2007). Given that blood supply to the brain infiltrates overlapping regions, aphasia can be accompanied by variety of cognitive, perceptual, and sensory-motor difficulties.

Table 11-1. Chronology of Classification Systems for Aphasia

Classification	*Perspective on aphasia*	*Aphasia test published*
Marie (1906)	Single unitary language disorder	No
Weisenberg & McBride (1935)	Dichotomy: receptive and expressive language	No
Schuell et al. (1964)	Single unitary language disorder	Minnesota Test of Differential Diagnosis of Aphasia (MTDDA)
Goodglass and Kaplan (1972)	Dichotomy: fluent and nonfluent	Boston Diagnostic Aphasia Examination (BDAE)

Classification

Several classification systems for aphasia have been described over the years. Some aphasiologists such as Marie (1906) and Schuell, Jenkins, and Jimenez-Pabon (1964) viewed aphasia as a single unitary language disorder, or a general language breakdown that crosses all language modalities (e.g., speaking, listening, reading, and writing; Chapey, 2008, p. 4), whereas others viewed aphasia as a dichotomy such as receptive vs. expressive language (Weisenberg & McBride, 1935) or fluent vs. nonfluent (originally proposed by Goodglass & Kaplan, 1972). See the historical chronology of classification systems in Table 11-1.

Current classification of aphasia involves a multifactorial approach to the underlying organizational systems involved in language comprehension and expression and specifies several types or syndromes of aphasia (Goodglass, Kaplan, & Barresi, 2000; Kertesz, 2006). The methods used for assessment of aphasia are linked to the clinician's view on aphasia and its classification. A syndrome approach to defining types of aphasia involves the consideration of brain localization. This approach can actually be linked to the original localizationist, Paul Broca (late 1800s, as cited in Brookshire, 2007). Broca defined aphasia based on the place in the brain where damage occurred, the anterior frontal lobe in the case of Broca's aphasia. At different points over the past 150 years or so, the localizationist view to classification of aphasia has been more or less popular. It is an approach that is viewed favorably, and it has grown to include several syndromes of aphasia (described originally by Goodglass & Kaplan, 1972). Localizationists associate a region of the cerebral cortex with a type of aphasia. There are eight types of aphasia defined by cerebral localization: Broca's aphasia, Wernicke aphasia, global aphasia, anomic aphasia, conduction aphasia, transcortical motor aphasia, transcortical sensory aphasia, and mixed transcortical aphasia. For example, a lesion in the posterior third frontal convolution of the left hemisphere (the lower portion of the premotor cortex) causes Broca's aphasia, whereas a lesion in the Wernicke area (the auditory association cortex within the temporal lobe) causes Wernicke aphasia. The aphasia syndrome classification system, the associated site of lesion for each type, and its **concomitant** assessment procedures are described in this chapter (Goodglass et al., 2000). An original description of these syndromes (Goodglass & Kaplan, 1972) was published by a group of researchers in an assessment instrument that has since been updated (Goodglass et al., 2000). In addition to this assessment instrument, other researchers use aphasia syndrome terminology in their assessments (e.g., Kertesz, 2006; Table 11-2).

Characteristics

Characteristics of aphasia involve assessment of naming, fluency, repetition, and comprehension.

Naming and Word-Retrieval Difficulties

A common characteristic of aphasia is **anomia** or word-finding problems, which refers to difficulty producing language content in terms of appropriate vocabulary in relation to objects, events, relationships, and content categories. For example, the patient may have a deficit in providing the spoken or written label for objects, actions, events, attributes, and relationships in response to highly structured tasks and during connected and spontaneous language. The following components of word retrieval need to be assessed: defining referents (e.g., "What does *bed* mean?); category naming (e.g., a rose, tulip, and carnation are flowers); confrontation naming (e.g., written or verbal naming of pictures, objects, actions); automatic closure naming (e.g., completing an open ended sentence or phrase such as "You sit on a _"; Bandur & Shewan, 2001). Because individuals with any and all types of aphasia usually present with some degree of naming or **word-retrieval difficulty**, naming is not a characteristic that allows one to determine the specific type of aphasia. Naming difficulty is common to all types of aphasia.

Table 11-2. Aphasia Syndromes

Aphasia Classification	*Compre-hension*	*Fluency*	*Naming*	*Spoken Language*	*Repeti-tion*	*Writing*	*Site of Lesion*
Broca's aphasia	Mild impairment; relative strength	Nonfluent	Impaired	Agrammatic; effortful speech; short phrase length	Poor	Poor mechanics; poor spelling	Posterior, inferior frontal lobe
Wernicke aphasia	Poor	Fluent	Impaired; many paraphasias	Effortless; lengthy utterances; jargon	Poor	Good mechanics; errors in content	Posterior, superior temporal lobe
Global aphasia	Poor	Nonfluent	Poor	Limited output	Poor	Poor	Anterior posterior left perisylvian
Anomic aphasia	Normal or mild impairment	Fluent	Poor; verbal paraphasias	Delayed initiation; circumlocution	Good	Good	Left temporal parietal lobes
Conduction aphasia	Mild to moderate impairment	Fluent	Impaired	Paraphasias	Good	Slow effortful; intact grammar	Left inferior parietal lobe
Transcortical sensory aphasia	Poor	Fluent	Impaired; many paraphasias	Effortless; lengthy utterances; jargon	Good	Good mechanics; errors in content	Posterior superior parietal lobe
Transcortical motor aphasia	Mild impairment; relative strength	Nonfluent	Impaired	Agrammatic; effortful speech; short phrase length	Good	Poor mechanics; poor spelling	Anterior, superior Broca's area

Adapted from Brookshire (2007).

Paraphasic Errors

When an individual with aphasia uses an inappropriate word for a target, the inappropriate word is termed a **paraphasic error**. A paraphasic error is defined as an unintended word or sound substitution. Subcategories of paraphasic errors include word substitutions: semantic paraphasic errors (when a semantically related word is substituted for the target, such as *table* for *chair*), **random paraphasic errors** (when an unrelated word is substituted for the target, such as *broom* for *sky*), **neologistic paraphasic errors** (when a nonword is substituted for the target, such as *schlan* for *book*), and sound substitutions: literal/phonemic errors (when an alternate phoneme is substituted for a target sound in a word, such as *tat* for *bat*).

Degree of Fluency

Speech fluency, the second characteristic on the list, is determined by the number of words connected in grammatically intact oral expressions. Fluent speech is defined as eight or more connected words, and nonfluent speech is defined as less than five connected words (Goodglass & Kaplan, 1972). This analysis may be misleading because, at times, patients with "fluent" speech experience many starts and stops due to word-retrieval difficulty. The clinician must take into account the number of connected words and the grammatical accuracy of the sentence when determining fluency. Patients with fluent speech in general express more accurate grammatical constructions than patients with nonfluent speech.

Repetition

Repetition is the ability to repeat words and sentences. In an aphasia assessment, repetition is helpful in determining a diagnosis.

Comprehension

Comprehension is the ability to understand spoken language, and comprehension is tested at simple and complex levels. See the aphasia classification chart in Figure 11-1.

Concomitant Disorders

Concomitant or associated disorders that may co-occur with aphasia include **agnosia**, **neglect**,

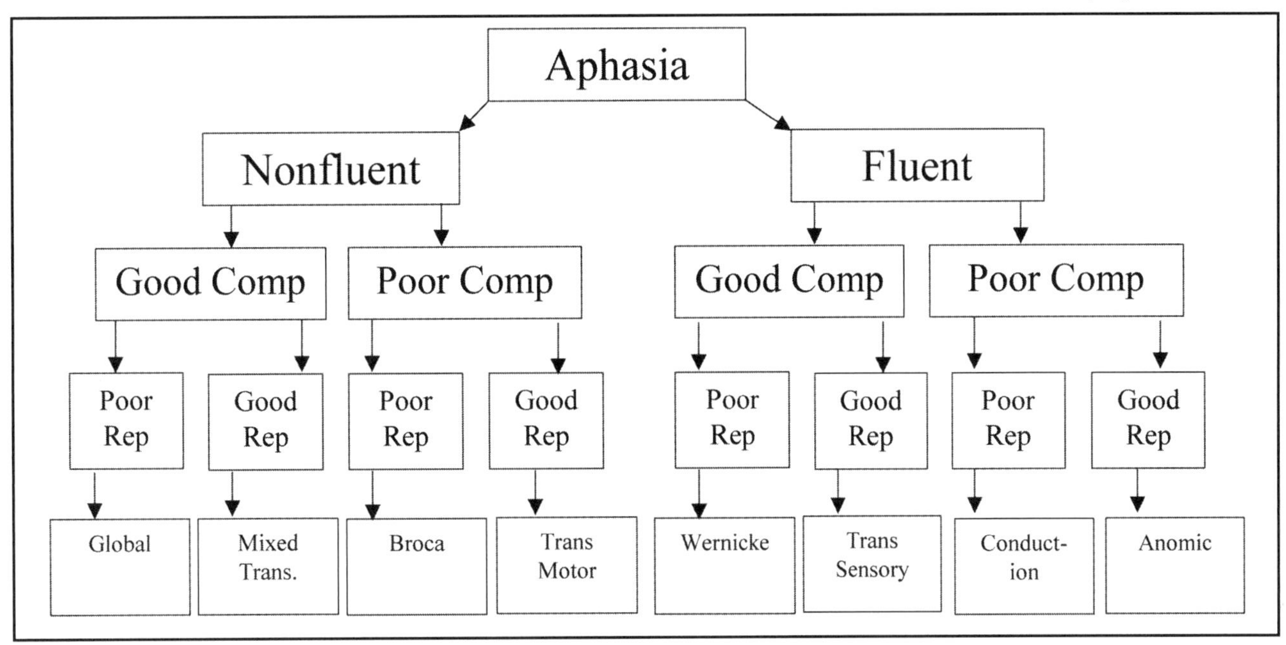

Figure 11-1. Aphasia classification. Comp = comprehension, Rep = repetition. (Adapted from Helm-Estabrooks & Albert, 2004.)

agraphia, **alexia**, **apraxia**, and **dysarthria**. Agnosia, or the inability to recognize familiar people, is typically present in right hemisphere brain damage but can be present with left hemisphere brain damage as well. Another syndrome that is more prevalent in right hemisphere damage is the neglect syndrome. A patient with neglect might bump into the doorway as he or she is walking out of a room, or might misread a paragraph because he or she does not attend to one side of space. Neglect has been reported in 15% to 65% of people with left hemisphere damage (Plummer, Morris, & Dunai, 2003), so it can be present concurrently with aphasia. Neglect is defined as the inability to perceive sensory information in the contralateral visual field, or difficulty with production of motor intentional acts in the space contralateral to the brain lesion. This phenomenon can have an effect on language assessment and intervention and is a major factor that correlates with prognosis for independence after experiencing a stroke. Neglect should not be confused with **hemianopsia**, a condition in which there is sensory loss of half of a field of view on the same side in both eyes.

Alexia (a reading disorder) and agraphia (a writing disorder) are concomitant disorders that are not part of the oral/auditory language modality. Rather, these syndromes are classified in the visual modality and reflect deficits in the areas of written language comprehension and expression. They can exist in isolation or in conjunction with an oral language disorder.

Apraxia of speech is a motor planning disorder that greatly affects communication. The site of lesion for the brain damage is the anterior frontal lobe, close to Broca's area. Apraxia of speech is often present with nonfluent Broca's aphasia, yet may also be present in isolation. Definitions of apraxia differ, with the common features including prosodic disturbance, slow rate, sound distortions, perceived sound substitutions, and consistency of errors (Wambaugh, Duffy, McMcneil, Robin, & Rogers, 2006).

Dysarthria refers to impaired speech production due to a disturbance in the muscular control of the speech mechanism secondary to damage in the central or peripheral nervous system. This disorder can involve difficulty with respiration, phonation, articulation, resonance, and prosody (Duffy, 1995). Dysarthria and or apraxia of speech often co-occur with aphasia. See differential characteristics of speech for dysarthria vs. apraxia in Table 11-3.

Aphasia Related to Right Brain Damage

Although this chapter focuses on left hemispheric damage, it is important to note that right hemispheric strokes can also occur. Right brain lesions involve cognitive communication problems and can present as difficulty sustaining attention, poor eye contact, diminished topic maintenance, impaired memory, prosody processing difficulties, poor reasoning and problem-solving skills, and visual and auditory agnosia, which

Table 11-3. Differential Diagnosis of Speech

Characteristic	*Dysarthria*	*Apraxia*
Etiology	Lesion in central or peripheral nervous system	Lesion in central nervous system
Type of error	Consistent and predictable	Inconsistent
Salient speech sounds affected	Consonants in any word position	Consonants in initial word position
Aspect of speech affected	All systems of speech production (articulation, respiration, resonance, prosody, phonation)	Mainly articulatory and prosodic systems affected
Effects of utterance complexity	Complexity does not have significant effect on degree of difficulty	Increased difficulty as complexity increases
Therapy	Top-down compensatory strategies are focus	Bottom-up stimulus driven treatments are focus

refers to the inability to recognize visual and auditory stimuli. Additionally, patients with right hemisphere brain damage often exhibit left-side neglect, which may result in difficulty attending to stimuli presented on the contralateral side of the stroke (Murray & Clark, 2006).

Parameters for Assessment

The main objective for the speech-language clinician assessing an adult who sustained a stroke is to determine the effect of the stroke on language and communication. Evaluation of an adult's language and communication skills can be conducted through the use of standardized tests (also called *norm-referenced measures*) and through the use of nonstandardized assessment. Dynamic assessment may occur as a part of the initial evaluation or at the initiation of treatment. It is a method that involves interaction and assessment of intervention strategies to consider potential intervention approaches by examining a person's response to a treatment technique. This may also be referred to as *modification stimulability*. On the basis of the patient's dynamic response to a modification assessed at the time of the evaluation, the therapist is able to identify initial intervention practices and initial treatment goals. Not every person who presents with a specific language profile will respond to treatment in the same ways, and dynamic assessment helps guide the clinician during the assessment process to design a treatment plan that will best fit with the patient.

The association of site of lesion to type of aphasia syndrome is the initial approach to determining the type of aphasia. Site of lesion information, however, needs to be coupled with the clinical assessment of language to allow for the diagnosis of the type of aphasia. It is possible for a clinician to assess a patient without prior access to his or her medical record information. In that case, the behavioral assessment alone leads the clinician to the aphasia diagnosis. In both cases, the clinician notes whether the individual presents with **fluent** or **nonfluent aphasia** and describes the receptive and expressive language of the patient.

Oral language evaluation involves both the assessment of auditory comprehension and verbal language expression. Auditory comprehension testing is assessed at the single word, sentence, and paragraph levels. The following are examples of such auditory comprehension testing:

- Single-word–level testing involves picture/object identification (e.g., present a group of objects or show a card with several pictures on the card and say, "Point to the _").
- Sentence-level comprehension testing includes answering yes–no questions (e.g., "Will a stone sink in water?") and following commands (e.g., "Point to the ceiling and then to the floor.").
- Paragraph-level comprehension testing involves the examiner reading oral paragraphs to the patient who is presented with questions that refer to the paragraph. In the BDAE-3 (Goodglass et al., 2000), the questions are presented in two forms, with both a "yes" and a "no" format for responses. Both questions must be answered correctly to receive credit. This format is designed to reduce the chance of a person guessing either "yes" or "no" for all responses and getting correct responses based purely on guessing. See the following example paragraph and questions.

  Example: A customer walked into a hotel carrying a coil of rope in one hand and a suitcase in the other. The hotel clerk asked, "Pardon me, sir, but will you tell me what the rope is for?" "Yes," responded the man, "that's my fire escape!" "I'm sorry sir," said the clerk, "but all guests carrying their own fire escapes must pay in advance."

- *Question*: Was the customer carrying a suitcase in each hand?
- *Question*: Was he carrying something unusual in one hand?

Oral expressive language is assessed at single-word, sentence, and discourse levels.

- Single-word–level responses are obtained in naming tasks (e.g., Show the patient a picture and say, "What's this?"; Boston Naming Test [Goodglass & Kaplan, 1983]; Northwestern Naming Battery [Thompson & Weintraub, 2014]).
- Fill in the blank tasks (e.g., "Please pass the _").
- Sentence-level responses are considered for grammatical accuracy and content within discourse tasks.
- Discourse tasks include an assessment of conversation. For the conversational task, the initial speech sample obtained when meeting the patient is often used. For the picture description discourse task, the clinician shows the patient a picture (as in the "Cookie Theft" picture from the BDAE-3 [Goodglass et al., 2000], and the "Picnic Scene" from the Western Aphasia Battery [WAB; Kertesz, 2006]). For a procedural discourse task, the clinician asks the patient to state a sequence narrative such as, "Tell me all the steps for _ (e.g., brushing teeth, making a salad, etc.)".

In addition, in the BDAE-3 (Goodglass et al., 2000), an aphasia severity rating scale is used to assign a severity of communication difficulty across patients. This is a zero- to five-point scale used to rate communicative effectiveness among participants. In the WAB (Kertesz, 2006), aphasia severity is determined by an Aphasia Quotient, which is determined by overall performance on all of the subtests of the WAB.

General parameters for assessment should include the following:

- Consideration of the patients' concerns and expectations
- Consideration of family members' concerns and expectations
- Consideration of vocational concerns and expectations
- Use of testing measures to determine the following:
  - Level of communication/socialization with peers
  - Interest level and level of engagement within environment
  - Level of comprehension of directives and questions
  - Ability to communicate needs and wants
  - Appropriate production of gestures to amplify communication
  - Comprehension and production of grammatical forms
  - Attention span, turn-taking skills, and degree of engagement in activities
  - Amount of support needed to complete activities

Key Clinical Interview Questions

The first part of an evaluation process entails an interview with the patient and a family member to obtain the patient's case history. This information is vital because it enables the clinician to understand the severity of the aphasia as relayed by the patient and family. In addition, the interview allows the clinician to gather information regarding lifestyle, expectations from family, culture, and the degree of communication handicap in daily living.

The patient and family interview is crucial because the patient's history has an impact on the efficacy and interpretation of the evaluation process. For example, if the patient has neglect, the clinician must make certain to place the stimuli in his or her field of vision when the patient is asked to point to a picture or object. If the stimulus is not perceived by the patient due to a sensory perceptual problem, the patient may not respond accurately, and the response may be misinterpreted as poor auditory comprehension. One can also obtain this information from the medical report. Learning which cues the patient responds to best (e.g., the type of cues the family uses) can facilitate the evaluation. Knowing the date of injury informs the speech-language pathologist (SLP) whether the patient is in a **spontaneous recovery** period. It should be noted that recovery is optimal within the first 3 to 6 months post-CVA. Recovery, however, is ongoing and people with aphasia make functional gains years after their stroke (Davis, 2000). In counseling patients and families, the early recovery period is sometimes interpreted as the timeframe that recovery can occur, when in actuality, recovery is lifelong.

It is important that the clinician engage with the individual in a respectful and patient manner. For example, if the patient comprehends spoken language but does not have the capacity to express him- or herself, the clinician should interview the patient directly in the presence of a family member. The clinician may consult with the family member as needed and include the patient in the discussion, informing the patient when he or she will proceed to consult the family member in the course of the discussion. Subsequently, the clinician should resume the interview with the patient. Suggestions for interview questions are listed in Table 11-4 in the first-person form.

Assessment Measures

There are several formal assessment measures (Table 11-5) and screening measures (Table 11-6) available for aphasia assessment.

A screening measure is designed to quickly evaluate a patient's language skills in order to determine if a formal evaluation is necessary. Some reasons for using screening measures are: (1) to determine whether a communication problem exists; (2) to help ascertain which standardized or norm-referenced measure would be most appropriate for evaluating the patient's language skills; (3) to ascertain the need for possible additional testing; (4) to allow for frequent assessment during the period following the injury because the symptoms can change rapidly during the critical time post injury. Additionally, a screening may be indicated when using a complete testing instrument is too time consuming (see Table 11-6 for screening measures for aphasia).

Many clinicians design their own screening measure instead of using one that is published. The clinician may want to elicit a spontaneous conversational sample and evaluate the patient's topic initiation, maintenance and closure, contextual appropriateness, ability to respond to wh- questions, length of utterance, grammatical complexity, vocabulary, word retrieval, and fluency. Additional tasks may include assessment of orientation to person, place, and time; automatic serial speech tasks such as reciting the days of the week, naming, identifying pictures, and/or objects; ability to follow directions; and simple writing tasks. These tasks may also be a part of informal testing.

Criterion-Referenced Measures

Criterion-referenced measures enable a clinician to explore a specific area in depth. These measures differ from norm-referenced tests in that their scores are not compared to age-matched peers. Often, scoring on criterion-referenced tests relies on a pass–fail score or a percentage correct. Of greater importance, however, is the nature of the errors in criterion-referenced tests, which provides the clinician with a better understanding of the patient's strengths and weaknesses. Criterion-referenced testing provides valuable baseline information on performance in a given area, prior to intervention as well. For adults, areas are frequently identified first in the standardized test, with further testing completed during criterion-referenced testing.

Advantages and Disadvantages of Standardized Testing

Standardized testing tends to be viewed by many as one of the most critical components of an evaluation. The standardization ensures that tests are as unbiased and consistent as possible in administration and scoring, so that scores can be accurately compared on test–retest within participants as well as compared among different individuals, which may help in determining groups for patients. It is important to keep in mind that standardized tests are not without limitations.

Although many tests purport to provide a general overview of level of linguistic functioning, the scope of these tests, though broad, rarely covers all areas of language, nor does it sufficiently target each specific area in depth. Therefore, not all areas of communication and language are always included in standardized assessments.

Additional Assessments

The advantage of informal testing is that the SLP can be flexible in terms of assessing patients who do not respond to certain tasks during formal testing. Many of the tasks are similar to the formal assessment tasks; however, the clinician can change the stimuli, materials, and application, as well as assess stimulability for certain techniques (e.g., cueing) to meet the patient's level of ability and go forward with the assessment, especially when the family has given input regarding certain modalities. The disadvantage is that the performance cannot be compared among patients, as in formal testing. Additionally, informal

Table 11-4. Interview Questions

Questions for Patient	*Clinician's Comments*
What languages do you speak? What is your first language? What is your primary language?	
Tell me what happened to you.	
What was the date of injury?	
What hand do you write with now? What hand did you write with before the stroke?	
Can you walk? Do you use a wheelchair or cane?	
Do you wear glasses?	
Do you have any visual problems (e.g., cataracts, visual field cuts)?	
Do you have a hearing loss or wear a hearing aid?	
How would you describe your current health?	
What medications do you take? List medications and dosages.	
Where do you live? Who lives in the home?	
Do you have any children?	
Did you go to high school? Up to what grade? How about college?	
What was your occupation before the injury?	
Are you currently working or employed?	
Do you use a computer, an iPad, or any other technology? How often?	
What are your interests and hobbies? Have these changed since your stroke?	
Do you like to read?	
Do you like to watch TV?	
How do you feel about your communication ability?	
Is there anything else you want to tell me?	
Questions for Family	*Clinician's Comments*
What is the medical diagnosis?	
How much does he or she talk right now?	
How much of the patient's speech or writing does the family understand?	
How has the patient's speech and language problem affected the family?	
Describe the patient's ability to communicate with family members and with non–family members.	
How does the patient feel about his or her communication skills?	
How does the patient react and respond when his message is not understood?	
What strategies have you found useful to help with the patient's communication?	
Does the patient have any other forms of communication (e.g., writing, gestures)?	
How would you describe the patient's personality?	
How has the patient's personality changed after the injury?	
Have you heard or read anything about aphasia? If yes, what did you hear and where did you hear it?	
Has the patient received prior speech-language evaluation services or speech therapy? Where?	
Has the patient received any other related services such as physical therapy or occupational therapy?	
Has the patient received psychological counseling or social work services?	

Table 11-5. Formal Measures for Aphasia Assessment

Name of Test	*Author*	*Standardization*	*Assessment Area*
Aphasia Diagnostic Profiles	Helm-Estabrooks (1992)	Norm-referenced	Social-emotional status of patient; speaking, listening, reading, writing and gestural communication; emphasizes conversational interaction
Aphasia Language Performance Scales (ALPS)	Keenan & Brassell (1975)	Norm-referenced	The examiner uses objects in pockets and around the room to assess language comprehension and expression
Assessment of Language-Related Functional Activities (ALFA)	Baines, Martin, & McMartin-Heeringa (1999)	Norm-referenced	Functional tasks such as writing a check, counting money, telling time
Bilingual Aphasia Test (BAT)	Paradis & Libben (1987)	Descriptive	Exists in 60 languages and tests all modalities
BDAE-3	Goodglass et al. (2000)	Norm-referenced	Auditory comprehension, conversational speech, fluency, naming, repetition, serial speech, reading, and writing
Boston Assessment of Severe Aphasia (BASA)	Helm-Estabrooks, Ramsberger, Morgan, & Nicholas (1989)	Norm-referenced	Identifies and quantifies preserved skills in patients with severe or global aphasia; areas assessed, for example, are gestural and verbal responses, refusals, affective responses, and perseverative responses.
Boston Naming Test	Kaplan, Goodglass, & Weintraub (1983)	Norm-referenced	Noun naming
Communicative Abilities in Daily Living-2 (CADL-2)	Holland, Frattali, & Fromm (1998)	Functional communication	Scores a patient's actual performance in an interview and in various simulated daily life activities; test is scored with regard to "getting the message across" rather than on how correct the message is
Communicative Effectiveness Index	Lomas et al. (1989)	Functional communication	A family member or friend rates the client's communicative skills for 16 situations deemed most important to them (e.g., getting someone's attention, communicating physical problems, giving appropriate yes–no answers)
Examining for Aphasia-3	Eisenson (1994)	Norm-referenced	Cognitive, personality, and linguistic changes, secondary to acquired aphasia, are examined Tests all the various modalities (e.g., verbal skills, comprehension, computations, reading)
Functional Assessment of Communication Skills for Adults (FACS)	Frattali (1995)	Functional communication	Examples of domains assessed are social communication of basic needs, daily planning, reading, writing, number concepts Patient is rated on a seven-point scale of communicative independence and on a five-point scale of qualitative dimensions of communication
Functional Communication Profile	Sarno (1969)	Functional communication	Patient is rated on five categories common in everyday life (i.e., movement, speaking, understanding, reading, and other)

(continued)

Table 11-5. Formal Measures for Aphasia Assessment (continued)

Name of Test	*Author*	*Standardization*	*Assessment Area*
MTDDA	Schuell (1972)	Norm-referenced Provides a list of signs for patients to be assigned into categories; few standardized procedures for interpreting patients' performance	Consists of 46 subtests and patients are assigned to one of five major categories and two minor categories of aphasia (e.g., simple aphasia, aphasia with visual involvement, aphasia with sensorimotor involvement)
Porch Index of Communicative Ability (PICA)	Porch (1981)	Norm-referenced	Verbal, gestural, and graphic modalities; does not assess spontaneous connected discourse
WAB-Revised	Kertesz (2006)	Norm-referenced	Auditory comprehension, spontaneous speech, repetition, naming, reading, writing, calculation, praxis and constructional abilities
Northwestern Naming Battery	Thompson & Weintraub (2014)	Norm-referenced	Noun and verb naming
Northwestern Assessment of Verbs and Sentences	Thompson (2011)	Norm-referenced	Verb naming, verb comprehension, argument structure production, sentence production, sentence comprehension
Reading Comprehension Battery for Aphasia (RCBA)	LaPointe & Horner (1998)	Norm-referenced	Reading comprehension, writing

Adapted from Brookshire (2007), Davis (2000), and Helm-Estabrooks et al. (1989).

Table 11-6. Screening Measures for Aphasia Assessment

Name of Test	*Author*
Acute Aphasia Screening Protocol (AASP)	Crary, Haak, & Malinsky (1989)
ALPS	Keenan & Brassell (1975)
Aphasia Screening Test	Whurr (1997)
Bedside Evaluation and Screening Test for Aphasia	Fitch-West & Sands (1987)
Bedside WAB-Revised	Kertesz (2006)
BDAE-3—Short Form	Goodglass et al. (2000)
Frenchay Aphasia Screening Test (FAST)	Enderby, Wade, & Wood (1987)
Quick Assessment for Aphasia	Tanner & Culberston (1999)
Mississippi Screening Test	Nakase-Thompson (2004)
Multimodal Communication Screening Task for Persons with Aphasia	Garrett & Lasker (2005)
Sklar Aphasia Scale (SAS)	Sklar (1983)

Adapted from Haynes & Pindzola (2008).

testing may not uncover all of the strengths and weaknesses because the stimuli are not as comprehensive as in formal testing. Often, informal testing occurs as part of dynamic assessment or diagnostic therapy, once the patient has completed an initial standardized assessment and has been referred for intervention (see various approaches to therapy in Helm-Estabrooks and Albert [2004] and Chapey [2008]).

Before assessing a patient informally, information gained from the patient during formal testing should be considered. For example, if a patient uses verbal rehearsal as a strategy to promote auditory comprehension, in an informal assessment, use of this strategy can be considered. Also, it is crucial to obtain information from the family during the interview with regard to which modalities are the strongest for the patient (e.g., oral expression, comprehension, gestural); the cues the family uses to facilitate language production (e.g., a semantic cue such as "a sport where there is a ball and a bat" vs. a phonemic cue such as "b" for the target "baseball"); and the patient's likes, dislikes, and interests. The family's information can facilitate the language assessment as the SLP can use the information to obtain responses, which may otherwise not be possible at the time.

These areas will also be revealed during informal testing.

Informal Measures

A. Examination of Oral-Motor Mechanism: It is important to determine whether the structure and function of the oral mechanism are adequate or if it in any way interferes with the client's speech production and need to be addressed. The oral-motor assessment is important for differential diagnosis purposes.

B. Language Sample: If possible (depending on the deficit), initially obtain a language sample (including responses to examiner's interview questions) to assess general comprehension of questions asked and expressive language such as word retrieval, syntax, morphology, and prosody (tape record for assessment). The language sample is also used for determining speech fluency. The language sample consists of the interview questions as well as a picture description.

C. Comprehension Tasks: These are simple to complex tasks to determine the level of comprehension and to determine the most facilitating place to begin therapy.

- Identifying real objects or pictures of common objects named by the examiner. (One can modify the number of items or positioning [e.g., pictures vertically presented on the one side due to neglect vs. two pictures in front of the patient]. This aspect is also important, especially if visual-perceptual difficulties as well as attentional deficits are suspected in addition to aphasia.)
- Identifying action pictures
- Identifying spatial and temporal relationships
- Following one to three part directions
- Answering simple and complex yes–no questions (Because patients with aphasia have word-finding difficulties, avoid using wh- questions when assessing comprehension because the results you are getting will be difficult to interpret—comprehension issues vs. word-finding difficulties.)
- Testing patient comprehension of simple/complex conversation and paragraphs
- Testing comprehension of questions with increasing length and complexity

D. Visual Comprehension Tasks: These tasks are to determine ability to comprehend language presented visually, which can facilitate language.

- Match object to object
- Categorization tasks: Client to match picture to correct picture or category
- Sequencing pictures in proper order

E. Expressive Tasks: These determine level of ability to facilitate appropriate place to begin therapy and areas to address.

- Automatic tasks (counting 1 to 21, days of the week, months of the year, singing songs, responding to greetings)
- Completing sentences (closure tasks): high probability (e.g., "You sleep in a _") and low probability (e.g., "In the store you buy _") and comparing performance on high vs. low probability sentence fill in the blank tasks
- Naming objects or pictures of common objects to assess word retrieval (e.g., implementation of semantic cues and training internal semantic self-cueing hierarchy before provision of external phonemic cue; implementing theme-based materials with overlapping content for materials to stimulate internal stimulus cues)
- Naming object function (use of related objects vs. unrelated objects)
- Providing category name when given a small list of category members to assess word retrieval
- Responding to close-ended wh- questions (e.g., "What time do you go to _?")

- Describing simple action pictures to assess word retrieval, syntax, morphology, and prosody for expressive language
- Describing sequencing pictures to assess procedural discourse as well as word retrieval, syntax, morphology, and prosody for expressive language
- Generating responses to simple problem-solving questions (e.g., "What would happen if you put ice on the sun?") to assess patient ability to organize appropriate responses as well as to assess reasoning skills
- Observe patient's behavior to assess reasoning/problem-solving skills in nonverbal tasks
- Divergent thinking tasks (e.g., "Tell me three things you can do with a scarf."), verbal fluency naming task (e.g., "Tell me all the animals you can think of.")
- Repetition tasks: Client to repeat words, phrases, sentences

F. Reading Tasks: These determine reading level for comprehension and determine whether reading aloud aids speech.

- Patient to match words and sentences to corresponding pictures
- Patient to point to the letter, word, or sentence named by examiner
- Patient to read letters, words, sentences, and paragraphs aloud
- Patient to answer questions based on his or her reading (by pointing to an answer or verbalizing it)

G. Writing Tasks: These determine level of writing and determine if the writing modality facilitates speech and comprehension.

- Patient to write his or her name and address
- Patient to write letters dictated by examiner
- Patient to write words dictated by examiner
- Patient to write phrases and sentences dictated by examiner
- Patient to write self-generated words, sentences, narratives

H. Cognitive Tasks: These assess orientation, problem-solving pictures and questions, and reasoning and inference.

- Patient to answer orientation questions referring to person, place (state, city, current location, floor, room), time (month, date, year, day, time, season)
- Patient to complete reasoning tasks (e.g., analogies; deductive reasoning scenarios)
- Patient to complete long-term memory tasks (e.g., biographical and historical questions)
- Patient to complete short-term memory tasks (immediate [e.g., word repetition, digit repetition] or delayed [e.g., recall of three unrelated words after 10 minutes] recall)
- Working memory (e.g., spell the word world backward)
- Attention (e.g., count backward by sevens, starting at 100)
- Problem solving (e.g., identifying problems and possible outcomes on the "Cookie Theft" picture from the BDAE-3 [Goodglass et al., 2000]; coming up with multiple solutions to household problems; prioritizing solutions to common household problems)
- Thought organization (e.g., verbal sequencing, e.g. how to make a pot of coffee)

As noted earlier, neglect refers to the patient's failure to respond to people or objects presented opposite the brain lesion. The patient has difficulty perceiving sensory information on the contralateral visual field or demonstrating motor intentional acts in the space contralateral to the brain lesion. For example, in a right-sided CVA, when present, the neglect will occur on the left side of space, contralateral to the lesion. If there is a left-sided lesion, neglect will occur on the right side of space. There is evidence that unilateral neglect occurs most often after a right CVA or lesion. However, as noted earlier, neglect has been reported in 15% to 65% of people with left hemispheric damage (Plummer et al., 2003).

One test for unilateral neglect consists of a line bisection task. For example, in right-sided brain lesions, neglect patients bisect lines far rightward of center whereas normal subjects usually bisect lines with a slight leftward bias (Metehan, Deouell, & Knight, 2009).

Pragmatics Language Skills and Rating Scales

This area of language involves rules that govern the use of language in context in that meaning is created from the combination of the utterance and the social setting in which it occurs (Pence & Justice, 2008). Pragmatics also includes the study of speaker and listener interactions, and it covers the rules of conversation, narrative and conversational discourse, and repair. Assessment of pragmatic skills poststroke may take the form of clinician judgment or may take the form of a rating instrument (e.g., social communication section of the ASHA FACS; Frattali, 1995).

Self-assessment measures provide information regarding a patient's awareness of deficits and ability to judge communication strengths and weaknesses. These are considered to be within the patient-reported outcome category of assessment and can provide clinicians with important information that is relevant to the ICF and how activities and participation as well as the environment interface with the ICF impairment domain. Although impairment is measured using formal assessment instruments such as the BDAE-3 or the WAB, the Aphasia Communication Outcome Measure (ACOM; Doyle et al., 2013) is a patient- and surrogate-reported communicative outcome measure that addresses an individual's activities and participation in life with regard to his or her aphasia.

Case History for the Sample Report

Mrs. X is a 70-year-old woman referred by her physiatrist (Dr. Joe Brown) for a speech and language evaluation secondary to a stroke suffered on March 1, 2010. The daughter reported that the brain injury occurred in the left frontal lobe in Broca's area subsequent to an aortic heart replacement. At present, Mrs. X experiences difficulty retrieving words, **agrammatism** (telegraphic speech) in that she omits function words (e.g., prepositions, articles), and her speech is often labored, all of which are typical of Broca's aphasia (Karg Academy, 2010). Comprehension was reported to be generally good. Past medical history is significant for cataracts removed approximately 3 months ago. Mrs. X wears corrective glasses.

Assessment Procedures and Rationale

The following assessment measures were selected for this case history. A corresponding rationale is provided for each assessment selection.

- Audiological screening
  - Rationale: To rule out the influence of hearing loss on language performance (Hearing loss is more prevalent in older adults, making the audiological screening and/or evaluation important for the accurate language diagnosis.)
- Neglect screening
  - Rationale: To rule our sensory perceptual or motor intentional neglect
- Oral-motor-speech mechanism examination
  - Rationale: To assess the structural and functional integrity of the speech mechanism
- Patient/family interview
  - Rationale: To obtain full case/medical history
  - Rationale: To determine patient and family concerns and perception of problem
  - Rationale: To determine family involvement attitude and motivation
- A narrative/picture description
  - Rationale: To help determine degree of speech fluency, word retrieval, and grammar (A language sample analysis is an essential component of a speech-language evaluation.)
- The BDAE-3 or the WAB
  - Rationale: To formally assess auditory comprehension and expressive language skills
  - To obtain an aphasia severity level

Instructional Writing Rubric for Formal Language Section of the Diagnostic Report

The following outline may assist the reader in formatting the formal language assessment portion of the written diagnostic report.

☐ Introductory statement to include name of test in full (underlined) and in abbreviated form in parentheses (not underlined)

Example: Language was formally assessed through the administration of the Boston Diagnostic Aphasia Examination-3 (BDAE-3).

☐ Test construct (what it purports to measure)

Example: The BDAE-3 is a test of aphasia and assesses auditory comprehension and expressive language skills in adults; it utilizes *z* scores to make relative comparisons among performance on different subtests. The BDAE-3, however, does not purport to represent all individuals with aphasia.

☐ Elicitation procedures (describe where appropriate)

Example: The Auditory Comprehension subtests require the adult patient to demonstrate comprehension by pointing to pictures, following simple and complex directives while using familiar objects and pictures, answering yes–no simple questions, and questions based on auditory paragraphs. The Expressive Communication subtests have the adult complete automatic tasks (e.g., counting), label pictures and objects, respond to simple questions and engage in spontaneous speech. (Refer the reader to the table with a numbered and named reference to follow.)

☐ Quantification of results in paragraph form (derived scores from test)

Example: Mrs. X scored 10/12 on the auditory paragraphs section of the Auditory Comprehension subtest. This score is at the 80th percentile, indicating she scored at or above the level of 80% of her peers and that she has some auditory comprehension difficulty. On the Expressive Communication automatic sequences section, she scored a raw score of 3/3. This score is at the maximum and is within 1 standard deviation of the mean, indicating a relative strength in performance in this area.

☐ Quantification of results in table form

BDAE-3: Summary of Scores

Subtest	*Score*	*Percentile*
Auditory Comprehension—Complex Ideational Material	10/12	80th
Expressive Communication—Automatized Sequences	8/8	100th

☐ Qualification in narrative form

Example: Results of the Auditory Comprehension, Auditory Paragraphs and Expressive Communication, and Automatic Sequences subtests of the BDAE-3 indicate adequate auditory comprehension at the paragraph level. Oral expressive language was characterized by adequate production of automatic sequences. The patient's narratives and conversational speech, however, were characterized by telegraphic, labored speech, as well as word-finding difficulty. Interpret results and compare informal to formal in terms of strength and weakness.

Sample Report

Jane X
123 Main Street
New York, NY 10016

D.O.E.: 7/1/2010
D.O.B.: 7/10/1940
Language: English

I. Reason for Referral

Mrs. X reports "difficulty finding words and producing speech" since the time of her stroke in March 2010. In addition, she noted people find her "difficult to understand."

II. Tests Administered/Procedures

- Case History/Interview
- Audiological Screening
- Neglect Screening
- Oral-Motor-Speech Mechanism Examination
- Boston Diagnostic Aphasia Evaluation-3 (BDAE-3)
- Informal measures and clinical observations

III. Background Information

Mrs. X sustained an anterior frontal lobe CVA in March 2010 and received inpatient speech-language intervention poststroke. She was discharged from the Smith Rehabilitation Unit in NYC 2 months ago and was seen in the outpatient department of the Smith Hospital for a speech-language evaluation at that time. She was referred for this assessment by her physiatrist, Dr. Joe Brown, and was accompanied to this evaluation by her daughter, Mary X.

IV. Clinical Observations

Audiological Screening

Mrs. X received an audiological screening in August 2010. She passed the screening, and hearing was determined to be within normal limits. She responded appropriately to speech delivered at a typical conversational level.

Neglect Screening

Mrs. X did not demonstrate neglect on the line bisection task.

Oral-Motor-Speech Mechanism Examination

Facial structures were asymmetrical with a slight right facial droop. Range of motion of oral motor structures was adequate, with reduced strength bilaterally, right-side structures weaker than left.

Articulation and Language

Intelligibility of Mrs. X's speech was judged to be fair. Initiation of oral expression was difficult; she struggled to initiate the words and demonstrated labored, telegraphic speech (omitting function words), all of which had a negative effect on intelligibility.

Communication Skills

The BDAE-3 was administered.

Auditory Comprehension

Auditory Comprehension		
Subtest	*Score*	*Percentile*
Word discrimination	37	100
Commands	15	90
Complex ideational material	10	80

On the Auditory Comprehension sections of the BDAE-3, Mrs. X demonstrated adequate auditory comprehension in conversation and for single words, sentences, and paragraph-level material. Auditory comprehension is judged to be within functional limits.

Expressive Communication

Expressive Communication		
Subtest	*Score*	*Percentile*
Repetition words	6	20
Repetition sentences	4	50
Responsive naming	13	30
Boston Naming Test	33	50
Phrase length	4	20

Oral Expressive Language

Spontaneous oral language was nonfluent, with a repetition deficit and naming difficulty in spontaneous language contexts and in testing. As noted, she presented with telegraphic speech, omitting function words, and presenting with word finding difficulties. She also produced occasional semantic paraphasic errors in conversation and in oral picture description tasks.

Voice

Vocal parameters were subjectively assessed to be within functional limits.

Mrs. X made several attempts to initiate speech in verbal descriptions and demonstrated frustration at times, pounding her fist on the table when she was unsuccessful at producing the word. Semantic paraphasias were produced in place of the target on many occasions.

V. Summary

Mrs. X, a 70-year-old woman, was seen for an aphasia assessment secondary to a left hemisphere anterior frontal stroke. She presents with nonfluent Broca's aphasia characterized by labored, telegraphic speech (omitting function words) and word-retrieval difficulty. The aphasia was also characterized by poor repetition and difficulty initiating speech in the presence of relatively preserved auditory comprehension.

In addition, Mrs. X appears to be frustrated with her difficulty expressing herself, as indicated by her use of nonverbal gesture (e.g., hitting the table) and facial expressions.

It is strongly recommended that Mrs. X receive outpatient speech-language services twice weekly for 12 weeks to address these issues with special emphasis on increasing oral expressive language with the following goals: (a) increase word retrieval by implementation of compensatory word finding strategies (synonyms, antonyms) given minimal assistance, (b) increase length of utterance to include S-V-O sentence structure using a modified VNeST treatment approach given moderate assistance, and (3) increase fluency and prosody of speech answering questions using complete sentences 8/10x. A stimulus-driven approach to intervention is recommended.

I certify that I personally evaluated the above-mentioned patient, employing appropriate instruments and procedures as well as informed clinical opinion. I further certify that the findings contained in this report are an accurate representation of the patient's level of functioning at the time of my assessment.

____

(Name of clinician or clinical supervisor and credentials)

Speech-Language Pathologist

Practice Exercises

The following practice exercises provide an opportunity to integrate what you have learned in this chapter. Take advantage of the instructional writing rubric and sample report when completing your exercises.

Practice Exercise 1

Read the "Cookie Theft" (from the BDAE-3, Goodglass et al., 2000) picture description sample of speech that follows. Determine the average number of words for this sample of speech, and classify the speech sample as representing fluent or nonfluent aphasia. What types of paraphasic errors are demonstrated?

There's a lady drying dishes and the water is overflowing onto the dloor. And the bloy is on the thing and reaching for it and the girl is telling him not to let her hear them at all. The girl-no mother-is not seeing the kids and the wasimer is running over. She is looking out the bawindel the kids keep on eating.

Practice Exercise 2

Write up the following assessment findings (formal and informal) in standard report writing format. Be sure to look for areas of strength as well as weakness and to make comparisons between subtests as well as between formal and informal assessment findings. The patient is a 45-year-old male with past medical history of hypertension and is status post left CVA with no hemiparesis/**hemiplegia**.

The BDAE-3 was administered.

Auditory Comprehension		
Subtest	*Score*	*Percentile*
Word discrimination	24	10
Commands	10	20
Complex ideational material	5	20

Expressive Communication		
Subtest	*Score*	*Percentile*
Repetition words	3	10
Repetition sentences	3	40
Responsive naming	13	30
Boston Naming Test	33	50
Phrase length	7	90

Informal Assessment

- Oral motor examination: oral motor examination within normal limits; no oral motor weakness
- Long-term memory: 4/10 (40%)
- Short-term memory (immediate 1/3 words; delayed 1/3 after 10 minutes)
- Problem solving: provided multiple solutions to verbal problems 1/5 (20%)
- Reasoning: 0/5 analogies (0%)
- Thought organization/sequencing: reduced (stated two steps to activity when coached to state five steps)
- Attention: adequate for testing
- Neglect: 3/3 line bisection within normal limits
- Discourse production: poor for conversation, reduced for picture description and discourse tasks; production of literal/phonemic paraphasias as well as neologisms throughout the narrative

Practice Exercise 3

N.P., a 55-year-old male, presents with fluent aphasia characterized by difficulty following directions, difficulty answering yes–no questions appropriately, failure to identify pictures and objects named by the examiner, inappropriate answers to WH questions. Speech is fluent but often nonsensical with paraphasic errors. There is also a tendency for the patient to speak at the same time the examiner spoke.

Glossary

Agnosia: The inability to recognize stimuli in a sensory modality despite intact sensation in the modality (e.g., visual agnosia).

Agrammatism (telegraphic speech): The production of short utterances that consist primarily of content words such as nouns and verbs with the omission of function words such as articles, conjunctions, and prepositions.

Agraphia: An acquired disturbance in writing (excludes penmanship).

Alexia: An acquired disturbance in reading.

Aneurysm: An out-pouching of a blood vessel.

Anomia: Word finding and naming difficulties.

Aphasia: Communication disorder caused by an impairment of the language modalities: speaking, listening, reading, and writing, pragmatics.

Appendix 11-A. Cognitive Assessments for Individuals With Aphasia

Test	*Author (year)*	*Assessment area*
Behavioral Inattention Test	Wilson, Cockburn, & Halligan (1987)	Visual neglect
Cognitive Linguistic Quick Test	Helm-Estabrooks (2001)	Attention, memory, executive functions, language, and visuospatial skills
The Montreal Cognitive Assessment	Nasreddine et al. (2005)	Attention and concentration, executive functions, memory, visual spatial skills, conceptual thinking, calculations, and orientation
Ross Information Processing Assessment-2	Ross-Swain (1996)	Cognitive-linguistic processing following traumatic brain injury
Scales of Cognitive Ability for Traumatic Brain Injury	Adamovich & Henderson (1992)	Perception and discrimination, orientation, organization, recall, and reasoning
Wisconsin Card Sorting Test	Heaton, Chelune, Talley, Kay, & Curtiss (1993)	Perseveration and abstract reasoning

Apraxia: Difficulty making volitional movement sequences in the absence of sensory loss or paralysis (e.g., apraxia of speech, limb apraxia, and ideational apraxia).

Arterial-venous malformation (AVM): An out-pouching of a vessel.

Cerebrovascular accident (CVA): Event that deprives the brain of its blood supply.

Cognition: The processes involved in thinking; includes attention, memory, concentration, problems solving, reasoning, sequencing skills.

Concomitant: Associated disorders that may co-occur with aphasia, such as agnosia, neglect, agraphia, alexia, apraxia, and dysarthria.

Dysarthria: Impaired speech production due to a disturbance in the muscular control of the speech mechanism secondary to damage in the central or peripheral nervous system

Embolic stroke (embolism): An artery is suddenly occluded by material that moves through the vascular system.

Fluent aphasia: Aphasia with ability to connect eight or more words.

Hemianopsia: Sensory loss of half of a field of view on the same side in both eyes.

Hemiplegia: Paralysis of an arm and/or leg on one side of the body.

Hemorrhagic stroke: Stroke caused by rupture of a cerebral blood vessel, and blood fills the brain; this type of stroke may be due to weakness in the vessel wall.

Infarct: Death of tissue caused by interruption of its blood supply for more than 3 to 5 minutes.

Ischemic stroke: Deprivation of blood (80% of strokes); an artery is blocked, and there is a loss of blood to part of the brain served by that artery; can be thrombotic (cerebral thrombosis) or embolic.

Neglect: Inability to perceive sensory information in the contralateral visual field or demonstrate motor intentional acts in the space contralateral to the brain lesion.

Neologistic paraphasic error: Substituting a made-up word in place of the target word.

Nonfluent aphasia: Aphasia with ability to connect to connect fewer than five words.

Paraphasic error: Unintended sound or word substitution—literal (phonemic); semantic (verbal) substitution of words for intended words.

Random paraphasic error: An unrelated word is substituted for the target.

Speech fluency: Articulatory agility, speech rate, phrase length, and grammatical form; less than five connected words exemplifies nonfluent speech, and more than eight connected words demonstrates fluent speech.

Spontaneous recovery: Critical period when recovery begins to take place after a CVA: 3 months to 1 year.

Stroke: See cerebrovascular accident.

Thrombotic stroke: An artery is gradually occluded by a plug of material.

Word-retrieval difficulty: Difficulty producing language content in terms of using the appropriate vocabulary words in relation to objects, events, relationships, and content categories.

References

Adamovich, B. B., & Henderson, J. (1992). *Scales of cognitive ability for traumatic brain injury* (SCATBI). Chicago, IL: Riverside.

Baines, K. A., Martin, A. W., & McMartin Heeringa, H. (1999). *Assessment of language-related functional activities.* Austin, TX: Pro-Ed.

Bandur, D. L., & Shewan, C. M. (2001). Language-oriented treatment: A psycholinguistic approach to aphasia. In R. Chapey (Ed.), *Language intervention strategies in aphasia and related neurogenic communication disorders* (4th ed., pp. 629-662). Baltimore, MD: Lippincott, Williams & Wilkins.

Brookshire, R. H. (2007). *Introduction to neurogenic communication disorders.* Philadelphia, PA: Mosby.

Chapey, R. (Ed.). (2008). *Language intervention strategies in aphasia and related neurogenic communication disorders* (5th ed.). Baltimore, MD: Lippincott, Williams & Wilkins.

Crary, M. A., Haak, M. J., & Malinsky, A. E. (1989). Preliminary psychometric evaluation of an acute aphasia screening protocol. *Aphasiology, 2*, 67-78.

Davis, G. A. (2000). *Aphasiology: Disorders and clinical practice.* Boston, MA: Allyn & Bacon.

Doyle, P. J., Hula, W. D., Hula, S. N. A., Stone, C. A., Wambaugh, J. L., Ross, K. B., & Schumacher, J. G. (2013). Self-and surrogate-reported communication functioning in aphasia. *Quality of Life Research, 22*, 957-967.

Duffy, J. R. (1995). *Motor speech disorders: Substrates, differential diagnosis, and management.* St. Louis: Mosby.

Eisenson, J. (1994). *Examining for Aphasia (EFA-3): Assessment of aphasia and related impairments* (3rd ed.). Austin, TX: Pro-Ed.

Enderby, P. M., Wade, D. T., & Wood, V. (1987). *Frenchay aphasia screening test (FAST).* London, England: NFER_NELSON.

Ferrand, C. T., & Bloom, R. L. (1997). *Introduction to organic and neurogenic communication disorders of communication.* Boston, MA: Allyn & Bacon.

Fitch-West, J., & Sands, E. (1987). *Bedside evaluation and screening test of aphasia.* Rockville, MD: Aspen.

Frattali, C. (1995). *Functional Assessment of Communication Skills for Adults (ASHA FACS).* Rockville, MD: American Speech-Language-Hearing Association.

Garrett, K. L., & Lasker, J. (2005). Multimodal communication screening task for persons with aphasia. Retrieved from http://aac.unl.edu/screen/screen.html

Goodglass, H., & Kaplan, E. (1972). *The assessment of aphasia and related disorders.* Philadelphia, PA: Lea & Febiger.

Goodglass, H., & Kaplan, E. (1983). *Boston diagnostic aphasia examination (BDAE).* Philadelphia, PA: Lea & Febiger

Goodglass, H., Kaplan, E., & Barresi, B. (2000). *Boston diagnostic aphasia examination* (3rd ed.; BDAE-3). Philadelphia, PA: Lippincott, Williams & Wilkins.

Haynes, W. O., & Pindzola, R. H. (2008). *Diagnosis and evaluation in speech pathology* (7th ed.). New York, NY: Pearson.

Heaton, R. K., Chelune, G. J., Talley, J. L., Kay, G. G., & Curtis, G. (1993). *Wisconsin Card Sorting Test manual: Revised and expanded.* Odessa, FL: Psychological Assessment Resources.

Helm-Estabrooks, N. (1992). *Aphasia diagnostic profiles.* Rolling Meadows, IL: Riverside.

Helm-Estabrooks, N. (2001). *Cognitive linguistic quick test (CLQT).* San Antonio, TX: The Psychological Corporation.

Helm-Estabrooks, N., & Albert, M. A. (2004). *Manual of aphasia and aphasia therapy.* Austin, TX: Pro-Ed.

Helm-Estabrooks, N., Ramsberger, G., Morgan, A. R., & Nicholas, M. (1989). *Boston assessment of severe aphasia.* Chicago, IL: Riverside.

Holland, A. L., Frattali, C. M., & Fromm, D. (1998). *Communication activities in daily living (CADL)* (2nd ed.). Austin, TX: Pro-Ed.

Kaplan, E., Goodglass, H. & Weintraub, S. (1983). *The Boston naming test (BNT).* Philadelphia, PA: Lea & Febiger.

Karg Academy. (2010). Broca's aphasia. Retrieved from http://www.kargacademy.com/disability-research-and-resources/broca-s-aphasia

Keenan, J. S., & Brassell, E. G. (1975). *Aphasia language performance scales.* Murfreesboro, TN: Pinnacle Press.

Kertesz, A. (2006). *Western Aphasia Battery—Revised (WAB-R).* San Antonio, TX: Harcourt Assessment.

LaPointe, L. L., & Horner, J. (1998). *Reading comprehension battery for aphasia* (2nd ed.). Tigard, OR: C.C. Publications.

Lomas, J., Pickard, L., Bester, S., Elbard, H., Finlayson, A., & Zoghaib, C. (1989). *The Communicative Effectiveness Index: Development and psychometric evaluation of a functional communication measure for adult aphasia.* Rockville, MD: American Speech-Language-Hearing Association.

Marie, P. (1906). Revision de la question de l'aphasie: L'aphasie de 1861 a 1866: Essai de critique historique sur la genese de la doctrine de Broca. *La Simaine Medicale, 26*, 565-571.

Metehan, C., Deouell, L. Y., & Knight, R. T. (2010). Brain activity during landmark and line bisection tasks. Retrieved from http://www.ncbi.nlm.nih.gov/pmc/articles/PMC2694675

Murray, L. L., & Clark, H. M. (2006). *Neurogenic disorders of language: Theory driven clinical practice.* Clifton Park, NY: Delmar Cengage Learning.

Nakase-Thompson, R. (2004). Introduction to the Mississippi aphasia screening test. *The Center for Outcome Measurement in Brain Injury.* Retrieved from http://www.tbims.org/combi/mast

Nasreddine, Z. S., Phillips, N. A., Bedirian, V., Charbonneau, S., Whitehead, V., Collin, I. ... Chertkow, H. (2005). The Montreal Cognitive Assessment, MOCA: A brief screening tool for mild cognitive impairment. *Journal of the American Geriatrics Society, 53*, 695-699.

Paradis, M., & Libben, G. (1987). *The assessment of bilingual aphasia.* Mahwah, NJ: Erlbaum.

Pence, K. L., & Justice, L. M. (2008). *Language development from theory to practice.* Upper Saddle River, NJ: Pearson Education.

Plummer, P., Morris, M. E., & Dunai, J. (2003). Assessment of unilateral neglect. *Physical Therapy, 83*, 732-740.

Porch, B. E. (1981). *Porch index of communicative ability* (3rd ed.). Palo Alto, CA: Consulting Psychologists Press.

Ross-Swain, D. (1996). *Ross information processing assessment* (2nd ed.). Austin, TX: Pro-Ed.

Sarno, M. T., & New York University, Institute of Rehabilitation Medicine. (1969). *The functional communication profile.* New York, NY: Institute of Rehabilitation Medicine, New York University Medical Center.

Schuell, H. (1972). *Minnesota test for differential diagnosis of aphasia.* Minneapolis: University of Minnesota Press.

Schuell, H., Jenkins, J. J., & Jimenez-Pabon, E. (1964). *Aphasia in adults: Diagnosis, prognosis, and treatment.* London: Harper Row.

Sklar, M. (1983). *Sklar aphasia scale—Revised.* Los Angeles, CA: Western Psychological Services.

Strauss, M. H., & Pierce, R. S. (1986). Pragmatics and treatment. In R. Chapey (Ed.), *Language intervention strategies in adult aphasia* (3rd ed., pp 248-272). Philadelphia, PA: Williams & Wilkins.

Tanner, D., & Culbertson, W. (1999). *Quick assessment for aphasia.* Oceanside, CA: Academic Communication Associates.

Thompson, C. K. (2011). *The Northwestern assessment of verbs and sentences.* Evanston, IL: Northwestern University.

Thompson, C. K., & Weintraub, S. (2014). *The Northwestern naming battery.* Evanston, IL: Northwestern University.

Wambaugh, J. L., Duffy, J. R., McMcneil, M. R., Robin, D. A., & Rogers, M. A. (2006). Treatment guidelines for acquired apraxia of speech: Treatment descriptions and recommendations. *Journal of Medical Speech-Language Pathology, 14*(2), xxxv-xxxvii.

Weisenberg, T. H., & McBride, K. E. (1935). *Aphasia: A clinical and psychological study.* New York, NY: Commonwealth Fund.

Whurr, R. (1997). *Aphasia screening test* (2nd ed.). Milton, Australia: Wiley.

Wilson, B., Cockburn, J., & Halligan, P. (1987). Development of a behavioral test of visuospatial neglect. *Archives of Physical Medicine and Rehabilitation, 68*, 98-102.

World Health Organization. (2001). *International Classification of Function, Disability, and Health: ICF.* Geneva, Switzerland: Author.

Website Resources

Academy of Neurologic Communication Disorders and Sciences: www.ancds.org

American Brain Tumor Association: www.abta.org

American Heart Association/American Stroke Association: www.heart.org/HEARTORG/

American Speech-Language-Hearing Association: www.asha.org

Aphasia Hope Foundation: http://aphasiahope.wpengine.com/

Aphasia Institute: www.aphasia.ca

Brain Injury Association of America: www.biausa.org

National Aphasia Association: www.aphasia.org

12

Assessment of Voice Disorders

Natalie Schaeffer, DA, CCC-SLP

Key Words

- abduction
- adduction
- airflow rate
- aphonia
- breathy
- coarticulation
- diplophonia
- dysphonia
- easy onset
- expiratory reserve volume
- fundamental frequency
- glottal attack
- glottis
- harsh voice
- hoarse voice
- hyperfunctional voice
- hypernasality
- hyponasality
- intensity (loudness)
- jitter/relative average perturbations
- maximum phonation time
- monopitch
- phonation
- phonation breaks
- phonotrauma
- pitch
- pitch breaks
- pitch variation
- pressed voice
- resonance (oral and nasal)
- resting expiratory level
- S/Z ratio
- shimmer
- subglottal pressure
- tidal volume
- vital capacity
- vocal noise
- vocal strain

Introduction

A complete assessment of voice disorders incorporates the use of laboratory instrumentation, informal vocal tasks, client observation, client monologue, and an extensive client interview. Depending on the facility, instrumentation is not always available for student clinicians and speech-language pathologists (SLPs). As a result, students and professionals may not have had the opportunity and training to use instrumental equipment for conducting that aspect of vocal assessment. Thus, it is the goal of this chapter to demystify the process of vocal analysis, provide relevant background information, and walk the student clinician and SLP step-by-step through the process. This chapter provides the reader with an understanding of the following aspects:

- The general components involved in vocal production (i.e., quality, **pitch**, **intensity** or loudness, and **resonance**) and how to evaluate these areas in relation to their influence on voice

Stein-Rubin, C., & Fabus, R. *A Guide to Clinical Assessment and Professional Report Writing in Speech-Language Pathology, Second Edition (pp 265-294).*

- Specific parameters (e.g., pitch, intensity) to assess in a vocal analysis
- The interview and questions that pertain specifically to this population
- Formal assessment measures, including instrumental measurement and the corresponding graphic read-outs or figures
- Informal assessment measures (e.g., **maximum phonation time** (MPT), **S/Z ratio**, counting from a soft to loud voice [i.e., dynamic range])
- Stimulability and trial therapy techniques
- A case history for a corresponding sample report that includes information based on the client interview and formal and informal measures
- An instructive writing rubric
- A model report on an adult voice client
- A novel case history as a practice exercise
- Key words at the beginning of the chapter that may be used as a guide for technical vocabulary
- A glossary at the conclusion of the chapter

The chapter focuses on **hyperfunctional voice** or **phonotrauma**. Throughout the chapter, the terms *hyperfunctional voice* and *phonotrauma* are used interchangeably. This voice disorder, which is associated with abnormal laryngeal tension, occurs in 88% of the adult population (Koufman, 2010). This **dysphonia** refers to vocal disorders associated with misuse, overuse, or abuse of the voice. Dysphonias stemming from other conditions or etiologies are listed, classified, and described briefly in this chapter, along with resources where further information may be found. A detailed overview regarding methods for these other dysphonias are beyond the scope of this chapter. In addition, refer to Andrews (1999), Andrews and Summers (2002), and Boone, McFarlane, Von Berg, and Zraic (2010) for a discussion on voice disorders in children. Information on the anatomy and physiology of the vocal mechanism can be found in Boone et al. (2010) and Colton and Casper (1996).

Characteristics of Voice

In producing voice, there is a synergistic relationship between **phonation** (voice production) and respiration (inhalation and exhalation). When breathing for speech/voice, phonation originates in the larynx, which houses the vocal folds. Phonation refers to the rapid vibration or opening and closing of the vocal folds, the latter on the exhaled air stream. The larynx is suspended from the hyoid bone and attaches superiorly to the trachea (the windpipe between the larynx and lungs). Moreover, voice production encompasses four main parameters, which include vocal quality, intensity (loudness), pitch, and resonance, as described in Boone et al. (2010).

1. Vocal quality refers to movement or vibration of the vocal folds (i.e., the opening and closing of the vocal folds for phonation). The vocal folds can vibrate symmetrically or periodically, like mirror images of each other with regard to proper **abduction** (opening of the vocal folds) and **adduction** (closing of the vocal folds), reflecting a voice within normal limits. If vocal fold vibration is asymmetrical or aperiodic, **vocal noise** (e.g., roughness) can result. If the vocal folds do not adduct sufficiently, breathiness can occur because there is air leakage through the **glottis**. For example, vocal noise and breathiness are often perceived as a **hoarse voice**, vocal noise can be perceived as rough or **harsh**, and **strain** can be perceived as pressed (overadducted), although **breathy** voices can also sound strained.
2. Intensity refers to vocal loudness (normal, too loud, too weak, or without variation); a voice that is too loud or too weak can be related to the improper coordination of respiration and phonation (speech breathing).
3. Pitch refers to how high or low the voice can ascend or descend and depends on the lengthening and shortening of the vocal folds. A pitch that is too high or too low may have a negative effect on voice or be inappropriate for the speaker. **Pitch variation** is a component of pitch, and some disorders are characterized by excessive pitch variation, while other disorders reflect **monopitch** (little or no pitch variation).
4. Resonance refers to where and how the laryngeal sound is amplified or dampened by the vocal tract or supralaryngeal system (e.g., nasal cavity, oral cavity, pharyngeal cavity). For example, the nasal sounds, /m/, /n/, /ŋ/ are resonated in the nasal cavity, whereas all of the other sounds are resonated in the oral cavity (Boone et al., 2010).

Classification According to Etiological Origin

There are alternate ways of defining and classifying voice disorders. For example, a voice disorder may be defined as a problem in any one or more of the parameters of voice already described (loudness, quality, pitch, and resonance) as related to the individual's age, gender, situational context, and message intent (Haynes & Pindzola, 2004). In addition to classifying and assessing voice based on perceptual signs (the four preceding components), vocal disorders are typically classified according to etiology or causative origin as follows: functional, organic (e.g., structural/anatomical and neurological), psychogenic (psychologically based origin), and resonance or nonphonatory/nonvibratory disorders (i.e., not specifically related to vocal fold vibration). See Haynes and Pindzola (2004) for additional classification paradigms used to describe dysphonia.

Functional Voice Disorders

Functional vocal disorders have no organic or neurogenic etiology but arise from improper use of the voice (e.g., an individual who screams excessively or uses the voice without breath support). Nevertheless, persistent misuse of the voice may result in the development of structural laryngeal changes such as benign lesions (e.g., nodules, polyps, thickened vocal folds that can be reflected in, for example, a breathy, hoarse, or strained voice). Structural changes, which are behavioral in origin, will be classified as functional because the client's use of voice is contributing to his or her disorder (Boone et al., 2010; Morrison & Rammage, 1993).

Hyperfunctional Dysphonia

Hyperfunctional voice, or phonotrauma, refers to excessive laryngeal tension when phonating or during voice production. It can be related to shouting, excessive loudness, squeezing and straining the vocal folds, excessive force or muscle tension during speech production (e.g., muscle tension dysphonia), attempts to speak on inadequate expiration, insufficient inspiratory phase for the phonatory task, improper use of exhalation for voice/speech, chest and abdominal muscles in competition with each other, and anxiety or tension, all of which may contribute to failure to provide sufficient breath support for speech (Aronson, 1980; Boone et al., 2010; Hixon & Hoit, 2005; Sapienza, Stathopoulos, & Brown, 1997). Benign vocal fold lesions, secondary to phonotrauma, may develop and are associated with abnormal vocal characteristics.

The Relationship of Vocal Fold Lesions to Abnormal Vocal Characteristics

As previously explained, phonotrauma is associated with benign vocal fold lesions (defined next), which can result in abnormal vocal characteristics. These lesions may prevent the vocal folds from adducting sufficiently, thus allowing a leakage of air through the glottis with resultant breathiness or noise (aperiodic vocal fold vibration in which the vocal folds are not moving as mirror images of each other).

Benign Lesions Associated With Hyperfunctional Voice

The following benign lesions may occur secondary to prolonged vocal abuse or phonotrauma:

- Nodules are whitish protuberances on the anterior middle third of the vocal folds, are usually bilateral, and become hard with continued abuse.
- Polyps are typically unilateral in the same area as nodules and often precipitated by a single event (e.g., screaming at a ball game), which may result in a hemorrhage. Polyps can occur with one incident (broken blood vessel in which a polyp forms out of a hemorrhage), and continued phonotrauma maintains them. Polyps are soft and fluid filled (Boone, McFarlane, & Von Berg, 2005).
- Contact ulcers occur on the posterior glottal margins of the vocal folds. They are related to slamming together the arytenoid cartilages during the production of low-pitched phonation, hard **glottal attacks**, possible increased loudness, and frequent throat clearing and coughing. Gastroesophageal reflux disease is often associated with contact ulcers. When reflux is involved, the disorder can become organic (Boone et al., 2005).
- Thickening and reddening of the vocal folds (Reinke edema) refers to a swelling of the vocal folds and is usually seen bilaterally. A gelatinous material develops on the vocal folds and is not localized as in polyps and nodules.
- Traumatic laryngitis refers to swelling of the vocal folds as a result of excessive shouting, often at a ball game or other spectator event. The vocal folds increase in size and mass (Boone et al., 2005).

Continued abusive vocal behaviors may result in a possible exacerbation of the benign lesions and dysphonia. See Boone et al. (2010) for in-depth descriptions of changes in vocal fold tissue associated with the aforementioned conditions.

Vocal Characteristics

The following vocal characteristics may typically occur as a result of the aforementioned benign vocal lesions (see Boone et al., 2010):

- Breathiness: As noted previously, breathiness refers to air leakage through the glottis during phonation

- Hoarseness: Vocal noise and breathiness
- Harshness: Pressed voice with noise and/or over-adducted vocal folds
- Strain: Tense, stiff use of the vocal folds
- **Phonation breaks**: Loss of voice on syllables, words, phrases
- **Aphonia**: Speaking in a whisper or loss of voice
- **Pitch breaks**: Excessively high or low pitch that breaks upward or downward
- Inappropriate intensity: An excessively loud or weak/soft voice
- Ventricular phonation: Using both the false and true vocal folds secondary to excessive tension
- **Diplophonia**: Two vocal frequencies heard simultaneously (e.g., may result from a polyp on one vocal fold or ventricular phonation)
- Hard glottal attacks: Banging together the vocal folds, usually on initial vowels
- **Pressed voice**: Overadduction of the vocal folds characterized by severe strain
- Weak voice: Related to speaking in noisy environments and loudly, and relates to vocal overdoers (Titze, 2017). (According to Boone et al. [2010], weak, soft voices may develop secondary to prolonged hyperfunctional use of the vocal mechanism, which may cause the eventual breakdown of vocal adduction, resulting in breathiness/vocal nodules.)

Environmental and Physical Contributory Factors

Additional factors may contribute to misuse of the vocal mechanism. These can promote compensatory use of the voice, or vocal hyperfunction, as the patient attempts to adjust his or her voice in a maladaptive manner.

Smoking, medications such as antihistamines (may dry the mouth and the laryngeal mucosa), excessive alcohol, use of caffeine (drying effects), and insufficient hydration are all environmental factors that can negatively affect the vocal folds and, thus, the use of the vocal mechanism. Conditions such as allergies, asthma, and acid reflux may also be detrimental to the voice. When the folds are dry or have mucous from allergies, there is a tendency to clear the throat, which can be abusive to the vocal folds. Noisy and smoke-filled environments can give rise to speaking above noise, yelling, forceful singing, coughing, and throat clearing and can also have a negative effect on the vocal folds. For a more in-depth discussion, see Andrews and Summers (2002); Colton and Casper (1996); and Columbia University Medical Center (n.d.). Specific vocal hygiene steps are outlined in Appendix 12-A).

A variety of physical factors can also affect vocal function. For example, reflux disease—the passage of gastric juices from the stomach to the esophagus (i.e., gastroesophageal reflux disease) or from the esophagus to the larynx (laryngopharyngeal reflux)—can contribute to voice problems (Boone et al., 2010; Columbia University Medical Center, n.d.; Lombard & Popovich, 2008; Vocal Health, 2009). Symptoms of acid reflux are heartburn, excessive mucous, throat clearing, a feeling of a lump in the throat, sore throat, choking incidents, wheezing, a sense of a postnasal drip, and hoarseness. In children, persistent vomiting, bleeding from the esophagus, respiratory symptoms, choking spells, and swallowing problems can occur. Some foods will create stomach acids (e.g., alcoholic drinks, citrus drinks, highly spicy foods), contributing to reflux.

Excessive weight can also promote reflux. It is important to sleep on a bed with the head elevated. Avoiding foods that contribute to reflux and maintaining a normal weight should also help reduce the symptoms (Boone et al., 2010; Columbia University Medical Center, n.d.; Vocal Health, 2009). For a more in-depth discussion on reflux disease, see Chapter 14). The gastric juices, as a result of reflux, make the vocal folds vulnerable. According to Aronson and Bless (2009), esophageal reflux irritates the laryngeal tissues and sets up an environment conducive to laryngeal pathology. This situation suggests that, as the patient abuses the vocal folds in the presence of reflux, the voice problem may be exacerbated.

Organic Voice Disorders

Organic voice disorders include those with a structural or neurological etiology. Voice disorders that are related to structural problems are anatomically based (e.g., a laryngeal web), and dysphonias that stem from a neurological component are secondary to malfunctioning of the cranial nerves or the central nervous system (e.g., paralyzed vocal fold, spastic dysarthria).

Structurally Based Voice Disorders

Refer to Table 12-1 for a summary of organic voice disorders that are anatomical or structural in origin.

Neurologically Based Voice Disorders

The following neurological disorders are discussed in detail in Boone et al. (2010), Duffy (1995), and Freed (2000). As previously noted, other populations, aspects, and etiologies with dysphonia are beyond the

TABLE 12-1. STRUCTURALLY BASED VOICE DISORDERS

Disorder	*Definition*
Bowing of the vocal folds	Refers to an elliptical glottal shape during phonation secondary to loss of tissue mass or laryngeal scarring (Aronson & Bless, 2009).
Contact ulcers-laryngeal reflux	Unilateral or bilateral erosions that develop on the medial aspect of the vocal processes of the arytenoid cartilages. They result from one or a combination of hard glottal attacks, throat clearing, coughing, and laryngopharyngeal reflux. See Sasaki (2008) for further information.
Cysts	Often caused by an abnormal blockage of the ductal system of laryngeal mucous glands and can be congenital or acquired. Surgical intervention is often necessary. See Boone et al. (2010) and Eastern Virginia Medical School (2009) for further discussion.
Endocrine disorder	Endocrine changes (e.g., hypofunction of the pituitary gland; excessive or insufficient hormone secretion) may affect the developing larynx and cause an excessively high or low pitch (Boone et al., 2010).
Granulomas	A firm granulated sac on the vocal folds, usually occurring on the posterior glottis. Granulomas are often associated with intubation during surgery, but they are also related to glottal trauma from abuse/misuse and gastric reflux (Boone et al., 2005).
Hemangioma	Refers to a soft, pliable, blood-filled sac which occurs on the posterior glottis. It is often associated with laryngeal hyperfunction or intubation (Boone et al., 2010).
Hyperkeratosis	A pinkish, rough lesion that can occur secondary to continued tissue irritation (e.g., secondhand smoke). These lesions may be either malignant or nonmalignant (Boone et al., 2010).
Infectious laryngitis	This disorder can occur as a symptom of a severe cold or upper respiratory infection. Voice may be hoarse (breathiness and noise) or aphonic (loss of voice; Boone et al., 2010).
Laryngeal web	Grows across the glottis (space between the vocal folds) between the two vocal folds, and a high-pitched, rough voice occurs. The airway may also be compromised. A congenital web can be seen at birth with symptoms of shortness of breath and stridor (inhalation noise); immediate surgery is required. Acquired webs can result from bilateral trauma to the medial edges of the vocal folds, and the inner margins grow together. Surgery is the treatment for webbing (Boone et al., 2010).
Leukoplakia	White patches; represent precancerous lesions on the vocal folds and negatively affect phonation because they increase the mass of the vocal folds. Heavy smoking is often the cause (Boone et al., 2010).
Papillomas	Wartlike growths that are viral in origin and occur in the airway, usually in young children. They contribute to dysphonia as well as obstruction of the airway and need to be removed surgically (Boone et al., 2010).
Pubertal changes	As the vocal folds are changing, boys may experience temporary dysphonia and occasional pitch breaks (Boone et al., 2010).
Sulcus vocalis	A groove or infolding of mucosa along the surface of the vocal fold. The mucosa is scarred down to the underlying vocal ligament (in the area of the sulcus). Hoarseness, vocal fatigue, and weak phonation with increased effort are characteristics (Sulica, n.d.).
Trauma	Damage to the larynx from neck injuries such as choking, car accidents, gunshot wounds, or accidents (e.g., waterskiing, motorcycling; Aronson & Bless, 2009).

scope of this chapter. Refer to Table 12-2 for a summary of neurologically based dysphonias. See also Murry and Carrau (2006) for a discussion on swallowing disorders that may accompany neurological disorders.

Psychogenically Based Voice Disorders

Psychogenic voice disorders are a result of psychological stress, which can be a single traumatic event, social causes, or living in long-term stressful situations (Aronson & Bless, 2009; Boone et al., 2010). Please refer to Table 12-3 for a summary of these disorders.

Resonance Disorders

A resonance disorder refers to the function of the resonating cavities (e.g., the nasal, oral, and pharyngeal cavity) and includes nonphonatory and nonvibratory disorders.

Table 12-2. Neurologically Based Voice Disorders

Disorder	*Definition*
Ataxic dysarthria	In some clients, phonation is hoarse with mild tremors, the latter related to cerebellar damage; additionally, inhalation and exhalation may be dyscoordinated and can interrupt respiratory function.
Essential tremor	Characterized by voice breaks and stops with rhythmic regularity that occur in all types of voice activity: speech, singing, sustained vowels.
Flaccid dysarthria	Often involves the cranial nerves (e.g., the laryngeal branches of the vagus nerve) and can result in a paralyzed vocal fold. In this case, the voice is breathy with noise, with instances of diplophonia (double voice) because the vocal folds (the paralyzed and nonparalyzed vocal fold) are moving at two frequencies.
Hyperkinetic movement disorders	Related to the basal ganglia and involve excessive laryngeal or articulatory movements (e.g., adductor spasmodic dysphonia). Spasmodic dysphonia is a hyperkinetic disorder characterized by momentary periods of uncontrolled vocal spasms of muscles of the vocal folds, causing an abnormal voice. The most common type is adductor spasmodic dysphonia (tight laryngeal adduction). An abductor type has also been identified in which voices are suddenly interrupted by temporary abduction of the vocal folds (Boone et al., 2010). Huntington chorea is another example of a hyperkinetic disorder in which excessive articulatory movements affect phonation.
Myasthenia gravis	A chronic autoimmune neuromuscular disease characterized by varying degrees of weakness of the skeletal (voluntary) muscles of the body. The muscle weakness increases during periods of activity and improves after periods of rest (National Institute of Neurological Disorders and Stroke, n.d.). According to Boone et al. (2010), the client's voice deteriorates after use, particularly with other symptoms (e.g., drooping eyelid).
Parkinson disease	A hypokinetic disorder in which the voice is weak, breathy, monotone, and monopitch, secondary to a disorder of the basal ganglia (subcortical structure of the brain) in which there is an insufficiency of the neurotransmitter dopamine.
Spastic dysarthria	The voice is strained and sounds strangled, accompanied by hypernasality and imprecise articulation, secondary to bilateral (both sides of brain) upper motor neuron disease (e.g., amyotrophic lateral sclerosis).

Table 12-3. Psychogenically Based Voice Disorders

Disorder	*Definition*
Falsetto (puberphonia, mutational falsetto)	Refers to the high-register or high-pitched voice produced by the male adolescent or adult, even though the maturational changes from prepubertal to postpubertal have taken place; individual speaks in an inappropriately high pitch; can also occur in girls and women
Conversion/hysterical voice disorder	Any loss of voluntary control over muscular action as a consequence of environmental stress; patient is convinced these unconscious simulations of illness are organic in nature
Conversion dysphonia or muteness	Patient neither whispers nor articulates
Conversion aphonia	Involuntary whispering despite a normal larynx
Conversion dysphonia	Voice problem that has no physiological basis (normal larynx)

Once a sound is generated at the level of the vocal folds, it passes through a series of cavities (noted previously), which dampen or enhance the sound (Stemple, Glaze, & Gerdeman, 1999). The following are examples of resonation problems, which relate to the difficulty with the resonating structures. Certain resonation problems can have an organic basis (e.g., cleft palate) or a neurological cause (e.g., damage to the nerves which innervate the velopharyngeal structures).

Hypernasality

Hypernasality is a resonance problem in which sound escapes from the nasal cavity on non-nasal sounds (e.g., /p/, /d/, /l/, vowels), and the voice is perceived as over-nasalized. This dysphonia may be attributed to velar insufficiency (e.g., cleft palate, bifid uvula, or paralysis to the vagus nerve, which innervates the soft palate); the soft palate is not making contact with the posterior pharyngeal wall, or throat, to prevent air from escaping into the nasal cavity.

Cleft Palate

Children born with a cleft palate are often hypernasal secondary to velar insufficiency. A cleft is an opening in an anatomical part that is normally not open. Cleft palate frequently, but not necessarily, occurs in conjunction with a cleft lip. The voice is hypernasal because the soft palate is not occluding the posterior pharyngeal wall to block the upcoming air from going through the nasal cavity on nonnasal sounds. Hypernasality may also occur with a submucous cleft (the hard palate did not fuse and is covered by mucosa). Without therapy, persons with cleft palates can develop compensatory substitutions because of difficulty building up intraoral air pressure secondary to the cleft palate. The following are examples of compensatory substitutions: pharyngeal fricatives, producing fricatives with the posterior tongue against the pharyngeal wall; pharyngeal stops, producing stop plosives with the posterior tongue against the pharyngeal wall; and glottal stops, producing sounds, especially fricatives and plosives, by occluding the vocal folds. These substitutions, as well as weak production of consonants, further compromise voice production. Surgical treatment and prostheses are used to facilitate velar efficiency. See Boone et al. (2005, 2010) and Shprintzen and Bardach (1995) for further discussion of cleft palate and velar insufficiency.

Hypernasality Related to Neurological Disease

- Flaccid dysarthria, unilateral upper motor neuron lesions: Unilateral paralysis of the soft palate on the opposite of the lesion can cause hypernasality, related to cortical or subcortical lesions.
- Spastic dysarthria: Hypernasality is related to slowness of velopharyngeal movement, not paralysis of the soft palate.
- Dystonia refers to relatively slow, uncontrolled, nonrhythmic contractions of the velopharyngeal muscles as well as other muscle groups (e.g., tongue, mandible, lips). (For discussion on hypernasality related to neurological disease, see Aronson & Bless, 2009; Boone et al., 2010.)
- Basal ganglia lesions: Hypernasality in these lesions is connected to the longer duration of the velopharyngeal opening (e.g., dystonia).

Functional Nasality

Functional or assimilative nasality refers to resonance patterns that are not necessarily pathological. Assimilative nasality affects vowels and voiced consonants, which occur immediately before and after nasal consonants and become nasalized. For example, the word *time* has the bilabial nasal /n/ in the word that may affect the vowel. At times, the velar openings begin too soon or are maintained for too long.

Assimilative nasality can occur in regional accent, such as nasal twang, or exposure to faulty speech patterns. Additionally, functional nasality may simply relate to a reduced effort to produce normally vigorous speech when the velopharyngeal structures are intact (Aronson & Bless, 2009; Boone et al., 2010). The author of this chapter has clinically seen clients with assimilative nasality related to imprecise articulation and very rapid rate.

Organic Hyponasality

Organic **hyponasality** is a resonance problem in which there is reduced nasal resonance for the three nasalized phonemes /m/, /n/, and /ŋ/. This problem can be associated with a cold, nasal polyps, deviated septum, and hypertrophied adenoids, all of which may prevent the resonance of sufficient air through the nose on the three phonemes. See Boone et al. (2010) and Aronson and Bless (2009) for further information on hyponasality. Although the literature suggests that hyponasality is organic and associated with an obstruction, the author of this chapter has seen cases of functional hyponasality related to imprecise articulation or insufficient range of articulatory movement.

Dysphonia in Special Populations

The following groups present with characteristics of dysphonia that are unique to their population.

Laryngectomy

Total laryngectomy (often secondary to cancer of the larynx) is a surgical procedure that involves removal of the entire larynx and separates the airway from the mouth, nose, and esophagus. The laryngectomee client breathes through a stoma, which is an opening in the neck/trachea. The main goal of therapy is to help establish another method of speech or sound production to restore communicative ability.

There are three current methods for speech rehabilitation after total laryngectomy: the electrolarynx, esophageal speech, and tracheoesophageal (TEP) speech. The electrolarynx is an electronic device that is placed on a compliant surface (e.g., neck, cheek, under the chin) and creates a vibration. The vibration creates a sound, and the person uses his or her articulators to shape words and sentences—that is, articulate speech.

A second method is esophageal speech. The speaker traps air in the mouth and forces it down to the esophagus and upper pharynx. The pharyngoesophageal segment (segment between the pharynx and esophagus) vibrates, creating a low-pitch sound that is brought up in a belch; speech is produced on the belched or exhaled air.

A third method is the TEP puncture. A puncture is made between the esophagus and trachea by a surgeon, and a prosthesis is placed in this puncture (fistula). Air is provided by the lungs. As the air comes up from the lungs, it vibrates the pharyngoesophageal segment and speech is formed on the upcoming air. That is, TEP speech occurs when the air is directed through the prosthesis to the mouth, and the person forms speech on the air. Precise articulation is essential for clients who have had a laryngectomy to obtain good speech intelligibility, considering the new voice production. See Boone et al. (2010), Keith and Darley (1994), and Lombard and Popovich (2008) for further discussions on laryngectomy.

Dysphonia Related to Aging

Some of the physiological changes related to aging are lengthening of the vocal tract, a reduction in pulmonary function, laryngeal cartilage ossification (fixed rigidity), increased vocal fold stiffening, and diminished vocal fold closure. Specific characteristics found in the aging voice are tremor, hoarseness, breathiness, voice breaks, a decrease in loudness, change in habitual pitch (raises in men and lowers in women; Zraick, Gregg, & Whitehouse, 2006, p. 252).

Dysphonia Related to Deafness and Hearing Impairment

This population exhibits an elevated **fundamental frequency** (pitch), excessive pitch variation, and excesses in vocal intensity (too loud or too soft) because of limitations in hearing which result in difficulty self-monitoring (Boone et al., 2010).

Parameters of Assessment

Because dysphonia may be the result of, or result in, a medical problem, all clients must be evaluated before the initiation of therapy (and preferably before the diagnostic assessment) by an otolaryngologist or ear, nose, and throat physician (ENT). The ENT determines the condition and functioning of the vocal folds, as well as the velopharyngeal structures (soft palate and pharyngeal wall) and makes recommendations. This examination is essential to rule out serious conditions (e.g., cancer) to inform the clinician of the status of the client's vocal folds, and to recommend whether voice therapy is appropriate. The physician may also determine whether a medical procedure is necessary prior to initiating voice therapy. The status of the client's vocal folds should be monitored by the otolaryngologist, followed by a period of voice therapy and recommendations for vocal hygiene (author's clinical experience).

Other members of the Voice Team can include the following professionals when the need to consult them arises in relation to the client's dysphonia:

- A psychologist, should there be a psychological component related to voice
- An audiologist, if the person's voice is affected by a hearing problem
- A pulmonologist, if the client's lungs or breathing has a negative impact on voice
- An allergist to determine whether allergies or asthma are affecting the voice
- A neurologist who can advise on the contribution of neurological difficulties related to voice
- An endocrinologist with regard to a hormonal impact on voice (e.g., aging)
- An oncologist, should certain treatments for cancer affect voice
- The SLP

The parameters of assessment delineated in the list that follows are crucial to understanding how they affect the voice and interact with each other. For example, a rapid speech rate and limited articulatory movement may have a negative effect on voice in terms of reducing appropriate vocal projections, limiting pitch variation, diminishing speech intelligibility, and negatively affecting resonance. Poor speech rhythm (e.g., choppy speech) may interfere with appropriate continuous flow of speech. Failure to pause appropriately to replenish breath supply may result in losing the voice, particularly at the ends of utterances.

For effective assessment, it is crucial that the SLP have a thorough knowledge of normal anatomy and physiology of the laryngeal and respiratory system, as well as an understanding of the wide range of vocal pathologies (Stemple et al., 1999). Additionally, assessment and treatment of the total person is important because vocal function and emotionality are closely connected (Boone et al., 2005).

The following aspects should be taken into consideration as part of a complete voice evaluation:

- Hearing screening: A hearing screening should be conducted to rule out any hearing loss that may affect voice and speech.
- Oral-peripheral mechanism examination: Refer to Chapter 6 for a detailed discussion of examination of the speech mechanism.
- Vocal parameters: These include vocal quality, fundamental frequency (pitch) and pitch variation, intensity (loudness), and resonance.
- Suprasegmental: Prosody of the voice is related to intonation, stress, and speech rate and rhythm and contributes to the melody and intentionality of the message. Individuals with the disorders described previously often have diminished prosody, particularly some of the dysarthrias (e.g., spastic dysarthria, Parkinson disease). A person may have either a hyperfunctional or hypernasal voice and still maintain appropriate prosody. Often, however, improper vocal fold vibration or abusive vocal patterns result in reduced prosody (author's clinical experience; see also Aronson & Bless, 2009).
- Intelligibility: Intelligibility is the understandability of speech. Assess the impact of the client's dysphonia on speech clarity. Note any other factors that may be impeding intelligibility such as articulation and/or rapid speech rate.
- Hydration: To maximize efficacy of treatment, it is important to determine whether the client drinks a sufficient amount of water on a daily basis. Sufficient hydration is related to the health of the laryngeal system and is an important parameter of assessment.
- Attitude and motivation: It is important to assess the client's attitude toward his or her dysphonia and motivation to improve vocal quality (see Key Clinical Interview Questions section).
- Response to stimulability and trial therapy: The client's ability to imitate facilitating techniques, as in all communication assessment, is a prognostic indicator for improvement during therapy and may indicate a starting point and a course of action for voice therapy. Demonstrating how his or her voice may be improved in trial therapy may increase motivation and interest.

Vocal Hygiene

It is important to facilitate awareness of vocally abusive behaviors and to provide a baseline for therapy. Therefore, specific vocal hygiene charts should be assigned to the client immediately after the evaluation. The client should maintain a record that keeps track of when he or she screamed or spoke above noise, when he or she refrained from screaming or speaking above noise, and when he or she corrected him- or herself at different times of the day. Different symbols should be given to apply to these categories (e.g., a star to represent refraining from shouting, an X to represent vocal abuse, and a check for self-correction). Over the course of treatment, the client should be able to see an increase in stars and a decrease in Xs. Additionally, the amount of hydration (e.g., six glasses of water per day) should be included in this chart. This procedure fosters the client's ability to immediately take proactive steps following the first meeting and is, therefore, empowering. Refer to the vocal hygiene program in the Appendix 12-A for a handout to share with your clients.

Many of the parameters for assessment may be probed during the client interview. The following section outlines this essential portion of the vocal assessment.

Key Clinical Interview Questions

It is important for the SLP, who is conducting a voice evaluation and a diagnostic interview, to understand the client's three domains of development, which are cognition, physical, and social/emotional development (CPSED; discussed in Chapter 1 in the Introduction to Assessment section). The interview provides an opportunity to observe these three critical domains in the dysphonic client and to determine how they interact with each other and impact upon vocal function. Through the client's CPSED interaction, the SLP has the opportunity to learn about and address the total person, as previously highlighted by Boone et al. (2005). For example, the interview provides the setting for the diagnostician to observe the client's posture and any physical tension of the body parts (e.g., head, neck, and shoulders), as well as oral posture and any accompanying tension; to observe the client's temperament, presence of anxiety, and attitude toward his or her dysphonia; and to obtain an idea of how well the client understands and follows through on direction.

The interview process is crucial with regard to disclosing a number of components that must be taken into account when planning therapy. These areas, which include the following important examples, can then be effectively addressed in terms of moving the therapeutic process forward: the client's use, abuse, and misuse of voice in a variety of contexts; the client's attitude, compliancy, and motivation, which can impact progress negatively or positively (e.g., a motivated client will eliminate abuse, practice, and make progress, whereas a client who is resistant may not move forward in the therapeutic process); use of medications or overuse of alcohol, cigarettes, or caffeine, which can have an effect on the vocal folds (e.g., dry out the vocal folds); hospitalizations that may have affected the vocal folds (e.g., intubation); and chronic disorders such as asthma or neurological problems that must be considered and addressed in the evaluation and therapeutic process. In these cases, it is in the best interest of the client, with his or her written consent, to maintain an open dialogue with the physician.

In addition, the clinician would also wish to know whether the client has a history of previous evaluations or therapy and whether the therapy was successful (or unsuccessful) and incorporate this knowledge into planning therapy for success (author's clinical experience). Similarly, the presence of a family history of speech or voice disorders should be determined.

The client with dysphonia, however, must recognize the problems and be motivated to improve his or her voice. Frequently, clients with phonotrauma are not motivated to correct their vocal problems because they perceive that having a breathy or hoarse voice sounds glamorous or unique, reinforced by people who comment that they like the sound of the client's voice. Additionally, voice clients are often intelligible and usually get their message across, unlike the difficulties experienced by people who stutter; thus, these voice clients may not feel the need to engage in the therapeutic process. Furthermore, confounding motivation in this population is the fact that clients referred for a voice evaluation are frequently referred by a physician or by a university speech screening, not self-referred. As one may surmise, motivating these clients may prove to be a challenge because they might not be inclined to enroll in therapy or to practice sufficiently once involved in therapy.

Motivated clients who wish to correct their vocal problems are usually those who depend on their voices for their careers or jobs (e.g., a teacher, a singer, salesperson, performing telephone work). In these cases, the clients are not only motivated to improve their voice, but are very concerned as well.

The following interview questions are useful in disclosing relevant information regarding the client's voice with respect to the various aspects of his or her life: a history of communication problems, health, previous evaluations and therapy, lifestyle, vocal habits, and attitudes (Table 12-4; see also Appendix 12-B).

Most Relevant Formal Assessment Measures (Instrumental Measurements)

Instrumentation to assess voice is not available in all clinics or offices. However, informal measures, when properly used, can provide pertinent data regarding the client's voice (see Informal Assessment and Behavioral Measures on p. 281). Formal assessment measures that are free or less costly than those discussed in this section can be found later in this chapter.

The advantage of instrumental measures is that much of the data obtained are objective and may confirm informal testing. The disadvantage is that the voice output of the client is often limited to vowel production or does not measure dynamic speech/voice.

Acoustic Measures (Used With a Microphone)

Sona Speech Multidimensional Voice Program

The rationale for using Sona Speech, version 2.70 (Pentax Medical, n.d.; previously Kay Elemetrics) is that it gives a rapid, quantitative assessment of the severity of dysphonia (in terms of periodicity of vocal-fold movement), which can be compared with perceptual findings. This Multidimensional Voice Program (MDVP) is used mainly with adults, which is the population with which it was normed.

The client is instructed to take in a normal breath through the mouth, immediately produce the vowel /a/ into the microphone (held 6 inches from client's mouth) at a comfortable pitch and loudness level, and sustain the vowel from the beginning to the end of the indicated area on the screen. The clinician presses the space bar to register the completed waveform. The clinician can also isolate a particular area of the

Table 12-4. Interview Questions

History and Characteristics of Voice Problem	*Clinician's Comments*
Who referred you and why?	
With whom do you live?	
When did you first notice the voice problem? How has it progressed?	
Was your voice problem present in childhood (if an adult)?	
Has your voice changed since you first noticed the hoarseness?	
Have you ever lost your voice?	
When is your voice best, morning, noon, night?	
Does your voice change with any particular time of year/season?	
Why are you coming for an evaluation now?	
Medical History	*Clinician's Comments*
What is your medical history (e.g., hospitalizations, swallowing, operations)?	
Have you had a hearing test?	
What were the results of the doctor's examination (doctor's report)?	
Do you have reflux, asthma, allergies (or other voice related health issues)?	
Do you take medication (name, dosage, purpose)?	
Do you smoke, drink alcohol, or caffeine (frequency)?	
How many glasses of water do you drink in a day?	
History and Family History of Speech-Voice-Hearing Evaluation/Therapy	*Clinician's Comments*
Have you had any previous evaluations or therapy?	
Have you ever had your hearing tested?	
Does anyone in your family have a voice problem?	
Does anyone in your family have a hearing problem?	
Educational/Occupational History and Hobbies	*Clinician's Comments*
What is your educational history?	
What type of work do you do?	
What are your hobbies, interests, activities?	
How would you describe yourself?	
Do you shout, talk continuously, engage in frequent and prolonged telephone conversation, sing, act, yell from room to room, speak over background noise?	
Attitude and Motivation	*Clinician's Comments*
How do you feel about your voice problem?	
Does anyone else notice your voice problem?	
What would you like to accomplish in this evaluation?	

waveform to be analyzed. The clinician presses the appropriate keys on the key board for the instrument to display a graphic readout representing the voice and to designate the following values: **jitter/relative average perturbations** (RAP; cycle-to-cycle variability in terms of the duration of vocal fold vibration—pitch); **shimmer** (cycle-to-cycle variability in terms of vocal-fold opening and amplitude); noise-to-harmonic ratio (the ratio of noise to the vocal signal); and voice turbulence index (condition where noise is created by the airstream from the glottis). In the graphic display, the green circle indicates that the voice is within normal limits. Figures 12-1 and 12-2 display results from the MDVP; they would ordinarily be displayed using

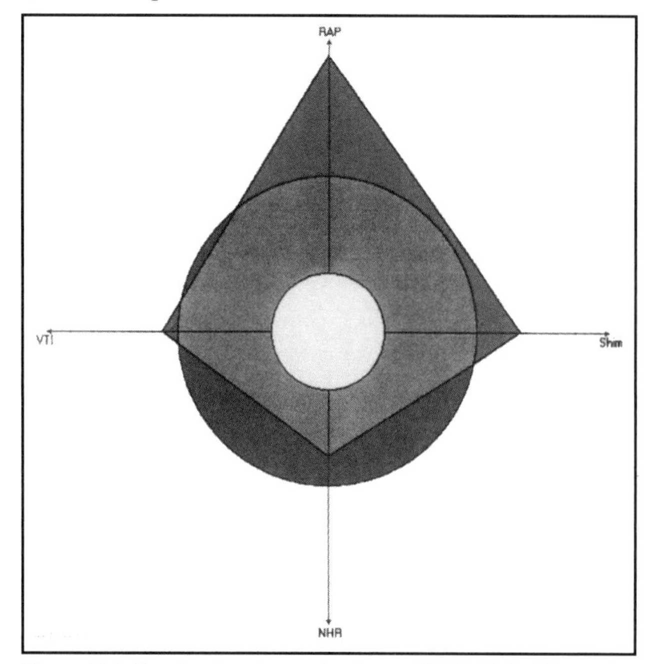

Figure 12-1. Dysphonic voice production on MDVP (clinical illustration by the author of this chapter).

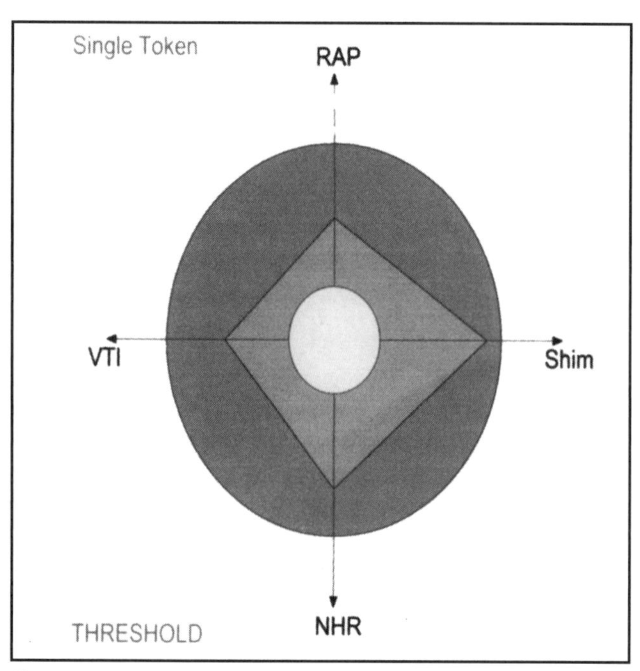

Figure 12-2. Normal voice production on MDVP (clinical illustration by the author of this chapter).

Table 12-5. Sona Speech Multidimensional Voice Program (Pentax Medical, n.d.)

	Adults (Pentax Medical)		*Children (Campisi et al., 2002)*
	Norms %	**Threshold %**	**Threshold %**
Jitter			
Relative average			
Perturbations (RAP)	.378	.680	.75
Shimmer	1.997	3.810	3.35
Noise-to-harmonic ratio	.112	.190	.11
Voice turbulence index	.046	.061	
Fundamental Frequency (Fo)	**Norms as per MDVP (Hz)**		
	Female 243.973		
	Male 143.233		

the colors red and green but are represented here in differing shades of gray. The shading, which is outside of the circle, indicates jitter/RAP, shimmer, noise-to-harmonic ratio, and/or voice turbulence index. The threshold values obtained are in accordance with the levels of green or red (now in grayscale) on the graphic display (see Figures 12-1 and 12-2). The task should be performed three times for consistency. Table 12-5 displays values that are within normal limits (norms and threshold data) for adults (Pentax Medical). See the Pentax Medical (n.d.) website for further information. Campisi et al. (2002) established norms for children aged 4 to 18 years old.

Sono Speech: Visipitch

The Visipitch (Pentax Medical) can obtain fundamental frequency value, a pitch range, and a display an intonation pattern. The rationale for using this instrument is that the quantitative data obtained can be compared with pitch obtained from informal tasks and provide hard evidence to support perceptual analysis. The client is instructed to take in a normal breath and produces the vowel /a/ into a microphone (held 2 inches from client's mouth) at a comfortable pitch and loudness level. The waveform appears on the computer screen as the client is sustaining the vowel. The clinician presses the space bar to the end of the phonation, and the instrument calculates the fundamental frequency (Fo) after the clinician presses analysis on the screen. The pitch range can also be assessed by the Visipitch. For pitch range, the client will produce the vowel at decreasing and then increasing pitch levels (lowest to highest). According to Boone et al. (2005), Fo averages are as follows: female 225 Hz; male 125 Hz. Andrews (1999) found that mean Fo average for children aged 5 to 11 years is 231.88 Hz.

Sona Speech: Spectrograph

The spectrograph displays a graphic representation of the frequency and intensity of the sound wave as a function of time (spectrogram) of the client's voice (Boone et al., 2010). The rationale for using this instrument is that it allows the clinician to specifically view the function of the vocal folds (represented by the vertical striations on the spectrogram—one vertical striation is one vocal fold cycle, which is the opening and closing of the vocal folds for one cycle), as well as the frequency and intensity of the client's voice. The client is instructed to produce a vowel or sentence into a microphone (held 2 inches away from the mouth) at a normal pitch and intensity. In a normal voice, the vertical striations are connected and indicate regularity in terms of vocal fold vibration. Disconnected vertical striations represent aperiodic movement of the vocal folds. Pitch characteristics can be seen in the closeness of the vertical striations. The closer the striations are to each other, the more rapidly the vocal folds vibrate and the higher the pitch. The spectrogram also displays the formant frequencies (bands of energy shaped by the resonating cavities), represented by the horizontal bars on the spectrogram. Lack of breathiness will show strong formant frequencies (Yasui, 2004), and weak or light formant frequencies represent breathiness. See Boone et al. (2005, 2010) and Behrman (2007) for spectrographic illustrations and discussion. The displays may visually confirm the quantitative findings from the MDVP and electroglottograph (EGG; which follow), giving hard evidence and depth to the voice evaluation.

Vibratory Instruments

Electroglottograph/Laryngograph

The rationale for using the EGG (Pentax Medical) is that it is noninvasive and provides a visual representation (waveform) and a numerical value of the ratio of open phase to closed phase during a glottal cycle, thus assessing percentage of vocal fold contact. Symmetry

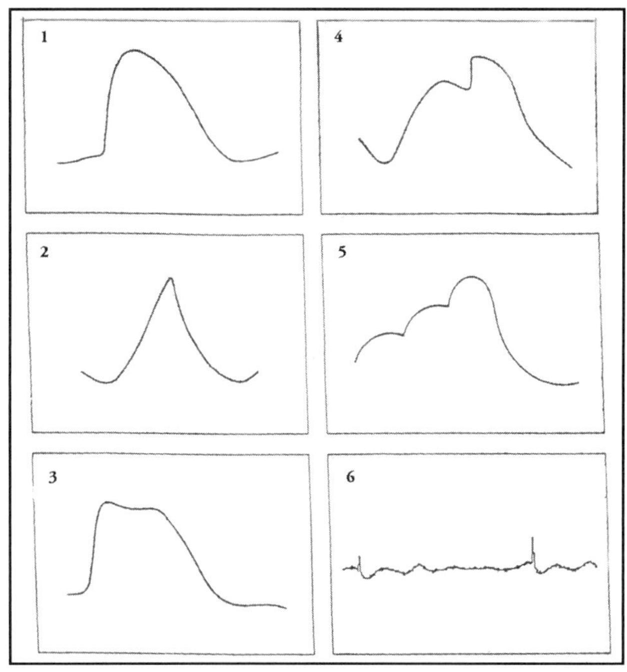

Figure 12-3. Normal and dysphonic cycles on the EGG (Motta et al., 1990; Orlikoff, 1991). (1) Normal opening and closing of the vocal folds. (2) Vocal folds not completely closed (Parkinson disease). (3) Excessive closure of the vocal folds (hyperkinetic dysarthria). (4) Notch in the closing faze of the vocal folds (nodules). (5) Double notch in the closing faze (swelling of the local folds). (6) Irregular waveform (minimal glottal closure, left paralyzed vocal fold).

of vocal fold movement may also be measured by obtaining a contact index. According to Orlikoff (1991), the contact index or speed quotient (SQ) is the ratio of the durational difference between the contact closing and the contact opening phases, divided by the duration of the contact phase.

In the normal voice, there is a steep vertical rise for the closing phase (voice onset), closure of the vocal folds is at the top of the waveform, a sloping return to indicate the opening of the vocal folds, and an open phase (baseline; Figure 12-3, number 1). The waveform is also periodic (Figure 12-4A) in that the vocal folds are vibrating as mirror images of each other. In the breathy voice, there is a sloping voice onset (i.e., not a steep closing phase), a peak for contact quotient (reduced vocal fold closure), and a long open phase (Figure 12-3, number 2 and Figure 12-4B). Figure 12-4C displays an aperiodic waveform in that the vocal folds are not moving as mirror images of each other. Overadducted vocal folds (long closed phase) can be seen in Figure 12-3, number 3. In a paralyzed vocal fold, there is minimal vocal fold contact (shown in peaks; Figure 12-3, number 6; Motta, Cesari, Lengo, & Motta, 1990; Orlikoff, 1991, 1998). To use the EGG, surface electrodes (conducts electrical current, which

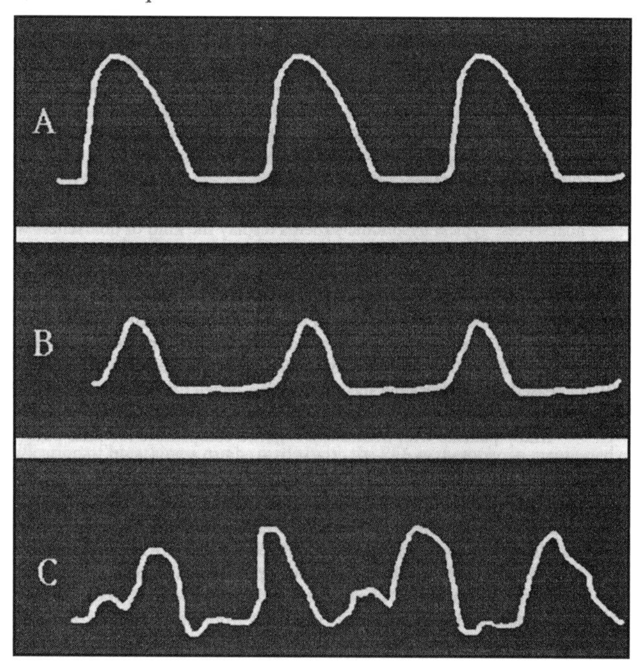

Figure 12-4. Normal and dysphonic waveforms on the EGG (Boone et al., 2005). (A) Normal waveform. (B) Breathy waveform. (C) Aperiodic waveform.

is noninvasive) are placed on either side of the thyroid cartilage. The client is instructed to phonate a vowel or connected speech into a microphone at a comfortable pitch and loudness level. A waveform is seen on the computer screen, and the electrograph analyzes the signal in terms of vocal fold contact and contact index. These values are obtained by pressing analysis. Because air causes a higher resistance to the electrodes than tissue does, the highest resistance occurs when the glottis (space between the vocal folds) is open, and there is the largest volume of air between the folds. Resistance is smallest when the glottis is closed and the volume of air between the vocal folds is at a minimum. The current from the electrodes can therefore achieve better flow between the folds when there is the most vocal fold contact (Boone et al., 2005). A normal voice could have from 40% to 60% vocal fold contact (see Table 12-6 for normal values), whereas percentages lower than 40% can indicate laryngeal pathology (e.g., nodule, polyp), with an excessive air leakage through the glottis (breathy voice). Values greater than 60% can indicate excessive glottal adduction in a pressed voice.

Motta et al. (1990) found that the EGG wave showed a particularly sharper peak and reduced amplitude (abbreviated vocal fold contact) in 93% of the cases of hypokinetic dysphonia, where the glottis was not completely closed. In contrast, patients with hyperkinetic dysphonia showed a plateau-like EGG wave (prolonged vocal fold contact) in 95% of the cases.

Table 12-6. Electroglottograph/Laryngograph

	Norms (Orlikoff, 1998)
Contact quotient (CQ; relative degree of vocal fold contact)	40% to 60% contact (no significant sex effect)
Contact index (CI; degree of contact symmetry; 0 = perfect contact symmetry)	-0.6 to -0.4

The following research illustrates the findings of contact index or SQ using the EGG: Jilek, Marienhagen, and Hacki (2004) used the contact index to determine vocal fold periodicity between hypertonic and healthy voices. These authors determined that, although large standard deviations existed, the hypertonic voices had higher perturbation levels or asymmetry (a higher contact index or SQ) than the healthy voices. In their study, Chen, Robb, and Gilbert (2002) found that both female and male speakers displayed significantly higher SQ values in vocal fry register than in their model registers, particularly males. The authors suggest that the SQ can be used as a means of diagnosing vocal fry when it has been viewed as a voice disorder. For example, Vieira, McInnes, and Jack (2002) compared acoustic and EGG jitter in creaky-like vibrations (glottal fry) in some of their patients. These authors associated "creaky voice" with the findings of Isshiki, Tanabe, Ishizaka, and Broad (1977), who studied effects of asymmetrical vibratory patterns in terms of tension and mass of the vocal folds. Vieira et al. (2002) concluded that EGG signals may detect laryngeal asymmetry, findings that were consistent with their acoustic data. See Aronson and Bless (2009) for more recent information on EGG.

Videostroboscopy (Rigid Endoscope)

This instrument provides a close-up, magnified view with a high-quality image of the vocal folds. One can observe laryngeal anomalies (including subtle lesions), vocal fold vibration, (symmetrical or nonsymmetrical movement), the mucosal wave (waves or undulations of the vocal folds during vibration), and glottal closure (whether the vocal folds are adducting properly). One can also see the vocal folds elongating as pitch raises or increases and shorten as pitch decreases (video tapes). The client sits upright with the head and upper body extended forward. A topical anesthetic is provided to patients who need it. The doctor draws the tongue forward as the rigid scope (a tube) is placed in the oral cavity to the oropharynx. The client phonates a vowel (e.g., /i/) and also raises and lowers his or her pitch on the vowel. The disadvantage of the scope is that vowels only can be used. See Aronson and Bless (2009) for further information.

Fiber Optics (Flexible Endoscopic)

Use of this endoscope allows for observation of vocal fold movement observed during dynamic speech. The function of the arytenoids cartilages, epiglottis, and false vocal folds and their interaction can be seen as the person speaks. Lesions are also evident, but there is not a close-up as with the rigid endoscope. The patient sits upright, and anesthesia is sprayed into both nostrils; subsequently a flexible tube is placed in one nostril to view vocal fold function/vibration as the patient speaks in relation to the doctor's questions. See Aronson and Bless (2009) for further information on fiberoptics.

Aerodynamic Measures

Spirometer

The spirometer measures **vital capacity** and **tidal volume**. Vital capacity refers to the maximum amount of air that can be expired after a maximum inspiration. Tidal volume is a typical inspiration and expiration. The average vital capacity is 5 L, whereas the average tidal volume is .5 L with variations depending on weight, height, and other factors (Boone et al., 2010). These norms come from the American Thoracic Society (1987). If respiratory volume is not within normal limits (as in some neurological diseases), voice production efficiency may be reduced. For vital capacity, the patient sits or stands upright; the nose is closed with a nose clip. He or she is instructed to inhale and exhale three breaths through a tube to obtain tidal volume. The patient immediately takes a maximum inspiration followed by a maximum expiration (through the same tube) for vital capacity measurements. This procedure is performed three times for the best measurement. Handheld spirometers are lower in cost than the standard nonportable spirometers.

Pneumotachograph MS-100

According to Boone et al., "laryngeal airflow is the volume of air passing through the glottis in a fixed period of time" (2010, p. 159). Airflow is measured in millimeters to reflect an **airflow rate** when phonating. Excessive airflow may result in a breathy voice, while insufficient airflow may reflect a tight, pressed voice. Hirano (1981) found that normal range of airflow rate is 40 mL/s (low end) to 200 mL/s (high end). According to Baken (2010), however, normal airflow rate is 100 mL/s. To use a pneumotachograph, a Rothenberg mask is placed over the client's nose and mouth, and the client is instructed to take in a breath and sustain a vowel at a comfortable pitch and loudness level. Airflow is recorded on a computer attached to the pneumotachograph (Subglottal Pressure Monitor Suite; Glottal Enterprises).

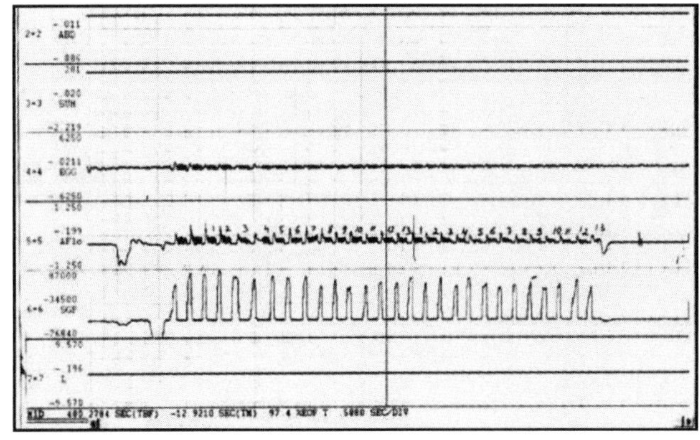

Figure 12-5. Pneumotachograph MS-100 and Pressure Transducer MS-100. Graph of normal airflow (AFLO) through the glottis and normal estimate of subglottal pressure (SGP) during repeated production of syllable /pi/ (clinical illustration by the author of this chapter).

Pressure Tranducer MS-100

The purpose for using the Pressure Transducer MS-100 (Glottal Enterprises) is to obtain an estimate of **subglottal pressure** (pressure under the vocal folds obtained through oral pressure). Excessively high pressure may reflect vocal strain and a pressed voice (overadducted) because normal airflow is being restricted by the high glottal pressure. A breathy voice may be the result of low pressure, where the vocal folds are not adducting properly to build up subglottal pressure, thus allowing excessive airflow. To obtain an estimate of subglottal pressure, the client sits upright, and a Rothenberg mask is placed over the client's nose and mouth. The client is instructed to take in a breath and repeat the sounds /pi, pi, pi/ at a comfortable pitch and loudness level. An oral pressure level is registered from the plosive sound /pi/ and recorded on the computer (see Figures 12-5 and 12-6 for normal and dysphonic waveforms of airflow and estimates of subglottal pressure waveforms). Compare the height of the airflow and pressure illustrations on normal and dysphonic readouts. The height of these parameters is greater on the dysphonic waveforms. An estimate of subglottal pressure is 4 to 8 cm of $H_2 0$ (Netsell, Lotz, Duchane, & Barlow, 1991). As noted, airflow can be observed during pressure tasks. A U-tube manometer

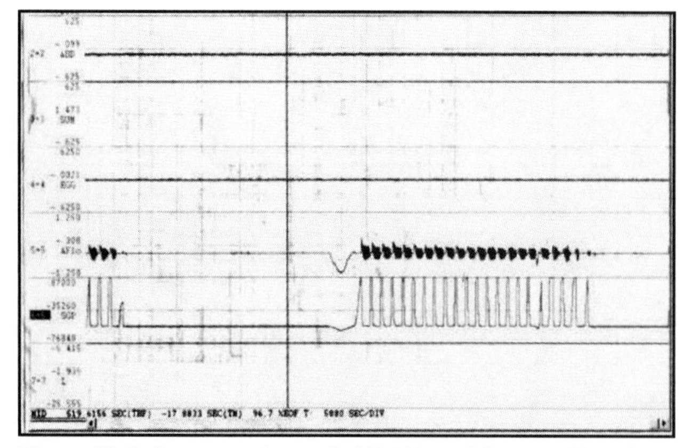

Figure 12-6. Pneumotachograph MS-100 and Pressure Transducer MS-100. Graph of excessive AFLO through the glottis and excessive SGP estimate during repeated production of syllable /pi/ (clinical illustration by the author of this chapter).

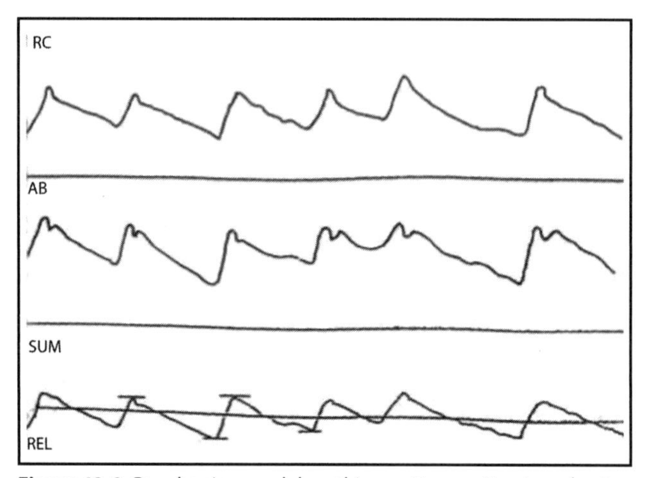

Figure 12-8. Dysphonic speech breathing pattern on Respigraph—termination of speech below REL (clinical illustration by the author of this chapter, Schaeffer et al., 2002). See third waveform, SUM section (the expiratory limb extends below the REL line).

measures static oral pressure (Baken & Orlikoff, 2000) and is low in cost.

Respigraph or Respitrace

The Respigraph (noninvasive monitoring system [NIMS]) is used to obtain an estimate of speech breathing. The instrument provides an estimate because the mouth and nose are not closed. One transducer band (changes one form of energy to another) is placed around the client's abdomen and one around the rib cage. The client must stand against a wall or stable object to keep from moving the transducer bands. The client is instructed to breathe quietly for 1 minute (to obtain tidal volume), which is a typical inspiratory and expiratory cycle(s) during quiet breathing (seen as the SUM of the rib cage and abdomen on the readout).

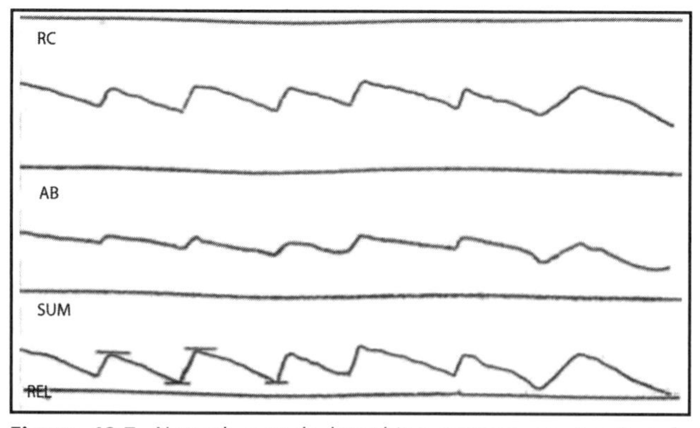

Figure 12-7. Normal speech breathing pattern on Respigraph. Termination of speech above REL (clinical illustration by the author of this chapter; see also Schaeffer et al., 2002). See third respiratory waveform, SUM section (the expiratory limb is above the REL line).

Tidal volume must be obtained to calibrate the instrument with the spirometer and to determine **resting expiratory level** (REL; resting expiration obtained during quiet tidal breathing). The client is then instructed to speak or read connected speech (e.g., a paragraph) at a comfortable pitch for the purpose of measuring speech breathing volume and its relationship to REL. If the client consistently extends speech volume into his or her **expiratory reserve volume** (the volume which extends below REL), he or she is not properly replenishing breath supply for breath support, especially if inspiration (which can also be seen on the readout) is inadequate. The literature has shown that participants with normal voices (both men and women typically terminate speech above REL; Figure 12-7), whereas participants with dysphonia tend to terminate speech below REL and exhibit lower end expiratory levels than participants with normal voices (Hixon & Putman, 1983; Hodge & Rochet, 1989; Koufman & Blalock, 1988; Schaeffer, Cavallo, Wall, & Diakow, 2002; Sperry, Hillman, & Perkell, 1994; Figure 12-8).

Low-cost or free software for voice analysis is the following: PRAAT software for voice analysis; RT Pitch; American Speech-Langugage-Hearing Association (ASHA) website for free or low-cost voice analysis software. Use a Google search to determine available choices. PRAAT has many of the evaluation aspects as the MDVP. As noted, a handheld spirometer is also available to measure vital capacity. Inexpensive speech breathing instruments may not be available. Pentax Medical in New Jersey has a computer program with regard to the Respitrace.

Informal Assessment and Behavioral Measures

The SLP can obtain pertinent data from informal measures, which in many cases confirm one another. The advantage of informal measures is that the clinician obtains a clinical and realistic impression of what the client can perform vocally as well as how the voice can be modified. The disadvantage of this assessment is that some of the measures are subjective (e.g., analysis of the speech sample). Results from informal and formal measures should confirm each other. For example, if the client has been judged to have a hoarse voice with informal measures, he or she would probably exhibit an aperiodic waveform on the EGG or a high jitter/RAP and/or shimmer value on the MDVP. If the client has a low MPT (cannot sustain a vowel to normal values, indicating air leakage through the glottis), he or she would probably exhibit a high airflow rate on the pneumotachograph.

Informal vocal tasks encourage the evaluator to listen for and record various aspects of the client's voice (e.g., glottal efficiency, pitch variation, intensity) and compare the results with normal values as well as with results derived from laboratory assessment. The SLP may obtain pertinent data from informal measures, which in many cases confirm formal measures. For example, a low MPT (i.e., sustaining a vowel for 8 seconds during informal testing, when 15 to 25 seconds are within normal range) correlates with a long opening phase and 30% peak closure on the EGG. Both the MPT and peak closure results indicate breathiness.

The advantage of informal measures is that the clinician obtains a clinical and realistic impression of what the client can perform vocally as well as how the voice can be modified. The disadvantage of this assessment is that some of the measures are subjective (e.g., analysis of a speech sample). As noted, results from informal and formal measures should confirm each other. For example, if a client has been judged to exhibit a hoarse voice on informal measures, he or she would probably demonstrate an aperiodic waveform on the EGG, or a high jitter/RAP and/or shimmer value on the MDVP. Similarly, if a client has a low MPT (cannot sustain a vowel to normal values, indicating air leakage through the glottis), he or she would probably exhibit a high airflow rate on the pneumotachograph.

If possible, it is ideal to evaluate a client's voice with both formal and informal measures (even if only one formal instrument is available) to obtain a complete and valid assessment of the client's vocal function.

Informal Measures

Oral-Peripheral Mechanism Examination

The rationale for performing this examination is to assess the adequacy of the oral structures and functions (e.g., strength and range of articulatory motion) for normal voice production, including assessment of the velopharyngeal movement. If the structures are inadequate or show reduced range or precision of movement, the voice may be negatively affected during speech. It is important for the clinician to be aware of these aspects, recognize their impact on voice production, note the implications for therapy, and make appropriate referrals. For example, if the client exhibits a reduced range of articulatory movement when speaking, feels pain when attempting to increase that range, or exhibits a tongue thrust and reverse swallow (which can affect speech and dentition), the SLP can make a referral to a dentist to further assess the problem.

Sample of Spontaneous Speech

The purpose of obtaining this uninterrupted monologue sample is to evaluate vocal quality, articulation, speech rate, speech breathing, prosody, intensity, resonance, and resulting intelligibility. These factors should be evaluated for patterns in terms of where the dysphonia occurs most often and how they interact and affect phonation.

It is important to tape record a running speech sample or narrative (without clinician interruption) using a high-quality recording instrument. When the client speaks without interruption, his or her vocal patterns can emerge (e.g., producing glottal attacks on initial vowels, losing voice at the ends of sentences, squeezing the voice at the ends of sentences, speaking without pausing to replenish breath supply).

Sample of Oral Reading (Tape Recorded for Assessment)

It is important to compare the client's vocal quality in varied linguistic contexts to determine if one speech situation enhances vocal quality in comparison to another context. For example, the client should read a passage aloud to determine if the visual guidance of punctuation markers has a positive effect on vocal quality.

Maximum Phonation Time

The purpose of MPT is to measure the duration of a maximally sustained vowel to assess glottal closure or efficiency. The client takes a deep breath/maximum inspiration (following the clinician's model) and sustains the vowel /a/ three times at a comfortable pitch and loudness level for as long as possible. A stopwatch is used to determine how many seconds the client can sustain the sound and whether the performance is within normal limits. The longest of the three trials is reported (Andrews, 1999; Behrman, 2007; Boone et al., 2010). Normal values are 15 to 20 seconds for adults (or higher) and 10 seconds for children. Any value lower than the data noted here suggests air leakage through the glottis or improper breath support for voice. For further clinical information, the client can sustain three different vowels such as /a/, /i/, and/u/ to determine which vowel facilitates the longest phonation.

S/Z Ratio

The purpose of the S/Z ratio task (Eckel & Boone, 1981) is to assess the integrity of glottal closure upon phonation. The /s/ and /z/ are produced in the same manner and place in the oral cavity; however, the /s/ is voiceless and the /z/ is voiced. The client is asked to take a deep breath and prolong /s/ as long as possible and then to follow through with sustaining /z/. The procedure is repeated three times. A stopwatch is used to time each prolongation, and then the longest /z/ is divided into the longest /s/ (e.g., $15 \div 9 = 1.6$, which is below the acceptable ratio). A ratio of 1 to 1.4 indicates that expiration time for /s/ closely matches the MPT of /z/. A ratio of 1.1 is perfect. Any value higher than 1.4 indicates a marked reduction in vocal duration and air leakage through the glottis on /z/ (the voiced phoneme; Behrman, 2007; Boone et al., 2010). For children, a ratio of 1 suggests a normal value (Pindzola, 1987). A sample chart is as follows:

S/Z Ratio Chart	
Age Range (Years)	*Duration (Seconds)*
7;0 to 10;0	8
11;0 to 15;0	12
16;0+ (women)	15
16;0+ (men)	20

Instructions for Obtaining the S/Z Ratio

1. Ask the client to take a deep breath and then to sustain the sound "s" for as long as possible at a comfortable pitch and loudness on one exhalation, without straining. Using a stopwatch, time (in seconds) how long the client can sustain the sound. Record the time in a table such as the sample under "duration of first /s/."
2. Repeat this procedure, this time using the sound "z." Record the time as "Duration of first /z/."
3. Repeat Step 1 and record the time under "Duration of second /s/."
4. Repeat Step 2 and record the time under "Duration of second /z/."
5. Calculate the S/Z Ratio by dividing the time of the longest /s/ by the time of the longest /z/ (see https://www.sltinfo.com/sz-ratio/).

Singing Up and Down the Musical Scale

The reason for this task is to determine the client's pitch range or variation, the efficiency of the voice on different notes, and the note on which the voice sounds best or is the least effortful. See the Andrews Protocol for various pitch range assessments (Andrews & Summers, 2002).

Dynamic Range (Counting)

Assessing vocal intensity helps to determine whether the client can use his or her voice efficiently and appropriately (not too loud or too soft) and vary the intensity without straining the voice, as well as to rule out any physiological problem. If the client's voice is too soft or weak, one of the difficulties may be related to insufficient mouth opening. In addition, varying loudness provides the examiner with the opportunity to examine changes in vocal quality with respect to alterations in loudness. Instruct the client to count from a high intensity to a low intensity and from a low intensity to a high intensity. See the Andrews Protocol in Andrews and Summers (2002).

Resonance Testing

If a resonance problem is suspected, testing is appropriate to rule out hyponasality and/or hypernasality. Have the client produce or read words beginning with nasals (e.g., nine, no, more, make, going) to specifically assess hyponasality or nasal resonance and words without nasals (e.g., pop, popeye, take, cup, sit) to further evaluate hypernasality or oral resonance. Pictures of words with nasals and without nasals can also be presented. See the Andrews Protocol (Andrews & Summers, 2002) for further resonance assessment tasks.

Additional Assessment Measures

- Voice Assessment Protocol (Pindzola, 1987): This protocol is organized to rate vocal quality, pitch, intensity, vocal effort, resonance, breath features, rate of speech, MPT, S/Z ratio, and diadochokinetic rate. This protocol is excellent because it delineates various choices to describe the parameters (e.g., hoarse, harsh, breathy) as well as different degrees of deviant production (e.g., severe, moderate, intermittent). The choices allow clinicians specificity in their assessments.
- *Guide to Vocology* (Verdolini, 1998): This manual describes various voice disorders, causes, and treatment in a concise practical format.
- *The Source for Voice Disorders Adolescent & Adult* (Schwartz, 2004): This manual provides an overview of anatomy and physiology of the vocal mechanism, vocal assessment tools (instrumentation and informal measures), descriptions of various dysphonias, a vocal hygiene questionnaire, and therapeutic strategies.
- Andrews Protocol (Andrews & Summers, 2002): This protocol provides specific tasks and parameters to measure respiration (speech breathing), vocal quality, onset of phonation, loudness, resonance, and pitch.

Stimulation or Facilitating Techniques (Performed After Informal Testing)

Stimulating the client with various facilitating techniques, or trial therapy, helps determine prognosis as well as which methods are most efficient in achieving the optimum voice. Trial therapy also guides the clinician to the starting point for treatment and in making appropriate recommendations in the diagnostic report.

The following tasks may facilitate improved voice production by having the client move out of his or her habitual manner of voice production. These tasks are provided to determine whether any of the vocal parameters improve upon production of these tasks. With certain exceptions, similar vocal techniques can initially be used for both abuse-related dysphonia and dysphonias associated with other types of disorders. For example, a similar method may benefit a person who is abusively overadducting his or her vocal folds, as well as someone whose dysarthria (e.g., spastic dysarthria) results in overadduction of the vocal folds. Conversely, a technique to facilitate vocal fold adduction in a person whose voice is severely breathy (secondary to a paralyzed vocal fold) could be too extreme for an individual with abuse-related breathiness (author's clinical experience).

Facilitating Techniques

1. Producing a phrase in a loud voice: This task may determine whether speaking in a loud voice (e.g., on a phrase) improves quality in terms of using increased breath support or if it increases the strain.
2. Producing a phrase in a soft voice: This task may determine whether speaking in a soft voice decreases strain in the vocal quality or causes increased breathiness.
3. Singing, to determine whether singing improves vocal quality and pitch variation (e.g., client sings "Happy Birthday" or "Good Morning to You").
4. Producing sentences with rising inflections (which elicit yes–no answers) to determine improved quality on rising inflection and ability to vary pitch. Questions should be short so that the client can focus on the ability to raise the pitch at the end of the sentence. *Examples*: Do you want to go?↑ Do you like pie?↑ Can you ski?↑ Are you hungry?↑ Will you see him?↑
5. Producing sentences with falling inflections (which elicit an answer, not a yes–no response) to determine improved quality on the falling inflection and ability to vary pitch. Questions should be short to focus on the falling inflection. *Examples*: What's your name?↓ Who came late?↓ When are they coming?↓ How do you feel?↓ Where are you going?↓ For these sentences, the pitch is usually higher on the first word.
6. Sustaining nasal sounds in single words (e.g., no, more, meat) and phrases (e.g., make meat, more milk) for clients with breathy voices to assess a decrease in breathiness. Ending the phrase with a plosive reduces continued breathiness. Other voiced sounds may be tried (e.g., good, good girl).
7. Producing words or phrases with voiceless consonants (e.g., cup, take, take time, pick two) for clients with pressed, strained voices to determine whether content with voiceless phonemes reduces over adduction.

Speech Breathing

1. Inhalation: To obtain an appropriate amount of air for inhalation, take a small breath through the mouth (not excessive for speech), without raising the shoulders. The diaphragm descends and the

abdomen extends (moves outward) to make room for the air.

2. Exhalation: For voice production, the abdomen moves inward allowing the air to be expelled and used for phonation in the exhalation phase of speech.

Because speech breathing is an essential component of supported voice, trial therapy is implemented during the evaluation to initiate the process of coordinating respiration (inhalation and exhalation) without voice, and then respiration (inhalation and exhalation) with phonation.

Trial Therapy (as Explained Under Speech Breathing)

- Respiration without phonation (trial therapy)
  - Take in (sip in) a little air and feel the abdominal muscles go out or extend.
  - Exhale (blowing out the air) and feel the abdominal muscles go in without phonation.
- Coordination of respiration with phonation on the vowel /u/
  - Sip in a little air.
  - Feel the abdominal muscles go out.
  - Upon exhalation, produce the vowel /u/ (with phonation) using a similar lip position to blowing out air without phonation.
  - Release body completely to get ready for the next task.
- Coordination of respiration and phonation on words and phrases for breathy voices
  - Initial voiced consonants are used to aid in adducting the vocal folds. Repeat speech breathing Steps 1 and 2 and, upon exhalation (Step 3), phonate words first and then phrases, beginning with voiced consonants (e.g., more, milk, blue moon, more milk) to gently adduct vocal folds "with support" to reduce breathiness. Release completely after each production of content to get ready for the next task or words.
- Coordination of respiration and phonation on words and phrases for pressed voice or over adducted vocal folds
  - Repeat the speech breathing steps (Steps 1 and 2) and, upon exhalation (Step 3), produce words and phrases beginning with voiceless consonants (take, pick, cake, take time) to reduce overadduction of the vocal folds. Release/pause completely after production of content to get ready for next task or words. The voiceless consonants that begin the word(s) can reduce the overadducted patterns of the client.
- Actively pulling in abdominal muscles for additional support and to take pressure off the larynx:
  - Actively pull in the abdominal muscles without phonation (without raising the shoulders) to feel the execution of this technique.
  - Repeat speech breathing (Step 1) inhalation and, upon exhalation (Step 2), engage or pull in the abdominal muscles simultaneously with phonation on a vowel. Extend this technique to appropriate words or phrases (e.g., words beginning with voiced or voiceless consonants) depending on whether the client's voice is breathy or pressed. In certain cases, the clinician may try both types of phonemes. Pause or release the body completely after producing the content, and inspiration may occur automatically to obtain breath for the next words or group of words. Closing the lips completely after each group of words or content aids in the release of the body or complete pausing after speaking.

In the spirit of addressing the whole person, all voice therapy is tailored to the individual's vocal needs (see the interview questions in Table 12-4). The following case history and example of a voice evaluation illustrate the reasons for the instruments and informal measures: (1) obtaining appropriate information from the client regarding voice background, (2) evaluating the client with appropriate measures/instrumentation to determine the points of difficulty, and (3) to recommend the most relevant goals for treatment.

Case History

N.D., a 25-year-old female, was seen for a voice evaluation in June 2008, after a referral from Dr. John Sanders, otolaryngologist, in April 2008. She was referred by a friend because of vocal hoarseness. N.D. was cooperative and served as her own informant. Medical history was significant for allergies and occasional migraine headaches.

Dr. Sanders viewed the client's vocal folds through both flexible and rigid endoscopic procedures. He reported bilateral vocal fold nodules, secondary to vocal abuse, and recommended voice therapy. He also noted acid reflux and prescribed Zantac (ranitidine). Medical history was otherwise uneventful. N.D. stated that her voice has been hoarse on and off for 5 years.

She is a third grade teacher and often speaks loudly to maintain the children's attention. She reported that she sings with the children and tends to run out of breath during this activity. N.D. also noted that she speaks continuously, and often above noise at home, to get her children's attention. She does not smoke or drink. Her voice is best in the morning and worse at the end of the day. She said the inconsistent hoarseness did not really bother her until she could "no longer talk." Additionally, she reported that she drinks one glass to no water each day.

Formal and Informal Procedures Selected With Rationales for the Choices

The following instruments were chosen because they provide acoustic values (e.g., degree of hoarseness—jitter/RAP and shimmer), vibratory information of the vocal folds (e.g., EGG to determine if the vocal folds are movement symmetrically), and respiratory and speech breathing information (aerodynamic measures). See areas explaining these instruments later in this chapter. If these instruments are not available, informal testing, implemented properly, can also measure the parameters of voice.

Formal Measures: Instrumental Assessment

- Acoustic Measures (used with a microphone)
  - MDVP will be used to obtain jitter/RAP and shimmer values by having N.D. produce the vowel /a/ into a microphone, as well as to determine her fundamental frequency.
  - Visipitch will be used to observe N.D.'s pitch range. The client will (a) phonate /a/ into a microphone and (b) subsequently increase and decrease range of phonation (pitch) from the lowest note to the highest note and from the highest note to the lowest note, respectively. Fundamental frequency will be obtained on the MDVP (as noted above) but can also be seen on the Visipitch (values may not be exactly the same).
  - Spectrograph will be used to obtain a visual display of (1) vocal fold vibration as per the vertical striations and (2) the quality of the client's formant frequencies.
- Vibratory Instruments
  - EGG will be used to obtain (a) a percentage of vocal fold contact, (b) to visualize the opening and closing phases of the waveform, and (c) to assess periodicity of the waveform.
  - Videostroboscopy (rigid endoscope) will be used by an otolaryngologist or a trained SLP to visualize the condition and function of the vocal folds upon phonation of the vowel /a/.
  - Fiber optics (flexible endoscopic) will be used by the otolaryngologist or trained SLP to visualize the condition and function of the vocal folds and arytenoid cartilages during dynamic speech.
- Aerodynamic Measures
  - Spirometer will be used to obtain the client's vital capacity and tidal volume.
  - Pneumotachograph will be used to measure the client's airflow rate.
  - Pressure transducer will be used to obtain an estimate of subglottal pressure.
  - Respitrace or Respigraph will be used to observe the client's speech breathing volume in relation to resting expiratory level.

Informal Measures

- Oral-peripheral mechanism examination is performed to determine the condition and function of the oral and velopharyngeal structures.
- Sample of spontaneous speech (where client speaks without interruption) will be taken to obtain a pattern of her voice as well as articulation and prosody aspects. The sample is tape recorded for analysis.
- Sample of client's oral reading is tape recorded for analysis/assessment.
- MPT is obtained to determine whether client can sustain a vowel within a normal number of seconds.
- S/Z ratio is obtained to determine if client can sustain /z/, a voiced sound, as long as she can sustain /s/, which is voiceless, for a normal S/Z ratio.
- Singing up and down the musical scale will be used to determine the client's pitch range and the note on which the voice is most efficient.

Stimulation or facilitating techniques to determine if voice improves:

- Reading aloud to be guided by punctuation to determine appropriate pausing
- Producing a phrase in a soft voice

- Producing a phrase in a loud voice
- Producing sentences with rising inflections
- Producing sentences with falling inflections
- Sustaining nasal sounds in single words (e.g., no, more, meat) (Because N.D. has vocal fold nodules, her voice is most likely breathy with noise.)
- Producing phrases with voiceless consonants (e.g., take time, pick two) for clients with pressed, strained voices.

Recommendations for Therapy

A. Therapy is recommended for 1 hour once a week.

1. Long-Term Goals
   - Client will eliminate all voice abuse and misuse.
   - Client will increase hydration to at least six glasses of water per day.
   - Client will use an efficient voice in all situations and with all persons.
2. Short-Term Goals
   - Client will monitor and eliminate abusive vocal behavior by keeping track on a chart.
   - Client will drink at least 6 to 8 glasses of water per day.
   - Client will increase coordination of inspiration and exhalation on (a) vowels, (b) words beginning with voiced sounds, (c) eventually words beginning with voiceless sounds, (e) phrases, and (e) sentences.
   - Client will pause appropriately between phrases and sentences to replenish breath supply.
   - Client will use an appropriate speech rate.
   - Client will (a) use **easy onset** on initial vowels and (b) **coarticulation** of final consonants with initial vowels to eliminate glottal attacks (e.g., come on).
   - Client will increase pitch variation.
   - Client will use all learned behaviors during sentence production, rhythmic verse, paragraph reading, structured spontaneous speech, and spontaneous speech (narratives and conversation).

B. Return to otolaryngologist after therapy to determine status of the vocal folds.

C. Client to use all learned techniques to maintain an efficient voice outside the therapy situation.

D. Marshfield Clinic-Vocal Hygiene Program (1995–2008; see Appendix 12-A).

Sample Report

Identifying Information

Name: N.D. **D.O.E.**:
Address: *(street)* **D.O.B.**:
(city, state, zip code) **Phone**:
Diagnosis: Voice disorder Age 25, female
Referred by: Dr. Natalie Schaeffer

Presenting Problem

N.D., a monolingual 25-year-old woman, is currently enrolled in her first semester at the Diana Rogovin Davidow Speech-Language and Hearing Center (DRDSLHC) at Brooklyn College, where she receives group voice therapy once weekly. She was referred by Dr. Natalie Schaeffer because of dysphonia characterized by a rapid rate, vocal noise, and a low pitch.

Background Information

Medical History

Medical history was significant for allergies and occasional migraine headaches. With regard to voice, the client was seen by Dr. John Sanders for an ENT evaluation in April 2008. The vocal folds were assessed through both flexible and rigid endoscopy. Dr. Sanders reported large bilateral vocal fold nodules, secondary to vocal abuse and recommended voice therapy. He also noted acid reflux and prescribed Zantac (ranitidine). Medical history was otherwise uneventful.

Voice History

N.D. stated that her voice has been hoarse on and off for 5 years. She is a third-grade teacher and often speaks loudly to maintain the children's attention. She also sings with the children and tends to run out of breath when she sings. N.D. also noted that she speaks continuously and often above noise at home to obtain her own children's attention. She does not smoke or drink. Her voice is best in the morning and worse at the end of the day. She said her voice did not really bother her until she could "no longer talk or get her voice out." Additionally, she reported that she drinks one glass to no water each day.

Family, Occupational, and Social History

N.D. lives with her husband and two children, a daughter age 2 years and a son age 4 years. She speaks English and Hebrew. As noted, she teaches third grade in the public school. N.D. described herself as a very social person who has long conversations on the telephone and gives speeches at social events.

Educational History

N.D. has a master's degree in education and plans on pursuing her doctorate in the future.

Voice Evaluation

Behavior

The client was cooperative during the entire evaluation and participated in all of the tasks presented.

Formal Testing

Multidimensional Voice Program

This program measures jitter (instability of pitch or fundamental frequency) and shimmer (instability of vibration of vocal fold amplitude). Normal and threshold jitter data are .345% and .680%, respectively, and normal and threshold shimmer values are 2.523% and 3.810%, respectively. N.D.'s jitter and shimmer values were higher than the foregoing data. Her threshold jitter value was 1.077%, and her threshold shimmer value was 4.821% (higher than normal and threshold values), indicating aperiodicity of vocal fold vibration or noise in the vocal signal. Fundamental Frequency was 180 Hz, which is low for a female (normal is 243 Hz), possibly related to increased mass of the vocal folds secondary to large bilateral vocal fold nodules.

Spectrograph

N.D.'s spectrogram reflected disconnected vertical striations (aperiodicity of vocal fold vibration and thus vocal noise) as well as weak bands of energy, indicating breathiness.

Visipitch

The client had difficulty increasing and decreasing her pitch range, and her waveform was a line with very little inflection.

Electroglottograph

The EGG readout showed reduced steepness of the closing phase, 30% vocal fold contact (average normal is 40% to 60%), a long opening phase and open phase.

Rigid and Flexible Endoscopy

The vocal folds were assessed with both flexible and rigid endoscopy. Dr. Sanders reported large bilateral vocal fold nodules (secondary to vocal abuse), incomplete glottal closure, and asymmetrical vocal fold vibration. He recommended voice therapy

Spirometer

N.D.'s vital capacity and tidal volume were within normal limits (5 liters and .5 liters, respectively).

Respigraph

N.D. read a paragraph while attached to the Respigraph. The results indicated that her end-expiratory values were all significantly below resting expiratory level.

Airflow Rate

The client's airflow rate was 400 mL/s, reflecting excessive airflow through the glottis. Normal airflow rate for most individuals is between 100 and 150 mL/s upon phonation.

Estimate of Subglottal Pressure

Although N.D. demonstrated excessive airflow rate, indicating incomplete glottal closure, estimate of subglottal pressure was high at 9 cm/H_2O, secondary to vocal fold strain (normal range of pressure is 4 to 8 cm/H_2O).

Informal Testing

Oral-Peripheral Speech Mechanism

Structures and functions of the oral and velopharyngeal mechanisms were adequate for normal voice and speech production.

Perceptual Assessment of Voice During Conversation

The client presented with a moderate-to-severe dysphonia characterized by strain, breathiness, noise, glottal attacks, and occasional phonation breaks. She spoke at the lower end of her pitch range (with limited pitch variation), squeezing her voice at the ends of sentences. She spoke with a rapid rate and did not pause to replenish her breath supply; both behaviors contributed to the dysphonia. Resonance was within normal limits, and vocal intensity (loudness) was reduced secondary to breathiness. Articulation per se was adequate for voice production.

Maximum Phonation Time

N.D. sustained the vowels /a/, /i/, and /u/ for 10 seconds each, indicating a leakage of air through the glottis (vocal folds); normal MPT is 15 to 20 seconds.

S/Z Ratio

N.D.'s S/Z ratio (the longest /s/ divided by the longest /z/) was 2.1, whereas the normal ratio is 1 to 1.4. She sustained the voiceless /s/ for 21 seconds and the voiced /z/ for 10 seconds. These results indicated a leakage of air through the glottis on the voiced sound /z/.

Singing Up the Musical Scale

N.D. had difficulty singing up the musical scale. Her voice lacked pitch variation and she did not reach the higher notes.

Dynamic Range (Loudness Level)

N.D.'s loudness level was within normal limits during spontaneous speech (between 65 and 70 dB SPL) on the sound pressure level meter, but she had difficulty obtaining increased intensity when attempting to produce a louder voice on the dynamic range test (counting from softer voice to louder voice).

Stimulability/Trial Therapy

N.D. responded well to the following tasks, demonstrating improved vocal production: sentences with rising inflections; sustaining nasals in single words (e.g., more, no, meat); reading aloud where she stopped at the comas and periods; singing; and when pulling in her abdominal muscles during voice production. She was also able to coordinate respiration and phonation on vowels and on words with nasals during trial therapy.

Clinical Impressions

The client presented with a moderate-to-severe dysphonia characterized by strain, breathiness, noise, glottal attacks, and occasional phonation breaks. N.D. spoke at the lower end of her pitch range (with limited pitch variation), squeezing her voice at the ends of sentences. She spoke with a rapid rate and did not pause to replenish her breath supply; both behaviors contributed to the dysphonia. Resonance and vocal intensity during conversation were within normal limits. Informal and formal testing revealed that numerical values were consistent with the perceptual assessment of dysphonia (e.g., breathiness and vocal noise). Additionally, formal values confirmed informal results.

Prognosis

Prognosis with voice therapy is good because N.D. responded well to trial therapy and appeared motivated to improve her voice.

Recommendations

Voice therapy two times per week, for 45-minute sessions, with the following goals:

- Long-Term Goals
    - Eliminate all voice abuse.
    - Increase hydration.
    - Use an efficient voice in all situations and with all persons.
- Short-Term Goals
    - Monitor and eliminate abusive vocal behavior by keeping track on a chart.
    - Drink at least six glasses of water per day.
    - Increase coordination of inspiration and exhalation without phonation.
    - Increase coordination of respiration and phonation on vowels; words beginning with voiced sounds; eventually words, phrases, and sentences beginning with voiced and voiceless sounds; and phrases and sentences with voiced and voiceless sounds.
    - Pause appropriately between phrases and sentences to replenish breath supply.
    - Use an appropriate speech rate.
    - Use easy onset of initial vowels and coarticulation of final consonants with initial vowels to eliminate glottal attacks.
    - Increase pitch variation.
    - Use all learned behaviors during rhythmic verse, paragraph reading, structured spontaneous speech, and spontaneous speech (narratives and conversation).
    - Return to otolaryngologist after therapy to determine status of the vocal.
    - Carry over new vocal behaviors outside of the therapy situation.

______________________________ Date ________

(Name of supervisor and credentials)
Speech-Language Pathologist

______________________________ Date ________

(Name of case manager writing this report and credentials)

______________________________ Date ________

Graduate Student Clinician

Case History

Read the following case history and create a list of formal and informal assessment tools as well as any other relevant assessment information. Write the list with a rationale regarding why you selected these particular instruments.

M.G., a 50-year-old woman, presented with a moderate-to-severe dysphonia characterized by overadducted vocal fold production, which resulted in a harsh, strained voice with noise and little or no pitch variation. She spoke very rapidly and did not pause to replenish her breath supply. She exhibited glottal attacks and often lost intensity at the end of her utterances.

Appendix 12-A. Marshfield Clinic Vocal Hygiene Program

A vocal hygiene program is important in terms of maintaining healthy laryngeal function. The following is reproduced from the Marshfield Clinic Vocal Hygiene Program with permission.

Vocal Hygiene Program

Dos

- **Use good breathing.** Abdominal-diaphragmatic breathing provides good support for singing and voice projection. When at rest, breathe through your nose with your lips closed, so that the air can be filtered and warmed.
- **Maximize relaxation throughout the body.** Do not use strained vocal productions. Use a good rate of speech and an open relaxed mouth and throat.
- **Talk in an easy manner and initiate vocal tones smoothly and effortlessly.** Hold your head straight when you talk. Do not strain the muscles of the face, throat, neck, and shoulders, particularly when talking and singing.
- **Use your optimal pitch and loudness.** Speaking at extremes of any dimension creates additional strain.
- **Rest your voice or pace yourself.** Talk when you wish but avoid singing or speaking for excessive amounts of time.
- **Do vocal warm-ups before singing or using the voice in unusual ways.** Take a few minutes to build from normal tone to the more forceful. This attracts blood to the larynx for more power.
- **Reduce general voice use before a performance.** Think conservation.
- **Use amplification when necessary.**
- **Drink at least four 8-ounce glasses of water daily.** By drinking fluids, which add water to the body, you enhance the mucus production of the throat and lessen vocal stress. Acceptable beverages:
  - Water
  - Decaffeinated soft drinks
  - Fruit juices
  - Decaffeinated coffee
  - Herbal tea
- **Have proper humidity in your house and classrooms, especially in the winter.** Ideal relative humidity is 40% to 50%. Avoid breathing through your mouth in cold weather.
- **Stay in good health.** Eat a balanced diet, exercise regularly, and get plenty of rest.
- **See a doctor if you think you have allergies.** These conditions can cause the vocal folds to swell and become inflamed, which creates more mucus and irritation on the folds. Milk and chocolate are common food allergies.
- **Know your medicines and their effects on your throat, mouth, and nose.** Antihistamines and diuretics will dry the vocal folds. Aspirin can promote their bruising.
- **Wear seat belts and shoulder straps when riding in a car.** Use of these devices may minimize laryngeal trauma in case of an accident.

Don'ts

- **Do not sing with a sore throat.** Avoid talking and singing when you have an upper respiratory infection such as a cold.
- **Do not cough, clear your throat, or sneeze with forceful voicing.** When you must, sneeze gently without voicing and use the method of silent coughing/throat clearing so that it is gentle and easy. Foods and liquids that tend to thicken saliva, such as whole milk and chocolate, should be avoided before a speaking or singing engagement.

- **Do not smoke or use tobacco products.** Avoid smoky or dusty places and breathing other airborne laryngeal irritants.
- **Do not abuse alcohol or caffeine.** Alcohol and recreational drugs have an adverse effect on your throat and breathing tract. Alcohol may interfere with your perception. Caffeine can cause the vocal folds to vibrate faster, leading to vocal fatigue.
- **Do not shout and scream.** Avoid loud laughing and cheering excessively.
- **Do not make strange noises with your voice, like using reverse phonation, abrupt glottal attack, or strained vocalizations.**
- **Do not yell.** Avoid speaking in places such as: around machinery, power lawn mowers, farm equipment; a stereo, hair dryer, or car radio; in a cafeteria, auditorium, or swimming pool. Avoid speaking loudly into the telephone. Avoid talking while using noisy transportation such as buses, trains, cars at high speed, motorcycles, and snowmobiles. When we shout, the vocal folds are knocked together and become irritated and sore.

Symptoms of Vocal Abuse

- Vocal fatigue after a period of voice use
- Throat irritation or soreness while talking
- Dryness, tickling, or choking sensation while talking
- Fullness or "lump" in throat
- Excess mucus in nose and throat
- Raspiness and/or hoarseness after use
- Loss of vocal range
- Volume disturbance
- Persistent hoarseness or inability to sing or speak with a clear voice after 24 to 48 hours of voice rest

Causes of Vocal Abuse

- Throat clearing and coughing
- Throat dehydration
- Voice strain (while talking and/or singing)
    - Too loudly
    - Too long
    - With a cold
    - Whispering
    - Over a throat irritation
    - When physically fatigued
- Smoking, breathing airborne irritants
- Drinking in excess
    - Alcohol
    - Caffeinated drinks

Appendix 12-B: Sample Intake Form

Name: ______________________ Today's Date: ______________________
Address: ______________________ Telephone: ______________________
Date of Birth: ______________________ Age: ______________________
Reason for Evaluation: ______________________ Referred by: ______________________

I. Family/Educational/Employment History

Family members with whom client lives (please note age and gender of children): ______________________

____

Languages spoken at home: ______________________

____

Describe any family history of speech/language voice problems: ______________________

____

Describe your present/previous employment/school: ______________________

____

II. Medical History

Have your ever been hospitalized? Yes ☐ No ☐
If yes, please explain, giving dates and location: ______________________

____

Do you have any chronic medical problems? Yes ☐ No ☐
If yes please explain: ______________________

____

Do you take medications regularly (other than vitamins?) Yes ☐ No ☐
If yes, indicate type and reason: ______________________

____

Do you have difficulty swallowing? Yes ☐ No ☐
If yes, please explain: ______________________

____

Do you or any member of your family have a hearing problem? Yes ☐ No ☐
If yes, please explain: ______________________

____

Have you had a complete audiological evaluation? Yes ☐ No ☐
If yes, please explain, giving dates, locations, and results: ______________________

____

III. Voice/Speech History

Describe your present speech/language/voice problem: ______________________

____

Describe the onset of the problem: ______________________

____

Was this problem present in childhood? Yes ☐ No ☐
Explain the suspected cause of the problem: ______________________

____

Why have you sought treatment at this time? ______________________

____

Does the problem bother you? Yes ☐ No ☐
If so why? ______________________________

____

Are other people aware of this problem? Yes ☐ No ☐
Explain: ______________________________

____

Please add any additional information related to the problem you feel is important for the evaluation.

____
____
____
____

Please answer the following questions with "yes" or "no." If "yes," explain the circumstances and frequency.
Do you have reflux? Yes ☐ No ☐
If yes, please explain when it first started and the doctor's report: ______________________________

____
____

Do you have allergies? Yes ☐ No ☐

____

Do you clear your throat often? Yes ☐ No ☐

____

Do you shout? Yes ☐ No ☐

____

Do you talk continuously? Yes ☐ No ☐

____

Do you sing? Yes ☐ No ☐

____

Do you act in plays? Yes ☐ No ☐

____

Do you smoke? Yes ☐ No ☐

____

Do you take drugs? Yes ☐ No ☐

____

Describe your voice before the present problem: ______________________________

____
____

Describe your present voice: ______________________________

____
____

Time of the day your voice is best: ______________________________

____

Time of the day your voice is worst: ______________________________

____

Attitude about voice: ______________________________

____
____

Glossary

Abduction: Open vocal folds, away from the midline.

Adduction: Closed vocal folds, toward the midline.

Airflow rate: The rate of air that flows through the glottis in a fixed period of time.

Aphonia: Without voice.

Breathy: Audible escape of air through the vocal folds (glottal insufficiency).

Coarticulation: Connecting the final consonant with a following word that begins with a vowel.

Diplophonia: Voice vibrating at two different frequencies (double voice).

Dysphonia: Voice disorder in terms of deviant quality, pitch, intensity, and resonance.

Easy onset: Easy phonation of words, especially on words with initial vowels.

Expiratory reserve volume: Maximum volume of air that can be expired beyond the end of a tidal expiration.

Fundamental frequency: Perceptual correlate of pitch, which is the rate of vocal fold vibration.

Glottal attack: Extremely abrupt, hard glottal closure, usually heard on initial vowels.

Glottis: Space between the vocal folds.

Harsh voice: Voice that is characterized roughness and noise.

Hoarse voice: Voice that is characterized by noise (aperiodicity) and breathiness.

Hyperfunctional voice: Characterized by excessive force, effort and strain.

Hypernasality: Excessive nasal resonance on nonnasal sounds.

Hyponasality: Insufficient nasal resonance on nasal sounds.

Intensity: Perceptual correlate of loudness.

Jitter/relative average perturbations (RAP): Instability of pitch or fundamental frequency regarding vocal fold vibration.

Maximum phonation time (MPT): Vowel prolongation for a measure of airflow rate during phonation, or the longest time that phonation can be sustained for a vowel sound.

Monopitch: Little or no pitch variation.

Phonation: Refers to voice production.

Phonation breaks: A temporary loss of voice on a syllable, word, phrase or sentence (related to prolonged hyperfunction of the voice).

Phonotrauma: Associated with abuse.

Pitch: Refers to the rate of vibration of the vocal folds, which should be normal for age and gender.

Pitch breaks: The voice may break an octave or two upward or downward; that is, the voice ascends or descends inappropriately (upward or downward).

Pitch variation: Refers to a normal range and inflection of voice/pitch.

Pressed voice: Voice characterized by over-adduction of the vocal folds and strain during phonation.

Resonance: The work of the resonating cavities (e.g., pharynx, oral cavity, nasal cavity), which amplify or dampen certain frequencies in the voice signal. See also *hypernasality* and *hyponasality*.

Resting expiratory level: The end of an expiratory cycle during tidal breathing.

S/Z ratio: A measure which obtains a ratio of voiced /z/ and voiceless /s/ in terms of the number of seconds each can be prolonged.

Shimmer: Instability of amplitude regarding vocal fold vibration.

Subglottal pressure: Pressure under the vocal folds which blows the folds apart.

Tidal volume: The amount of air inspired and expired during a typical respiratory cycle.

Vital capacity: The total volume of air that can be expired from the lungs following a maximum inhalation.

Vocal noise: Aperiodic or random distribution of acoustical energy, that is, noise in the vocal signal (roughness in the voice). A hoarse vocal quality incorporates noise and breathiness, whereas harshness incorporates strain and noise. However, a combination of these factors can exist in the various labels of voice.

Vocal strain: Effortful, tense vocal quality.

References

American Thoracic Society. (1987). Standardization of spirometry—1987 update. *American Review of Respiratory Disease, 136*, 1285-1289.

Andrews, M. L. (1999). *Manual of voice treatment: Pediatrics through geriatrics* (2nd ed.). San Diego, CA: Singular.

Andrews, M. L., & Summers, A. C. (2002). *Voice treatment for children and adolescents*. San Diego, CA: Singular.

Aronson, A. E. (1980). *Clinical voice disorders: An interdisciplinary approach*. New York, NY: Thieme-Stratton.

Aronson, A. E., & Bless, D. (2009). *Clinical voice disorders* (4th ed.). New York, NY: Thieme Medical.

Baken, R. J. (2010). Voice evaluation. In D. R. Boone, S. C. Von Berg, & R. I. Zraick. *The voice and voice* (8th ed., pp. 133-179). New York, NY: Allyn & Bacon.

Baken, R. J., & Orlikoff, R. G. (2000). *Clinical measurement of speech and voice* (2nd ed.). San Diego, CA: Singular.

Behrman, A. (2007). *Speech and voice science.* San Diego, CA: Plural.

Boone, D. R., McFarlane, S. C., & Von Berg, S. L. (2005). *The voice and voice therapy* (7th ed.). New York, NY: Allyn & Bacon.

Boone, D. R., McFarlane, S. C., Von Berg, S. L., & Zraick, R. I. (2010). *The voice and voice therapy* (8th ed.). New York, NY: Allyn & Bacon.

Campisi, P., Tewfik, T. L., Manoukian, J. J., Schloss, M. D., Pelland-Blaise, M., & Sadeghi, N. (2002). Computer assisted voice analysis. *Archives of Otolaryngology Head and Neck Surgery, 128*, 156-160.

Chen, Y., Robb, M. P., & Gilbert, H. R. (2002). Electroglottographic evaluation of gender and vowel effects during modal and vocal fry phonation. *Journal of Speech, Language and Hearing Research, 45*, 821-829.

Colton, R. H., & Casper, J. K. (1996). *Understanding voice problems: A physiological perspective for diagnosis and treatment* (2nd ed.). New York, NY: Lippincott, Williams & Wilkins.

Columbia University Medical Center. (n.d.). Voice and Swallowing Institute. Retrieved from http://entcolumbia.org/our-services/voice-and-swallowing-institute

Duffy, J. R. (1995). *Motor speech disorders: Substrates, differential diagnosis and management.* St. Louis, MO: Mosby.

Eastern Virginia Medical School. (2009). Vocal fold nodules and cysts. *EVMS Ear, Nose and Throat Surgeons.* Retrieved from http://www.evmsent.org/cysts_or_polyps.asp https://www.evms.edu/patient_care/specialties/ent_surgeons/services/laryngology/voice_disorders/vocal_fold_nodules_and_cysts/

Eckel, F., & Boone, D. R. (1981). The s/z ratio as an indicator of laryngeal pathology. *Journal of Speech and Hearing Disorders, 46*, 147-149.

Freed, D. (2000). *Motor speech disorders: Diagnosis and treatment.* San Diego, CA: Singular.

Haynes, W. O., & Pindzola, R. H. (2008). *Diagnosis and evaluation in speech pathology* (7th ed.). New York, NY: Pearson.

Hirano, M. (1981). *Clinical examination of voice.* New York, NY: Springer-Verlag.

Hixon, T. J., & Hoit, J. D. (2005). *Preliminaries. Evaluation and management of speech breathing disorders: Principles and methods.* Tucson, AZ: Redington Brown.

Hixon, T. J., & Putnam, H. B. (1983). Voice disorders in relation to respiratory kinematics. *Seminars in Speech and Language, 4*, 217-231.

Hodge, M. M., & Rochet, A. P. (1989). Characteristics of speech breathing in young women. *Journal of Speech and Hearing Research, 32*, 466-480.

Isshiki, N., Tanabe, M., Ishizaka, K., & Broad, D. (1977). Clinical significance of asymmetrical vocal cord tension. *Annals of Otolaryngology, Rhinology, and Laryngology, 86*, 58-66.

Jilek, C., Marienhagen, T., & Hacki, T. (2004). Vocal stability in functional dysphonia versus healthy voices at different times of voice loading. *Journal of Voice, 18*, 1-23.

Keith, R. L., & Darley, F. L. (Eds.). (1994). *Laryngectomy* (3rd ed.). Austin, TX: Pro-Ed.

Koufman, J. (2010). Vocal decompensation: A model of voice disorders. *Voice Institute of New York.* Retrieved from http://www.voiceinstituteofnewyork.com/vocal-decompensation-how-and-why-people-get-voice-disorders

Koufman, J. A., & Blalock, P. D. (1988). Vocal fatigue and dysphonia in the professional voice user: Bogart-Bacall syndrome. *Laryngoscope, 98*, 493-498.

Lombard, L. E., & Popovich, A. A. (2008). Laryngectomy rehabilitation. *Medscape.* Retrieved from https://emedicine.medscape.com/article/883689-overview

Marshfield Clinic. (1996). Vocal hygiene program. Retrieved from https://www3.marshfieldclinic.org/proxy///mc-cattails_vocalhygieneprogram.1.pdf

Morrison, M. D., & Rammage, L. A. (1993). Muscle misuse voice disorders: Description and classification. *Acta Otolaryngol (Stockh), 113*, 428-434.

Motta, G., Cesari, U., Lengo, M., & Motta, G., Jr. (1990). Clinical application of electroglottography. *Folio Phoniatrica, 42*, 111-117.

Murry, T., & Carrau, R. L. (2006). *Clinical management of swallowing disorders.* San Diego, CA: Plural Publishing.

National Institute of Neurological Disorders and Stroke. (n.d.). Myasthenia gravis information page. Retrieved from https://www.ninds.nih.gov/Disorders/All-Disorders/Myasthenia-Gravis-Information-Page

Netsell, R., Lotz, W., Duchane, A. S., & Barlow, S. M. (1991). Vocal tract aerodynamics during syllable production: Normative data and theoretical implications. *Journal of Voice, 5*, 1-9.

Orlikoff, R. F. (1991). Assessment of the dynamics of vocal fold contact from the electroglottogram: Data from normal male subjects. *Journal of Speech and Hearing Research, 34*, 1066-1072

Orlikoff, R. E. (1998). Scrambled EGG: The uses and abuses of electroglottography. *Phonoscope, 2*, 37-53.

Pentax Medical. (n.d.). Sona speech. Retrieved from http://www.pentaxmedical.com/pentax/en/99/1/Multi-Speech-Model-3700-Sona-Speech-II-Model-3650

Pindzola, R. H. (1987). *Voice assessment protocol for children and adults.* Austin, TX: Pro-Ed.

Sapienza, C. M., Stathopoulos, E. T., & Brown, W. S., Jr. (1997). Speech breathing during reading in women with vocal nodules. Journal of *Voice, 11*, 195-201.

Sasaki, C. T. (2008). Vocal cord contact ulcers. Merck manual: Consumer version. Retrieved from http://www.merckmanuals.com/home/ear-nose-and-throat-disorders/mouth-and-throat-disorders/vocal-cord-contact-ulcers

Schaeffer, N., Cavallo, S. A., Wall, M., & Diakow, C. (2002). Speech breathing behavior in normal and moderately to severely dysphonic subjects during connected speech. *Journal of Medical Speech-Language Pathology, 10*, 1- 18.

Schwartz, S. K. (2004). *The source for voice disorders: Adolescent & adults.* East Moline, IL: LinguiSystems.

Shprintzen, R. J., & Bardach, J. (1995). *Cleft palate speech management: A multidisciplinary approach.* St. Louis, MO: Mosby.

Sperry, E. E., Hillman. R. E., & Perkell, J. S. (1994). The use of inductance plethysmography to assess respiratory function in a patient with vocal nodules. *Journal of Medical Speech-Language Pathology, 2*, 137-145.

Stemple, J. C., Glaze, L. E., & Gerdeman, B. K. (1999). *Clinical voice pathology* (2nd ed.). San Diego, CA: Singular.

Sulica, L. (n.d.). Sulcus vocalis. Voice medicine. Retrieved from http://voicemedicine.com/disorders/sulcus-vocalis

Titze, I., (2017). Overcoming a worn out voice: Advice from a top voice scientist. *Voice Council Magazine.* Retrieved from http://www.voicecouncil.com/worn-out-voice-advice-from-voice-scientist-ingo-titze/

Verdolini, K. (1998). *Guide to vocology* (pp. 2-63). Salt Lake City, UT: National Center for Voice and Speech.

Vieira, M. N., McInnes, F. R., & Jack, M. A. (2002). On the influence of laryngeal pathologies on acoustic and eletroglottographic jitter measures. *Journal of the Acoustical Society of America, 11*, 1045-1055.

Vocal Health. (2009). Patient information. Retrieved from http://www.med.umich.edu/oto/vocalhealthcenter/patient/reflux.htm

Yasui, A. (2004). Objective study of vocal disorders using spectrograph. *Bulletin of Central Research Institute Fukoka University. Humanities, Series A, 4*, 35-46.

Zraick, R. I., Gregg, B. A., & Whitehouse, E. L. (2006). Speech and voice characteristics of geriatric speakers: A review of the literature and a call for research and training. *Journal of Medical Speech Language Pathology, 14*(3), 133-142.

13

Assessment of Fluency Disorders

Naomi Eichorn, PhD, CCC-SLP, TSSLD and Renee Fabus, PhD, CCC-SLP, TSHH

Key Words

- accessory behaviors
- avoidance behaviors
- blocks
- between-word disfluencies
- broken words
- cluttering
- clusters
- core behaviors
- covert stuttering
- disfluency
- dysfluency
- escape behaviors
- incipient stuttering
- interjections
- locus of control of behavior
- prolongations
- real-time analysis
- repetitions
- revisions
- running starts
- spontaneous recovery
- stutter-like disfluencies
- tremors
- within-word disfluencies

Introduction

Among the diverse speech and language disorders we work with as clinicians, fluency disorders seem to maintain a sense of ambiguity and challenge. We have certainly made great strides in understanding various potential causes of stuttering; nevertheless, a definitive notion of its etiology continues to elude researchers. By its very nature, stuttering is a condition of inherent contrasts. It involves surface features that are easily accessible for measurement and analysis, but is almost always complicated by a vast underlying set of emotions that are more difficult to label and organize but that are critical to our assessment and treatment. Sheehan (1970, p. 14) aptly described overt characteristics of stuttering as "the tip of the iceberg," an analogy that highlights the need for clinical protocols that take into account both symptoms that are perceptible as well as those that may be more challenging to observe but that play a critical role in driving the development of this disorder.

Our aim in this chapter is to present clinicians with an accessible assessment guide that, in the tradition of Sheehan's metaphor, considers both surface and underlying symptoms associated with stuttering. It is our hope that clinicians reading this chapter will feel empowered to help clients and parents through the diagnostic process more effectively and be able to mitigate the confusion and frustration often complicating this journey. Like many other challenging experiences,

Stein-Rubin, C., & Fabus, R. *A Guide to Clinical Assessment and Professional Report Writing in Speech-Language Pathology, Second Edition (pp 295-334).*

the process of understanding and treating stuttering often spurs a deep and ultimately rewarding form of self-exploration in which individuals who stutter discover, examine, and learn to change certain attitudes and psychological tendencies. It is a unique experience to be a catalyst for and to be a part of this process.

In the sections that follow, we provide an overview of stuttering disorders and describe a number of key parameters considered during the assessment process. We then review the specific components of an evaluation for three age groups: preschool children, school-age children, and adults. Our discussion focuses primarily on stuttering disorders rather than related fluency disorders such as **cluttering**, neurogenic stuttering, or psychogenic stuttering, although we do briefly consider the differential diagnosis of stuttering and cluttering. For more information on any of these topics, see the suggested reading list and websites provided at the end of this chapter.

Defining Stuttering

Most laypeople describe stuttering as chronic interruptions in the rhythm, flow, or fluency of speech. Researchers, too, have traditionally defined stuttering based on these general parameters (Andrews et al., 1983; Cordes, 2000; Sommer, Koch, Paulus, Weiller, & Buchel, 2002). What complicates this understanding is that a number of the behaviors observed in the speech of stutterers are, to some extent, observed in all speakers (Ambrose & Yairi, 1999; Wingate, 1964; Yairi, 1997). Ultimately, much of what we call "stuttering" is based on listener perceptions of what constitute "typical" or "atypical" types of interruptions in the flow of speech as well as listener-defined norms for the frequency with which these can occur before they become exceedingly distracting. As stated by Bloodstein, stuttering may be defined as "whatever is perceived as stuttering by a reliable observer who has relatively good agreement with others" (1995, p. 10).

Despite an ongoing lack of consensus, certain aspects of stuttering have been identified as critical to its definition and diagnosis. In one description of stuttering provided by the American Speech-Language-Hearing Association (ASHA, n.d.), emphasis is placed on specific types of **disfluency** that are present: "Stuttering... is an interruption in the flow of speaking characterized by **repetitions** (sounds, syllables, words, phrases), sound **prolongations**, blocks, interjections, and revisions, which may affect the rate and rhythm of speech. These disfluencies may be accompanied by physical tension, negative reactions, secondary behaviors, and avoidance of sounds, words, or speaking situations." According to Starkweather and Givens-Ackerman (1997), stuttering refers to discontinuities in speech that are not only excessive in frequency and duration, but that also add an unusual amount of physical and mental effort to the act of speech production. In his classic definition, Van Riper (1982) suggested that stuttering "called attention to itself" and distracted listeners from the intended message. Certain researchers (Perkins, Kent, & Curlee, 1991) have emphasized the need to look beyond all objective speech and nonspeech behaviors and defined stuttering as disruptions of speech in which the speaker experiences a loss of control. In the case of interiorized or **covert stuttering**, little to no overt stuttering behavior may be observed, and a speaker will outwardly "pass" as fluent by avoiding sounds, words, or situations in which stuttering is anticipated (Murphy, Lafayette, Quesal, & Gulker, 2007). Attempts to evaluate stuttering must consider surface features that may or may not be available for direct observation as well as deeper beliefs and fears that are more difficult to access and examine. This chapter attempts to integrate the various notions of stuttering described in the literature and is based on the understanding that stuttering involves not only a characteristic set of measurable behaviors, but also certain subjective experiences and perceptions that take on increasingly greater significance as a child grows and his or her stuttering evolves.

This perspective is reflected in the *International Classification of Functioning, Disability, and Health* developed by the World Health Organization (WHO; 2001), which recognizes that complex disorders, such as stuttering, involve not only physical impairment in structure or function, but also limitations on an individual's activities and restrictions on his or her participation in life. This more holistic approach encourages us to look beyond superficial behaviors observed in people who stutter and consider the broader health experience and real-life, everyday challenges associated with this disorder. This concept has been used as the basis for a number of assessment profiles and scales and is discussed further in our review of specific assessment measures later in this chapter.

Shapiro (2011, pp. 9 to 12) identifies three broad categories of stuttering definitions: (1) descriptive definitions, which focus on visible and/or audible stuttering behaviors; (2) explanatory definitions, which emphasize feelings and attitudes in the person who stutters; and (3) combined descriptive and explanatory definitions, which include both aspects of the disorder. The sections that follow describe an approach to the assessment of stuttering disorders that represents a combined descriptive and explanatory perspective to stuttering; that is, we present methods for measuring and understanding both overt and covert symptoms that may be present.

In defining stuttering, it is also useful to differentiate between the terms *disfluency* and **dysfluency**. Although the words are sometimes used interchangeably (often incorrectly), they are distinct in meaning. The prefix *dis-* implies a lack of something or the opposite of something; disfluency thus refers to speech that is simply not fluent. The prefix *dys-* has a more clearly negative connotation and refers to something atypical, difficult, or bad. Dysfluency thus implies that the lack of fluency is deemed abnormal. In general, it is preferable to use the term *disfluency* because this term encompasses both speech interruptions that are normal as well as those that may be abnormal. Referring to speech behaviors as "normal dysfluency" is obviously incorrect because the phrase represents an inherent contradiction of terms (for further detail on this topic, see Guitar, 2014, p. 5; Quesal, 1988; and Shapiro, 2011). In this chapter, we use the word disfluency to refer to all discontinuities in speech production, whether typical or atypical. Disfluencies that clearly represent a fluency disorder are referred to as stuttering.

Onset and Prevalence of Stuttering

Although a great deal of vagueness persists in how we define stuttering, there is much that we do know about the disorder and that has been confirmed consistently over years of research. First, a large number of typically developing young children demonstrate normal speech disfluencies between the ages of 2 and 5 years (Ambrose & Yairi, 1999), when they are experiencing rapid growth in the areas of speech and language. Early signs of stuttering, or **incipient stuttering**, are most likely to occur during this same period, when children are beginning to combine three or more words together (Bloodstein, 2006), and are differentiated from normal disfluencies based on specific speech characteristics that will be described in more detail below. The prevalence of stuttering is also highest among preschool children compared to school-age children and adults, with estimated prevalence rates of approximately 2.4%, 1%, and less than 1% for the three age groups, respectively (Andrews et al., 1983; Beitchman, Nair, Clegg, & Patel, 1986; Bloodstein & Bernstein Ratner, 2008, p. 79). Overall, the prevalence of stuttering is considerably higher before age 6 years than it is at later periods in life (Yairi & Ambrose, 2013). This consistent finding underscores the need for focused clinical training in dealing with specific concerns related to this age group, such as evaluating children's risk for persisting stuttering, counseling parents, and determining the need for direct or indirect forms of treatment, as appropriate.

These age-based variations reveal another important fact about stuttering that becomes critical in the diagnostic process, which is that a large number of preschool children who stutter experience "natural" or **"spontaneous" recovery** without any formal intervention or treatment. A prospective study by Kloth, Kraaimaat, Jansssen, and Brutten (1999), for example, found that stuttering symptoms subsided in 70% of young stuttering children followed over a 6-year period. Certain researchers (Ramig, 1993) have suggested that recovery rates may be somewhat more modest; however, most recent studies point to a more positive prognosis, with recovery rates as high as 88% or 91% (see Yairi & Ambrose [2013] for review). It is well accepted that a young child who stutters is by no means destined to a lifetime of stuttering, and the likelihood of a favorable outcome is high. Some children, however, will go on to develop chronic stuttering. To direct resources and effort where they are most needed, it is imperative for researchers and clinicians to identify factors that might help predict the likelihood of stuttering recovery or persistence.

Of all the child-related and speech-related variables examined in the literature, the factor most reliably associated with recovery is the child's gender, with girls being far more likely to outgrow early stuttering and boys being more likely to persist. Male-to-female ratios appear to be approximately equal at or near the onset of stuttering (Kloth et al., 1999) but steadily increase as children get older, with ratios ranging from 3:1 to 5:1 during school years, and higher ratios in adulthood (Andrews et al., 1983; Bloodstein & Bernstein-Ratner, 2008, p. 79; Curlee, 1999). This pattern is consistent with gender differences reported for a variety of other neurodevelopmental disorders (Baron-Cohen, 2008; Halpern, 1997; Shaywitz et al., 1995). Research in the area of early stuttering has identified a number of additional factors associated with greater likelihood of persistence or recovery (Ambrose, Yairi, Loucks, Seery, & Throneburg, 2015; Spencer & Weber-Fox, 2014; Ward, 2013); these are reviewed later in our sections on Key Assessment

Parameters (Related Measures) and Assessment of Stuttering in Preschool Children later in the chapter.

Characteristics of Stuttering: General Symptoms

Reported rates of spontaneous recovery vary widely in the literature, but it is clear that a considerable number of young children with disfluencies will develop chronic stuttering. This section provides an overview of general symptoms and characteristics of stuttering disorders and outline details to help clinicians differentiate between typical and atypical forms of disfluency. Three critical groups of symptoms are reviewed: **core behaviors** of stuttering, **accessory behaviors**, and emotional reactions.

Core Behaviors

The key feature of stuttering is the presence of involuntary discontinuities in the flow of speech. These are traditionally called *core behaviors* (Van Riper, 1982) and consist of three basic symptoms: repetitions, prolongations, and **blocks**.

Of all the core behaviors, repetition is the most common form of disfluency observed in both typically developing children as well as children who are demonstrating early stuttering (Ambrose & Yairi, 1999; Bloodstein & Bernstein Ratner, 2008, p. 31). Repetitions may occur at the phrase, single word (single syllable word and multisyllabic words), syllable, or sound level. The size of the speech unit affected plays an important role in classifying the disfluency as typical or atypical. In general, the smaller the unit being repeated, the more likely it is that the behavior represents stuttering. This concept is considered further in our later discussion of **stutter-like disfluencies** (SLD).

Prolongations are disfluencies in which sound or air flow continues but movement of the articulators is stopped and can occur on continuant consonants (s, f, th, sh, v, z, w, r, l, y) or vowels. Prolongations are generally judged by listeners to be an atypical form of disfluency (Cordes, 2000) and are most often observed later than repetitions, although they are sometimes reported at the onset of stuttering as well (Yairi, 1997).

Blocks involve stopping of both airflow and sound during the production of speech. Blocks are usually the last core symptom to be observed in the development of stuttering and are almost always perceived by listeners as an abnormal type of disfluency. Some researchers (Schwartz, 1974) have suggested that blocking is caused by inappropriate tensing of muscles at the level of the glottis; however, others believe this obstruction may occur at the respiratory, laryngeal, and/or articulatory levels of speech production (Guitar, 2014, p. 15).

Two additional behaviors may be observed in individuals who stutter. Both tend to be somewhat less common and are generally perceived as atypical (Cordes, 2000). **Broken words** are blockages in the middle of a vowel, during which there is audible laryngeal tension, followed by abrupt reinitiation of the vowel. **Tremors**, often observed in individuals with advanced forms of stuttering, involve rapid fasciculations (small involuntary contractions or twitching) of the speech muscles.

A final group of disfluencies includes behaviors that are less likely to be considered atypical based on listener perceptions (Cordes, 2000; Zebrowski & Conture, 1989), but that may occur with excessive frequency in the speech output of people who stutter. These behaviors are sometimes categorized as forms of **avoidance** (discussed in more detail below) rather than core behaviors since they may represent attempts on the part of the speaker to gain control of his or her speech or avoid an anticipated block. These disfluencies include **interjections** (often called *fillers*), in which speakers insert extraneous, meaningless words or phrases such as "um," "you know," or "like" into the flow of connected speech; **running starts**, in which speakers return once or several times to the beginning of a thought or sentence in an attempt to regain fluency; and **revisions**, in which phrases or whole sentences are reformulated, often to avoid anticipated difficulties on specific words or sounds.

Because many of the preceding disfluencies are observed in normal speakers, a great deal of effort has been made by both researchers and clinicians to distinguish between those behaviors that are more or less likely to represent symptoms of stuttering. One classification system reviewed by Zebrowski and Kelly (2002) divides disfluencies into two broad categories: **between-word disfluencies**, which include all difficulties that occur while a speaker is attempting to link words together (phrase repetitions, interjections, running starts, revisions), and **within-word disfluencies**, which include all discontinuities that interfere with the smooth transitioning between sounds or syllables within a word (sound repetitions, syllable repetitions, prolongations, blocks, broken words).

Table 13-1. Types of Disfluency

Core Behavior	*Example*	*Between- vs. Within-Word Disfluency*	*Stutter-Like Disfluency*
Phrase repetition	"I want–I want to go now"	Between	No
Word repetition (multisyllabic)	"Cinnamon-cinnamon-cinnamon and sugar"	Between	No
Word repetition (single syllable)	"He-he-he wants some water"	Within	Yes
Syllable repetition	"The par-par-party is at 6:00"	Within	Yes
Sound repetition	"My name is D-D-D-David"	Within	Yes
Sound prolongation	"I fffffeel good"	Within	Yes
Block	"Do you [tense pause, often with fixed articulatory posture for subsequent sound] want some?"	Within	Yes
Broken word	"Gi-[silent pause]-ive it to me"	Within	Yes
Interjections	"I, um, like to travel"	Between	No
Running start	"She wants to go with us to the-she wants to go with us to the fair"	Between	No
Revision	"I really like to-I really love ice-cream"	Between	No

Within-word disfluencies are sometimes called SLD (Yairi, 1997) and are generally understood to be more closely associated with chronic forms of stuttering. Accurate classification of monosyllabic whole-word repetitions is somewhat ambiguous and has been the subject of ongoing debate (Howell, 2013; Riley, 2009; Wingate, 1964, 2001; Yairi & Ambrose, 2013). Developmental data by Yairi and his colleagues (Ambrose & Yairi, 1999; Throneburg & Yairi, 2001) indicate that monosyllabic word repetitions occur significantly more frequently in children who stutter than in fluent children and represent a large proportion (33% to 39%) of the total SLDs produced by children whose stuttering persists. In keeping with recommendations by this group and others (Yaruss, 1998), we recommend categorizing repetitions of single-syllable words as within-word disfluencies or SLDs and repetitions of multisyllabic words as a form of between-word disfluency. However, clinicians should note recent findings by Howell (2013), who found that Stuttering Severity Instrument-3 (SSI-3) scores more accurately classified stuttering and fluent school-age children when data were analyzed without including single-syllable whole word repetitions. Table 13-1 summarizes the various forms of disfluency along with examples of each behavior and their classification based on the two systems presented.

Accessory Behaviors

As disfluencies persist, the person who stutters begins to develop an awareness of his or her difficulties. It is at this point that the disorder starts to become more complex and often more severe, as layers of perceptions, expectations, feelings, and attitudes begin to take root beneath the surface symptoms. The emergence of accessory behaviors is often one of the first signs that a child's stuttering is probably not developmentally typical (Zebrowski & Kelly, 2002, pp. 15-16) and that it has progressed from its earliest form. These behaviors, sometimes referred to as *secondary behaviors*, *secondary stuttering characteristics*, *secondary mannerisms*, *extraneous behaviors*, or *concomitant behaviors*, represent the reaction of the person who stutters to his or her speech difficulties and usually begin as a random struggle, through which the speaker tries to push out of involuntary repetitions, prolongations, and blocks.

Over time and with repetition, these behaviors are reinforced and become learned patterns that accompany core disfluencies. These behaviors may take the form of speech-related movements such as lip pressing, lip pursing, or teeth clenching; extraneous body movements such as eye blinking, head jerking, fist clenching, or stamping; or stereotypic speech utterances such as interjections, running starts, or circumlocutions, in which the speaker uses evasive or wordy substitutions to avoid an anticipated disfluency. According to Guitar (2014, p. 16), accessory behaviors can be described as either **escape behaviors** or avoidances. Escape behaviors represent the speaker's attempt to release him- or herself from the block (e.g., by blinking, moving head, or stamping feet). Avoidance behaviors, on the other

Table 13-2. Categories of Accessory Behaviors		
	Escape Behaviors	*Avoidance Behaviors*
Purpose	Terminate block	Circumvent anticipated disfluencies
Examples	Blinking, moving head, stamping feet	Word substitutions, stalling, using starters

hand, are used to circumvent the moment of disfluency altogether and may include behaviors previously used as escapes or new behaviors such as substituting words, postponing feared words, or using starters. As mentioned earlier, covert stutterers may use avoidance strategies so extensively that they are unable to speak without habitually avoiding sounds and words and uncontrolled moments of disfluency will rarely be available for observation altogether. Table 13-2 summarizes these categories of accessory behaviors.

Emotional Reaction

Ongoing struggle in the production of speech gradually results in deep-rooted feelings of shame, frustration, anger, anxiety, fear, negative self-perceptions, and, eventually, habitual avoidance of speaking situations. Young children may already manifest strong emotional reactions to their stuttering by 5 years of age, or even earlier (Bloodstein, 1995, p. 49), and there is evidence that individual differences in children's temperament may be a contributing factor to early stuttering and its likelihood of persistence (Kefalianos, Onslow, Block, Menzies, & Reilly, 2012; Jones, Choi, Conture, & Walden, 2014). Some children may stop talking for several days or develop a habit of asking parents to speak for them. Older children may avoid oral presentations or voluntary participation in class. Adults may avoid the telephone and begin withdrawing from social situations. Starkweather and Givens-Ackerman (1997, p. 34) described a startling form of avoidance in which individuals who stutter may "lose touch" with their surroundings and what they are doing, presumably to block out the pain and negative experience associated with their stuttering.

Key Assessment Parameters

This section outlines key parameters to be considered in the assessment of a client who stutters. These parameters form the basis for many of the formal and informal measures designed for evaluating stuttering. Although the availability of published protocols makes it possible for clinicians to evaluate stuttering using standardized materials and scoring, we hope the details provided in this section will help clinicians understand the basic components from which these measures are derived as well as the criteria used to arrive at specific clinical decisions.

Certain components of stuttering disorders, such as the presence and severity of disfluencies, are relatively simple to measure and quantify. Other aspects of stuttering, such as the extent to which an individual may be reacting to his or her disfluencies, may be more difficult to analyze. Ideally, assessment of fluency must examine core behaviors as well as attitudes, perceptions, and reactions to stuttering. Following is a list of general areas explored in most fluency evaluations. When available, we include normative data so that clinicians can determine whether certain observed behaviors are atypical.

Measurement of Core Behaviors

Because certain core behaviors are present in the speech of fluent speakers, a key clinical question is how to differentiate typical disfluencies from those that signify a stuttering disorder. This can be accomplished by looking at specific characteristics of the core behaviors:

- Disfluency types: In the preceding section on core behaviors (see Table 13-1 for a summary), we identified specific types of disfluencies (e.g., phrase repetitions, interjections) that are more likely to be considered normal disfluencies, and other types (e.g., sound repetitions, prolongations, blocks, broken words) more likely to be perceived by listeners as atypical. Recording the types of disfluencies observed helps the clinician determine the presence and severity of a stuttering disorder. A useful worksheet is provided later in the section on core assessment procedures. Specific questions to consider are as follows:
    - Do disfluencies primarily comprise typical disfluencies or atypical disfluencies?
    - What is the proportion of within-word disfluencies to between-word disfluencies? The same question can be framed using the terms SLDs and other disfluencies (ODs). How much of the total number of disfluencies do the SLDs represent? Occasional SLDs may be present in speech produced by nonstuttering children; however, the proportion of SLDs to ODs will

differ significantly between children who do and do not stutter. According to Yairi (1997), the proportion of SLDs to the total number of disfluencies will typically be 36% to 50%. Children who stutter, on the other hand, tend to show an average of at least 65% SLDs.

  - What is the specific frequency of within-word disfluencies (or SLDs)? On the basis of data reviewed by Yairi (1997), we know that preschool children who stutter produce at least three to four SLDs per 100 syllables, whereas nonstuttering children produce fewer than three SLDs for the same total number of syllables.

- Frequency of disfluencies: Examining the amount of disfluency present can provide information about the presence and severity of a stuttering disorder and is usually measured as the number of disfluencies per 100 words or syllables. In general, it is preferable to use measurements based on syllable counts in order to capture multiple disfluencies that may occur on multisyllabic words and to be able to form accurate comparisons between disfluency counts obtained during the preschool years, when single syllable words predominate, to later years, when use of multisyllabic words increases.

  It is well-established that, as a group, children who stutter produce more disfluencies than nonstuttering children; however, there tends to be some degree of overlap between groups. This fact makes it difficult to differentiate stuttering from normal disfluency on the basis of frequency alone. Nevertheless, considerable data for both children and adults who stutter suggest that the presence of more than 10 disfluencies per 100 words is a valid cause for concern (Adams, 1980; Bloodstein & Bernstein Ratner, 2008, p. 318; Yairi, 1997; Yaruss, 1998). Similar findings are reported for frequency counts that are based on syllables rather than words. Yairi (1997) found an average of 17 disfluencies per 100 spoken syllables in preschool children who stuttered, and 19 to 20 disfluencies per 100 syllables in slightly younger children who were closer to the onset of stuttering. In contrast, nonstuttering children produced only 6 to 8 disfluencies for the same total number of syllables. Other researchers (Pellowski & Conture, 2002) focus specifically on SLDs and suggest that the presence of more than three SLDs per 100 words represents incipient stuttering rather than typical developmental disfluencies. This criterion is similar to Yairi's (1997) findings related to the frequency of SLDs in stuttering preschoolers, as described earlier. For additional information on counting the frequency of disfluencies, readers are referred to the sample worksheet provided later in this chapter in the section on assessment aims and procedures. The worksheet is designed for a 100-syllable speech sample; however, clinicians can design their own tables to accommodate any number of syllables and follow instructions provided to derive the percentage of stuttered syllables (or percentage of stuttered words).

- Presence of **clusters**: Clusters are defined as the occurrence of two or more disfluencies on the same word or utterance (e.g., "I-I-I went to the b-b-beach"). Several researchers have suggested that clusters may be a useful marker of early stuttering based on studies showing a much greater prevalence of clusters in the speech of stuttering children compared to nonstuttering children (Hubbard & Yairi, 1988; LaSalle & Conture, 1995; Logan & LaSalle, 1999). According to Zembrowski and Kelly (2002), children with three or more clusters of disfluencies in a 100-syllable sample should be considered to be stuttering or "at risk" for stuttering. Findings by Robb, Sargent, and O'Beirne (2009) indicated that disfluency clusters continue to be a feature of stuttering in adults and that the frequency of clusters is positively correlated with overall percentage and severity of disfluency.

- Duration of disfluencies: The duration of certain disfluencies, such as repetitions, can be measured as the number of reiterations (repetitions beyond the initial production); however, the duration of most other forms of disfluency is described as a length of time (typically in seconds). According to Bloodstein and Bernstein-Ratner (2008, p. 3), measurements of duration have limited usefulness for describing the severity of stuttering in adults because most adults who stutter do not vary very much from each other in this particular feature. Nevertheless, the duration of disfluency is recommended by a number of researchers (Yairi & Lewis, 1984) for the differential diagnosis of typical vs. atypical disfluency in young children and can be quite helpful in clinical practice. These findings are summarized in Table 13-3.

- Weighted SLD: This measure is helpful in distinguishing stuttering from normal disfluency and reflects the combined dimensions of frequency of

Table 13-3. Differentiating Incipient Stuttering and Normal Disfluency Based on Duration

Disfluency	*Incipient Stuttering*	*Normal Disfluency*	*References*
Within-word repetitions (sound, syllable, or single-syllable words)	More than two reiterations (e.g., "b-b-b-ball")	Fewer than two reiterations (e.g., "b-ball")	Adams (1980), Curlee (1980), Van Riper (1982), Yairi & Lewis (1984)
Prolongations	Longer than 1 second	Less than 1 second	

disfluency, extent of repetitions, and disfluency type (Ambrose & Yairi, 1997). As demonstrated by these authors, a score of 4 weighted SLDs per 100 syllables can reliably differentiate the two forms of disfluencies, with stuttering children falling above this boundary and nonstuttering children falling below. Specific guidelines for calculating the weighted SLD are described later (see Assessment Aims and Procedures).

Observation of Accessory Behaviors

The presence of accessory behaviors reflects the child's growing awareness of his or her stuttering and is evidence of increasing struggle. Most often, accessory behaviors emerge during early elementary years and gradually become part of the child's chronic stuttering pattern. Some children, however, display associated behaviors as early as 1 month following the onset of stuttering (Zembrowski & Kelly, 2002). Either way, the presence of these symptoms unequivocally differentiates between typical disfluency and stuttering because nonstuttering children do not produce secondary characteristics when they are disfluent. To measure these characteristics, the clinician must carefully note extraneous behaviors that occur specifically during moments of disfluency (general movements or behaviors that are observed during both fluent and nonfluent speech production, such as nervous tics or habits, are excluded). Accessory behaviors may include one or more of the following:

- Closing eyes
- Blinking rapidly
- Squeezing eyes shut
- Looking around
- Moving eyes vertically or laterally
- Consistent loss of eye contact
- Throwing head back
- Torso or limb movements
- Foot, hand, or finger tapping
- Audible inhalation or exhalation
- Gasping
- Visible tension around face or mouth
- Facial grimacing
- Lip pursing or pressing
- Tongue clicking
- Sudden changes in vocal pitch, loudness, or quality
- Word substitutions or circumlocutions
- Stalling

It is important to keep in mind that stuttering can sometimes be almost entirely covert, with no observable symptoms at all. In such situations, the person who stutters has become so adept at substituting words and avoiding disfluencies that he or she does not actually appear to be stuttering. This is the portion of the "iceberg" that is completely hidden from view but that may be a powerful negative force within the person who stutters. In such situations, a diagnosis of stuttering may be based on the individual's perception of him- or herself as a person who stutters and the shame, anxiety, fear, and avoidance behaviors that typically accompany this perception. For further information related to the evaluation of covert symptoms associated with stuttering, see the later discussion on assessment of psychological reaction and avoidance behaviors.

Assessment of Variability

An important but sometimes confusing aspect about stuttering is the inconsistencies with which symptoms are observed, particularly in young children. Near onset, parents will often report that the child's stuttering "comes and goes" or that it fluctuates in severity, depending on a variety of factors such as the child's fatigue, level of excitement, familiarity with the listener, or other specific characteristics related to the setting or the nature of the interaction. To some degree, fluctuations in disfluency are typical for all individuals who stutter; however, it is helpful to determine the extent to which the disorder may vary in a particular speaker and whether there are specific factors or situations that precipitate greater fluency or disfluency. Perhaps most critical is to establish whether the level of disfluency observed during an

Table 13-4. Sources and Examples of Variability

Sources of Variability	*Examples*
Setting	Home, clinic, school
Speaking task	Free-play, play with pressures imposed, story retell, picture description, monologue, dialogue, reading
Conversational partner	Parent, clinician, friend, teacher, employer, spouse
Number of conversational partners or listeners	1:1 vs. group interaction
Conversational medium	In person, over telephone, in presence of a recording device
Conversation topic	Factual vs. personal/emotional
Time	Different times of day, weekday vs. weekend, typical schedule vs. vacation
Nature of speaking situation	Casual conversation, argument, interview, formal presentation

Adapted from Yaruss (1997).

evaluation is typical for that individual. In Table 13-4, we list a number of factors associated with variability in stuttering severity. Although it is not practical or even desirable to measure all of these factors, we encourage you to consider how each potential source of variability may affect specific clients and to measure this variability directly when appropriate.

Assessment of Psychological Reaction and Avoidance Behaviors

Most people with chronic forms of stuttering gradually begin to try avoiding disfluencies. Paradoxically, the struggle to avoid stuttering only serves to intensify the disorder by adding layers of accessory behaviors and anxiety, which can become quite pervasive. Many theories of stuttering, such as Bloodstein's (1995, pp. 63-67) anticipatory struggle hypothesis, emphasize the ways in which negative perceptions and beliefs exacerbate and complicate stuttering disorders. Even individuals with mild forms of stuttering may react significantly to disfluencies, showing very negative attitudes about their stuttering, extreme forms of self-criticism, and hypervigilance about their speech production (Leith, Mahr, & Miller, 1993). Gaining insight into these beliefs and attitudes is therefore an integral component of the diagnostic process.

Over the past several decades, many protocols have emerged to help clinicians examine different attitudinal and emotional reactions to stuttering. Although there is no single instrument that provides a comprehensive assessment of all of the possible psychological sequelae of stuttering, each protocol will help clinicians learn about specific ways in which a client may perceive and feel about his or her stuttering, communicative abilities, and social situations in general. Table 13-5 lists some of the broad areas considered in these scales with sample questions that might be presented to the person who stutters, often in written form. Typically, scales are developed by administering sets of questions or statements to both people who stutter and people who do not. Participants indicate whether individual statements or questions are characteristic of them. These responses provide the basis for profiles that are considered typical of individuals who stutter or typical of nonstutterers. Later in the chapter, we present references and details regarding specific protocols available for clinical use.

Assessment of Locus of Control of Behavior

A concept closely related to attitudes and perception is that of **locus of control of behavior** (LCB). This idea was popularized by social psychologist Julian Rotter (1966) through his development of a published scale to measure this construct. His original scale has since been adapted to evaluate perceptions of control in people who stutter (e.g., Locus of Control of Behavior developed by Craig, Franklin, & Andrews, 1984). Locus of control refers to the extent to which an individual attributes the outcome of events to external circumstances, such as luck, coincidence, and environmental factors, vs. internal factors, such as personal abilities and effort. In general, individuals who locate control outside of themselves believe that they have less control over their fate and tend to be more stressed and depression-prone as a result. A

Table 13-5. Measuring Psychological Reaction to Stuttering

Psychological Reaction to Stuttering	*Sample Statements and Questions*
Expectancy (anticipating difficulty)	• Do you help yourself get started talking by laughing, coughing, clearing your throat, or gesturing? • Do you anticipate difficulty on particular words or sounds? • Do you repeat a word or phrase preceding the word on which stuttering is expected? • Do you substitute a different word or phrase for the one you intended to say? • Do you make your voice louder or softer when stuttering is expected? • Do you whisper words to yourself or practice what you will say before you speak?
Attitudes about communication and perceptions of self as a communicator	• I usually feel that I am making a favorable impression when I speak. • It is easy to speak with anyone. • I socialize and mix with people easily. • My speaking voice is pleasant. • I have confidence in my speaking ability. • I dislike introductions. • I cannot speak to aggressive people. • People's opinions about me are based primarily on how I speak. • How much does stuttering interfere with your sense of self-worth or self-esteem?
Avoidance	• Do you respond briefly to questions using as few words as possible? • Do you withdraw from situations requiring verbal participation? • Do you avoid use of the telephone? • Do you give excuses to avoid talking (e.g., feigning fatigue or lack of interest in topic)? • Do you ask others to speak for you in difficult situations (e.g., have someone order food for you in a restaurant)? • Do you use gestures as a substitute for speaking (e.g., nodding your head instead of saying "yes" or smiling to acknowledge a greeting)?
Social anxiety or phobia	• I'm of no use in the workplace. • People will think I'm incompetent. • I'm hopeless. • People will think I'm strange. • Everyone will think I'm an idiot. • No one would want to have a relationship with someone who stutters. • I embarrass the people I speak with. • People will laugh at me. • Everyone hates it when I start to speak.

Sample questions and statements adapted from Perceptions of Stuttering Inventory (Woolf, 1967); Unhelpful Thoughts and Beliefs about Stuttering (UTBAS) scale (St. Clare et al., 2009); S-24 Scale (Andrews & Cutler, 1974); and Overall Assessment of the Speaker's Experience of Stuttering (Yaruss & Quesal, 2006).

number of researchers have examined LCB in people who stutter with somewhat equivocal findings. First, it is unclear whether people who stutter actually differ from nonstutterers in LCB, particularly when measuring overall LCB rather than locus of control beliefs related specifically to speech production (McDonough & Quesal, 1988). Moreover, LCB scores may not be associated with treatment outcome in any predictable way (De Nil & Kroll, 1995), although certain researchers have provided evidence to the contrary (Craig & Andrews, 1985). Nevertheless, one's belief that he or she is a victim of his or her stuttering and has no control over the disorder is certainly an important assumption to be aware of and to examine in fluency assessment. Table 13-6 lists several statements and questions drawn from the Mastery-Powerlessness

Table 13-6. Sample Questions and Statements to Assess Locus of Control of Behavior
*Locus of Control Scale**
• If you had a job that did not have automatic pay raises, would you: (1) ask for one when you thought you deserved it or (0) wait until it was offered to you?
• When you have an accident at home or at work, do you usually blame it on: (0) bad luck or the carelessness of others or (1) your own negligence?
• At a social gathering, who usually takes the lead in choosing the topics of conversation: (0) the person I'm talking with or (1) myself?
• If you were driving in a strange city and got lost, would you first: (1) look at a map and try to figure it out yourself or (0) pull into a gas station and ask for directions?
• Choose the statement that is closest to what you believe: (0) What is going to happen will usually happen, no matter what I do. (1) Taking definite actions has usually worked out better for me than trusting fate.
*Low score indicates external locus of control of behavior; high score indicates internal locus of control of behavior.
Sample items adapted from the Mastery-Powerlessness Scale (Hoehn-Saric & McLeod, 1985, as cited by Leith et al., 1993).

Scale (Hoehn-Saric & McLeod, 1985, as cited by Leith et al., 1993). Additional protocols for evaluating LCB in people who stutter are listed in Table 13-14 later in this chapter in the section on formal and informal assessment measures. For further information about LCB and how the clinician can facilitate its shift from an external to internal source, please see Chapter 2.

Measurement of Speech Rate

Speech rate may reflect the severity of an individual's stuttering, with severe forms of stuttering often resulting in significant reductions in speaking and reading rate (Bloodstein, 1995, p. 7). Very rapid speech rates, particularly when accompanied by irregular pacing, may also indicate the presence of a cluttering rather than stuttering disorder. Speaking rate is typically measured as either the number of syllables or words produced per minute, with syllable counts being the preferred method (see earlier discussion on counting the frequency of core behaviors or refer to Guitar, 2014). All disfluencies are included in the speaking time total; however, extra repetitions of phrases, words, or syllables are excluded from the syllable count so that the final syllable total reflects only those syllables in which meaningful information is being conveyed to the listener. For example, "My my my name is um Da-Da-David" would be counted as five syllables. A related measure, known as *articulatory rate*, focuses specifically on fluent speech. Analysis of articulatory rate includes only syllables that are produced fluently, excluding all disfluencies, long pauses, and the time during which these occur. Below are several suggestions (based on Guitar [2014] and Riley [2009]) to make the task of syllable counting as efficient and accurate as possible:

- Use graph paper or a table that you have prepared with a predetermined number of cells. Place a dot in individual cells for each syllable or word that is spoken.
- Use a commercially available counter that can be pressed rapidly for each spoken syllable or word.
- Press a specific key on a standard keyboard for each syllable spoken. (A separate key can be used simultaneously to indicate moments of disfluency.)
- Using a standard calculator, press 1+ for the first syllable, then continue pressing the = button for each subsequent syllable to keep a running total.
- Regardless of the counting method, a stopwatch should be used to obtain a precise measurement of the total length of time for the speech sample. If speaking rate is being measured during conversation, the stopwatch must be stopped for turns taken by participants other than the speaker of interest. To measure articulatory rate, the stopwatch must be stopped during disfluent speech and during pauses so that only continuous runs of fluent speech are being considered in the final results.

Results of speaking rate calculations are interpreted with reference to normative data reported for specific age groups and speech contexts. Following is a list of expected speaking and reading rates for fluent individuals based on the findings of several studies (Tables 13-7 through 13-9).

Table 13-7. Speaking Rates for Fluent Speakers by Age

Age (years)	*Range (spm)*
3	116 to 163
4	117 to 183
5	109 to 183
6	140 to 175
8	150 to 180
10	165 to 215
12	165 to 220
Adults	162 to 230

spm = syllables per minute.

Adapted from Pindzola et al. (1989) and Guitar (2006, p. 193).

Table 13-8. Range of Speaking Rates in Fluent Speakers by Context

Age Group	*Context*	*Range (wpm)*
Children (7 to 11 years)	Conversation	92 to 161*
Children (7 to 11 years)	Narrative	87 to 178^
Adults	Conversation	116 to 164
Adults	Monologue	114 to 173
Adults	Reading	148 to 190

wpm = words per minute.

*Rate in spm: 109 to 195; ^Rate in spm: 100 to 216.

Adapted from Andrews & Ingham (1971), Shapiro (2011), and Sturm & Seery (2007).

Table 13-9. Average Speaking Rates for Fluent Adults by Age and Context

Age (years)	*Conversation (wpm)*	*Monologue (wpm)*	*Reading (wpm)*
21 to 30	182.7	151.4	219.9
45 to 54	153.7	133.7	182.1
55 to 64	168.7	141.7	190.1

wpm = words per minute.

Adapted from Duchin & Mysak (1987).

Assessment of Environmental Demands and Expectations

Many theorists have discussed the role of the environment in the development of stuttering disorders. Wendell Johnson's original notion that stuttering may begin "in the parent's ear" has been largely discredited (Meyers, 1986; Yairi & Lewis, 1984); however, this idea set the stage for other hypotheses that have been more widely accepted and that have inspired specific clinical approaches to stuttering intervention. Sheehan (1970, p. 286) believed that children who stutter have probably had too many demands placed on them while receiving too little support to meet those demands. The "Demands and Capacities" model (Starkweather & Gottwald, 1990) similarly attributes stuttering to an imbalance between a child's developing capacities in skill areas required for communication and the demands, standards, or expectations imposed on the child by his or her environment. Environmental demands may take the form of rapid questioning, frequent interruptions, use of overly complex sentences or vocabulary, impatience with developmentally typical disfluency, or high standards for achievement and performance in general. These sorts of challenges are alluded to in Marty Jezer's book about his own stuttering, in which he wrote: "To be heard I had to force my way into a conversation (something I rarely had the confidence to do) and then say what I had to say as fast as I could in order not to be interrupted" (1997, p. 60). Interestingly, a recent longitudinal study reported by Reilly and colleagues (2010) has identified higher levels of maternal education as a predictive factor for the emergence of stuttering before age 3, which suggests that parents' standards may be influenced by their own educational experiences and achievements and that these standards may be either implicitly and/or explicitly relayed to very young children.

Environmental pressures can be evaluated by considering several specific questions (for further details, see Guitar [2014, pp. 241-242] and Starkweather & Givens-Ackerman [1997, pp. 91-92]). These factors are most often discussed with relation to young children who stutter; however, many remain relevant for older children, adolescents, and adults.

- What is the speaking rate of the parents or other significant speakers in the child's environment? How do these rates compare with the rate of the child's speech? (There is no established norm for measuring the difference between the speaking rates of a child and adults in his or her environment; however, Zebrowski and Kelly [2002] suggested that a difference of 100 syllables per minute may be significant.) Adults, too, are affected by the speech rate of their listeners and will often report more difficulty speaking when conversational partners use a particularly rapid rate of speech (Starkweather & Givens-Ackerman, 1997, pp. 91-92).

- Do parents use overly complex sentences or difficult vocabulary when speaking with the child? Young children who stutter may be more likely to persist when parents use syntax or vocabulary that is beyond the child's level (Kloth et al., 1999).
- How do parents react to the child's disfluency? Are they supportive or critical? Empathetic or anxious? For an older individual who stutters, how do teachers, employers, or colleagues react?
- What type of communication style is used by the child's family or in the adult speaker's workplace? Are there frequent interruptions, or is there consistent turn-taking during conversations?
- What is the general atmosphere of the household? Is it typically rushed and busy, or is it relaxed and calm? Is there a consistent daily schedule, or is there frequent change and lack of predictability?
- Is the individual often in social situations that involve significant time pressure (e.g., ordering in a store or restaurant where customers are waiting behind him or her, speaking to customer-service representatives over the telephone)?
- Does the family have very high standards for academic, athletic, social, or verbal performance? Does the child feel inadequate in comparison to his or her siblings?

Related Measures

As for most speech and language disorders, assessment of fluency involves not only consideration of features related directly to stuttering, but also evaluation of other systems and abilities that contribute to the production of speech. These include the following:

- Oral-motor strength, coordination, and control: Measures of articulatory control and diadochokinetic rate may help the clinician rule out speech production difficulties related to dyspraxia or apraxia. Assessment of oral-motor function can also provide important information about the speaker's ability to control articulatory structures in the absence of verbal demands (i.e., in simple speech contexts such as isolated sounds or syllables). For more information on this topic, see Chapter 6.
- Receptive and expressive language skills: Just as rapid growth in the verbal system accounts for normal disfluency in typically developing children, persisting difficulties in receptive and/or expressive language may contribute to or exacerbate stuttering disorders (Anderson & Conture, 2000). Difficulties with word retrieval and sentence formulation, in particular, can cause disfluencies in speech production (Boscolo, Bernstein Ratner, & Rescorla, 2002) but may not represent a stuttering disorder at all and would require a very different type of treatment approach. Additionally, cluttering disorders often involve difficulties in organizing and formulating thoughts, whereas stuttering disorders do not (Van Zaalen, Wijnen, & De Jonckere, 2009). The presence of deficits within the language system, therefore, can be an important consideration for differential diagnosis. For a complete discussion on the evaluation of language disorders, please refer to Chapters 8 and 10, which cover assessment of preschool language disorders and assessment of school-age language and literacy disorders, respectively.
- Articulation and overall speech intelligibility: Articulatory proficiency (measured via the Consonant Inventory subtest of the Bankson–Bernthal Test of Phonology [BBTOP; Bankson & Bernthal, 1990]) was recently found to predict eventual recovery status for stuttering preschoolers (Spencer & Weber-Fox, 2014). On the basis of this finding, it may be useful to administer formal measures of phonology as part of the diagnostic workup in young children who stutter. Careful evaluation of articulatory rate, accuracy, and intelligibility is also critical for differential diagnosis of cluttering and stuttering. Rapid and/or irregular articulatory rate is a key feature of cluttering, as are excessive coarticulation (deletion of sounds or syllables in multisyllabic words), indistinct articulation, and reduced overall speech intelligibility (St. Louis, Myers, Bakker, & Raphael, 2007). Differential diagnosis of stuttering and cluttering is considered in more detail later in this chapter. Further information on the assessment of articulation can be found in Chapter 7.
- Nonword repetition ability: Recent data reported by Spencer and Weber-Fox (2014) showed that children who eventually recovered from or persisted in their stuttering differed in their ability to accurately repeat nonsense words administered from the Nonword Repetition Test (Dollaghan & Campbell, 1998). Group differences were most apparent at the longest nonword length (four syllables), whereas shorter lengths resulted in more overlap between groups. The use of such processing-dependent measures may add important prognostic information for young children who stutter and can be easily incorporated into the assessment process.

- Voice: Basic aspects of vocal function, such as vocal intensity, pitch, and quality, should be considered and can typically be evaluated informally using the same speech samples obtained for fluency analyses. Readers are referred to Chapter 12 for further information on this topic.
- Hearing: A basic hearing screening should be included in all standard speech and language evaluations. For more information, see Chapter 5.
- Nonverbal intelligence: Assessment of intelligence is not typically included in fluency assessment; however, higher nonverbal IQ is associated with greater likelihood of spontaneous recovery from early stuttering (Yairi, Ambrose, Paden, & Throneburg, 1996) and may be a useful prognostic indicator, particularly when evaluating preschool children.
- Temperament: Several recent studies have shown an association between children's temperament and the emergence of stuttering during preschool years (see Kefalianos et al. [2012] for review). These data suggest that stuttering children tend to be less adaptable to change, exhibit heightened negative affect, and are less capable of regulating attention and emotions than their fluent peers. Although there is some debate regarding the precise clinical significance of these findings (Alm, 2014), the value of considering temperament is generally acknowledged. Ambrose and colleagues (2015) found that children with persisting stuttering had higher ratings than recovered stutterers on temperament subscales related to negative affect (mothers tended to rate these children as more fearful and less easily soothed). Others suggest that understanding a child's temperament can help guide treatment decisions. For example, indirect forms of therapy (in which speech fluency is not directly modified) may be more effective than direct treatment for emotionally reactive children with limited resilience (Jones, Conture, & Walden, 2014). The most widely used protocol in research on temperament and stuttering is the Children's Behavior Questionnaire (Putnam & Rothbart, 2006). Temperament can also be assessed by using the various Carey Temperament Scales (Carey & McDevitt, 1995), available at the Behavioral Developmental Initiatives website (www.b-di.com). Measures of children's temperament are generally completed by parents or caregivers and consist of questions related to the child's behavior, as described in more detail later in the chapter (see Assessment of Preschool Children).

Assessment Aims and Procedures

The primary aim of assessment is usually to determine the presence of a disorder, as well as to describe the nature and severity of the problem before initiating treatment. In addition to these goals, Shenker (2006) emphasizes the importance of using continuous outcome measures in order to monitor progress while a client is in therapy and to measure maintenance of fluency following the termination of treatment. Shenker further encourages the establishment of self-measurement as a specific treatment goal. Training clients to measure their own outcomes and overall success can facilitate their acceptance of responsibility for treatment and help them become a more active participant in the therapeutic process.

The following general procedures form the basis for all fluency evaluations, regardless of the client's age:

- Case history: Before beginning any evaluation, it is essential to obtain background information related to prenatal and birth circumstances, family structure, general motor and speech-language development, academic performance, social history, medical/surgical history, and employment information, if relevant. It is helpful to mail paperwork to parents or clients and have them send this information back before the scheduled evaluation so that you can form certain expectations and prepare accordingly.
- Interview the parent and/or client: The interview provides clinicians with the opportunity to review the case history, obtain a general impression of the client, and explore questions that can provide important information about the stuttering and its effect on the client's life. Sample questions are provided in the sections covering assessment for specific age groups.
- Direct interaction with the child, teen, or adult in order to obtain speech samples for further analysis: This may be accomplished through spontaneous play, structured speech tasks, and/or conversation and is discussed in more detail for specific age groups subsequently.
- Recording speech samples: Video recording is strongly recommended for all fluency evaluations to capture both core stuttering behaviors as well as accessory behaviors, and to ensure precise quantification of these symptoms. Significant differences have been reported between severity ratings based on audio recordings vs. audiovisual recordings, with audio-based ratings being much less reliable and tending to underestimate the frequency

of disfluencies and related symptoms (Rousseau, Onslow, Packman, & Jones, 2008). Use of video samples can also be an extremely effective way to help clients understand, monitor, and measure their stuttering behaviors.

- Informal analysis of stuttering behaviors: Experienced clinicians may be able to perform **real-time** disfluency counts, using prepared charts and forms that are based on clinic-specific methods. This form of analysis can also be completed later by reviewing recorded speech samples obtained during the evaluation. Examples and details related to such methods can be found in Yaruss (1998). Following is a sample form to demonstrate analysis of disfluencies in 100 syllables.
- The 100-syllable sample: Place a dot in one box for each fluent syllable or word spoken. Use the following abbreviations to indicate disfluencies. (Multiple reiterations of the same disfluency can be noted by placing a superscript above the symbol, such as R-p^{2}, but should not be indicated by multiple abbreviations in separate boxes.)

R-p (phrase repetition) P (prolongation)
R-w (whole word repetition) B (block)
R-sy (syllable repetition) I (interjection)
R-sd (sound repetition) R (revision)

R-w	•	•	•	•	B	•	B	•	•
•	R-sy	•	•	B	•	•	•	•	•
•	•	•	•	•	R-p	P	•	•	•
•	•	P	•	•	•	•	R-sd	•	R-w
•	•	•	•	I	•	•	•	•	•
R-sd	•	•	P	•	•	I	•	•	•
•	B	•	•	•	•	•	•	•	R-p
•	•	•	•	B	•	•	R	•	•
•	P	•	•	•	•	•	•	•	•
•	•	P	•	•	R-w	•	•	P	•

Results can then be organized to reflect the frequency of each disfluency type and relative proportion of within-word to between-word disfluencies:

Within-Word Disfluencies		*Between-Word Disfluencies*	
Syllable repetitions	1	Phrase repetitions	2
Word repetitions (single syllable)	3	Word repetitions (multisyllabic)	0
Sound repetitions	2	Revisions	0
Prolongations	6	Interjections	2
Blocks	5		
Total	**17**	**Total**	**4**

Informal analyses may also involve computing speaking rate, percent of stuttered syllables, and specific proportions represented by each type of disfluency. These calculations will require the use of a stopwatch, as well as some method for counting syllables and time (in seconds), as discussed earlier in the sections on counting frequency of disfluencies and the section on measuring speaking rate. Use of an Excel spreadsheet (Microsoft) with basic formulas may simplify the task of deriving an overall percentage of syllables stuttered (%SS) as well as individual frequencies (expressed in %SS) for each disfluency type and disfluency category (within- vs. between-word), which may be required for certain assessment protocols. A sample table may be organized as follows:

	Disfluency Type	**Total**	**Within**	**Between**	**%SS**
Between-Word	Phrase repetition	0		0	0
	Word repetition (multisyllabic)	5		5	1.67
	Interjections	2		2	0.67
	Running start	3		3	1
	Revision	1		1	0.33
Within-Word	Word repetition (single syllable)	6	6		2
	Syllable repetition	4	4		1.33
	Sound repetition	5	5		1.67
	Sound prolongation	3	3		1
	Block	5	5		1.67
	Broken word	0	0		0
	Totals	**34**	**23**	**11**	**11.33**
	Category %		67.65	32.35	
	% SS	11.33	7.67	3.67	
Syllable Number 300					

Clinicians may also wish to calculate a weighted SLD, a more complex measure that reflects the frequency, type, and extent (units of repetition beyond first intended production) of disfluencies in a single score, and that can help distinguish stuttering from normal disfluency. As described by Ambrose and Yairi (1999), the weighted SLD is calculated by (1) adding the frequency of part-word and single-syllable word repetitions per 100 syllables (PW + SS); (2) multiplying this sum by the mean number of repetition units (RU); and then (3) adding twice the frequency of disfluencies that involve dysrhythmic phonation (DP; blocks and prolongations) per 100 syllables. The resulting formula is $[(PW + SS) \times RU] + (2 \times DP)$. As an example, suppose we have collected a 100-syllable speech sample from a child and observe disfluencies on the following utterances:

I wwwwant the red one. (1 DP)
R-r-r-r-reading a book. (1 PW with 4 units)
Sometimes it it it does that. (1 SS with 2 units)

On the basis of conventional disfluency counts, SLD frequency would be 3 per 100 syllables. In contrast, the weighted SLD calculation results in a total of $[(1 + 1) \times 6/2] + (2 \times 1) = (2 \times 3) + 2 = 6 + 2 = 8$, which more accurately quantifies the child's stuttering and more clearly differentiates it from normal disfluency.

- Use of formal and informal assessment measures to quantify symptoms and rate stuttering severity: A large number of scales and protocols have been published to measure specific aspects of stuttering behavior, describe psychological reactions to stuttering, and predict stuttering chronicity. These are listed and described in further detail later in this chapter under the section "Formal and Informal Assessment Measures for Stuttering Disorders."
- Stimulability testing: An important part of the assessment process is determining the client's responsiveness to specific treatment techniques that are demonstrated by the clinician. A complete discussion on the various forms of treatment available for stuttering are beyond the scope of this chapter. However, the evaluation should involve brief trials of strategies such as easy onsets, continuous phonation, or pullouts for older children and adults; and slow, relaxed forms of speaking for young children. Clients may express a preference for certain methods over others, may be able to imitate certain techniques more easily than others, or may be able to imitate techniques only in specific speech contexts (e.g., single words beginning with vowels). These considerations are essential for effectively bridging assessment findings to practical treatment planning.

Remaining sections in this chapter are subdivided by age group because stuttering disorders tend to evolve in fairly predictable ways over the course of development. As a child with stuttering matures, we often see changes in the specific types of disfluencies that predominate, as well as emergence of physical tension and accessory behaviors, development of negative attitudes, emotions, and self-perceptions, and often an increasing assortment of avoidance behaviors and situational fears (for details on the development of stuttering disorder, see Guitar, 2006, pp. 137-169). The assessment process varies somewhat based on the individual's age and the level to which his or her stuttering has progressed.

Assessment of Preschool Children

The evaluation of stuttering in preschool children is driven by two key questions: (1) Is this child stuttering (i.e., are the child's disfluencies developmentally typical, or do they represent a stuttering disorder)? (2) If the child is stuttering, is the disorder likely to be outgrown naturally, or is it more likely to persist?

The clinician will typically begin by interviewing the child's parent(s) or guardian and reviewing background information provided. During this interaction, the clinician may seek answers to specific questions regarding the nature and history of the fluency disorder but should also be prepared to listen, answer questions, and provide information. Open-ended questions are generally the most effective means of learning about the child, the child's environment, and the stuttering problem. Initial questions may consist of the following:

- Tell me about your child's speech; what are your concerns?
- Describe your pregnancy with this child. Were there any complications during the birth?
- How would you describe this child's motor development?
- What was the child's early speech and language development like? Does the child have any difficulties producing specific sounds, understanding what others are saying to him or her, or expressing himself or herself?
- Is there any family history of stuttering or other speech-language problems?

Additional inquiries may focus more specifically on the child's disfluencies:

- How does the stuttering sound? Can you describe or demonstrate it?

- When were disfluencies first noted? How did the disfluencies sound at that time? Have the disfluencies changed since then?
- Was anything unusual occurring in the child's life at the time of onset? Was anything going on in the family or at school?
- Does the child seem aware of his stuttering in any way? If so, how does he or she react?
- Does the child ever avoid speaking due to disfluencies? Does the child ask others to speak for him or her, say "Forget it," or change a word when it is difficult?
- Describe the child's personality: Is he or she sensitive, anxious, timid, and introverted; or more self-confident, resilient, and outgoing?
- What is the family structure? Are there siblings? How does the child relate to them?
- What is the child's schedule like? Are there situations or settings that seem to make the stuttering worse or better?
- What is the atmosphere like at home? Is it fast-paced, stressful, or noisy? Are there often several people talking at once?
- Do the parents have ideas about what caused the problem?
- How do the parents typically react to the child's stuttering? What do they say or do?
- Has the child been evaluated or treated? What advice were the parents given? What was the nature of the intervention?

Responses to these questions will guide the clinician's decisions throughout the rest of the diagnostic process. If the child's fluency is highly variable or the child is described as sensitive and shy, the clinician may have parents record multiple speech samples outside of the clinic to supplement the one obtained during assessment. Details about the child's family and home environment may indicate the need for more direct observations of these interactions and for specific management recommendations. Reported concerns about speech and language development would clearly indicate the need for more in-depth assessment of these skill areas and the ways in which language difficulties may be interfering with the child's ability to express himself fluently. Finally, reports of emotional trauma, motor difficulties, or academic problems may indicate the need for referrals to other professionals to clarify the nature of the fluency disorder and its potential causes.

To evaluate fluency in young children, clinicians typically arrange two types of interactions: one in which the clinician observes parents or guardians interacting with the child, and one in which the clinician interacts with the child directly. Parent–child interaction involves 10 to 15 minutes of natural play or conversation and provides an opportunity for the clinician to observe whether there are specific communicative behaviors contributing to the child's disfluencies. These may include the following:

- Frequent interruptions
- High proportion of questions vs. comments
- Use of rapid speaking rate
- Use of complex vocabulary
- Use of lengthy or syntactically complex sentences
- Asking a second question before the initial one was answered
- Poor turn-taking
- Frequent correction of child's behavior (verbal/nonverbal)
- Filling in words or finishing the child's sentences

The primary aim of the clinician's interaction with the child is to obtain a representative speech sample. This may be accomplished through one or more of the following tasks:

- Spontaneous speaking during play (e.g., blocks, play figures, dolls, Play-Doh)
- Describing pictures scenes
- Telling a story based on a wordless picture book
- Narrating a recent event or familiar story
- Play with pressure: the clinician interrupts, speaks rapidly, challenges or disagrees with the child, and imposes pressure to induce disfluencies (see Gregory & Hill, 1999, for further detail)

Although speech samples of 300 words or syllables are often considered adequate for fluency analysis (Riley, 2009), it is recommended that clinicians record longer speech samples (e.g., 600 syllables) for preschool-age children, particularly when the child is demonstrating relatively low levels of disfluency, since the additional information can be critical for correct diagnosis. As demonstrated by Sawyer and Yairi (2006), the frequency of SLDs tends to increase for most children as sample sizes become longer, and a diagnosis of stuttering may be missed when only 300 syllables are considered. According to Curlee (1999), the use of word counts is satisfactory for 2- to 3-year-old children because words produced by young children generally do not consist of many syllables;

Table 13-10. Classification of Disfluencies as Normal, Borderline, or Beginning Stuttering

Normal Disfluency	*Borderline Stuttering*	*Beginning Stuttering*
• Fewer than 10 disfluencies per 100 words • Disfluencies consist primarily of non-SLDs • Repetitions consist of two or fewer reiterations • Repetitions are slow and regular in tempo • SLDs comprise less than 50% of the total disfluencies	• More than 10 disfluencies per 100 words • Loose, relaxed disfluencies • SLDs and non-SLDs may be present • Repetitions may have more than two reiterations • More than 50% of disfluencies are SLDs • Clusters may be present	• Disfluencies are marked by tension • Repetitions are rapid and rushed • Rises in pitch during repetitions and prolongations • Struggle with airflow or phonation • Facial tension • Awareness, possible frustration • May use escape behaviors to terminate blocks (e.g., eye blink) • Possible avoidance (e.g., word substitution)

however, syllable measures are preferred for children who use a greater percentage (more than 25%) of multisyllabic words. Another important factor to consider is the great deal of variability typically present in the stuttering of young children. Obtaining several speech samples in different settings (e.g., home, preschool, clinic), with different speakers (e.g., mother, father, clinician), and during different activities (spontaneous play, picture description, play with pressure) often provides the best representation of the child's typical speaking pattern as well as important information about environmental influences on the child's fluency levels.

Once speech samples are obtained and key assessment parameters have been analyzed, these results can be used by the clinician to determine the presence of a stuttering disorder, the severity of the disorder, and its likelihood to persist. A number of general criteria are provided in the literature in addition to various formal and informal protocols to help clinicians with these decisions. Following are several examples of these criteria as well as an overview of the scales and protocols that are available for this age group.

According to Guitar (2006, pp. 138-156), young children's disfluencies can be classified as developmentally normal, borderline stuttering, or beginning stuttering based on the characteristics in Table 13-10.

Curlee (1999) further described five potential diagnostic conclusions that may be reached as a result of the young child's fluency assessment. These profiles may help clinicians integrate various observations and information from the evaluation to form specific recommendations (Table 13-11).

Specific results of the child's speech sample analysis are also used to complete available protocols that can provide information regarding the severity level of the disfluency and help the clinician assess the likelihood that stuttering will persist. A full list of measures used for preschool children and details regarding each measure can be found later in this chapter in the section on Formal and Informal Assessment Measures for Stuttering Disorders. Perhaps the most commonly used protocol is the SSI-4 by Riley (2009), which provides percentile scores and severity ratings (very mild, mild, moderate, severe, very severe) based on the frequency and duration of core behaviors as well as the presence and nature of associated behaviors. When used for older children or adults, the SSI-4 combines samples obtained in both speaking and reading tasks; however, normative data are also provided for nonreaders. The Pindzola Protocol for Differentiating the Incipient Stutterer (Pindzola & White, 1986) can help the clinician determine whether a child's disfluencies are developmentally typical or more consistent with childhood stuttering based on specific speech characteristics such as disfluency type, frequency, duration, and the presence of associated behaviors or avoidances. Yairi and Ambrose (2005) suggested simply using a cutoff score of 4 for differentiating normal from stuttered disfluency based on the weighted SLD calculation. The Stuttering Prediction Instrument for Young Children (Riley, 1981) is a formal measure that provides prognostic information about the likelihood of chronic stuttering. The Children's Behavior Questionnaire (Putnam & Rothbart, 2006) and various Carey Temperament Scales, such as the Behavioral Style Questionnaire (BSQ; McDevitt & Carey, 1995) consist of questions administered to parents to obtain information about the child's temperament. Although these measures do not assess stuttering behaviors directly, it can help the clinician identify constitutional characteristics such as behavioral inhibition,

Table 13-11. Disfluency Profiles and Diagnostic Conclusions

Disfluency Profile	*Conclusion*	*Recommendation*
• May be highly disfluent, but SLD frequency falls below 2% to 3% of total words or syllables • No excessive muscle tension or effort • Normal speech and language skills	Minimal or no signs of childhood stuttering	No intervention or ongoing follow-up needed; reassess with any significant change
• Initial stuttering described as severe; however, few SLDs present in sample	Inconsistent signs of childhood stuttering	Further observation and testing; ensure that low frequency of disfluency during evaluation represents child's typical fluency level
• SLDs on 3% to 10% of total syllables/words • Accessory behaviors may be present • Evidence of muscle tension during disfluencies • Emerging awareness of stuttering; may seem frustrated when having unusual difficulty • Symptoms present less than 1 year	Signs of childhood stuttering present, but for less than 1 year	Regular follow-up and monitoring of fluency for 1 year post-onset; direct intervention if no reduction in symptoms over this time
• Early signs of stuttering along with possible articulatory, phonological and/or language disorder	Evidence of childhood stuttering as well as speech and/or language problem	Direct intervention addressing both disorders
• Frequent disfluencies with SLDs present on 15% or more of total syllables/words • Tense, effortful disfluencies • Associated behaviors (e.g., lip tremor, blinking) • Frustration, avoidance • Symptoms present for one year or more	Consistent evidence of childhood stuttering for 1 year or longer	Immediate intervention

adaptability to change, and ability to self-regulate, which may contribute to the development of stuttering (Guitar, 2014, pp. 125-130), predict stuttering persistence (Ambrose et al., 2015), and help inform clinical decisions (Jones, Choi, et al., 2014), as discussed earlier.

A number of factors have been associated with greater likelihood of either chronic stuttering or natural recovery (Ambrose et al., 2015; Brosch, Haege, Kalehne, & Johannsen, 1999; Curlee, 1999; Kloth et al., 1999; Rommel, Hage, Kalehne, & Johannsen, 2000; Spencer & Weber-fox, 2014; Yairi et al., 1996; Yairi & Ambrose 1999). These should be carefully considered by the clinician and are outlined in Table 13-12.

Assessment of School-Age Children

Assessment of the school-age child includes most of the same procedures used for the preschool child, with several considerations and modifications. First, it is important to remember that disfluencies at this stage in development are no longer likely to be spontaneously outgrown (Guitar, 2006, p. 246). The key questions guiding the evaluation are as follows: (1) Is this child stuttering? (2) If so, what is the nature and severity of the stuttering? (3) To what extent is the child affected by or reacting to his stuttering? (4) What forms of treatment may be most appropriate?

For this age group, information about the stuttering can be obtained not only from the child's parents, but also from the child and, if possible, classroom teachers. As with most interviews of this nature, open-ended questions are often most effective, with more specific inquiries as necessary. The following questions are provided as guidelines.

Child Interview

- Do you find it difficult to speak? What usually happens?
- How often does this happen? Does your speech usually sound the same or does it sound different at different times?

Table 13-12. Factors Associated With Persistent Stuttering Versus Spontaneous Recovery

	Associated With Persisting Stuttering	*Associated With Spontaneous Recovery*
Gender	Male	Female
Family History	Relatives with persisting stuttering	No family history of stuttering
Handedness	Left-handedness	Right-handedness
Speech/Language	Presence of articulation and/or language difficulties	Age-appropriate speech and language abilities
Nonword Repetition	Difficulty repeating long nonsense words (particularly four-syllable)	Strong nonword repetition abilities
Nonverbal Intelligence	Low nonverbal intelligence scores	High nonverbal intelligence scores
Parental Speech	Complex language and syntax	Short sentences with simple vocabulary
Age of Onset	Later age of onset	Earlier age of onset
Time Since Onset of Disfluencies	Disfluencies present 1 year or longer	Disfluencies present less than 1 year
Changes in Disfluencies	No change in SLDs or worsening SLDs 1 year post-onset	Decreased SLDs within 12 to 15 months post-onset
Escape/Avoidance Behaviors	Presence of accessory behaviors, tension, struggle, word substitutions	No accessory behaviors, tension, struggle, or avoidance
Speaking Rate	Fast speaking rate	Slower speaking rate
Temperament	High negative affectivity rating (more fearful, difficult to soothe)	Lower negative affectivity rating

- Is it more difficult to speak in certain situations than in others?
- Are certain words or sounds more difficult than others?
- Do you ever avoid speaking because of the way you sound?
- How do other people react to your speech?
- How does your speech make you feel?
- Do you use any "tricks" to get hard words out?

Parent Interview

- How is your child doing academically? Socially?
- Does your child avoid any speaking situations because of his or her stuttering?
- Does your child feel ashamed? Is he or she being teased?
- Has your child learned any strategies to manage his or her stuttering?

Teacher Interview

- Does the child participate in class?
- Is the child teased by classmates?
- How do you typically react to the child's disfluencies?

Unlike preschoolers, school-age children are able to provide samples of their speech in both speaking and reading tasks, and separate analyses of stuttering behaviors and speech rates are completed for each context. Speaking tasks for this age group should include both monologue (e.g., retelling a book/movie, describing recent event, describing sequenced picture cards) and dialogue. Reading samples are based on reading material below the child's reading level to ensure that disfluencies are due to stuttering rather than decoding difficulties. The SSI-4 (G. D. Riley, 2009) includes reading samples at the third-, fifth-, and seventh-grade levels that can be used for this purpose. Additional measures for determining the presence and severity of stuttering in school-age children can be found in Table 13-13 in the section on formal and informal fluency measures.

Although some information about the child's attitudes and feelings may emerge from the case history, interview, and speaking tasks, the clinician may want to measure this aspect of stuttering more directly using paper and pencil tasks. A variety of measures have been developed to assess children's perceptions

TABLE 13-13. MEASURES AND SCALES FOR PRESCHOOL AND/OR SCHOOL-AGE CHILDREN WHO STUTTER

Measure/Scale	*Author*	*Age (years)*	*Behaviors Assessed*
Overall Assessment of the Speaker's Experience of Stuttering-School Age (OASES-S)	Yaruss, Coleman, & Quesal (2010)	7 to 12	Perception of stuttering; reactions to stuttering; impact of stuttering on communication and quality of life
A-19 Scale for Children Who Stutter	Andre & Guitar (cited in Guitar, 2006)	School age	Attitudes about communication
BSQ	McDevitt & Carey (1978)	3 to 7	Temperamental characteristics in children (based on parent report)
Behavior Assessment Battery (BAB): combination of Behavior Checklist (BCL), Communication Attitude Test (CAT), and Speech Situation Checklist (SSC)	Brutten & Vanryckeghem (2007)	6 to 15	Anxiety ratings for different situations; coping responses for dealing with disfluencies; attitudes toward communication
BCL	Brutten & Vanryckeghem (2007; part of BAB)	School age	Coping responses of the child
Cognitive, Affective, Linguistic, Motor, and Social (CALMS) Rating Scale for School-Age Children Who Stutter	Healey, Scott Trautman, & Susca (2004)	School age	Cognitive, affective, linguistic, motor, and social factors
CAT	Brutten & Dunham (1989); revised version by Brutten & Vanryckeghem (2007; part of BAB)	School age	Speech-related attitudes
Communication Attitude Test for Preschool and Kindergarten Children Who Stutter (KiddyCAT)	Brutten & Vanryckeghem (2007)	Preschool and kindergarten children	Communication attitudes
The Cooper Chronicity Prediction Checklist	Cooper (1973)	Preschool	Predicts children who will recover with and without treatment
Crowe's Protocols	Crowe, DiLollo, & Crowe (2000)	Children, adolescents, adults	Affective, behavioral, and cognitive aspects of stuttering; stuttering severity; stimulability
Pindzola Protocol for Differentiating the Incipient Stutterer	Pindzola & White (1986)	Preschool	Frequency, type, and duration of disfluency; audible effort; rhythm and rate; secondary behaviors; awareness and reaction
Rosenberg Self-Esteem Scale (RSE)	Rosenberg (1979)	Fifth grade and up	Self-esteem
SSC-ER and SSC-SD	Brutten & Vanryckeghem (2007; part of BAB)	School age	Emotional reactions to disfluencies
Stuttering Prediction Instrument for Young Children (SPI)	Riley (1981)	3 to 8 years	Core stuttering behaviors and reactions; used to rate severity and predict chronicity
SSI-4	Riley (2009)	2;10 to adult	Frequency and duration of disfluencies; physical concomitants
Test of Childhood Stuttering-3 (TOCS-3)	Gillam, Logan, & Pearson (2009)	4 to 12	Child's speech fluency skills and stuttering-related behaviors

of their stuttering, psychological reaction to stuttering, and avoidance behaviors. Most are developed based on responses that have been found to differentiate children who stutter from fluent peers (De Nil & Brutten, 1991) and provide normative data for each group. Several sample measures for this age group include the A-19 scale (Guitar & Andre, as cited in Guitar, 2006), CAT (Brutten & Dunham, 1989; revised by Vanryckeghem & Brutten, 2007b), and OASES-S (Yaruss, Coleman, & Quesal, 2010). A full list of available protocols for measuring attitude, perceptions, and LCB in school-age children is provided in the section on formal and informal measures. Reports from teachers can also be useful in determining a child's reactions to stuttering and possible avoidance behaviors. Information can be obtained through telephone conferences, meetings, or through written scales and forms, such as the Teachers Assessment of Student Communicative Competence (Smith, McCauley, & Guitar, 2000), in which teachers rate the child's communicative functioning in the classroom.

As for preschool children, stimulability testing is an important part of the evaluation for this age group. Brief trials of stuttering modification techniques and simple fluency shaping strategies can be attempted to determine which treatment approach may be better suited for a particular child.

Assessment of Adolescents and Adults

Adolescents and adults with stuttering disorders typically have an extensive history of stuttering. The key diagnostic questions for individuals in this age group is usually not whether a stuttering disorder exists, but rather the following:

- What is the nature and severity of this individual's stuttering?
- How severely is this individual reacting to his or her stuttering?
- What specific fears or avoidance behaviors are present?
- How has stuttering affected and limited this individual's life?

As mentioned earlier in this chapter, ongoing struggle to produce speech often creates many layers of negative emotions. These may be quite pervasive in the adolescent or adult who stutters but difficult to observe and measure. Although pretreatment measures of stuttering severity may ultimately be the most reliable predictor of treatment outcome (Block, Onslow, Packman, & Dacakis, 2006), the development of learned helplessness and confirmed self-perception as a poor communicator can be serious impediments to successful fluency intervention and must be explored during an initial evaluation. Sometimes, experienced stutterers may negotiate anticipated disfluencies so skillfully that core behaviors will not be observed at all, and assessment will need to tap into hidden emotions, attitudes, and fears to uncover any evidence of a stuttering disorder.

Interview questions for the adult who stutters will be similar to those presented for younger populations, but rather than focusing primarily on the "tip of the iceberg" (i.e., observable speech disfluencies), equal emphasis is placed on aspects of the disorder that lie beneath the surface. The following are suggested areas of inquiry:

- When did your stuttering start? How has it changed since then?
- How does your stuttering feel, physically and emotionally?
- How do different situations and/or listeners affect your stuttering?
- Do you have specific "tricks" that you use to get out of difficult blocks?
- Have you had prior therapy? Describe these treatment experiences. Are there any specific strategies or techniques that have been helpful?
- Do you avoid speaking or social situations? Has your stuttering contributed to certain decisions that you have made in your life (e.g., relationships, career choices)?
- What do you aim to achieve in therapy? What is your primary goal?
- Why have you decided to pursue treatment now?

As described for preschool and school-age children, the clinician can use a combination of formal and informal measures to describe the nature and severity of an adult's stuttering disorder. Assessment procedures must include tasks to measure the frequency, duration, and types of disfluencies present in monologue, dialogue, and reading contexts; along with qualitative measurement of associated behaviors and calculation of speech rate. Results of these analyses can be used to complete a protocol such as the SSI-4, which will provide diagnostic information about stuttering severity. Of equal importance, however, will be the inclusion of measures that provide information about other aspects of the stuttering disorder. The Perceptions of Stuttering Inventory (PSI; Woolf, 1967), for example, may help the clinician understand the extent of struggle perceived by the client who stutters, the client's anticipation of failure during attempts to speak, and the extent to which he avoids speaking situations. The Modified Scale of Communication Attitude (S-24) developed by Andrews and Cutler (1974) and Communication Attitude Test for Adults (BigCAT) by Brutten and Vanryckeghem (2003) both reflect the client's self-perceptions as a communicator and his or her attitude toward communication in general. Locus of control measures, such as the Locus of Control of Behavior (LOC-B) developed by Craig et al. (1984) or Speech Locus of Control Scale (Sp-LOC) by McDonough and Quesal (1988) provided specific information about whether the client views life circumstances as the result of external forces or internal control. Understanding the way an individual views events or approaches change can be essential in designing and planning appropriate stuttering intervention. A number of more recent protocols explore stuttering disorders from a more holistic perspective. These protocols provide measures of core behaviors as well as information about the ways in which an individual may be reacting to his stuttering and the overall impact of stuttering on the individual's life. Examples of such measures include Yaruss and Quesal's OASES for Teenagers and Adults (Yaruss & Quesal, 2010; Yaruss, Quesal, & Coleman, 2010, respectively) and the Wright and Ayre Stuttering Self-Rating Profile (WASSP; 2000).

Stimulability testing for adolescents and adults can provide insight into the client's level of behavioral self-awareness (i.e., the client's ability to identify moments of disfluency or anticipated moments of disfluency). Poor performance may suggest the need to heighten the client's attention to the physical sensations associated with stuttering to eventually help him or her control disfluencies through stuttering modification techniques. Reluctance or refusal to participate in such tasks may indicate the need to focus on desensitization in therapy or to consider initiating treatment with a fluency shaping approach. In general, trial techniques drawn from different treatment approaches can help guide the clinician in planning intervention that will be most appropriate for the individual client and most likely to succeed.

Formal and Informal Assessment Measures for Stuttering Disorders

See Tables 13-13 and 13-14 for measures and scales for children and adults who stutter.

Differential Diagnosis of Stuttering and Cluttering

In this final section, we briefly consider the differential diagnosis of stuttering and a closely related fluency disorder, cluttering. Detailed information related to the assessment of cluttering is beyond the scope of this work; however, a number of books, websites, and journal publications on this topic are listed at the end of this chapter. Cluttering is classified as a disorder of fluency but is distinct from stuttering based on certain key features that include abnormal fluency that is not consistent with stuttering, rapid and/or irregular speech rate, disorganized language formulation, excessive coarticulation and reduced speech intelligibility, and poor self-monitoring (St. Louis & Myers, 1997). An important difference between the two disorders is that stuttering consists primarily of atypical forms of disfluency, such as prolongations or blocks, whereas cluttering involves typical disfluencies such as interjections, revisions, or phrase repetitions that usually occur without visible struggle or tension (Guitar, 2006, p. 445). According to Daly and Burnett (1999), individuals with cluttering may present with difficulty in five communicative dimensions including cognitive, linguistic, pragmatic, speech, and motor abilities. Several possible impairments in each dimension are listed in Table 13-15.

The Predictive Cluttering Inventory (PCI), originally developed by Daly and Cantrell (2006) and recently revised (Van Zaalen et al., 2009), may be helpful for identifying symptoms associated with cluttering; however, it is not a reliable or sensitive measure in its current form (Van Zaalen et al., 2009). In Table 13-16, we compare characteristics of stuttering and cluttering to assist clinicians in this differential diagnosis.

Table 13-14. Measures and Scales for Adolescents and Adults Who Stutter

Measure/Scale	*Author*	*Age*	*Behaviors Assessed*
Adult BAB: combination of BCL for Adults, BigCAT, and SSC for Adults	Brutten & Vanryckeghem (2003)*	Adults	Anxiety ratings for different situations; coping responses for dealing with disfluencies; attitudes toward communication
BAB: combination of BCL, CAT, and SSC	Vanryckeghem & Brutten (2007a)	6 to 15 years	Anxiety ratings for different situations; coping responses for dealing with disfluencies; attitudes toward communication
BCL for Adults	Brutten & Vanryckeghem (2003)*	Adult	Coping responses
BigCAT	Brutten & Vanryckeghem (2003)*	Adults	Speech-related attitudes
Crowe's Protocols	Crowe et al. (2000)	Children, adolescents, adults	Affective, behavioral, and cognitive aspects of stuttering; stuttering severity; stimulability
LOC-B	Craig et al. (1984)	Older children, adolescents and adults	Extent to which a person perceives outcome of events to be under internal or external locus of control
Modified Scale of Communication Attitudes (S-24)	Andrews & Cutler (1974)	Adolescents and Adults	Feelings, attitudes, and self-esteem
OASES-Teenager (OASES-T)	Yaruss, Quesal, & Coleman (2010)	Adolescents (12 to 17 years)	Perception of stuttering; reactions to stuttering; impact of stuttering on communication and quality of life
OASES-Adult (OASES-A)	Yaruss & Quesal (2010)	Adult	Perception of stuttering; reactions to stuttering; impact of stuttering on communication and quality of life
Perceptions of Stuttering Inventory	Woolf (1967)	Adolescents and adults	Speaker's perception of the struggle, avoidance, and expectancy of stuttering
Rathus Assertiveness Schedule (RAS)	Rathus (1973)	Adults	Assertiveness
RSE	Rosenberg (1979)	Fifth grade and up	Self-esteem
SSC-ER and SSC-SD	Brutten & Vanryckeghem (2003)*	Adults	Emotional reactions to disfluencies
Stuttering Problem Profile	Silverman (1980)	Adults	Identifies behaviors to be modified in therapy
SSI-4	Riley (2009)	2;10 to adult	Frequency and duration of disfluencies; physical concomitants
Stuttering Severity Scale	Lanyon (1967)	Adults	Severity of stuttering behaviors; attitudes and feelings
Subjective Screening of Stuttering (SSS)	Riley, Riley, & Maguire (2004)	Adults	Stuttering severity, locus of control, avoidances
Unhelpful Thoughts and Beliefs about Stuttering (UTBAS)	St. Clare et al. (2009)	Adults	Speech-related social anxiety
WASSP	Wright & Ayre (2000)	18 to adult (14 to 18 with clinical judgment)	Speaker's perceptions of stuttering behaviors; negative thoughts and feelings; avoidances and "disadvantage" due to stuttering

*Adult SSC, BCL, CAT, and BAB commercially published in Belgium and the Netherlands; not yet available in the United States.

Table 13-15. Communicative Dimensions Affected in Cluttering Disorders

Cognition	*Language*	*Pragmatics*	*Speech*	*Motor*
• Poor self-monitoring • Impulsivity • Memory difficulties • Poor attention span	• Difficulty organizing thoughts • Sentence fragments • Oral and written language difficulty • Difficulty listening and/or following directions	• Inappropriate turn-taking • Verbose or tangential • Poor eye contact • Inappropriate introduction or maintenance of conversational topics	• Excessive repetitions of words and phrases • Omission of sounds or syllables • Syllable transpositions	• Prosody problems • Poor penmanship • General clumsiness, poor coordination

Table 13-16. Cluttering Versus Stuttering

	Cluttering	*Stuttering*
Onset	Often not diagnosed until school years	Onset typically between age 2 and 5 years
Disfluencies	Excessive normal disfluencies (between-word)	Atypical disfluencies (primarily within-word)
Awareness/Concern	Frequently unaware of problem	Highly aware, frustrated and embarrassed
Articulation	Slurred, imprecise	No articulation difficulty
Reaction to Pressure	Improved performance under pressure or on demand	Poorer performance under pressure
Language Skills	Disorganized discourse, word-finding difficulties, grammatical errors	Language skills generally age-appropriate
Written Expression	Disorganized, parallels verbal expression	Normal writing skills
Attention	More frequent diagnosis of attention deficit	Attention deficits less frequent
Pragmatic Skills	Impatient listening, difficulty processing nonverbal cues, poor conversational skills	No pragmatic deficits
Associated Behaviors	Generally absent	Generally present
Tension/Struggle	Generally absent	Generally present
Avoidance Behaviors	Generally absent	Generally present

Adapted from Daly & Burnett (1999) and Guitar (2006, pp. 451-452).

Summary

This chapter began with an allusion to Sheehan's well-known comparison of observable stuttering symptoms to the "tip of an iceberg." We hope that details provided in the chapter will help clinicians explore beneath this surface and feel comfortable measuring and interpreting not only core behaviors, but also underlying perceptions, attitudes, and beliefs in the person who stutters. The chapter also illustrated the need for broadening the diagnostic scope to consider how various environmental features may contribute to a stuttering disorder. Approaching the assessment process from this more holistic perspective will enable the clinician to appreciate the complex interactions that ultimately determine the way a stuttering disorder is manifested in a particular individual. Specific age groups were considered individually, based on certain patterns in the way stuttering develops and evolves over time, as well as important differences in the diagnostic questions relevant for each age group. In line with this general structure, we now present a case history and model report for each of the age groups discussed to demonstrate and apply some of the key concepts reviewed in the chapter.

Case History and Model Reports

Writing Rubric for Sample Reports

The following guidelines may be useful in preparing the fluency section of a diagnostic report:

- ☐ Describe the specific contexts in which speech samples were obtained (e.g., play interaction with parent, play with pressure, monologue, dialogue, reading).
- ☐ Provide a summary of informal analyses that includes: total number of syllables in sample; speech rate; total frequency of disfluencies (typically expressed as a percent of total syllables or words); frequencies or relative proportions of between-word and within-word disfluencies; list of disfluency types observed with examples for each; average duration of longest disfluencies (number of reiterations and/or in seconds); occurrence of clusters; and presence or absence of accessory behaviors.

  Example: "Informal analyses were based on speech samples obtained during monologue, dialogue, and reading, with a total of 300 syllables in each sample. Speaking rate was measured as the number of syllables per minute (spm). The frequency of disfluencies in each context was measured as the percentage of total syllables stuttered (%SS), with results as follows:

Context	*Speaking Rate (spm)*	*Frequency of Disfluencies (%SS)*
Monologue	190	11
Dialogue	196	12.5
Reading	183	9

  "Disfluencies generally occurred in clusters and consisted primarily of SLDs) which included sound repetitions (e.g., M-m-my name is M-M-Michael), prolongations (e.g., I like the ssssummer), and tense blocks. Several non-SLDs were observed (interjections, revisions); however, these did not represent the majority of disfluencies. When results were combined across speaking contexts, SLDs represented 83% of total disfluencies; non-SLDs represented only 17% of total disfluencies. The average duration of the three longest disfluencies was approximately 2.5 seconds. Frequent accessory behaviors were observed, including finger tapping, head movements, and obvious facial tension."

- ☐ For formal measures, provide an introductory statement that includes the full test name, abbreviated test name in parenthesis, and a brief description.

  Example: "The Stuttering Severity Instrument-4 (SSI-4) was completed based on speech sample results. This measure provides a severity rating based on quantification of core stuttering behaviors and accompanying physical symptoms."

- ☐ Provide a summary of derived scores in a table form followed by a paragraph that interprets and explains these results.

  Example: "Overall scores obtained on the SSI-4 fell between the 61st to 77th percentile, which means that this child demonstrated greater disfluency than 61% to 77% of children his age. These results indicate a moderate stuttering disorder."

- ☐ To report results of scales measuring perceptions, attitudes, or feelings, provide the scale name, authors, year of publication, and what the scale purports to measure. In paragraph form, describe the client's responses and how these compare to original findings reported by the author(s) for stuttering and nonstuttering individuals.

  Example: "The S-24 (Andrews & Cutler, 1974) was administered to assess the client's general attitude toward communication. The client's total score was 18, which indicates distinctly negative reactions toward disfluencies and communication overall. This score corresponds to normative data obtained for stuttering adults (Mean = 19.22) rather than nonstuttering adults (9.14), suggesting that the client strongly identifies with perceptions and attitudes that are typical of people who stutter."

- ☐ Describe stimulability testing and results.

  Example: "Brief trials of pullouts were attempted with the client following an explanation and demonstration; however, the client had significant difficulty identifying discrete moments of disfluency."

Case History (Preschool)

Eric is a 3;2-year-old boy who began showing signs of childhood stuttering several months ago when his family moved to a new apartment. On the basis of his mother's description, disfluencies increased approximately one month following onset and now consist of frequent repetitions of phrases, whole words, and sounds. Eric's mother has also noticed tension around his face and mouth when he is struggling to produce certain words. She is especially concerned because there is a history of stuttering in Eric's father's family.

Selection of Assessment Procedures (Preschool)

Several types of interactions were planned and recorded to obtain representative samples of Eric's speech: play interaction with Eric and his parent at the clinic; play interaction with Eric and the clinician; and conversational interaction with Eric and his parent at home. An informal analysis of all speech samples was completed to determine the overall frequency of disfluencies and individual frequencies of SLDs vs. ODs. Two measures were used to interpret speech sample results. The SSI-4 was selected as an age-appropriate standardized measure of stuttering severity and the Pindzola Protocol for Differentiating the Incipient Stutterer was selected to determine whether Eric's disfluencies were developmentally typical or not. Core subtests of the Clinical Evaluation of Language Fundamentals Preschool-2 (CELF Preschool-2) were also administered to screen language skills and confirm that disfluencies were not related to weaknesses in language processing.

Sample Report (Preschool)

Speech/Language Evaluation

Name: Eric Taylor
Address:
Date of Birth: 2/13/04
Date of Evaluation: 4/30/07

I. Background Information

Eric is a 3;2-year-old boy who was seen for a fluency evaluation due to parental concern regarding stuttering. Eric was accompanied by his mother, Ms. Taylor, who served as a reliable informant. Presenting problem, as described by Eric's mother, was increasing disfluency over the past several months, along with emerging frustration.

Eric was the product of a full-term pregnancy and caesarian delivery with no reported complications during pregnancy or birth. Birth weight was 8 pounds, 10 ounces. Medical history includes asthma (since age 3 years) and an allergic reaction to penicillin at 9 months. Eric currently takes albuterol for asthma as needed.

Motor milestones were achieved at age expectancy with sitting occurring at 4 months, crawling at 6 months, standing at 8 months, and independent walking at 12 months. Eric began feeding himself at approximately 9 months, dressed independently between 1;6 to 2 years, and was toilet trained at 2 years. Early speech and language development was grossly within normal limits with single words emerging at around 18 months and word combinations at 2 years.

Eric resides with his mother, Ms. Taylor, age 25 years, and his sister, Bridget, who is 2 years old. His father resides elsewhere but sees Eric several times per week. English is the only language spoken at home and by the child. Eric attends a local preschool program where he is reportedly doing well both academically and socially. He was described by his mother as a "shy" child who warms up slowly to people who are familiar to him. Eric enjoys building, drawing, and coloring but also plays and interacts appropriately with neighborhood friends and relatives.

II. Speech-Language History

Onset of stuttering was several months ago, coinciding with a move to a new apartment. Disfluencies increased in frequency approximately 1 month following onset. As described by his mother, stuttering is characterized by repetitions of phrases, words, and sounds and becomes noticeably worse when Eric is upset or excited. Disfluencies occur throughout the day and are accompanied by visible tension around the face, which has become somewhat more pronounced over the past several weeks. There is a family history of stuttering (Eric's father and paternal uncle received speech therapy for stuttering when they were children; both still stutter). Eric has not received any previous speech-language services.

III. Tests Administered/Procedures

- Oral-peripheral examination
- Clinical Evaluation of Language Fundamentals Preschool-2 (CELF Preschool-2)
- Goldman-Fristoe Test of Articulation-3 (GFTA-3)
- Speech sample analysis (play with clinician, play with parent, home sample)
- Informal fluency analysis
- Protocol for Differentiating the Incipient Stutterer
- Stuttering Severity Instrument-4 (SSI-4)

IV. Clinical Observations

Eric presented as a playful, friendly child who was easily engaged in interactive play. He showed affect readily, maintained appropriate eye contact, and was cooperative throughout assessment.

Hearing Mechanism

Complete audiological evaluation at this facility on 4/21/07 revealed hearing thresholds within normal limits at all test frequencies (250 to 8000 Hz) for both ears. Immittance testing revealed normal middle ear function bilaterally. Acoustic reflexes were elicited at expected levels.

Peripheral Speech Mechanism

Cursory inspection of the oral peripheral mechanism revealed no gross structural deviations. Strength and function of all oral and facial musculature were within normal limits for both speech and nonspeech purposes.

Language

Language skills were assessed via screening subtests of the CELF Preschool-2 with the following resulting scores:

CELF Preschool-2	
Subtest	*Standard Score*
Sentence Structure	13*
Word Structure	13*
Expressive Vocabulary	11*
Core Language Score	114** (82nd percentile)
*Mean = 10; standard deviation ± 3 **Mean = 100; standard deviation ± 15	

Standard scores for individual subtests all fell within the average to high-average range for Eric's age level. Eric's core language score was 114, which falls at the 82nd percentile and indicates high-average overall language ability.

Informal assessment of language (based on unstructured play and a picture description task) corroborated formal test findings. Eric responded appropriately to questions and directions during play and expressed himself in short but complete sentences with age-appropriate vocabulary and syntax.

Articulation

Assessment of articulation skills via the GFTA-3 revealed age appropriate speech sound production. Overall intelligibility was good at the single-word level as well as in connected speech, for both known and unknown contexts.

Voice

Vocal pitch, quality, and volume were appropriate for age and gender.

Rate, Fluency, and Rhythm

Three spontaneous speech samples were obtained: one during a play interaction with the clinician; one during a play interaction with the parent at the clinic; and one during a conversational interaction with the parent at home. Results were analyzed individually but then combined due to consistency of findings across contexts. Analysis of core stuttering behaviors was based on a total of 800 syllables and revealed the following:

Number of disfluencies per 100 syllables (% stuttered syllables)	19
Number of stutter-like disfluencies (within-word) per 100 syllables	15
Number of developmentally typical disfluencies per 100 syllables	4

Overall frequency of disfluencies was approximately 19% of total syllables with the majority of disfluencies occurring in clusters (multiple disfluencies per utterance). Disfluency types consisted primarily of within-word disfluencies (also known as SLD), which are generally considered atypical. These included blocks, sound prolongations, sound repetitions, syllable repetitions, and monosyllabic word repetitions. Some between-word disfluencies were observed (e.g., phrase repetitions, interjections, revisions); however, the majority of disfluencies in the sample did not fall in this category.

Disfluency types and frequency of each type (expressed as a percentage of total syllables in the sample, or %SS) were as follows:

Between-Word Disfluencies (More Typical)		*Within-Word Disfluencies (Less Typical)*	
Disfluency type	**Frequency (%SS)**	**Disfluency type**	**Frequency (%SS)**
Phrase repetition	2	Single-syllable word repetition	1
Interjection	1	Syllable repetition	1
Revision	1	Sound repetition	3
		Prolongation	4
		Block	6
Total	**4**	**Total**	**15**

When disfluencies involved repetition, the typical number of reiterations was two or three; the average duration of the three longest disfluencies in the sample was approximately 3 seconds. Several emerging secondary behaviors were observed, including occasional rise in pitch, audible vocal tension, visible tension around the mouth and eyes, and frequent loss of eye contact during moments of disfluency. Two standardized stuttering measures were completed based on Eric's sample and are described next.

The Protocol for Differentiating the Incipient Stutterer (Pindzola & White, 1986) is designed to identify preschool children whose stuttering is likely to persist based on specific disfluency parameters. Total score is based on measurement of auditory behaviors (frequency, type, and duration of disfluencies) as well as visual evidence of accessory behaviors. Eric's results were as follows:

Protocol for Differentiating the Incipient Stutterer	
Total Score	35
Interpretation	Probably atypical*
*1 to 20 = probably typical; 20 to 42 = probably atypical.	

The SSI-4 provides a severity rating based on quantification of a child's core stuttering behaviors (frequency, duration) and physical concomitants. Results for Eric were as follows.

SSI-4		
Individual Scores	*Sample Data*	*SSI-4 Score*
Frequency (calculated for nonreader)	15% total syllables (non-SLDs excluded)	16
Duration	3 seconds	10
Physical concomitants	Visible tension (eye, face), pitch rise, poor eye contact	5
Total Overall Score	16 + 10 + 5	31
Percentile		89th to 95th
Severity		Severe

Combined results of the Pindzola Protocol and SSI-4 indicate a severe stuttering disorder that is most likely atypical; that is, more consistent with stuttering than with typical developmental disfluency. Speech and language therapy is strongly recommended to help Eric learn to use slow/relaxed forms of speech and to help parents implement communication styles that will support and enhance fluency at home. Eric was able to imitate several trials of slow and easy speech at the single word level but will need further practice with longer and more spontaneous speech contexts.

V. Clinical Impressions

Eric Taylor, a 3;2-year-old boy, was seen for a speech and language evaluation to assess parental concerns regarding stuttering. Findings revealed a severe stuttering disorder marked by excessive disfluencies that were primarily atypical and that were frequently accompanied by visible tension around the face and eyes, an audible rise in pitch, and loss of eye contact, all of which indicate emerging awareness, tension, and struggle. Language skills, articulation, and vocal function were age-appropriate.

VI. Recommendations

Parent was informed of findings and demonstrated awareness of the following:

1. Indirect strategies for fluency management were discussed with parent with specific recommendations including: parental use of slower speech rate; regular one-on-one time with Eric, during which specific methods for reinforcing fluency can be implemented; avoiding negative reactions such as anxiety, fear, or sadness in response to Eric's disfluencies; use of consistent turn-taking during conversation with care to avoid "talking over" each other.
2. Direct fluency treatment: teach Eric to use slow/easy speaking patterns, implement fluency-supporting patterns of conversation
3. Home therapy program to reinforce treatment goals: specific exercises to practice treatment targets, inclusion of siblings

____

(Name and credentials)
Speech-Language Pathologist

Case History (School-Age)

Emily is a 7-year-old child who briefly stuttered at age 2 years and is now showing reoccurrence of stuttering symptoms. On the basis of her mother's description, disfluencies fluctuate in frequency and severity but are consistently observed on most days. Disfluencies reportedly consist of word and syllable repetitions with no obvious signs of tension or struggle. Emily is an outgoing and popular child and does not seem to avoid speaking situations; however, her mother was concerned that Emily may be privately self-conscious or ashamed about her stuttering and that this might eventually limit her either academically and/or socially.

Selection of Assessment Procedures (School-Age)

Three tasks were selected to obtain representative samples of Emily's speech: monologue, dialogue, and reading. For the monologue sample, Emily summarized the plot of a movie she had recently seen. The reading task was based on a simple storybook at the first-grade level. An informal analysis of each speech sample was completed to determine the overall frequency of disfluencies and relative frequencies of SLDs vs. ODs. The SSI-4 was selected as an age-appropriate standardized measure of stuttering severity. The A-19 (Andre & Guitar, 2006) was administered to assess Emily's underlying attitudes about her speech and about communication. The Expressive and Receptive One-Word Picture Vocabulary Tests were selected as age-appropriate standardized measures of vocabulary skills to compare receptive and expressive word knowledge and rule out possible word retrieval difficulties.

Sample Report (School-Age)

Speech/Language Evaluation

Name: Emily Ross
Address:
Date of Birth: 2/13/01
Date of Evaluation: 4/30/08

I. Reason for Referral

Mrs. Ross requested a speech and language evaluation for her 7-year-old daughter, Emily, due to concerns about fluency. Emily was previously evaluated for stuttering at approximately age 2 years. At that time, stuttering was intermittent with accompanying behaviors (hitting mouth with hand) occurring for a short period of time. Direct therapy was not recommended, however, indirect management strategies were implemented at home and disfluency eventually resolved.

Recent re-emergence of stuttering symptoms was noted just after the summer and has been consistently observed since then both at home and school. Disfluency appears to fluctuate in frequency and severity without any identifiable triggers. As described by Mrs. Ross, disfluencies consist of word and syllable repetitions with no signs of visible tension or struggle. Emily seems to be aware of the problem but does not show any specific fears or anxiety related to speaking. Family history is significant for several relatives with stuttering, some with persisting severe disfluency into adulthood.

II. Background Information

Emily is the third of four children born to John and Pamela Ross. Pregnancy, birth, and medical history were uncomplicated; developmental milestones were achieved at age expectancy.

Early language and academic skills were described as above average. Emily currently attends P.S. 23, where she is in a regular-education second-grade class. She is described as a very verbal child and highly motivated student. There are no academic concerns. Emily speaks English as her primary language.

III. Tests Administered/Procedures

- Oral-peripheral examination/articulation
- Receptive One-Word Picture Vocabulary Test (ROWPVT)
- Expressive One-Word Picture Vocabulary Test (EOWPVT)
- Informal language analysis
- Speech sample analysis (conversation, monologue, and reading)
- Stuttering Severity Instrument-4 (SSI-4)

IV. Clinical Observations

Hearing Mechanism

Emily reportedly passed a recent hearing screening administered at school. Formal results were unavailable at the time of this evaluation.

Oral-Peripheral Mechanism and Articulation

Cursory inspection of the oral peripheral mechanism revealed no gross structural deviations. Strength and function of oral musculature were normal. No speech sound production errors were reported or observed throughout assessment.

Language

Formal Analysis

The ROWPVT and EOWPVT were administered to screen basic vocabulary skills and compare receptive and expressive word knowledge. The child is required to either point to the picture that corresponds to given word or provide labels for individual pictures or groups of pictures. Emily's results were as follows:

Emily's standard scores of 103 and 100 for the receptive and expressive vocabulary measures, respectively, both fell within the average range for age level,

Test	Standard Score	Percentile Rank
ROWPVT	103*	58th
EOWPVT	100*	50th
*Mean = 100; standard deviation ± 15.		

indicating that her word knowledge and word retrieval abilities are both age-appropriate.

Informal Analysis

Language skills were informally assessed in discourse level speech via question/answer exchange and a story retell task. Results were consistent with vocabulary scores described above. Emily used complete sentences that were grammatically correct and included detailed elaboration. Word specificity and range of vocabulary appeared generally appropriate for Emily's age level. During the story retell task, Emily sequenced events accurately and provided a coherent story with much description. Eye contact, turn taking, and other social conventions during conversation were all appropriate.

Fluency

Core Behaviors

Speech samples were obtained in several contexts including conversation, monologue, and reading. Reading sample was used for informal analysis but was excluded from formal analyses because data are not included for children reading below a third-grade level. Overall frequency of disfluency during speaking tasks was 9.3% of total syllables in conversation and 8.8% of total syllables during extended speaking (monologue). Disfluencies consisted of word ("and-and-and") and part-word repetitions ("pe-pe-pe-people"), usually with two to three reiterations. The longest duration of disfluencies was between 1.0 and 1.5 second. No obvious concomitant behaviors, such as unusual sounds, facial tension, or head/body movements were observed at moments of disfluency. Speech rate was generally average with occasional portions of more rapid speech, usually occurring when Emily was relating a lot of detail about a particular subject or event. Intonation and rhythm were normal during speech and reading tasks. Emily often self-corrected decoding errors during the reading task; however, these were all corrections of miscues rather than speech disfluencies. Overall calculations of stuttering behaviors were analyzed using the SSI-4 with the following results:

Combined scores yield a total task score of 20, which places Emily in the 24th to 40th percentile range for her age level. This corresponds to a severity rating of mild bordering on moderate stuttering.

SSI-4			
Measure	*Task Score*	*Percentile Rank*	*Severity*
Frequency of disfluency	14		
Duration of stuttering events	6		
Physical concomitants	0		
Total overall score	20	24th to 40th	Mild/moderate

Attitudes and Feelings

Emily's responses to questions about her speech suggested awareness of disfluencies and some sensitivity about her stuttering. She referred to her stuttering as "double talk" and stated that she is often advised by others to talk slowly, but that this does not seem to help her. She does not avoid speaking situations and openly discussed her stuttering during this evaluation. Emily's attitudes about her speech were further examined via the A-19 Scale for Children Who Stutter, a written scale that requires written yes–no responses to 19 statements about communication. Emily's total score was 4, which is quite low and is more consistent with the mean obtained for nonstuttering children (8.17) than for stuttering children (9.07). Overall, Emily appears to be somewhat self-conscious about her stuttering but has a healthy general attitude toward communication and is not reacting to disfluencies in any significant way at this point.

A brief telephone conference with Emily's classroom teacher, Ms. Thomas, on 5/2/10 corroborated A-19 findings already described. Ms. Thomas reported that Emily participates frequently in class discussions, volunteers to read aloud, and is popular among her peers. Overall, Emily is perceived by her teacher as a confident student who communicates freely despite occasional disfluency. No teasing or bullying was reported.

Stimulability

Stimulability was assessed via several trials of fluency shaping techniques including easy onsets (on single words), continuous phonation on short phrases (e.g., How are you), and rate control during a long sentence. Emily responded well to all methods following brief explanation and demonstration. Several trials of pullouts were attempted; however, these seemed more difficult for Emily because her disfluencies tended to have a short duration and her speech rate was often too rapid for her to identify and modify moments of disfluency effectively.

V. Summary and Recommendations

Emily is a 7;2-year-old child with a borderline mild-to-moderate fluency disorder. Her disfluencies generally consist of phrase, word, or part-word repetitions that occur fairly frequently but are not accompanied by any visible tension or other obvious physical behaviors. Emily is aware of her stuttering in a general sense and is somewhat self-conscious but has a healthy overall attitude toward communication. She is frequently told by others to speak more slowly, but she does not find this helpful and has no other effective means of managing disfluencies. Indirect and direct speech therapy is recommended, focusing on implementing methods to promote fluency at home and school, educating Emily and her family about stuttering, practicing strategies for fluent speech, and managing moments of disfluency as they occur. It is important for Emily to have an effective and reliable method of controlling her speech to avoid the development of compensatory methods, negative habits, and speech-related anxiety.

Speech therapy is recommended to address treatment goals described. Ongoing discussion of goals and progress with family members and teachers is also recommended in order to ensure that fluency is being properly supported at home and in school. Finally, Emily may benefit from joining support groups that have been formed for children who stutter in her community. Participation in support group activities may help Emily become less self-conscious about her stuttering and help her benefit from the experiences of other children with similar difficulties.

____

(Name and credentials)
Speech-Language Pathologist

Case History (Adult)

Amanda is a 22-year-old college student referred for a fluency evaluation by her college counselor. She is currently majoring in theatre and aspires to become a theatre director. Amanda began stuttering when she was 5 years old and has stuttered fairly consistently since then. She was evaluated previously but has never received intervention. Her stuttering is characterized by several types of disfluencies (repetitions, prolongations, interjections) in addition to certain accessory behaviors and avoidances. Amanda is comfortable speaking with most people and is not ashamed of her stuttering, but is anxious about how stuttering may affect her future career.

Selection of Assessment Procedures (Adult)

Representative samples of Amanda's speech were obtained in three contexts: monologue, dialogue, and reading. A timed monologue was also recorded to measure the effect of imposed pressure on disfluencies. Informal fluency analyses were performed on the three samples to determine speaking rate, disfluencies per minute, disfluency types, and disfluency durations. The LOC-B Scale was selected as an age-appropriate informal measure of attitudes and confidence level related to daily communication situations.

Sample Report (Adult)

Speech/Language Evaluation

Client: Amanda Rope **D.O.E**: 1/11/2010
Address: **Phone Number(s)**:
D.O.B: 1/11/1988 **Diagnosis**: Stuttering

I. Reason for Referral

Amanda Rope, a 22-year-old monolingual female, was seen at the Diana Rogovin Davidow Speech and Hearing Center (DRDSHC) at Brooklyn College for an evaluation on January 11, 2008. She was referred for an evaluation by her college counselor to improve her fluency. Amanda disclosed that she "wants to get some way to control" her stuttering. Amanda served as a reliable informant during the evaluation.

II. Tests Administered/Procedures

- Interview
- Oral-peripheral mechanism examination
- Audiological screening
- Locus of Control of Behavior Scale (LOC-B)
- Informal fluency assessment
- Stimulability assessment

III. Background Information

Medical/Health History

Amanda reported during the interview that she has an unremarkable medical history. No known allergies, illnesses, or hospitalizations were reported.

Family/Social History

Amanda was born in Nigeria and immigrated to the United States with her family in 2000. She currently resides in Bronx, New York, with her mother, brother, and two sisters. Amanda indicated that she feels comfortable speaking with her family and is not embarrassed when she stutters with them but is often shy and quiet when meeting new people. She enjoys singing in the church choir with her friends, watching television, writing, and reading novels.

Educational/Occupational History

Amanda attended high school in the United States and is currently in her fifth year at Brooklyn College. She is pursuing a bachelor's degree with a major in theater. She indicated that she is interested in directing theater productions.

Fluency History

Amanda reported that she does not hide her stuttering and has learned to "control" emotions related to her stuttering via specific techniques (i.e., controlling fears, relaxing in uncomfortable situations).

Amanda is motivated to improve her speech and indicated a desire to learn techniques for speaking fluently. She is anxious when producing new and long words and experiences the most difficulty at school, where she feels that her stuttering may be hindering her class work. She is also concerned that her disfluency may interfere with her ability to communicate effectively in her future role as a theatre director.

Amanda indicated that she exhibits secondary characteristics such as shaking her head and averting eye contact. During moments of stuttering, Amanda controls her speech by switching words.

Amanda reported a history of stuttering in her family. Amanda's maternal uncle stutters, but she is not in close contact with him because he lives in Georgia. Amanda stated that she first demonstrated stuttering behaviors at approximately age 5 years.

Therapeutic History

Amanda reported that she has no previous history of speech or language therapy. A diagnostic evaluation was conducted at the DRDSHC in September 2006. Therapy was recommended; however, Amanda did not pursue services at that time. Information obtained from the present evaluation corroborated previous assessment findings.

IV. Clinical Observations

Amanda presented as a pleasant young woman who was motivated and engaged in all required tasks during the evaluation. She reported that improving her speech would maximize her opportunities in school and help ensure future employment.

Oral-Peripheral Mechanism Examination

An oral-peripheral examination was conducted to assess structural and functional integrity of the speech mechanism. Normal facial tone and symmetry were observed. Labial strength was observed to be within normal limits. Velopharyngeal movement upon phonation of /a/ was normal. Lingual mobility for lateralization, depression, and elevation appeared to be adequate for speech production. A diadochokinetic syllable task was administered to assess rapid movements of the speech musculature. Amanda was able to successfully produce the syllables /pʌ/, /tʌ/, and /kʌ/.

Audiological Screening

Amanda passed a hearing screening in which pure tones were presented bilaterally at 25 dB HL at the frequencies of 500, 1000, 2000, and 4000 Hz, suggesting hearing within normal limits.

Articulation and Phonological Skills

Articulation skills were informally observed throughout the evaluation. Observation revealed no articulation errors and overall intelligibility was judged to be good in both known and unknown contexts.

Language Skills

Language was informally assessed throughout the evaluation. Assessment revealed age-appropriate language skills. Cluttering was not suspected due to appropriate organization of expressive language skills and overall ability to communicate effectively.

Voice and Vocal Parameters

Amanda's vocal quality, pitch, resonance, and intensity were assessed through conversation and judged to be within normal limits.

Summary of Informal Results				
Context	*Rate of Speech (wpm)*	*Disfluencies per Minute*	*Duration (seconds)*	*Types of Disfluencies*
Oral reading	119	21	0.5 to 1.0	Repetitions, interjections, prolongations
Monologue	130	20	0.5	Repetitions, interjections
Conversation	93	23	0.5 to 1.0	Repetitions, interjections, prolongations

Fluency

Informal Assessment

Fluency skills were informally assessed to measure types of disfluencies, duration of disfluency, and speaking rate in a variety of linguistic contexts within the clinical setting, including oral reading, monologue, and dialogue.

Reading

Amanda read a 22-sentence passage ("Nicknames," by Shipley & McAfee, 2016) and a 1-minute sample was recorded. The average reading rate based on this sample was 119 words per minute (wpm). According to Shapiro (2011), the normal rate for oral reading in adults is 148 to 190 wpm. These results indicated that Amanda had a reduced speech rate for oral reading. She exhibited a total number of 21 disfluencies per minute, including initial sound repetitions (e.g.,"n-n-n-nicknames"), whole word repetitions ("nicknames, nicknames"), phrase repetitions ("some are not, some are not") interjections (e.g., "um"), and prolongations (e.g., a---apple"). Average duration of disfluencies was between 0.5 and 1.0 seconds during oral reading. Amanda exhibited some secondary characteristics including head jerking on first-syllable repetition.

Monologue

In a 1-minute monologue, Amanda spoke at an average rate of approximately 130 wpm. According to Shapiro (2011), the normal speech rate for monologue is 114 to 173 wpm. Compared with the speech rate in reading, Amanda spoke at an appropriate speech rate during monologue. She exhibited a total of 20 disfluencies, primarily initial sound repetitions and interjections. Duration of disfluencies was 0.5 seconds for monologue. A timed monologue was elicited to determine the effects of imposed time pressure on Amanda's fluency. Results of a 1-minute sample revealed no change in her fluency patterns.

Conversation

In conversation, Amanda spoke at an average rate of approximately 93 wpm. The average rate for conversational speech in adults is 115 to 165 wpm (Andrews & Ingham, 1971). Therefore, Amanda's speech rate in conversation falls slightly below average limits. On the basis of the clinician's perception, Amanda's speech rate during conversation was judged to be adequate for her age. During a 1-minute speech sample, Amanda exhibited a total of 23 disfluencies, including a combination of sound, whole-word and phrase repetitions, interjections (e.g., "umm"), and prolongations (e.g., "aaaand"). The duration of Amanda's disfluencies was between 0.5 and 1.0 seconds for conversation. During this task, Amanda exhibited some secondary characteristics, such as averting eye contact.

In summary, the duration of Amanda's disfluencies was between 0.5 and 1.0 seconds for oral reading, monologue, and conversation. Amanda's predominant core behaviors from most to least frequent were repetitions, (whole-word, phrase, and initial-sound repetitions), interjections, and sound prolongations. Accessory speech behaviors such as head jerks and decreased eye contact were exhibited throughout oral reading and monologue. Taped results of the informal assessment indicated that Amanda presents with a mild-moderate stuttering disorder. This is due to the types of disfluencies and secondary characteristics with which she presents, as well as the impact that stuttering has on her life, both socially and academically (see Summary of Informal Results).

Attitudes and Feelings Associated With Stuttering

The attitudes and emotions component of the evaluation assessed how Amanda feels about her stuttering in terms of self-esteem, locus of control, and assertiveness. The LOC-B Scale was administered and assessed Amanda's self-confidence and attitudes in daily communication situations. The test comprises 17 statements associated with speech-related behaviors and required Amanda to rate situations from 0 (strongly disagree) to 5 (strongly agree). Amanda did not present with confirmed attitudinal perception. For instance, she revealed that her stuttering "will not dominate" her life. In addition, she indicated that she is able to "anticipate difficulties and take action to avoid them."

Stimulability Testing

A trial of stuttering intervention was presented during the session. The tasks involved using various fluency shaping strategies (easy onset, light articulatory contacts, and continuous phonation techniques). Before the presentation of stimulus items, Amanda practiced each strategy while reading from a list of phrases and sentences. Amanda did not have practice implementing strategies during moments of stuttering. Amanda was stimulable for all the techniques; however, she was most comfortable applying easy onset.

V. Clinical Impressions

Amanda Rope, a 22-year-old English-speaking woman, presented with a mild-moderate stuttering disorder. Predominant core behaviors were repetitions (whole-word, phrase, and initial-sound repetitions), interjections, and sound prolongations. Duration of disfluencies was between 0.5 and 1.0 seconds for monologue, dialogue, and conversation. Physical accessory behaviors included loss of eye contact and head jerks during moments of disfluency. As evidenced by the locus of control scale, Amanda did not present with any confirmed attitudinal perceptions regarding her stuttering. Prognosis for improvement is good, given the client's motivation, awareness of disfluencies, positive perception of speaking abilities, and stimulability for using fluency shaping strategies (i.e., easy vocal onset and continuous phonation) when producing words and phrases.

VI. Recommendations

Individual therapy is recommended once per week in a structured therapeutic setting to address the following goals:

- Counseling to address fluency issues and goals related to future activities/plans. Amanda's intervention should emphasize stuttering education, self-awareness of disfluent behaviors, and desensitization.
- Long-Term Goal: Amanda will reduce anxiety and modify core behaviors and secondary characteristics associated with stuttering.
    - Short-Term Goals:
        - Amanda will identify primary and secondary characteristics of her stuttering (i.e., head jerking, word switching, poor eye contact) during a 1-minute conversation with 80% accuracy.
        - Amanda will express her feelings/attitudes toward her stuttering in relation to family, social, and school settings on 6 of 7 days of the week.
        - Amanda will perform desensitization activities (aimed at increasing awareness of stuttering and reducing associated anxiety) on 4 of 5 trials.
- Long-Term Goal: Amanda will produce fluent speech using easy vocal onset and continuous phonation strategies.
    - Short-Term Goals:
        - Amanda will produce easy vocal onset in words, phrases, and sentences with 80% accuracy.
        - Amanda will produce words, phrases, and sentences using continuous phonation with 80% accuracy.

____

(Name and credentials)
Speech-Language Pathologist

Novel Case Histories for Practice

Here, we present concluding paragraphs from two diagnostic reports. The first evaluation was conducted with Michael, a 2;5-year-old child who began showing questionable signs of childhood stuttering 13 months before assessment. The second evaluation was conducted with Julie, a 31-year-old female with a long history of stuttering. After reading each paragraph, select specific formal and informal procedures that could have led to the conclusions described. Explain how each procedure would have been implemented, how it would contribute to the diagnostic conclusion, and how specific findings from that procedure or analysis would be reported in the full text of the evaluation.

1. Case 1: Michael Davis, a 2;5-year-old child, was seen for a speech and language evaluation to assess parental concerns regarding stuttering. Findings revealed mild stuttering characterized by a relatively low frequency of disfluencies, brief duration of disfluencies, and no evidence of tension or struggle. Overall, results were more consistent with developmentally typical disfluency rather than beginning stuttering. Language skills, articulation, and vocal function were all age appropriate.

2. Case 2: Julie Russo, a 31-year-old female, was seen for a fluency evaluation to assess concerns relating to a long history of stuttering. Findings revealed a severe stuttering disorder marked by frequent, long blocks that occurred across speaking contexts and that were usually accompanied by significant facial tension, head movement, and/or audible gasping. Assessment of Julie's feelings related to her speech indicated significant negative reactions to her stuttering, strong identification with perceptions and attitudes that are typical of people who stutter, and a number of specific fears and avoidance behaviors.

Glossary

Accessory behaviors: Behaviors that begin as an attempt to push out of disfluencies but eventually become learned patterns that accompany core stuttering behaviors.

Avoidance behaviors: Attempts to circumvent moments of disfluency.

Blocks: A form of disfluency in which both airflow and sound are stopped during the production of speech.

Between-word disfluencies: Discontinuities interfering with smooth transitioning between words in an utterance (phrase repetitions, interjections, running starts, revisions).

Broken words: A form of disfluency involving a tense, silent pause in the middle of a vowel, followed by abrupt reinitiation of voicing.

Cluttering: A fluency disorder characterized by primarily typical forms of disfluency as well as possible abnormalities in speech rate, language formulation, articulation, and self-monitoring.

Clusters: The occurrence of two or more disfluencies on the same word or utterance.

Core behaviors: Involuntary discontinuities in the flow of speech that represent the key features of stuttering (e.g., repetitions, prolongations, blocks).

Covert stuttering: Form of stuttering in which the speaker shows little to no overt stuttering behavior and will outwardly "pass" as fluent by avoiding sounds, words, and situations in which stuttering is anticipated.

Disfluency: Speech that is not fluent (does not necessarily imply abnormality).

Dysfluency: A lack of fluency that is deemed abnormal.

Escape behaviors: Speaker's attempt to terminate a block (e.g., by blinking, stamping feet, moving head).

Incipient stuttering: Early signs of a stuttering disorder (vs. developmental disfluencies).

Interjections: Insertion of extraneous, meaningless words or phrases into the flow of connected speech (e.g., "um," "you know"); often called *fillers*.

Locus of control of behavior: The extent to which the outcome of events is attributed to external circumstances vs. internal factors.

Prolongations: A form of disfluency in which sound or airflow continues but articulatory movement is stopped.

Real-time analysis: Disfluency analysis performed while the speech sample is being obtained.

Repetitions: A typical or atypical form of disfluency that involves reiterations of a phrase, word, syllable, or sound.

Revisions: A form of disfluency (or escape behavior) in which phrases or sentences are reformulated, often to avoid anticipated difficulty on a particular word or sound.

Running starts: A form of disfluency (or escape behavior) in which the speaker returns once or several times to the beginning of a thought or sentence in order to regain fluency.

Spontaneous recovery: Recovery from childhood stuttering without any formal intervention or treatment.

Stutter-like disfluencies (SLD): Disfluencies associated with more chronic forms of stuttering, sometimes referred to as *within-word disfluencies*.

Tremors: Small, rapid muscle contractions.

Within-word disfluencies: Discontinuities that interfere with smooth transitioning between sounds or syllables within a word (sound repetitions, syllable repetitions, prolongations, blocks, broken words).

References

Adams, M. R. (1980). The young stutterer: Diagnosis, treatment and assessment of progress. *Seminars in Hearing, 1*, 289-299.

Alm, P. A. (2014). Stuttering in relation to anxiety, temperament, and personality: Review and analysis with focus on causality. *Journal of Fluency Disorders, 40C*, 5-21.

Ambrose, N. G., & Yairi, E. (1999). Normative disfluency data for early childhood stuttering. *Journal of Speech, Language, and Hearing Research, 42*, 895-909.

Ambrose, N. G., Yairi, E., Loucks, T. M., Seery, C. H., & Throneburg, R. (2015). Relation of Motor, Linguistic and Temperament Factors in Epidemiologic Subtypes of Persistent and Recovered Stuttering: Initial Findings. *Journal of Fluency Disorders, 45*, 12-26.

American Speech-Language-Hearing Association. (n.d.). Childhood fluency disorders: Overview. Retrieved from https://www.asha.org/Practice-Portal/Clinical-Topics/Childhood-Fluency-Disorders/

Anderson, J. D., & Conture, E. G. (2000). Language abilities of children who stutter: A preliminary study. *Journal of Fluency Disorders, 25*, 283-304.

Andre, S., & Guitar, B. (2006). A-19 scale for children who stutter. In: B. Guitar (Ed.), *Stuttering: An integrated approach to its nature and treatment* (pp. 196-197). Baltimore, MD: Lippincott Williams & Wilkins.

Andrews, G., Craig, A., Feyer, A.M., Hoddinott, S., Howie, P., & Neilson, M. (1983). Stuttering: A review of research findings and theories circa 1982. *Journal of Speech and Hearing Disorders, 48*, 226-246.

Andrews, G., & Cutler, J. (1974). Stuttering therapy: The relation between changes in symptom level and attitudes. *Journal of Speech and Hearing Disorders, 39*, 312-319.

Andrews, G., & Ingham, R. J. (1971). Stuttering: Considerations in the evaluation of treatment. *International Journal of Language & Communication Disorders, 6*(2), 129-138.

Bankson, N. W., & Bernthal, J. E. (1990). *Bankson-Bernthal Test of Phonology*. Austin, TX: Pro-Ed.

Baron-Cohen, S. (2008). Autism, hypersystemitizing, and truth. *The Quarterly Journal of Experimental Psychology, 61*, 64-75.

Beitchman, J. H., Nair, R., Clegg, M., & Patel, P. G. (1986). Prevalence of speech and language disorders in 5-year old kindergarten children in the Ottawa-Carleton region. *Journal of Speech and Hearing Disorders, 51*, 98-110.

Block, S., Onslow, M., Packman, A., & Dacakis, G. (2006). Connecting stuttering management and measurement: IV. Predictors of outcome for a behavioural treatment for stuttering. *International Journal of Language and Communication Disorders, 41*, 395-506.

Bloodstein, O. (1995). *A handbook on stuttering*. San Diego, CA: Singular.

Bloodstein, O. (2006). Some empirical observations about early stuttering: A possible link to language development. *Journal of Communication Disorders, 39*, 185-191.

Bloodstein, O. & Bernstein Ratner, N. (2008). *A handbook on stuttering* (6th ed.). Clifton Park, NY: Delmar.

Boscolo, B., Bernstein Ratner, N., & Rescorla, L. (2002). Fluency of school-aged children with a history of specific expressive language impairment: An exploratory study. *American Journal of Speech-Language Pathology, 11*, 41-49.

Brosch, S., Haege, A., Kalehne, P., & Johannsen, H. S. (1999). Stuttering children and the probability of remission—the role of cerebral dominance and speech production. *International Journal of Pediatric Otorhinolaryngology, 47*, 71-76.

Brutten, G., & Dunham, S. (1989). The Communication Attitude Test: A normative study of grade school children. *Journal of Fluency Disorders, 14*, 371-377.

Brutten, G., & Vanryckeghem, M. (2003). [*An evidence-based and multi-dimensional assessment instrument for children who stutter for the purpose of differential diagnostic and therapeutic decision making*]. Leuven, Belgium: Stichting Integratie Gehandicapten; The Hauge, the Netherlands: Acco.

Carey, W. B., & McDevitt, S. C. (1995). *Coping with children's temperament: A guide for professionals*. New York, NY: Basic Books.

Cooper, E. B. (1973). The development of a stuttering chronicity prediction checklist: A preliminary report. *Journal of Speech and Hearing Disorders, 38*, 215-223.

Cordes, A. K. (2000). Individual and consensus judgments of disfluency types in the speech of persons who stutter. *Journal of Speech, Language, and Hearing Research, 43*, 951-964.

Craig, A., & Andrews, G. (1985). The prediction and prevention of relapse in stuttering: The value of self-control techniques and locus of control measures. *Behavior Modification, 9*, 427-442.

Craig, A., Franklin, J. A., & Andrews, G. (1984). A scale to measure locus of control of behaviour. *British Journal of Medical Psychology, 57*, 173-180.

Crowe, T. A., Di Lollo, A., & Crowe, B. T. (2000). *Crowe's protocols: A comprehensive guide to stuttering assessment*. San Antonio, TX: The Psychological Corporation

Curlee, R.F. (1999). Identification and case selection guidelines for early childhood stuttering. In R. F. Curlee (Ed.), *Stuttering and related disorders of fluency* (2nd ed., pp. 1-21). New York, NY: Thieme Medical.

Daly, D. A., & Burnett, M. L. (1999). Cluttering: Traditional views and new perspectives. In R. F. Curlee (Ed.), *Stuttering and related disorders of fluency* (2nd ed., pp. 222-254). New York, NY: Thieme Medical.

Daly, D. A., & Cantrell, R. P. (2006). Cluttering characteristics identified as diagnostically significant by 60 fluency experts. In Proceedings of the Second World Congress on Fluency Disorders.

De Nil, L. F., & Brutten, G. J. (1991). Speech-associated attitudes of stuttering and nonstuttering children. *Journal of Speech and Hearing Research, 34*, 60-66.

De Nil, L. F., & Kroll, R. M. (1995). The relationship between locus of control and long-term stuttering treatment outcome in adult stutterers. *Journal of Fluency Disorder, 20*, 345-364.

Dollaghan, C., & Campbell, T. F. (1998). Nonword repetition and child language impairment. *Journal of Speech, Language & Hearing Research, 41*, 1136-1146.

Duchin, S., & Mysak, E. (1987). Disfluency and rate characteristics of young adult, middle-aged, and elderly males. *Journal of Communication Disorders, 20*, 245-257.

Gillam, R. B., Logan, K. J., & Pearson, N. A. (2009). *TOCS—Test of childhood stuttering*. Greenville, SC: Super Duper.

Gregory, H. H., & Hill, D. (1999). Differential evaluation—differential therapy for stuttering children. In R. F. Curlee (Ed.), *Stuttering and related disorders of fluency* (2nd ed., pp. 22-42). New York, NY: Thieme Medical.

Guitar, B. (2006). *Stuttering: An integrated approach to its nature and treatment* (3rd ed.). Baltimore, MA: Lippincott, Williams & Wilkins.

Guitar, B. (2014). *Stuttering: An Integrated Approach to Its Nature and Treatment* (4th ed.). Baltimore, MD: Lippincott Williams & Wilkins.

Halpern, D. F. (1997). Sex differences in intelligence: Implications for education. *American Psychologist, 52*, 1091-1102.

Healey, C. E., Scott Trautman, L., & Susca, M. (2004). Clinical applications of a multidimensional approach for the assessment and treatment of stuttering. *Contemporary Issues in Communication Science and Disorders, 31*, 40-48.

Howell, P. (2013). Screening school-aged children for risk of stuttering. *Journal of Fluency Disorders, 38*(2), 102-123.

Hubbard C. P., & Yairi, E. (1988). Clustering of disfluencies in the speech of stuttering and nonstuttering preschool children. *Journal of Speech and Hearing Research, 31*, 228-233.

Jezer, M. (1997). *Stuttering: A life bound up in words*. New York, NY: HarperCollins.

Jones, R., Choi, D., Conture, E., & Walden, T. (2014). *Temperament, Emotion and Childhood Stuttering. Seminars in Speech and Language, 35*, 114-131.

Jones, R. M., Conture, E. G., & Walden, T. A. (2014). Emotional reactivity and regulation associated with fluent and stuttered utterances of preschool-age children who stutter. *Journal of Communication Disorders, 48*, 38-51.

Kefalianos, E., Onslow, M., Block, S., Menzies, R., & Reilly, S. (2012). Early stuttering, temperament and anxiety: two hypotheses. *Journal of Fluency Disorders, 37*, 151-163.

Kloth, S. A. M., Kraaimaat, F. W., Jansssen, P., & Brutten, G. J. (1999). Persistence and remission of incipient stuttering among high-risk children. *Journal of Fluency Disorders, 24*, 253-265.

Lanyon, R. I. (1967). The measurement of stuttering severity. *Journal of Speech and Hearing Research, 10*, 836-843.

LaSalle, L. R. & Conture, E. G. (1995). Disfluency clusters of children who stutter: Relation of stutterings to self-repairs. *Journal of Speech and Hearing Research, 38*, 965-977.

Leith, W. R., Mahr, G. C., & Miller, L. D. (1993). The assessment of speech-related attitudes and beliefs of people who stutter. *ASHA Monographs, 29*, 1-32.

Logan, K. J., & LaSalle, L. R. (1999). Grammatical characteristics of children's conversational utterances that contain disfluency clusters. *Journal of Speech, Language, and Hearing Research, 42*, 80-91.

McDevitt, S. C., & Carey, W. B. (1995). *Behavioral Style Questionnaire.* Scottsdale, AZ: Behavioral-Developmental Initiatives.

McDonough, A. N., & Quesal, R.W. (1988). Locus of control orientation of stutterers and nonstutterers. *Journal of Fluency Disorders, 13*, 97-106.

Meyers, S. C. (1986). Qualitative and quantitative differences and variability in disfluencies emitted by preschool stutterers and nonstutterers during dyadic conversations. *Journal of Fluency Disorders, 11*, 293-306.

Murphy, B., Lafayette, W., Quesal, R. W., & Gulker, H. (2007, August). *Covert Stuttering*, 4-9.

Pellowski, M. W., & Conture, E. G. (2002). Characteristics of speech disfluency and stuttering behaviors in 3- and 4-year old children. *Journal of Speech, Language, and Hearing Research, 45*, 20-34.

Perkins, W. H., Kent, R. D., & Curlee, R. F. (1991). A theory of neuropsycholinguistic function in stuttering. *Journal of Speech and Hearing Research, 34*, 734-752.

Pindzola, R. H., Jenkins, M. M., & Lokken, K. J. (1989). Speaking rates of young children. *Language, Speech, and Hearing Services in Schools, 20*, 133-138.

Pindzola, R. H., & White, D. T. (1986). A protocol for differentiating the incipient stutterer. *Language, Speech, and Hearing in Schools, 17*, 2-15.

Putnam, S. P., & Rothbart, M. K. (2006). Development of short and very short forms of the Children's Behavior Questionnaire. *Journal of Personality Assessment, 87*, 102-112.

Quesal, R.W. (1988). Inexact use of "disfluency" and "dysfluency" in stuttering research. *Journal of Speech and Hearing Disorders, 53*, 349-350.

Ramig, P. R. (1993). High reported spontaneous stuttering recovery rates: Fact or fiction? *Language, Speech, and Hearing Services in Schools, 24*, 156-160.

Rathus, S. A. (1973). A 30-item schedule for assessing assertive behavior. *Behavior Therapy, 4*, 398-406.

Reilly, S., Onslow, M., Packman, A., Wake, W., Bavin, E. L., Prior, M., . . . Ukuomunne, O. C. (2010). Predicting stuttering onset by the age of 3 years: A prospective, community cohort study. *Pediatrics, 123*, 270-277.

Riley, G. D. (1981). *Stuttering Prediction Instrument for Young Children* (3rd ed.). Austin, TX: Pro-Ed.

Riley, G. D. (2009). *Stuttering Severity Instrument* (4th ed.). Austin, TX: Pro-Ed.

Riley, J., Riley, G., & Maguire, G. (2004). Subjective screening of stuttering severity, locus of control and avoidance: Research edition. *Journal of Fluency Disorders, 29*, 51-62.

Robb, M. P., Sargent, A., & O'Beirne, G. A. (2009). Characteristics of disfluency clusters in adults who stutter. *Logopedics Phoniatrics Vocology, 34*, 36-42.

Rommel, D., Hage, A., Kalehne, P., & Johannsen, H.S. (2000). Development, maintenance, and recovery of childhood stuttering: Prospective longitudinal data 3 years after first contact. In K.L. Baker, L. Rustin, & F. Cook (Eds.), Proceedings of the fifth Oxford disfluency conference (pp. 168-182).

Rosenberg, M. (1979). *Conceiving the self.* New York, NY: Basic Books.

Rotter, J. B. (1966). Generalized expectancies for internal versus external control or reinforcement. *Psychological Monographs: General and Applied, 80*, 1-28.

Rousseau, I., Onslow, M., Packman, A., & Jones, M. (2008). Comparisons of audio and audiovisual measures of stuttering frequency and severity in preschool-age children. *American Journal of Speech-Language Pathology, 17*, 173-178.

Sawyer, J., & Yairi, E. (2006). The effect of sample size on the assessment of stuttering severity. *American Journal of Speech-Language Pathology, 15*, 36-44.

Schwartz, M.F. (1974). The core of the stuttering block. *Journal of Speech and Hearing Disorders, 39*, 169-177.

Shapiro, D. A. (2011). *Stuttering intervention: A collaborative journey to fluency freedom* (2nd ed.). Austin, TX: Pro-Ed.

Shaywitz, B. A., Shaywitz, S. E., Pugh, K. R., Constable, R. T., Skudlarski, P., Fulbright, R. K., . . . & Gore, J.C. (1995). Sex differences in the functional organization of the brain for language. *Nature, 373*, 607-609.

Sheehan, J.G. (1970). *Stuttering: Research and therapy.* New York, NY: Harper & Row.

Shenker, R.C. (2006). Connecting stuttering management and measurement: I. Core speech measures of clinical process and outcome. International *Journal of Language and Communication Disorders, 41*, 355-364.

Shipley, K. G., & McAfee, J. G. (2016). *Assessment in speech-language pathology: A resource manual.* Independence, KY: Cengage Learning.

Silverman, F.H. (1980). The stuttering problem profile: A task that assists both client and clinician in defining therapy goals. *Journal of Speech and Hearing Disorders, 45*, 119-123.

Smith, A., McCauley, R. J., & Guitar, B. (2000). Development of the Teacher Assessment of Student Communicative Competence (TASCC) in grades 1 through 5. *Communication Disorders Quarterly, 22*, 3-11.

Sommer, M., Koch, M. A., Paulus, W., Weiller, C., & Buchel, C. (2002). Disconnection of speech-relevant brain areas in persistent developmental stuttering. *Lancet, 360*, 380-383.

Spencer, C., & Weber-Fox, C. (2014). Preschool speech articulation and nonword repetition abilities may help predict eventual recovery or persistence of stuttering. *Journal of Fluency Disorders, 41*, 32-46.

Spencer, C., & Weber-Fox, C. (2014). Preschool speech articulation and nonword repetition abilities may help predict eventual recovery or persistence of stuttering. *Journal of Fluency Disorders, 41*(C), 32-46.

St. Clare, T., Menzies, R.G., Onslow, M., Packman, A., Thompson, R., & Block, S. (2009). Unhelpful thoughts and beliefs linked to social anxiety in stuttering: Development of a measure. *International Journal of Language and Communication Disorders, 44*, 338-351.

St. Louis, K. O., & Myers, F. L. (1997). Management of cluttering and related fluency disorders. In R. F. Curlee & G. M. Siegel (Eds.) *Nature and treatment of stuttering: New directions* (pp. 313-332). Needham Heights, MA: Allyn & Bacon.

St. Louis, K.O., Myers, F.L., Bakker, K., & Raphael, L.J. (2007). Understanding and treating of cluttering. In E. G. Conture & R. F. Curlee (Eds.), *Stuttering and related disorders of fluency* (pp. 297-325). New York, NY: Thieme Medical.

Starkweather, C. W., & Givens-Ackerman. (1997). *Stuttering.* Austin, TX: Pro-Ed.

Starkweather, C. W., & Gottwald, S. R. (1990). The demands and capacities model II: Clinical applications. *Journal of Fluency Disorders, 15*, 143-157.

Sturm, J. A., & Seery, C. H. (2007). Speech and articulatory rates of school-age children in conversation and narrative contexts. *Language, Speech, and Hearing Services in Schools, 38*, 47-59.

Throneburg, R. N., & Yairi, E. (2001). Durational, proportionate, and absolute frequency characteristics of disfluencies: A longitudinal study regarding persistence and recovery. *Journal of Speech, Language, and Hearing Research, 44*(1), 38-51.

Tudor, H., Davis, S., Brewin, C. R., & Howell, P. (2013). Recurrent involuntary imagery in people who stutter and people who do not stutter. *Journal of Fluency Disorders, 38*(3), 247-259.

Van Riper, C. (1982). *The nature of stuttering* (2nd ed.). Englewood Cliffs, NJ: Prentice-Hall.
Van Zaalen, Y., Wijnen, F., & De Jonckere, P. H. (2009). Differential diagnostic characteristics between cluttering and stuttering—Part one. *Journal of Fluency Disorders, 34*, 137-154.
Vanryckeghem, M., & Brutten, G. J. (2007a). *Behavior Assessment Battery for School-Age Children Who Stutter.* San Diego, CA: Plural.
Vanryckeghem, M., & Brutten, G. J. (2007b). KiddyCAT: *Communication Attitude Test for Preschool and Kindergarten Children Who Stutter.* San Diego, CA: Plural Publishing.
Ward, D. (2013). Risk factors and stuttering: evaluating the evidence for clinicians. *Journal of Fluency Disorders, 38*, 134-40.
Wingate, M. E. (1964). A standard definition of stuttering. *Journal of Speech and Hearing Disorders, 29*, 484-489.
Wingate, M. E. (2001). SLD is not stuttering. *Journal of Speech, Language, and Hearing Research, 44*, 381-383.
Woolf, G. (1967). The assessment of stuttering as struggle, avoidance, and expectancy. *British Journal of Disorders of Communication, 2*, 158-171.
World Health Organization. (2001). *The International Classification of Functioning, Disability & Health.* Geneva, Switzerland: World Health Organization.
Wright, L., & Ayre, A. (2000). *Wright and Ayre Stuttering Self-Rating Profile.* Bicester, England: Speechmark.
Yairi, E. (1997). Disfluency characteristics of childhood stuttering. In R. F. Curlee & G. M. Siegel (Eds.), *Nature and treatment of stuttering: New directions* (pp. 49-78). Needham Heights, MA: Allyn & Bacon.
Yairi, E., & Ambrose, N. (1999). Early childhood stuttering I: Persistency and recovery rates. *Journal of Speech Language & Hearing Research, 42*(5), 1097-1112.
Yairi, E., & Ambrose, N. G. (2005). *Early Childhood Stuttering for Clinicians by Clinicians.* Austin, TX: PRO-ED.
Yairi, E., & Ambrose, N. (2013). Epidemiology of stuttering: 21st century advances. *Journal of Fluency Disorders, 38*, 66-87.
Yairi, E., Ambrose, N. G., Paden, E. P., & Throneburg, R. N. (1996). Predictive factors of persistence and recovery: Pathways of childhood stuttering. *Journal of Communication Disorders, 29*(1), 51-77.
Yairi, E. & Lewis, B. (1984). Disfluencies at the onset of stuttering. *Journal of Speech and Hearing Research, 27*, 154-159.
Yaruss, J. S. (1998). Real-Time Analysis of Speech Fluency: Procedures and Reliability Training. *American Journal of Speech-Language Pathology, 7*(2), 25-37.
Yaruss, J. S. (1997). Clinical implications of situational variability in preschool children who stutter. *Journal of Fluency Disorders, 22*, 187-203.
Yaruss, J. S. (1998). Real-time analysis of speech fluency: Procedures and reliability training. *American Journal of Speech Language Pathology, 7*, 25-37.
Yaruss, J. S., Coleman, C., & Quesal, R. W. (2010). *OASES-S: Overall Assessment of the Speaker's Experience of Stuttering—School-Age* (Ages 7-12). Bloomington, MN: Pearson Assessments.
Yaruss, J. S., & Quesal R. W. (2006). Overall assessment of the speaker's experience of stuttering (OASES): Documenting multiple outcomes in stuttering treatment. *Journal of Fluency Disorders, 31*, 90-115.
Yaruss, J. S., & Quesal, R. W. (2010). *OASES-A: Overall Assessment of the Speaker's Experience of Stuttering—Adult (Ages 18+).* Bloomington, MN: Pearson Assessments.
Yaruss, J. S., Quesal, R. W., & Coleman, C. (2010). *OASES-T: Overall Assessment of the Speaker's Experience of Stuttering—Teenagers (Ages 13-17).* Bloomington, MN: Pearson Assessments.
Zebrowski, P. M., & Conture, E. G. (1989). Judgments of disfluency by mothers of stuttering and normally fluent children. *Journal of Speech and Hearing Research, 32*, 625-634.
Zebrowski, P. M., & Kelly, E. M. (2002). *Manual of stuttering intervention (Clinical Competence Series).* Clifton Park, NY: Singular/Thomson Learning.

Additional Recommended Reading

Books

Bennett, E. (2006). *Working with people who stutter. A lifespan approach.* Hoboken, NJ: Pearson.
Bloodstein, O., & Bernstein Ratner, N. (2008). *A handbook on stuttering* (6th ed.). Clifton Park, NY: Delmar.
Bloom, C. M., & Cooperman, D. K. (1999). *Synergistic stuttering therapy. A holistic approach.* Woburn, MA: Butterworth Heinemann.
Conture, E. G. (2001). *Stuttering: Its nature, assessment and treatment.* Needham Heights, MA: Allyn & Bacon.
Curlee, R. F. (1999). *Stuttering and related disorders of fluency* (2nd ed.). New York, NY: Thieme Medical.
Curlee, R.F., & Siegel, G. (1997), *Nature and treatment of stuttering: New directions* (2nd ed). Needham Heights, MA: Allyn & Bacon.
Guitar, B., & McCauley, R. (2009). *Treatment of stuttering: Established and emerging interventions.* Philadelphia, PA: Lippincott.
Guitar, B. (2006). *Stuttering: An integrated approach to its nature and treatment* (3rd ed.). Baltimore, MA: Lippincott, Williams & Wilkins.
Manning, W.H. (2009). *Clinical decision making in fluency disorders* (3rd ed.). Clifton Park, NY: Delmar.
Murphy, W .P., Quesal, R.W., Reardon-Reeves, N., & Yaruss, J. S. (2013). *Minimizing bullying for children who stutter: A workbook for students.* McKinney, TX: Stuttering Therapy Resources, Inc.
Murphy, W. P., Quesal, R.W., Reardon-Reeves, N., & Yaruss, J. S. (2013). *Minimizing bullying for children who stutter: A workbook for parents.* McKinney, TX: Stuttering Therapy Resources, Inc.
Murphy, W. P., Quesal, R.W., Reardon-Reeves, N., & Yaruss, J. S. (2013). *Minimizing bullying for children who stutter: A workbook for teachers and administrators.* McKinney, TX: Stuttering Therapy Resources, Inc.
Parry, W. (2006). *The second edition—understanding & controlling stuttering. A comprehensive new approach based on the Valsalva hypothesis.* New York, NY: NSA.
Ramig, P., & Dodge, D. (2005). *Child and adolescent stuttering treatment and activity resource guide.* New York: Thomson-Delmar Learning.
Reardon, N. A., & Yaruss, J. S. (2004). *The source for stuttering: Ages 7-18.* East Moline, IL: LinguiSystems.
Reardon-Reeves, N., & Yaruss, J. S. (2013). *School-age stuttering therapy: A practical guide.* McKinney, TX: Stuttering Therapy Resources, Inc.
Reeves, N., & Yaruss, J. S. (2015). *Stuttering: How teachers can help.* McKinney, TX: Stuttering Therapy Resources, Inc.
Shapiro, D.A. (1999). *Stuttering intervention: A collaborative journey to fluency freedom.* Austin, TX: Pro-Ed.
Walton, P., & Wallace, M. (1998). *Fun with fluency: Direct therapy with the young child.* Imaginart.
Zebrowski, P.M. & Kelly, E.M. (2002). *Manual of stuttering intervention: Clinical competence series.* Clifton Park, NY: Singular-Thomson Learning.

Journals

American Journal of Speech-Language Pathology: A Journal of Clinical Practice
Contemporary Issues in Communication Science and Disorders
Journal of Speech, Language, and Hearing Research
Journal of Fluency Disorders
Journal of Communication Disorders
Language, Speech, and Hearing Services in Schools

Seminars in Speech and Language
The Journal of Stuttering Therapy, Advocacy and Research
Perspectives on Fluency and Fluency Disorders (ASHA Special Interest Division)

Website Resources

American Institute for Stuttering: www.stutteringtreatment.org
FRIENDS: www.friendswhostutter.org
International Stuttering Association: www.isastutter.org/
Judith Kuster Stuttering Homepage: www.mnsu.edu/comdis/kuster/stutter.html
National Stuttering Association: www.nsastutter.org
Stuttering Foundation: www.stutteringhelp.org
The Canadian Stuttering Association: www.stutter.ca
American Speech-Language-Hearing Association Special Interest Group 4 (Fluency and Fluency Disorders): www.asha.org/SIG/04/

14

Assessment of Feeding and Swallowing Disorders Across the Life Span

Patricia Kerman Lerner, MA, CCC-SLP, BCS-S and Tina M. Tan, MS, CCC-SLP, BCS-S

Key Words

- achalasia
- anterior faucial arches
- aspiration
- autonomic stress signals
- cervical auscultation
- cervical osteophyte
- dehydration
- eosinophilic esophagitis
- extubation
- failure to thrive
- gastric dysmotility
- gastroesophageal reflux disorder
- gastrostomy tube
- intubation
- laryngeal cleft
- laryngomalacia
- laryngopharyngeal reflux
- malnutrition
- mastication
- nasogastric tube
- nasopharyngeal regurgitation
- oral aversion
- orogastric tube
- oxygen desaturation
- penetration
- percutaneous endoscopic gastrostomy
- percutaneous endoscopic jejunostomy
- peristalsis
- phasic bite reflex
- pneumonia
- protrusion reflex
- pulse oximeter
- rooting reflex
- sensory integration dysfunction
- silent aspiration
- total parenteral nutrition
- tracheoesophageal fistula
- transverse tongue reflex
- upper esophageal sphincter
- valleculae
- Zenker's diverticulum

Adult Feeding and Swallowing Impairments

The ability to eat and swallow is a basic function essential to our health and well-being, affording us both pleasure and nutrition throughout our lifetime. Oral intake is intertwined in the daily fabric of life, with many occasions being celebrated with foods and liquids. The act of swallowing encompasses the interaction of multiple complex anatomic, neurological, and physiological systems. Even small alterations in these systems—the timing of events, variants in the anatomy, or changes in the physiology involved in swallowing—can have a profound effect on a person's health and significantly alter a person's quality of life.

Stein-Rubin, C., & Fabus, R. *A Guide to Clinical Assessment and Professional Report Writing in Speech-Language Pathology, Second Edition (pp 335-380).*

Swallow impairments, known as *dysphagia*, can affect people across the life span and are seen in a wide range of developmental, neurological, structural, behavioral, and medical etiologies. American Speech-Language-Hearing Association (ASHA, 2016) estimates that approximately 10 million Americans are evaluated each year in the United States with swallowing difficulties. **Malnutrition** and **dehydration**, aspiration pneumonia, compromised general health, chronic lung disease, choking, and even death may be a consequence of dysphagia.

Dysphagia can impair a person's ability to swallow saliva, liquids, and/or food of all consistencies. A person with dysphagia may swallow unsafely, causing food or saliva to enter his or her airway, termed **aspiration**. By definition, aspiration is the misdirection of foreign material including food, liquid, or gastric contents into the lungs. On the other hand, a person may have a weak or slow swallow, resulting in difficulty obtaining adequate food and liquids to insure proper nutrition. **Mastication** of foods, or chewing, may be impaired, and some individuals may experience drooling. Others may have difficulty propelling their foods through their mouth or pharynx and into the esophagus. These deficits create serious problems in sustaining a healthy body and satisfying quality of life. There may also be impairments with swallowing and airway protection in children; however, difficulties may also encompass delayed or disordered feeding skills including difficulty transitioning to age-appropriate textures due to oral motor or oral sensory deficits and refusal behaviors.

Consequences of dysphagia range from discomfort (e.g., throat pain) to coughing and choking or even life-threatening illness. Serious sequela include airway obstruction, aspiration pneumonia, pulmonary infection caused by material entering the airway, severe weight loss, dehydration, reduced fluids within the body and malnutrition, poor nourishment of the body, **failure to thrive**, decreased quality of life, and stress within the family unit.

The focus of this chapter is on oropharyngeal feeding and swallowing disorders, although the term *dysphagia* is sometimes used for disorders throughout the aerodigestive tract, the total swallowing mechanism, which includes the esophagus. Specifically, this chapter addresses the diagnostic decision-making process and the resources needed to evaluate and document a feeding or swallowing impairment in individuals of all ages with a variety of medical disorders.

Oropharyngeal swallowing problems may arise from various causes, including developmental disabilities, neurological diseases such as stroke, degenerative diseases, alterations of anatomy and physiology, traumatic brain injury, cardiovascular and other systemic diseases, congenital defects, failure to thrive, and damage arising from chemoradiation treatment or surgery for head/neck cancer. Dysphagia may also arise from mechanical problems of the swallowing mechanism or from gastrointestinal disorders (Murry & Carrau, 2006).

The field of diagnosis and management of the individual with feeding and swallowing disorders is relatively new, with the bulk of research and relevant literature being published during the past few decades. Initially, the focus was on varying symptoms of the disorder, evaluation of impairments, and the treatment of the adult with dysphagia. As the knowledge base developed and the information, skills, and success in managing this population expanded, health care professionals became aware of the large number of infants and children with feeding and swallowing difficulties that were seriously impeding their health and development.

In writing this chapter, the authors considered both the development of the field and the commonality of basic information needed to evaluate and treat individuals across both populations. In keeping with the development of this specialty, we are first presenting information that is useful to the diagnosis and treatment of both populations. This is followed by specific information germane to each population.

Basic to the evaluation of feeding and swallowing disorders is the understanding of the anatomy and physiology of the oropharyngeal swallow mechanism. Figure 14-1 provides a detailed depiction of the anatomical structures of the oropharyngeal swallow mechanism. Swallowing is a complex series of coordinated events involving the cerebral cortex, brainstem, six cranial nerves, and more than 30 facial and oral muscles working together to initiate the swallowing process. The swallowing mechanism and the fundamentals of swallow physiology are similar across the age span. Normal swallowing is rapid, safe, and efficient, taking an individual less than 2 seconds to move foods and liquids from the mouth, through the pharynx, and into the esophagus (Logemann, 1998).

Swallowing is usually thought of as occurring in three stages: oral, including oral preparatory and oral transit; pharyngeal; and then esophageal. The first stage is voluntary and is controlled by cortical centers

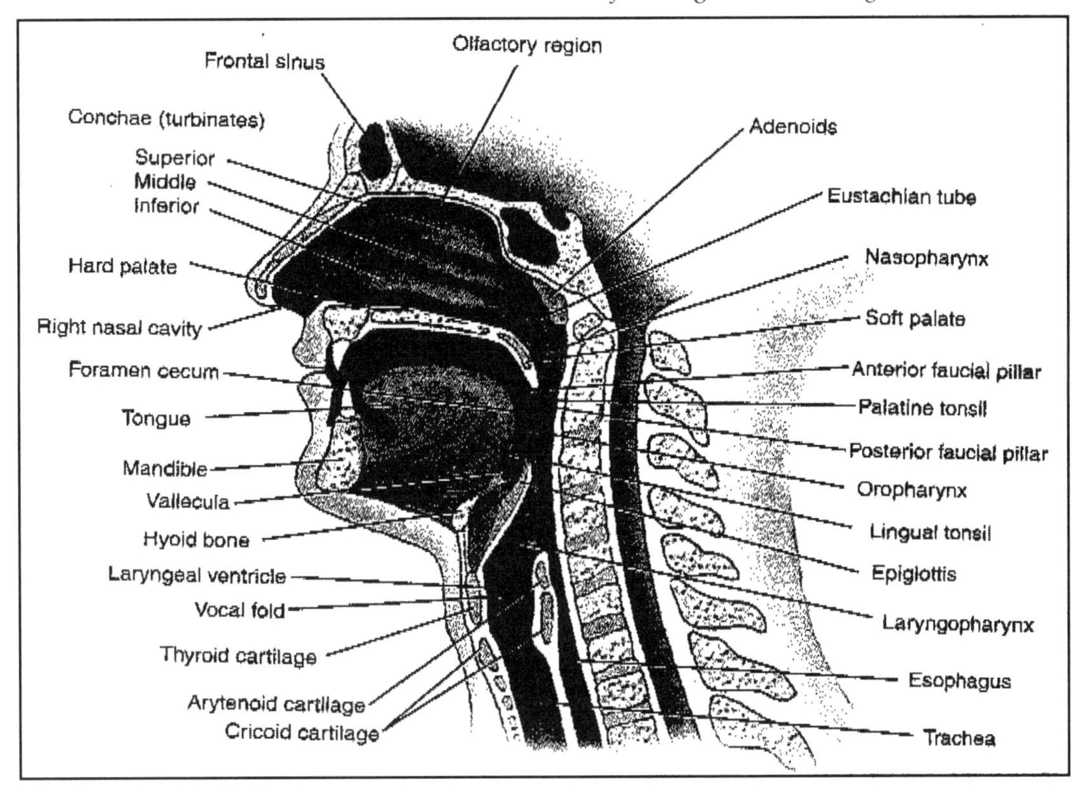

Figure 14-1. Adult oral, pharyngeal, laryngeal, and cervical esophageal structures.

located in the brain. The next two stages are involuntary and reflexive and primarily coordinated by brainstem centers.

Swallowing Stages

The following stages pertain to a normal swallow. See Figure 14-2 for a schematic of the process.

The Oral Preparatory Stage

Food is manipulated/prepared in the mouth as follows:

- Lips are closed.
- Food is mixed with saliva and formed into a bolus in the oral cavity.
- With liquids, the tongue cups around liquid with the sides of the tongue up against the lateral alveolar ridge.
- The velum (soft palate) usually makes contact with the back of the tongue.
- With solids, which require mastication, lateralization (side-to-side movement) and rotary action of the tongue and mandible takes place.
- The tongue repeatedly places material on the molars for mastication.
- After "chewing," foodstuff is prepared into a bolus or ball to be transported into the oropharynx.
- Foodstuff is held by the anterior portion of the tongue in a cupped position against the anterior alveolar ridge.
- Tension in the buccal musculature closes off lateral sulcus to decrease residue in the sulcus.
- The time this takes is variable, depending on viscosity.

The Oral Stage

- This stage is initiated when the oral tongue begins to move the material toward the oropharynx.
- Oral propulsion begins with the mid portion of the tongue sequentially squeezing material against the hard palate in a posterior direction.
- A grove created on the midline of the tongue acts as a ramp for food to pass. As food viscosity increases, greater oral tongue pressure against the palate is needed.
- The food is propelled backward in the mouth toward the oropharynx (Logemann, 1998).
- This process takes between less than 1 and 1.5 seconds.

The Pharyngeal Stage

This stage, which includes the pharyngal swallow and cricopharyngeal opening, is triggered as follows:

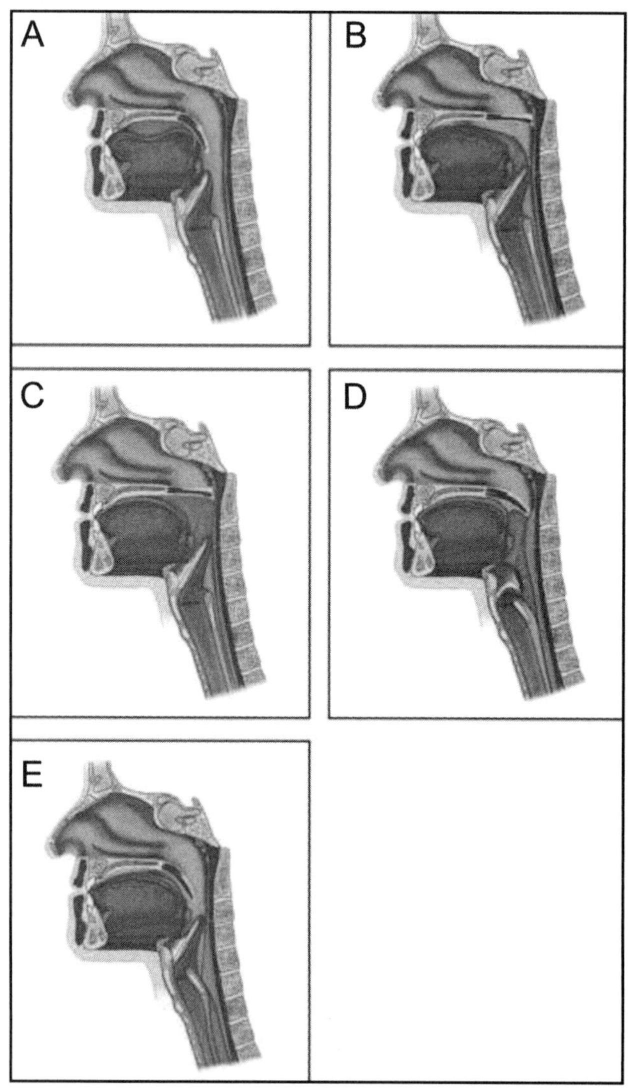

Figure 14-2. Schematic illustration showing oral, pharyngeal, and upper esophageal phases of a normal swallow (Shipley & McAfee, 2009). (A) Oral phase shows formed bolus contained within the oral cavity. (B) Head of the bolus is entering the oropharynx. (C) Pharyngeal swallow is initiated with elevated velum and beginning of posterior pharyngeal wall and tongue base contraction. (D) Movement of bolus through pharynx with protection of the airway. (E) Entry and movement of bolus into the UES and through the upper cervical esophagus.

- The pharyngeal stage of the swallow begins as the pharyngeal swallow is triggered.
- This initiation usually occurs when the head of the bolus passes a point where the tongue base crosses the lower edge of the mandible.
- In younger adults, the **anterior faucial arches** (separating the mouth from the pharynx) may be the anatomic point of trigger. In some older adults, the triggering of the swallow may not occur until material moves into the pharynx at the level of the **valleculae** (lateral recesses at the base of the tongue on each side of the epiglottis).

The Pharyngeal Swallow

After the swallow is triggered, the following occurs:

- The soft palate elevates and retracts, which results in closure of the velopharyngeal port.
- This closure prevents material from entering the nasal cavity.
- Both the hyoid and larynx elevate and move anteriorly, which is termed *hyolaryngeal excursion*.
- Closure of the larynx takes place from bottom up:
  - The true vocal cords approximate.
  - The laryngeal entrance closes (the false vocal cords close and the arytenoids tilt forward in a downward and inward rocking movement).
  - The base of the epiglottis thickens as the larynx rises and the arytenoids tilt forward.
  - The epiglottis moves into a horizontal position (epiglottic inversion).
- This closure prevents material from entering the airway (Logemann, 1998).

As material moves through the hypopharynx, the following occurs:

- The cricopharyngeal sphincter relaxes to prepare for material to be transported from the pharynx into the esophagus.
- The base of the tongue ramps and then bulges toward the posterior pharyngeal wall while the posterior pharyngeal wall contracts and moves in an anterior motion toward the tongue base.
- This tongue base contact with the posterior pharyngeal wall increases pharyngeal pressure generation.
- Marked shortening of the pharynx occurs during the bolus transport; the shortening of the pharynx also contributes to laryngeal elevation.
- The propulsive or stripping action generated moves the material through the pharynx and into the **upper esophageal sphincter** (UES) and through the cervical esophagus. The UES is a tonically contracted group of skeletal muscles separating the pharynx from the esophagus. The major muscle of this sphincter is the cricopharyngeus muscle, which is contracted except when food, liquid, or saliva is swallowed.
- Progressive top-to-bottom contraction of the pharyngeal constrictor muscles aids in the propulsion of material into the UES.
- Velopharyngeal closure occurs and enables the buildup of air pressure in the pharynx (Logemann, 1998).

Cricopharyngeal Opening

Cricopharyngeal opening (relaxation and opening of the cricopharyngeus muscle) occurs within the UES:

- Initial release of cricopharyngeal muscle tension
- Anterior and superior motion of the larynx pulling open the UES sphincter
- Pressure from the head of the bolus as it enters the upper cervical esophagus, which continues to open and widen the UES
- Timing of the pharyngeal stage is 1 second.

Esophageal Stage

The esophagus is a collapsed muscular tube approximately 23- to 25-cm long with a sphincter type valve at each end: the UES and the lower esophageal sphincter (LES).

- A peristaltic wave, a progressive esophageal muscular contraction, begins in the upper cervical esophagus and pushes the bolus ahead of it.
- **Peristalsis** continues in sequential fashion through the esophagus until the LES opens to allow the bolus to enter the stomach (Logemann, 1998).
- Esophageal transit times are usually from 8 to 10 seconds.

Oropharyngeal dysphagia is associated with an increased risk of airway obstruction, aspiration pneumonia, malnutrition, compromised general health, decreased quality of life, and, at times, death (ASHA, n.d.). If a feeding or swallowing impairment is suspected, a swallow evaluation should be performed to assess all stages of the swallowing mechanism to determine an initial comprehensive diagnosis and, as needed, a treatment and management plan.

Assessment of Feeding and Swallowing Disorders

Brief Clinical or Bedside Screen

Persons suspected of having a swallowing impairment may initially receive a "bedside screen" to grossly delineate oral, pharyngeal, and upper esophageal swallow functions. The bedside screen is usually brief and often administered as a pass–fail test. This screen of swallow function would be performed to determine the likelihood that a dysphagia exists. The screen provides valuable information for the patient's health care team and enables them to make an initial decision on whether the patient is cleared for oral intake. The clinical screen, however, does not define the disordered anatomy or physiology of the oropharynx and upper cervical esophagus, nor any resulting swallow impairments, nor a treatment regime (ASHA, n.d.).

The clinical or bedside screen may be performed by a trained health care professional (e.g., a nurse or other trained health care worker). Ideally, the brief screen would be completed during the initial hours of a patient's admission to a health care facility and would take place before foods or liquids are given to the patient. In some health care settings (e.g., hospital, nursing home, rehabilitation facility) where there are numerous patients whose medical history suggests a risk of an oropharyngeal swallow impairment, a brief "swallow screen" on admission is included in the patient's initial care.

ASHA recommends that individuals with suspected swallow impairments should be screened for swallowing deficits "as soon as they are alert and ready for trialing oral intake (e.g. medications, food, liquid)" (ASHA, n.d.). For possible screening protocols, see Antonios et al. (2010); Logemann, Veis, and Colangelo (1999); Martino et al. (2014); and the ASHA Portal: "Adult Screening."

Assessment: Full Clinical and Bedside Examination

If swallow difficulties are noted or suspected, a clinical examination of swallowing, performed by a speech-language pathologist (SLP), to assess signs and symptoms of swallow dysfunction and determine the status of the swallowing mechanism is often the first in-depth assessment. It usually includes a medical, feeding, and swallowing history and an assessment of the oral and anterior pharyngeal structures. It should note suspected aspiration events. It may also include the effect of any postures, maneuvers, or strategies that appear to improve the swallow. This clinical assessment may offer observations of swallow competence if test swallows are given (Goodrich & Walker, 2008). However, with the adult population, the clinical assessment does not fully define the disordered anatomy or physiology of the oropharynx and upper cervical esophagus nor the resulting swallow impairments. It usually does not contain the necessary information to initiate a treatment program and swallow management plan. It does, however, identify those patients who should receive an instrumental assessment to fully assess the patient's swallow mechanism and then, based on the findings of the clinical and instrumental assessments, initiate a swallow treatment and management plan.

Components of an In-Depth Clinical "Bedside" Assessment for Adults

1. Medical and Feeding and Swallow History: An in-depth clinical examination is usually initiated by obtaining a medical history including significant medical conditions and past surgeries, current medical diagnosis, patient's respiratory status, any respiratory diseases, and/or complicating medical factors. The clinical evaluation would also provide information for the initiation of swallow rehabilitation and, as appropriate, a suggested plan for oral intake.

   Obtaining a description of the feeding/swallowing difficulty is essential for diagnostic accuracy. The patient should describe the difficulties he or she is having when eating or drinking. Does the patient or caregiver describe coughing or choking, the sensation of food "stuck" in the throat, difficulty managing saliva, difficulty with foodstuffs entering the esophagus, nasal regurgitation, or material remaining in the mouth or pharynx after oral intake? What is the length of time the symptoms have occurred, and what is the severity of these symptoms?

- Current Nutritional and Feeding Status: What type of diet is the patient taking? Full oral diet? Modified diet? If any oral intake is taken, what are the diet modifications? Is the patient well nourished; is his or her weight within normal range, or is there a marked weight loss? If the patient is not eating by mouth, what type of nonoral feedings is he or she receiving? For further information, refer to the section, "Nonoral Feeding Options."
- Oral-Peripheral Mechanism: Assess symmetry of the face and smile and assessment of oral and facial sensation. Is there adequate jaw movement and is lip closure present? Can lip closure be maintained? Note the patient's dentition and secretion management. Is there control of saliva or is drooling present? Is the swallow reflex timely and intact?
- Behavioral Status: Is the patient alert, oriented, and cooperative, or is he or she lethargic, inattentive, distractible, or uncooperative? Does the patient show good endurance or fatigue easily? Is the patient aware of swallow difficulties?
- Respiratory System: Is the patient's respiratory system functional, with independent ventilation and adequate respiratory rate and rhythm, or is the patient on oxygen support using a ventilator, continuous positive airway pressure (CPAP), or a nasal canella? Does the patient have a tracheotomy for respiratory support? If so, is there a tracheostomy tube, cuffed or not cuffed, with or without a speaking valve?
- Swallow Screen With Liquid or Food Trials: If deemed appropriate, and if minimal risk to the patient's health, small trials of foods and/or liquids may be attempted in the examination. If oral trials are given, the following observations should be part of these trials:
  - Strength of lip seal
  - Appropriate tongue movement and coordination especially when attempting purees and solids
  - Tongue strength and range of motion during oral intake
  - Oral transit time, measured from entry point at lips to when swallow reflex is triggered (Mann, 2002)
  - Clearance of material from the mouth, including the presence or absence of residual material after the swallow is completed
  - Laryngeal elevation, both timing and completeness
  - Changes in vocal quality (e.g., from the patient's baseline to a wet, hoarse, or gurgly vocal quality after oral ingestion of small amounts of foodstuffs or liquid)
  - Coughing during or after ingestion of material; this may signal that material has been misdirected into the laryngeal airway entrance or into the airway itself

Risks of Oral Trials

There are risks associated with initiating oral trials without first completing a full diagnostic instrumental oropharyngeal swallow assessment. An instrumental assessment provides definitive information about the strength and safety of the oropharyngeal swallow mechanism. Using an instrumental assessment affords the clinician an evaluation that can provide definitive and reliable data about the safety of the oropharyngeal swallow. In addition, instrumental procedures can be used during testing to determine the appropriateness and the effectiveness of a variety of treatment strategies that can enhance swallow performance (ASHA, n.d.: "Adult Dysphagia").

High-risk factors for the patient when considering oral trials during a clinical assessment include the following:

- Acute illness
- Reduced pulmonary function
- Recent history of pulmonary infections
- Poor or weak cough
- Elderly or debilitated patient
- Presence of a tracheostomy
- Recent **extubation**, which involves removal of the airway tube previously placed into the trachea for breathing
- Reduced cognition
- Suspected pharyngeal swallow impairment

A trial of oral feeding given before an instrumental assessment is performed may be of high risk/low benefit when two or more of the factors listed previously are present especially when a swallow impairment is suspected. Refer to Daniels and Huckabee (2008), Groher and Crary (2010), and Mann (2002) for additional information on the clinical/bedside examination.

Additional Pertinent Medical Information

The following are brief descriptions of medical factors important to the master clinician when evaluating a person with feeding swallowing impairments.

The presence or absence of aspiration is often a critical part of an individual's assessment. By definition, aspiration is the passage of material into the airway below the level of the true vocal cords. Aspiration can interfere with effective air exchange and lead to asphyxiation, for example, or cause pulmonary inflammation and infection (e.g., aspiration pneumonia). Aspiration may occur before the actual swallow because of an unprotected larynx, during the pharyngeal swallow from overflow of residue remaining in the pharynx, or after the swallow from remaining laryngeal or upper esophageal residue or reflux of gastric contents (Perlman & Schulze-Delnieu, 1997).

Pneumonia is an acute infection and inflammation where efficient exchange of oxygen and carbon dioxide is compromised, affecting a person's health. Often, inflammation of the lungs is the body's response to handling the developing infection. Aspiration of foods, liquids, or even saliva can lead to pneumonia and damage the integrity of the immune system (Ashford, 2005).

Aspiration incidence that may precipitate pneumonia includes the following (Ashford, 2005):

- Frequent episodes of aspiration during oral intake or even with saliva swallows
- Volume of aspirated material
- Bacterial load, liquid vs. solid material
- pH level of the aspirated contents
- Frequency of aspiration events
- Integrity of immune system

The larynx is the gatekeeper of the lower respiratory system. Pneumonia may develop after one episode of aspiration or many small aspiration events over time, or pneumonia may develop as a secondary disease in a person who has an already established serious illness.

Smith and colleagues (1999) investigated the incidence of **silent aspiration** in a hospital population by analyzing all videofluoroscopic swallow studies performed over a 2-year period on patients with suspected signs of swallow difficulty in two major acute hospitals in the Chicago, IL area. Two thousand patients were reviewed, representing ages 3 to 98 years with a variety of medical diagnoses. Of that number, 1101 patients showed dysphagia and, of that group, 467 (44%) of the patients aspirated. Within the group of patients who showed aspiration, 276 (59%) had silent aspiration. Silent aspiration was noted when the patient showed no immediate overt signs that he or she was aspirating liquids or foods. In this carefully controlled investigation with a large study population, 59% of those patients who aspirated, aspirated silently. Smith and colleagues (1999) pointed out that these patients aspirated without showing any signs or symptoms that material had entered their airway. See Langmore, Skarupski, Park, and Fries (2002) for additional information on risk factors resulting in aspiration pneumonia.

Additional Clinical Assessments

Supplemental tests are available to provide other information on a patient's oropharyngeal swallow function. The use of **cervical auscultation** to hear breath sounds during swallow tasks, the **pulse oximeter** to measure adequacy of oxygen saturation during swallowing, and the blue dye test to determine the presence or absence of airway **penetration** during oral intake trials are several supplemental tests available to the clinician.

Cervical Auscultation

Cervical auscultation, an acoustic technique, allows the examiner to study the airway sounds produced by the patient during the swallowing task. A small microphone within a stethoscope is placed on the patient's neck, usually by the posterior portion of the thyroid cartilage or lateral portion of the larynx during the swallow. The examiner listens for specific sounds heard during the swallow. The literature reports some success in hearing a "click" associated with the opening of the Eustachian tube and a "clunk" associated with opening of the UES. Others find it valuable to listen to the inhalation and exhalation phases of respiration during the swallow. The change from quiet and clear breathing to a wet, gurgly breath quality can suggest swallowed material or secretions in the airway and, therefore, that aspiration has occurred. See Daniels and Huckabee (2008) for additional information.

Oxygen Saturation Test

A pulse oximeter attached to the individual is used to measure the patient's oxygen saturation level. Attaching the pulse oximeter to the patient (often to the finger or toe) can detect changes in oxygen saturation during the swallowing of foodstuffs. The rationale is based on the assumption that changes in the respiratory status may signal a change in airway protection during swallowing (Groher & Crary, 2010). Although the recent literature is mixed on its predictive value, Smith and colleagues (1999) noted that a 2% drop in oxygen saturation levels had an 86% sensitivity level in predicting aspiration. They advocated combining the standard clinical evaluation and oxygen saturation monitoring to improve the prediction of aspiration (Smith et al., 1999).

Sherman, Nisenboum, Jesberger, Morrow, and Jesberger (1999) studied 46 individuals who underwent a videofluoroscopic swallow study while being monitored by pulse oximetry. They found that patients who exhibited aspiration or penetration without clearance had a significant decline in oxygen saturation levels. The authors concluded that pulse oximetry could be a useful tool as part of a bedside examination of a person with symptoms of dysphagia.

Modified Evans "Blue Dye" Test

This test has been used to determine the presence of aspiration in a patient with a tracheotomy. The patient is given either foodstuff or liquid mixed with a few drops of food coloring to swallow. The coloring allows the examiner to distinguish any aspirated material from other secretions (ASHA, n.d.). After the patient swallows the test materials, suctioning is performed through the tracheostomy site. If there are colored foods or secretions suctioned out of the tracheostomy, one may suspect aspiration. Suctioning can be repeated at timed intervals; one protocol uses 15-minute intervals for the first hour after swallowing, and another protocol suctions at hourly intervals for at least 3 hours. If there are positive findings, it is common for precautions—no oral intake or specific dietary restrictions—to be put in place while the patient is receives further assessment (ASHA, n.d.).

The validity of the blue dye test has been called into question. Comments written by Steven Leder (1996) point out reduced sensitivity and specificity, resulting in aspiration not being detected in some patients, while false positives were noted in other patients. Furthermore, normal secretions often flow from the mouth into the pharynx. This can result in the food coloring mixing with normal secretions that gradually coat the upper trachea, allowing the trachea to remain moist. Therefore, when the patient is suctioned, the color-tinged normal secretions may appear as aspirated material. In addition to its limited validity, the blue dye test does not reveal the anatomical or physiological cause(s) of aspiration.

The Water Test

Various water tests used as part of a clinical assessment have been presented and discussed in the literature. Leder and Suiter (2010) studied 3000 patients admitted to the hospital with a variety of medical conditions. To screen their swallow function, each patient was asked to drink 3 oz of water from a cup using consecutive sips without stopping. Leder and Suiter relied on the patient showing visible signs of discomfort, exhibiting immediate voice changes or immediate coughs in response to the ingestion of water. Leder and Suiter considered this assessment an accurate measure of whether aspiration was present. The assumptions appear in direct contrast to other studies that show a high percentage of persons with suspected aspiration are aspirating silently. Those patients fail to cough or throat clear in response to the aspirated material (Smith et al., 1999).

Red-Flag Indicators of Pharyngeal Swallowing Difficulty

During a clinical swallowing assessment, certain signs, symptoms, medical conditions or history may suggest that the patient is at high risk for a swallowing problem. Examples include patients with the following:

- History of spiking fevers
- History of pneumonia, especially a recent episode or repeated pneumonia
- Frequent upper respiration infections/chronic lung disease
- Presence of tracheostomy
- Vocal cord paralysis
- Difficulty swallowing saliva
- Unexplained coughing or frequent episodes of coughing up mucous
- Unexplained throat clearing
- Vocal quality change
- Episodes of unexplained **oxygen desaturation**, especially when eating/drinking
- Diagnosis of a medical condition contributing to an increased risk of dysphagia (e.g., stroke, Parkinson disease, degenerative neurological diseases, dementia, recent cardiac surgery, or head and neck surgery)

With some patients at high risk for swallow impairments, a swallow screen may result in recommendations for rescreening or additional assessments before oral intake is initiated. The swallowing assessments allow the SLP to integrate information from the interview/case history, medical/clinical records, the physical examination, previous screening and assessments, and collaboration and input from physicians and other caregivers. During the assessment, the SLP can determine whether the patient is an appropriate candidate for treatment or management. This determination is based on findings that include medical stability; cognitive status; nutritional status; and psychosocial, environmental, and behavioral factors.

Esophageal Disorders That Can Affect Swallowing Function

The SLP should be familiar with common gastroesophageal disorders that may impact on the patient's swallowing function. Although gastroesophageal impairments are treated by a medical practitioner, the clinician should be aware of the effects that these conditions may have on the oropharyngeal swallow. Equally important are the occasions that the patient reports a swallowing problem when the symptoms actually originate within the esophagus. Several common esophageal disorders that can produce symptoms of an oropharyngeal swallow disorder include the following.

Gastroesophageal Reflux Disorder

Gastroesophageal reflux disorder (GERD) is the retrograde flow of gastric contents from the stomach through the LES and into the esophagus (and possibly into the upper airway.) People with GERD often complain of noncardiac chest pain, regurgitation of gastric contents, excessive salivary secretions, dysphagia and sometimes odynophagia (pain when swallowing). GERD is often associated with symptoms including pharyngitis, laryngitis, hoarseness, chronic cough, asthma, aspiration, and, at times, globus—the sensation of a lump in the throat (Murry & Carrau, 2006).

GERD is thought to occur through one of four mechanisms:

1. Inadequate or transient relaxation of the LES
2. Increased abdominal pressure or stress-induced reflux
3. Incompetent or reduced pressure of the LES valve between the esophagus and the stomach
4. Spontaneous reflux

GERD may be the underlying etiology of a globus sensation. **Laryngopharyngeal reflux** is similar to reflux but occurs when the stomach contents reach the larynx, frequently resulting in odynophagia, pain when swallowing, hoarseness, sore throat, a globus sensation, and/or chronic throat clearing (Groher, 2010a).

Motility Disorders Associated With Swallowing Difficulties

- **Achalasia**: Failure or incomplete relaxation of the LES and/or absent peristalsis of the esophagus
- Nonpropulsive tertiary contractions: Esophageal motility often seen in elderly people
- Diffuse esophageal spasm: Seen with intermittent dysphagia, chest pain, and repetitive contractions of the esophagus; on imaging, the esophagus may have a "corkscrew" appearance

Nonspecific Esophageal Disorders

Often seen in persons with symptoms of dysphagia without evidence of other systemic diseases:

- Presbyesophagus: Esophageal dysmotility related to the normal aging process; may include muscle weakness, muscle atrophy or reduced speed of movement of material through the esophagus (Murry & Carrau, 2006)
- Diverticulum: Esophageal out-pouching of one or more layers of the esophageal wall

- Webs/rings: Esophagus is narrowed by an extra band of tissue, often mucosal, that impedes the flow of material through the esophagus (Patients with intermittent dysphagia for solids may have an esophageal web or ring. A Schatzki ring, a lower esophageal mucosal ring seen when chronic gastroesophageal reflux is present, may be associated with a hiatal hernia.)

Instrumental Assessments of Swallow

An instrumental swallow examination should provide a complete picture of the oropharyngeal swallowing deficits observed. This information aids in formulating an evidence-based diagnosis, effective treatment, and a patient-specific plan of care. The most widely used instrumental assessments of swallow function available to the practitioner are the videofluoroscopic swallow study (VFSS), termed the modified barium study (MBS), and the fiberoptic endoscopic evaluation of swallowing (FEES; Langmore, 2001) and FEES with sensory testing (FEESST; Aviv et al., 1998).

Videofluoroscopic Swallow Study

VFSS is often the instrument of choice for practicing SLPs. It offers a comprehensive dynamic assessment of the oral, pharyngeal, and cervical esophageal phases of swallowing. VFSS is a radiographic procedure that provides a direct, dynamic view of oral, pharyngeal, and upper esophageal function (Logemann, 1993). An SLP completes VFSS by providing the patient with various consistencies of food and liquid mixed with barium, which allows the bolus to be visualized in real time, during the swallow via x-ray. VFSS uses videofluoroscopy to assess the swallow physiology during the oropharyngeal swallow examination by recording and viewing bolus formation, manipulation, and propulsion into the oropharynx and the aerodigestive track (Martin-Harris et al., 2008; Martin-Harris & Jones, 2008). VFSS is performed collaboratively by a radiologist or trained radiology technician and an SLP in a radiology suite.

The study allows for detection of the presence and timing of aspiration and provides information about the physiological causes of the aspiration. Martin-Harris and Jones (2008) pointed out that clinicians are able "to observe the effects of various bolus volumes, bolus textures, and compensatory strategies on the swallow physiology." It allows swallow modifications to be attempted during VFSS study that will reduce the observed swallow deficits.

VFSS is performed with the patient ingesting various consistencies of foods and liquids that are impregnated with a radiopaque contrast agent, usually barium. The consistencies chosen approximate the consistencies of foods and liquids that are common in daily oral intake. The recorded study can be viewed in regular speed, slow motion or frame by frame. This allows the clinician to obtain a detailed analysis of function, coordination, and timing of the swallow. It identifies the presence or absence of penetration and/or aspiration of material into the oropharynx and can observe the patient's attempts, if any, to clear the misdirected material.

If aspiration is seen, the study defines the etiology of aspiration as well as other swallow deficits noted (Logemann, 1998). It allows testing of multiple aspects of the oropharyngeal swallow, obtains real-time observations, and examines the effects of specific treatment procedures, compensatory strategies and swallow maneuvers (Murry & Carrau, 2006). VFSS is beneficial not only in identifying whether aspiration has occurred, but also the strategies that can be used during swallowing to decrease or eliminate the aspiration. VFSS can provide assessment of amount and timing of aspiration as well as assessment of anatomy and pathophysiology of swallow function in the oral and pharyngeal phases. It provides clinically useful information on the influence of compensatory strategies and diet changes (Martin-Harris et al., 2008).

Protocol for Performing VFSS

A standard protocol is recommended for VFSS because it allows the clinician to compare the test results against established criteria and ensures the consistency and reproducibility of examinations both within and across patients (Groher & Crary, 2010).

The protocol, originated by Jeri Logemann in her book, *Evaluation and Treatment of Swallowing Disorders* (1998) is easy to use, is widely accepted, and gives information that can be compared within the same patient, across patients, and across settings.

VFSS usually includes a variety of volumes, textures, and consistencies and visualizes the patient initially in a lateral plane. The patient is given discrete amounts of thin liquid starting with 1 mL and proceeding to 3, 5, and 10 mL and sips from a cup (average sip approximately 20 mL) as tolerated. If the patient cannot safely tolerate thin liquids, a thicker liquid (e.g., nectar-thick or honey-thick liquid) may be presented. This is followed by presentations of puree (pudding) and a solid to masticate, usually a cookie (e.g., a Lorna Doone [Nabisco]). After the lateral imaging view, the patient may be turned and viewed in the anterior-posterior plane to assess the symmetry of structures and function in the oral cavity and pharynx, cervical esophageal transport of material, and any pronounced residue in the oral cavity and cervical esophagus (Logemann, 1998).

During the evaluation, compensatory postures and/or swallow maneuvers may be attempted to improve swallow safety and efficiency. The effects of modifying the bolus viscosities can be also be examined. For more information, see Logemann (1993) and Groher and Crary (2010).

The Modified Barium Swallow Impairment Profile

In recent years, an enhanced modified barium swallowing radiographic assessment, the modified barium swallow impairment profile (MBSImp), was developed by Bonnie Martin-Harris and colleagues. The MBSImp was devised to perfect the clinician's ability to reliably quantify and report swallow impairments (Martin-Harris et al., 2008). It was designed to establish a new benchmark for swallow evaluation terminology, administration, and measurement. The tool attempts to provide a standardized evaluation protocol and an objective means of assessing swallow impairments using VFSS. The tool suggests a procedure for using universally accepted and standardized terminology and a protocol for administration and quantification of all major physiological components of the swallow mechanism (Martin-Harris et al., 2008, Martin-Harris & Jones, 2008; Sandidge, 2009).

Seventeen discrete swallow components are measured and "scored according to ascending levels of severity specific to observations of discrete variation in physiology inherent to each component" (Sandidge, 2009). These 17 components and their operational definitions comprise the MBSImp diagnostic tool. After VFSS (MBS) is administered to the patient, each of the 17 components is separately scored by a trained clinician using a short, ordinal, usually 3- to 5-point scale (Sandidge, 2009). Training on its use, protocol, and scoring system is available for clinicians using this tool either in continuing educational regional seminars or through Web-based modules. The following are the Physiological Components of the MBSImp:

1. Lip closure
2. Hold position/tongue control
3. Bolus preparation/mastication
4. Bolus transport/lingual motion
5. Initiation of pharyngeal swallow
6. Oral residue
7. Soft palate elevation and retraction
8. Laryngeal elevation
9. Anterior hyoid excursion
10. Epiglottic movement
11. Laryngeal vestibular closure
12. Pharyngeal stripping wave
13. Pharyngeal contraction
14. Pharyngoesophageal segment opening
15. Tongue base retraction
16. Pharyngeal residue
17. Esophageal clearance in the upright position

Fiberoptic Endoscopic Evaluation of Swallowing

FEES involves the passage of a fiberoptic endoscope through the nostril, into the nasopharynx, and then the pharynx to view the pharyngeal swallow during ingestion of various materials with varying consistencies. The examiner uses the flexible nasoendoscope for viewing and evaluates the larynx and pharynx while giving the patient small amounts of liquids and solids mixed with food dye or another coloring agent to swallow (Langmore, 2001). The study, which is also recorded, does not involve any radiation and is more sensitive than the MBS in detecting structural abnormalities of the pharynx and larynx. However, it does not assess the oral stage of swallowing, the cervical esophagus or, in some patients, view the actual swallow when it is occurring. This limits the examiner's information as to the oral, pharyngeal, and cervical esophageal deficits. The evaluation for aspiration during the swallow may also be limited because the aspiration is usually not seen at the moment of occurrence. Furthermore, depending on the endoscope's positioning, the examiner may not be able to observe additional aspects of the exam such as swallow modifications performed during the study (swallow postures, maneuvers, or changes in size or presentation of the bolus) to obtain improved swallow function. For further description and protocol, see Langmore's (2001) comprehensive textbook.

Fiberoptic Endoscopic Evaluation of Swallowing With Sensory Testing

FEESST, often used in conjunction with FEES, evaluates both the motor and sensory components of the swallowing mechanism by combining the basic endoscopic evaluation, FEES, with testing of the laryngopharyngeal sensory discrimination thresholds. Initially, FEESST testing delivers air pulse stimuli through a port in the flexible nasoendoscope to the mucosa innervated by the superior laryngeal nerve to elicit the laryngeal adductor reflex. For testing, air pulses (puffs of air) are delivered to the supraglottic larynx and pharynx.

The premise is this: By using a puff of air, the examiner can assess sensory thresholds. When the puff of air is presented, the "twitch" response of the laryngeal mucosa suggests sensory awareness. Therefore, FEESST can provide an accurate indication of sensory function or dysfunction of the aryepiglottic space. A positive response is thought to reflect an awareness of material in the oropharynx and the ability to protect the airway from aspiration (Aviv et al., 1998, 2000, 2002). For additional information, see Aviv et al. (2005), which reviews patient characteristics and patient safety in more 1300 consecutive patients examined with FEESST.

Comparing the Most Commonly Used Instrumental Assessments

FEES Versus VFSS

VFSS is a comprehensive examination that assesses the entire swallow including the oral, pharyngeal, and cervical esophageal phases. In contrast, FEES provides a partial viewing focused only on the laryngopharyngeal segment of the swallow. FEES infers events during the swallow because the actual pharyngeal swallow is often not visualized during the examination. There is often a lack of visualization of the pharynx because the epiglottis descends from a vertical to a horizontal position over the larynx. When that occurs, the laryngeal airway entrance may not be seen during the moment of the swallow. In contrast, VFSS views the pharyngeal and laryngeal impairments before, during, and after the actual moment of the swallow. With VFSS, the examiner is able to see all stages of the swallow.

The choice of which diagnostic tool to use depends on the medical questions raised, status of the patient, risk factors present, the diagnostic information needed, and whether treatment or a management regimen are desired as part of the patient's plan of care (Tables 14-1 and 14-2).

Additional and Supplemental Assessments

The following tests offer the clinician valuable additional information to aid in the diagnostic decision-making process and can be used in the creation of a treatment and management plan.

The Penetration and Aspiration Scale

The Penetration–Aspiration (P-A) 8-point scale developed by Rosenbek, Robbins, Roecker, Coyle, and Wood, first published in 1996, is a valuable tool to assess and quantify the deficits of penetration and aspiration. It offers the clinician important information that guides both treatment and patient management. The P-A scale is a validated ordinal equal-appearing interval scale that measures bolus direction by focusing on depth of airway invasion, clearance, and the patient's response (e.g., cough) to airway invasion. Used during the instrumental evaluation, the scale rates the severity of the penetration and/or aspiration and the patient's awareness of the misdirection detected during the exam (Robbins et al., 1999).

A score of 1 denotes no airway entrance of material (no laryngeal penetration or aspiration). Scores between 2 to 5 indicate laryngeal penetration using depth and clearance to determine the specific score. Scores 6 to 8 denote aspiration using the patient's response and clearance of the misdirected material to determine the specific score (Daniels & Huckabee, 2008, p. 135). Use of the scale can enhance the practitioner's diagnostic acumen and assist in integrating the diagnostic data into the patient's swallow management plan. As the patient's swallow improves, the patient will usually score higher on the P-A. This scale can enhance the practitioner's way of viewing swallow improvement and recovery (Table 14-3).

The SWAL–QOL Scale

The Swallowing Quality of Life (SWAL-QOL) scale was developed to assess the patient's feelings about his or her swallowing impairment and the effect of the disorder on the patient's day-to-day quality of life. It gives both the patient and the SLP insight into attainable goals for a meaningful swallow recovery. The standardized 44-item questionnaire covers 10 quality-of-life categories and requires 15 to 20 minutes

Table 14-1. Salient Differences Between FEES and VFSS (MBS)

FEES	*VFSS (MBS)*
Invasive	Noninvasive
No radiation exposure	Radiation exposure
Primarily views pharyngeal stage deficits	Views all stages of swallowing—oral, pharyngeal, and cervical esophageal
Excellent view of vocal cord function in motion	Limited view of vocal cord function
Excellent view of pharyngeal and laryngeal anatomy	Excellent view of oral, pharyngeal, laryngeal, and cervical esophageal physiology
Often cannot view the aspiration when it is occurring	Can see aspiration when occurring
Cannot determine the causation of the penetration or aspiration	Can measure and determine the causation of the penetration or aspiration
Examiner may have limited view of attempted techniques and compensatory strategies	Examiner has full view to determine effective techniques and compensatory strategies
Limited view while assessing specific techniques for aspiration clearance	Usually full view to determine successful techniques for aspiration clearance
Cannot visualize full UES function as view is limited to "top-down"	Visualize full UES function including opening, duration of opening, whether backflow exists, and why
Unable to view certain parameters (e.g., etiology of backflow into the hypopharynx, UES stricture, presence of a diverticulum)	Can analyze additional parameters not viewed by FEES (e.g., backflow, presence of a diverticulum, UES stricture)
Cannot time major components of the swallow	Can time major components of the swallow
No time limit to study; may use for patient training (e.g., biofeedback)	Clinician must have access to radiology equipment and space Limited examination time because of radiation exposure
Limited ability to assess impact of cervical osteophytes, **Zenker's diverticulum**, or other factors on swallow function	Can assess impact of cervical osteophytes, Zenker's diverticulum, etc.
Limited view of pharyngeal propulsion	Full view of pharyngeal propulsion
FEES is portable, can be performed bedside	VFSS needs radiology suite and radiology imaging equipment

to complete. The quality-of-life indicators include burden, eating duration, eating desire, food selection, communication, fear, mental health, social role, fatigue, and sleep. Administration of the SWAL-QOL before and during the course of swallow treatment may allow the clinician to document the effects of improved swallowing on a person's quality of life. Additional information including the test items and scoring can be found in McHorney et al. (2000, 2002).

There are some additional evaluation procedures performed on individuals with feeding and swallowing impairments to assist in the differential diagnosis of the etiology of the dysphagia. The clinician should be aware of these additional procedures, although they are outside of the scope of practice of the SLP and are usually performed by a specialized medical practitioner. Table 14-2 summarizes the most commonly ordered tests for both children and adults, provides a brief description, and outlines benefits and limitations of each.

Nonoral Feeding Options

Some patients are unable to take adequate nutrition by mouth. This may be temporary in patients who are recovering from an acute medical condition such as a stroke, or long term as with patients who have a neuromuscular degenerative disease and are no longer able to manage oral nutrition (Murry & Carrau, 2006). In those cases, nonoral feedings can provide a nutritiously balanced formula that bypasses the mouth, throat and esophagus. There are two types of nonoral feedings: enteral feedings that use a functional gastrointestinal (GI) tract, and parenteral feedings that

Table 14-2. Common Instrumental Assessments Used With Children and Adults Demonstrating Feeding and Swallowing Difficulties

Test/Procedure	*Adult or Pediatric*	*Description*	*Advantages*	*Disadvantages*
Barium esophagram	Both	Radiographic study performed by radiologist only Patient drinks liquid barium; structures are viewed while in supine, side-lying, or standing	Provides good visualization of the structures of the GI tract Detects anatomic defects such as TEF, strictures, vascular rings, and achalasia	Low sensitivity for detecting reflux and aspiration Exposure to radiation Child has to ingest unknown material
Endoscopy	Both	Performed by gastroenterologist Visualization of esophagus; able to obtain mucosal biopsy	Aids in differential diagnosis of GERD, EoE, and food allergies Used for foreign body removal	Invasive and requires sedation/general anesthesia
24-hour pH monitoring (can be combined with multichannel intraluminal impedance testing)	Both	Assesses the frequency and severity of acid reflux Insertion of nasoesophageal catheter with sensors placed just below the UES and right above the lower esophageal sphincter Single-, dual-, or four-channel monitoring	Variables such as presence of tube feedings, position of patient and the use of pharmacological agents can be manipulated to seek particular information Good detection of reflux Records data such as time of each episode, number of reflux episodes, length of episodes, and overall percentage of time that reflux is present	Invasive; remains in place for 24 hours
Esophageal manometry	Both	Quantifies the contractible activity and pressure dynamics of the pharynx, UES, and esophagus during swallowing Involves transnasal insertion of a catheter with a series of intraluminal solid-state transducers	Useful in diagnosis of motor disorders of esophagus such as achalasia or other disorders Can be used in combination with multichannel intraluminal impedance testing	Invasive
Nuclear Scintigraphy Procedures (various studies including swallow scintigraphy, milk scan, salivagram)	Both	Nuclear medicine test: Patient swallows food/liquid with radionuclide isotope Various temporal measurements can be obtained to track material through aerodigestive tract	Quantifies pharyngeal residue, aspiration (if occurs), and timing of bolus motility Can detect GERD and timing of stomach emptying in pediatrics Limited radiation exposure with minimal taste changes to food/liquid	Poor visualization of anatomic structures of swallowing Cannot diagnosis structural issues of GI tract Duration of study can be 1 to 2 hours

EoE = eosinophilic esophagitis; GI = gastrointestinal; TEF = tracheoesophageal fistula.

Additional pediatric material adapted from Arvedson & Brodsky (2002) and Vandenplas et al. (2009). Additional adult material adapted from Perlman & Schulze-Delnieu (1997).

Table 14-3. The Penetration-Aspiration Scale

Score	*Description of the Penetration–Aspiration Event*
1	Material does not enter the airway.
2	Material enters the airway, remains above the vocal folds, and is ejected from the airway.
3	Material enters the airway, remains above the vocal folds, and is not ejected from the airway.
4	Material enters the airway, contacts the vocal folds, and is ejected from the airway.
5	Material enters the airway, contacts the vocal folds, and is not ejected from the airway.
6	Material enters the airway, passes below the vocal folds, and is ejected into the larynx or out of the airway.
7	Material enters the airway, passes below the vocal folds, and is not ejected from the trachea despite effort.
8	Material enters the airway, passes below the vocal folds, and no effort is made to eject the material.

Adapted from Rosenbek et al. (1996).

support a patient who has a nonfunctioning gastrointestinal tract because of injury, disease, or developmental immaturity (Groher, 1997).

Enteral nonoral feedings are usually the preferred nutritional alternative rather than parenteral because enteral uses the stomach or intestines. The **nasogastric tube** (NG tube) is often used for short-term nonoral feedings because it is minimally invasive and easy to place. It is a small tube inserted through the nasal cavity, through the esophagus, and into the stomach. With infants and young babies, an **orogastric tube** (OG-tube) can be inserted through the oral cavity, through the esophagus, and into the stomach and used to supply partial or all nutrition and hydration.

The **gastrostomy tube** (G-tube) is a feeding tube surgically placed into the stomach and is preferred for longer-term use. The **percutaneous endoscopic gastrostomy** (PEG) is a G-tube placed endoscopically. This method involves an easier and less invasive surgical procedure for placement. If the stomach cannot be used as a site for placement, the **percutaneous endoscopic jejunostomy** (PEJ) is a feeding tube that is inserted into the second part of the small intestine known as the *jejunum*. For daily nutrition, formula is past into the tube and flows from the tube either by drip or by bolus feedings into the stomach or intestine.

When the GI tract cannot be used because of medical complications, then parenteral feedings may be given. **Total parenteral nutrition** (TPN) is a nonoral feeding administered through an intravenous line directly into the bloodstream via a central vein. A specialized highly digestible nutrient solution is administered directly into a central vein. It is a commonly used feeding choice, especially with hospitalized patients who cannot take nutrition into their digestive tract. The patient can obtain full nutrition and hydration through TPN. A second option of parenteral feeding is the peripheral parenteral nutrition (PPN), a less concentrated feeding given through a peripheral vein. PPN is usually a short-term solution as less daily nourishment can be administered in this manner.

Differential Diagnosis of Swallowing Impairments in Adults

Initially, difficulty with swallowing was thought of as a single disorder with little recognition of the variability of its presentation and its functional consequences. The many possible medical etiologies, the impaired anatomy and physiology, and the resulting deficits have been more fully realized in recent years. Currently, a wide range of adults with various medical etiologies and symptoms of dysphagia are referred to the SLP for an accurate differential diagnostic assessment. Upon the completion of the examination, the clinician will be expected to interpret the medical, anatomical, physiological, and symptomatic information to the patient. The clinician will also recommend a comprehensive and successful treatment and management plan based on efficacious data to both the patient's health care team and to the patient.

To provide a salient evaluation, the clinician will need to obtain all necessary history, perform relevant testing, and produce reliable and accurate results. In contrast to other areas of speech-language pathology practice, the swallow assessment must be based on science with exacting interpretation and analysis of the findings. Having a thorough history, including medical and swallow components; choosing the right questions to ask; and correctly interpreting the responses and analyzing the testing data gleaned from the diagnostic protocol(s) chosen are all essential to obtain valid and consistent results.

Special Populations

There are specific disorders and unique populations that may complete the swallow evaluation process but become exceptions to the guidelines that clinicians use to determine optimal swallow management regimes. This is especially prevalent with patients who are terminally ill, have an ongoing degenerative disease process including advanced dementia, are developmentally delayed or are receiving "comfort care," or palliative care—a plan of total care when the disease is not responsive to curative treatment (Yorkston, Miller, & Strand, 2004).

Management of the patient with a degenerative disease, for instance, is a challenge because of the diversity of symptoms and, depending upon the etiology, the progression of the disease. For instance, the person with amyotrophic lateral sclerosis might receive an evaluation with the goal of obtaining the best swallow function during a point in time during the disease's progression. The patient's optimal swallow function, however, will change over time as the disease progresses. The goal of intervention may just be to maintain the patient's present level of function for as long as possible. With others, the goal may involve using compensatory strategies to maximize the patient's ability to continue any oral intake. This might include modifying diet consistencies, amount of foodstuffs taken during one bite or sip, or altering the patient's speed of oral intake. The developmentally delayed individual may have different challenges including behavioral manifestations, communication limits, intellectual impairments and physical limitations.

Often, engagement during a meal between the caregiver and the developmentally delayed individual is a major socializing opportunity. The person assisting or feeding the patient provides nourishment as well as social interaction. The ingestion of foods can be an integral and pleasurable part of the individual's daily experience, not available if the patient is placed on nonoral nutrition. Another group, patients with advanced dementia, often have oral and pharyngeal swallow difficulties as well as difficulty following even simple directions. Therefore, the ability of the clinician to alter or enhance their swallowing function with helpful swallow strategies or maneuvers may be limited.

Practical solutions to the swallow impairments presented are paramount to the clinician's diagnostic and management approach with these special populations. The clinician must be flexible and understand that the swallow strategies chosen may need to be modified as the disease progresses. If the patient's quality of life is the principal factor, the SLP may be requested to modify your recommendations of a "safe" diet. Even though a swallow assessment shows that the person is clearly aspirating thin liquids, the clinician may be requested to suggest an oral diet that includes thin liquids. These difficult decisions are often made in collaboration with the patient, the patient's family or significant others, and the medical team. Of course, the patient and his or her significant others should be educated on the risks vs. benefits of the suggested diet. Guidance from the patient's medical team is important in determining the swallow management for the patient's medical and emotional well-being and as well as quality of life.

There are also those persons who have established an advanced directive that may include a statement made detailing his or her preferences for receiving or not receiving specific medical treatments (Groher & Crary, 2010, p. 309). Those individuals may seek to prevent any artificial means of feeding (usually a tube feeding). At other times, there may be no binding legal document spelling out the wishes of the patient, but rather the patient's family or legal guardian may specify the patient's wishes for diet modifications or whether nonoral nutrition/hydration may be administered. For a more complete discussion, refer to Groher (2010b).

Selected Case History

R.F. is a 67-year-old gentleman referred for an evaluation of his oropharyngeal swallowing mechanism because of his severe dysphagia. Medical history is significant for a brainstem cerebrovascular accident (CVA) 1 year ago with initial right-sided weakness, dysarthria, and dysphagia. The right-sided weakness and the dysarthria have subsequently cleared. Because the dysphagia was severe, a PEG feeding tube was placed within 10 days following the stroke. The patient has been NPO (nothing by mouth) since that time, with all nutrition and hydration being given via the PEG. Currently, the patient reports difficulty swallowing his saliva and frequently spitting out saliva in large napkins or a cup, episodes of drooling, several respiratory infections during the past year, and one diagnosed aspiration pneumonia. The aspiration pneumonia was treated successfully with antibiotics. It is suspected that he is aspirating his saliva. Because saliva aspiration can cause pneumonia, the patient was discouraged by his physician from swallowing his saliva. When he tried very small amounts of water, he swallowed and immediately coughed and choked.

Initially after his stroke, he received an evaluation of his oropharyngeal swallowing mechanism. This was followed by some inpatient and outpatient swallow treatment. The patient reported that the treatment was unsuccessful. He was employed before the stroke and expressed sadness of his need to retire after the onset of his illness. He articulated the desire to return to work but feels he cannot work with a feeding tube placed in his stomach.

Selected Assessments With Rationale

- Clinical History: Obtaining a pertinent medical history and swallow history from the patient and/or significant others is important to understanding the medical condition causing the severe dysphagia. Question any results from neurology, medicine, pulmonary, gastroenterology, otolaryngology, nutrition, and other special consultations or evaluations. Obtain a description of the swallow difficulties. Swallow history should include current nutrition, either oral or nonoral, methods of nutritional intake, episodes of coughing or choking. (See components of the Clinical Bedside Assessment for Adults for more detail.)
- Oral Motor and Vocal Examination: Assess current strength, range, and speed of movements of the tongue, mandible, mouth, lips, and palate. Palpate neck to determine laryngeal elevation during a requested swallow. Assess vocal phonation tone, vocal quality, and loudness level of voice to determine whether there might be vocal cord weakness resulting in reduced vocal cord approximation. This deficit could compromise airway entrance protection. Presence and strength of a volitional cough and adequacy of the patient's dentition for mastication should also be assessed.
- Assess respiratory sounds during breathing and attempted swallowing of saliva. May perform cervical auscultation to obtain more information on breath sounds during quiet breathing and when attempting saliva swallow. Observe the coordination of respiration and swallowing.

Choosing the Instrumental Assessment

- Videofluoroscopic Swallow Study: Performed to obtain complete physiological evaluation of patient's oral, pharyngeal, and upper cervical esophageal swallow function. Of particular interest are the patient's laryngeal and pharyngeal function, airway protection, presence of aspiration, and any physiological attempts to prevent or clear the aspiration. If deficits are seen, assess the patient's ability to improve his or her swallow through the use of modifications in bolus consistency or presentation manner and compensatory strategies including swallow postures and/or maneuvers. From the patient's medical and swallow history, one may suspect impairment of either the pharyngeal propulsion/stripping of the bolus or the relaxation and opening of the UES within the cervical esophagus.
- Fiberoptic Endoscopic Evaluation of Swallowing (FEES): Performance of FEES does not offer a full assessment of all stages of the oropharyngeal swallow mechanism; however, FEES will provide reliable basic information, including the presence or absence of aspiration. It will also give some definitive information on the overall function of the swallow and pertinent function of the vocal process. It may be easier to obtain because it does not require a radiology suite or specific radiographic equipment. Rather, FEES is portable and can be administered by a trained SLP who is credentialed to perform FEES. Independent administration of FEES must be within the scope of practice of the clinician's state's licensure law. FEES can also be performed by a SLP in conjunction with an otolaryngologist.

Instructional Writing Rubric for Formal Diagnostic Report (Clinical and/or Instrumental Assessment of Swallowing)

☐ Introductory Statement
- Provide an introductory statement to include which assessments were conducted, name and age of patient, date of examination, and reason for referral.

☐ Medical History
- In paragraph form briefly outline pertinent medical history, past swallow evaluations with summary of findings (if known), and treatments, if any. Comments on significant weight

loss, adequacy of dentition for mastication, appetite, fatigue factor during meals, length of meals, etc.

☐ Swallow History Including Symptoms Reported by Patient and/or Significant Others
  - Provide swallowing symptoms as gleaned from history and your own observations (e.g., copious drooling, frequent coughing, wet, hoarse sounding voice). Be specific to include types of food/liquids that are easiest or hardest to swallow, specific swallow difficulties detailed in the patient's interview, consistencies, portion sizes, time of day, and other factors. Provide information if difficulties arise during or after a meal, in the evening, when ingesting certain foods or liquids, etc.

☐ Results of Testing Performed
  - In paragraph form, provide the results of the instrumental assessment(s) completed during your evaluation. If VFSS is performed, the examiner should first summarize the protocol, which should include amounts and consistencies used during the test. The results should include information about all stages of the swallow and cover the major physiological events performed in each stage. For example, a comment about hyolaryngeal elevation/excursion and airway entrance protection would be appropriate when discussing the pharyngeal stage. This section should include sections on oral, pharyngeal and cervical esophageal, as indicated, and a statement about the presence or absence of penetration and aspiration.

☐ Impressions
  - Provide a diagnostic statement based on testing results, which includes the level of impairment (e.g., mild, moderate, severe, nonfunctional) when viewing the total oropharyngeal swallow. Provide pertinent information of the stages involved (e.g., "While the oral stage was grossly functional for all consistencies tested, the pharyngeal stage showed severe impairments in…").

☐ Recommendations
  - Summarize recommendations based on the patient's medical and swallow history, compliance, nutritional, respiratory and cognitive status, and assessments administered. What factors (e.g., the patient's motivation, living environment) will assist the patient's recovery, and can he or she obtain assistance in the oral intake as necessary. Recommend whether the patient is to remain on oral feedings or initiate nonoral feedings. Include statements on oral intake, types of foods/liquids including consistencies, amounts, modifications, swallow strategies, or liquid thickening, among others. Recommend swallow treatment, if appropriate, with goals for the treatment plan of care. In addition, if other medical or health care specialists should be suggested, detail the reason for your recommendation (e.g., a consultation to an otolaryngologist to assess vocal cord function may be beneficial).

Sample Report

Please note: Each area has been separated by a heading for ease of reading, practice, and developing the thought process. In an actual report, however, using only a few subtitles for major sections such as History, Assessment Results and Impressions, and Recommendations would allow the material to be read as a whole diagnostic summary.

Identifying Information

Patient's Name: R.F. **Date of Evaluation**:
Primary Diagnosis: **Date of Birth**:
Referred by: Dr. Harry Jones, Neurologist
Reason for Referral: Severe dysphagia; poststroke, nonoral feeder

Background Information

As per your request, R.F., a 67-year-old man was seen for a clinical evaluation and a videofluoroscopic assessment of his oropharyngeal swallowing mechanism.

Medical history is significant for a brainstem CVA 1 year ago with initial right-sided weakness, dysarthria, and dysphagia. The right-sided weakness and the dysarthria subsequently improved. Additional history, as reported by the patient, includes a past myocardial infarct followed by stent placement, chronic obstructive pulmonary disease, and severe respiratory infections during the past year with one episode of aspiration pneumonia.

Initially the patient was placed NPO and an NG tube for all nutrition and hydration was inserted. Several weeks later, a diagnostic swallowing assessment showed continued severe swallow impairments with aspiration. At that time, a PEG feeding tube was placed for all nutrition and hydration. Currently, the patient is NPO with nonoral nutrition and hydration via the PEG feeding tube.

Swallowing History

The patient reported difficulty swallowing both foods and liquids with occasional attempts at very small amounts of either consistency, resulting in coughing and choking. Even swallowing saliva is difficult, with frequent coughing episodes. After being diagnosed with aspiration pneumonia, he was encouraged to expectorate his saliva whenever possible instead of swallowing the material.

Testing

Clinical Assessment

An oral motor screening, performed to assess the structure and function of the oral mechanism, showed facial features to be symmetrical. Labial and mandibular range of motion, strength, and tone were functional. Lingual range of movement was adequate but strength appeared reduced. Articulation of speech was mildly imprecise but grossly functional; vocal quality was mildly hypernasal. Velar elevation was asymmetrical. Oral and facial sensation appeared intact. No pronounced deficit was noted in the coordination of respiration and swallowing. A strong cough reflex was elicited. The patient's dentition appeared adequate for mastication of foodstuffs.

Videofluoroscopic Assessment of Swallowing

A videofluoroscopic study of the oropharyngeal swallowing mechanism was performed with the patient seated upright. Both left-lateral and anterior-posterior views were taken. A variety of consistencies were administered in very small calibrated amounts, impregnated with barium including thin liquid, nectar-thick and honey-thick liquids, puree, and solid.

The results showed a functional oral stage when liquids were given. Oral bolus containment, manipulation, and anterior-posterior oral transport were adequate. With puree and solid, however, slow bolus manipulation, bolus formation, and mastication were noted. Efficiency of the tongue to propel the material into the oropharynx was reduced. Multiple attempts were needed to transport the material from the oral cavity into the oropharynx. Upon the completion of transport, some residue remained in the oral cavity.

When material entered the oropharynx, initiation of the pharyngeal swallow was mildly (1 to 2 seconds) delayed. During the delay, some material spilled into the pharynx to the level of the valleculae and, at times, into the pyriform sinuses. Upon swallow initiation, hyolaryngeal elevation and excursion and protection of the laryngeal airway entrance were markedly reduced, resulting in poor laryngeal vestibule closure. Material spilled over from the pyriforms and the valleculae into the laryngeal airway entrance (laryngeal vestibule). This penetration of material into the laryngeal vestibule was followed by aspiration.

Penetration and aspiration occurred with all consistencies but was most pronounced with thin and nectar-thick liquids where 10% to 15% aspiration was observed. With those consistencies, aspiration was "silent." The patient failed to spontaneously cough or clear the aspirate. Trace aspiration, 5%, was noted with the thicker consistencies of honey-thick liquid, puree, and solid. An attempted cough was noted intermittently with these consistencies, but aspiration clearance was not seen.

Pharyngeal propulsion and stripping of the bolus was mildly reduced with limited tongue base retraction and posterior wall contraction seen especially with the thicker consistencies. This resulted in moderate amounts of material remaining in the oropharynx and valleculae and on the tongue base.

The decrease in hyolaryngeal elevation and pharyngeal propulsion resulted in reduced relaxation/opening of the upper esophageal sphincter (UES). As material attempted to enter the UES, residual material remained in the pyriform sinuses. Additional trace, 5%, aspiration was noted after the swallow from the remaining valleculae and pyriform sinus residue. No spontaneous cough or clearance was observed.

A series of strategies, postures, and maneuvers were attempted to eliminate the aspiration and improve the pharyngeal contraction and stripping wave. Aspiration could be reduced but not eliminated with the use of a head turn to the right coupled with an effortful (hard) swallow when ingesting very small amounts, 1cc to 3cc, of nectar-thick liquid and puree.

Cervical osteophytes were noted at the level of C4 to C6, which did not interfere with the pharyngeal swallow.

Impressions

R.F. exhibits a severe oropharyngeal dysphagia with oral deficits in bolus manipulation and transport, and pharyngeal deficits including decreases in pharyngeal stripping of material, hyolaryngeal elevation and excursion, laryngeal airway entrance protection, and decreased opening of the UES. These deficits resulted in markedly reduced entry of material into the upper cervical esophagus and mild-to-moderate (5% to 15%) aspiration seen across all consistencies. The patient intermittently coughed in response to aspiration of liquids but failed to clear the aspiration. No cough was noted with aspiration of puree or solid. Suspect the patient continues to aspirate his saliva. These deficits are suggestive of oral, laryngeal, and pharyngeal muscular weakness.

Recommendations

Given the findings of the evaluation and the patient's recent pulmonary history, initiating an oral diet at this time would be high risk. It is suggested that he continue on nonoral feedings and hydration at this time.

It is recommended that the patient begin a swallow treatment program to remediate the deficits discussed with the goal of obtaining a safe and functional oropharyngeal swallow in order that oral intake can be safely resumed.

The results and recommendations for treatment were discussed with the patient who expressed understanding and agreed to initiate a swallow treatment regime.

____

(Name of clinician and credentials)

Practice Exercise

Read the following information, including medical and swallow information and data from VFSS that was performed on this patient. Write a diagnostic report using this information. The report will include medical and swallow history and findings from the clinical assessment and VFSS study. The report will conclude with impressions and recommendations including the final oropharyngeal swallow diagnosis and all recommendations. Recommendations should include the suggested mean of nutrition/hydration, oral or nonoral or a combination of both. If an oral diet is to be initiated or maintained, be specific on amounts; consistencies; and whether any modifications, compensatory strategies, or maneuvers are to be used. If needed, referrals for further testing and/or consultations, including medical consultations, should be explained and suggested.

Identifying Information

Name: S.S. **DOB**: 11/20/1948
Referred by: Dr K.P
Reason for referral: Dysphagia after cardiovascular surgery

Medical History

Significant for normal cognition and mental status s/p CABG × 4 followed by a mitrovalve replacement 7 days ago. This female patient was **intubated** for 5 days; extubated 2 days ago. Nasogastric tube is in place for all nutrition and hydration. When extubated, the patient showed decreased alertness with reduced cognition. At this time, the patient has shown some improvement in mental status, although it is still reduced.

Swallow History

Patient had a normal swallow before her surgery. While in a postoperative room, the physician gave the patient some water to drink; she coughed and choked in response. No further oral intake trials have been attempted. Patient expressed desire to eat and is feeling thirsty even though she is receiving liquids through the NG tube.

Testing: Clinical Assessment

- Evaluation of peripheral oral mechanism showed: normal range, strength and speed of oral and facial movements and tongue movements
- Velar elevation: Intact
- Swallowing of saliva: Appears adequate
- Speech articulation: Intact
- Voice: Patient's voice is very hoarse and breathy with low vocal volume
- Diadochokinetic movements of the articulators: Intact
- Mental status: Reduced; patient is aware of place but not aware of person or time of day
- Cognition and alertness: Reduced; patient has episodes of sleepiness and at times, appears very lethargic

- Standard protocol was administered starting with 1cc thin liquids and giving trials up to one-third teaspoon puree

Thin Liquid

- 1cc
  - Oral stage: Adequate bolus containment, oral transport and clearance
  - Pharyngeal stage: Delayed initiation of the pharyngeal swallow, pooling in the valleculae; material entered the hypopharynx and penetrated into the laryngeal vestibule
- 3cc
  - Oral stage: Continued as per 1cc trial
  - Pharyngeal: Same as 1cc, penetrated into the laryngeal vestibule; this was followed by mild 10% aspiration. Patient failed to cough/clear the aspirate
- 5cc
  - Oral stage: Remains the same as initial trial
  - Pharyngeal: Same as 3cc except aspiration increased to mild-moderate, 10% to 15% of the bolus presented; patient failed to cough/clear
- 5cc
  - Oral: Same as previous
  - Pharyngeal: Attempted a chin-to-chest head posture (chin tuck) to narrow the laryngeal airway entrance and move some of the pharyngeal structures in a posterior direction to aid in airway protection; patient was not able to perform the head posture consistently

Nectar-Thick Liquid

- 5cc
  - Oral stage: Same as previous
  - Pharyngeal: Same as previous with less aspiration, only 5% to 10%, but aspiration was seen during the swallow from uncleared penetrated material and after the swallow from residue throughout the pharynx, and specifically in the pyriform sinuse

    Again attempted the chin-tuck posture; patient was still unable to perform this strategy successfully and failed to cough/clear the aspiration

Honey-Thick Liquid

- 5cc
  - Oral: Same as previous
  - Pharyngeal: Aspiration in trace amounts, less than 5%. Attempted another posture; patient was requested to turn the head first to the left, and with the next trial, the patient was asked to turn to the right. Patient performed with repeated directions. With guidance and verbal prompts from the examiner, patient successfully used the head turn to the left. No aspiration was seen with left head turn while ingesting 5cc bolus.
- 10cc
  - Oral: Same as previous
  - Pharyngeal: Same as with 5cc

Sips From a Cup

- Oral: Same as previous
- Pharyngeal: Larger bolus size resulted in the occurrence of aspiration, less than 5 %. In addition, deficits in pharyngeal propulsion and stripping of material though the pharynx were noted. Attempted to teach patient the effortful swallow (hard swallow) maneuver to obtain more laryngeal airway entrance closure and enhance pharyngeal propulsion. Patient was unable to retain directions for the use of the effortful swallow during the trial but was able to use the head turn to the left posture.

One-Third Teaspoon Puree

- Using head turn to the left
  - Oral: Mild delays in oral bolus formation with prolonged bolus manipulation and anterior-posterior transport of the bolus through the oral cavity. Some oral residue noted to remain in the oral cavity after the swallow.
  - Pharyngeal: Delay in initiating the pharyngeal swallow 2 to 3 seconds. During the delay, material spilled into the pharynx to the level of the valleculae and pyriform sinuses. When swallow initiated, material moved inefficiently through the hypopharynx and entered the UES with some delay. Moderate-to-large amounts of residue remained throughout the pharynx. This residue placed the patient at aspiration risk after the swallow although no aspiration was observed. Second trial of puree showed same moderate-large amounts of pharyngeal residue. Again, the patient was unable to perform a chin tuck or an effortful swallow during swallowing, which could have lessened the pharyngeal residue.

The study was terminated with the assumption that results of solids would be similar to puree trials.

Pediatric Feeding and Swallowing Impairments

Assessment, treatment and management of pediatric feeding and swallowing disorders is best approached from a multidimensional view of the disorder as feeding and swallowing issues in children typically involve one or more of the following aspects: complex medical issues, oral motor delays, global motor impairments, physiological oropharyngeal swallow deficits, **sensory integration dysfunction**, or a variety of social and behavioral interferences (Arvedson, 2006; Prasse & Kikano, 2009). The components of the disorder all layer on and interact with each other as they affect the child's feeding and swallowing abilities. Deficiencies in any of these areas may have detrimental effect on the child's ability to be a successful oral feeder, gain weight, grow, maintain adequate nutrition/hydration, and experience the many pleasurable aspects associated with oral feeding. All areas of the disorder must be assessed and addressed, while being mindful of each area of involvement as it influences other areas and on the child. If the varied components of the disorder are treated in isolation, truly successful and optimal outcomes are not possible (Arvedson, 2008; Miller, 2009). The assessment process is often complex and varies depending on the age, medical status, and developmental abilities of the child and clinical setting of practice. A complex framework of decisions guiding the evaluation, treatment, and management process of these children is required. Clinicians who are interested in working with this population will benefit from supplementary reading, workshops, and hands-on clinical training focused on the various aspects of the disorder. Specific recommendations and referrals to the literature will be made throughout this section as they pertain to each specific topic. In-depth discussion of the clinical and instrumental evaluation process as they may pertain to specific age groups, developmental disabilities, and medical diagnoses is beyond the scope of this section.

Lefton-Greif and Arvedson (2007) summarize a number of studies that describe the prevalence of feeding and swallowing impairments. Reportedly, in normally developing children, the prevalence of feeding and swallowing problems are estimated to be up to 45%, with a higher range up to 80% among children with developmental delays. Feeding and swallowing problems may present in a variety of ways including, but not limited to, the following:

- Limited volume of foods and liquids accepted
- Repeated respiratory infections such as pneumonia
- Restricted weight gain and growth
- Failure to thrive (poor weight gain and growth in early infancy/childhood)
- Poor nutrition and hydration
- Aspiration
- Coughing, choking, gagging on foods/liquids
- Change in physiologic stability (particularly seen with pre-infants) such as change to heart rate, respiratory rate, or oxygen saturation
- Residual in the oral cavity or pharynx
- **Nasopharyngeal regurgitation**, regurgitation of food or liquid into the velopharyngeal port and up into the nasal cavity
- Hyper/hypo oral sensitivity
- **Oral aversion**, inability to tolerate stimulation to the oral/perioral area
- Insufficient mastication of solids or reduced chewing skills for age
- Negative mealtime or feeding refusal behaviors
- Severe food selectivity resulting in a limited oral diet repertoire

An SLP may assess feeding and swallowing skills in children through a clinical "bedside" assessment of feeding and swallowing and/or instrumental assessments. The process of a clinical assessment may occur in isolation if the examiner determines that an instrumental assessment is not indicated. An instrumental study of swallowing can provide valuable information beyond the clinical feeding and swallowing evaluation including the anatomy and physiologic function of the oropharyngeal swallow structures and aide in treatment and management decisions. This section on pediatrics first addresses the process of the clinical feeding and swallowing evaluation and then further discuss the indications, rationale, and options for an instrumental assessment of swallowing with children.

Norms and Developmental Considerations

As the field of pediatrics encompasses children of varying developmental abilities with age ranges from birth to 18 years and, in some facilities and schools, 21 years of age, it is important to be mindful of the child's developmental level when performing assessment regardless of chronological age. Clinicians must have a working and comprehensive knowledge of normal feeding and swallowing skill acquisition as well as understand this skill development within the larger context of cognitive, linguistic, motor, and social milestones (Delaney & Arvedson, 2008). Delaney and Arvedson (2008) noted that this knowledge is indispensible when evaluating children because the clinician needs to identify differences in the feeding and swallowing abilities observed in normal children and in those children demonstrating problematic skills. The following publications delineate the normal acquisition of feeding, swallowing, and oral motor skills in great detail as well as within the context of global development across an age-span of birth to 2 or 3 years. These resources provide samples of developmental feeding skill observation checklists or charts to use when conducting a feeding observation. Referring to these publications or similar ones may be useful in guiding clinicians to determine age-appropriateness of skills observed:

- Table 2-7 found in *Pediatric Swallowing and Feeding* (Arvedson & Brodsky, 2002)
- *The Pre-Feeding Checklist found in Pre-Feeding Skills* (Morris & Klein, 2000)
- *Development of Swallowing and Feeding: Prenatal Through First Year of Life* (Delaney & Arvedson, 2008)

Table 14-4 highlights the developmental progression of feeding and swallowing skill acquisition that is reviewed in greater detail in the preceding resources. In addition, refer back to the adult section of this chapter for an in-depth description of the stages of the normal swallow.

Anatomical and Physiological Changes With Maturation

In addition to thorough knowledge of feeding and swallowing skill development, the clinician must demonstrate understanding of the numerous changes that occur in the anatomy and physiology of the oropharyngeal swallow and its structures during maturation. Table 14-5 provides examples of some of the anatomical variations seen between the infant and the older child.

Figure 14-3 shows the anatomical structure of the infant. Note the close proximity of the soft palate and epiglottis and the elevated position of the larynx. This closeness of structures offers positional stability and a degree of inherent airway protection during the rapid, coordinated sequencing of sucking, swallowing, and respiration (Wolf & Glass, 1992).

Although the stages of swallowing as described in the adult section of this chapter are essentially the same for infants and children, there are differences that are important to note, particularly with respect to the oral phase in infants and very young children. In infancy, the oral stage is involuntary and reflexive, which is not the case in toddlers and older children in whom the oral phase involves cortical input for mastication of different textures. In infants, the oral phase primarily consists of nipple feeding with sucking and swallowing typically at a 1:1 ratio (Dodrill & Gosa, 2015). With infants and young toddlers, movements of the oral structures (tongue, lips, mandible, cheeks) change as the child's anatomy matures and different textures are presented (e.g., transition from vertical munching pattern to rotary diagonal pattern for chewing). Therefore, the functional characteristics of oral preparatory and oral phases of the swallow mechanism change over time.

Further detail regarding the differences in anatomy and physiology of the structures of the oral cavity, pharynx, and larynx in infants vs. older children; differences between breastfeeding and bottle-feeding; the mechanics of sucking; and discussion of the oral motor patterns at various stages of development can be found in *Feeding and Swallowing Disorders in Infancy* (Wolf & Glass, 1992) and *Pediatric Swallowing and Feeding* (Arvedson & Brodsky, 2002).

Specific Parameters for Assessment

It is important to note that evaluation of children with feeding and swallowing disorders can occur across a number of settings, including schools, outpatient clinics, hospitals, medical settings, or the home. Optimally, assessment of feeding and swallowing disorders in infants and children should be coordinated and conducted by a team of professionals. Consistent with a team approach, specialists on a pediatric feeding and swallowing team may include a combination of any of the following professionals: SLPs, pulmonologists, gastroenterologists, nurses, developmental pediatricians, otolaryngologists, nutritionists, occupational therapists, and psychologists (Miller et al., 2001). For school-age children, teachers, teaching assistants, and other school staff will also be integral members to developing and implementing a child's feeding and

Table 14-4. Normal Development of Feeding and Swallowing Skills

Age	Skill
Birth	• Bottle-feeding or breastfeeding initiated; suckles on nipple • Generally feeds every 2 to 3 hours; takes 2 to 5 oz per feeding • 1:1:1 suck/swallow/breathe ratio • Patterns of sucking bursts and rests
4 to 6 months	• Introduction of spoon-feeding of cereals and thin baby food purees • Sucking pattern used; pushes food out of mouth with tongue • Primary movements of tongue and jaw occur together • Tongue moves in vertical positions as well as protrusion/retraction
7 to 8 months	• Introduction of textured purees, mashed table foods, and small pieces of dissolvable and mashable solids • Sucking on solids with vertical jaw and tongue movements • Lateral movement of tongue emerges • Cup drinking may be introduced; unable to control volume of liquid; often loses liquid from mouth and coughs due to difficulty coordinating; takes 1 sip at a time • Swallows with lips closed and slight tongue protrusion • Self-feeds small pieces • Movements of the jaw, tongue, and lips become more precise
9 to 12 months	• Diagonal rotary movement chewing emerges • Demonstrates increased jaw stability for biting through solids • Actively removing food from the spoon with lips • Tongue-tip elevation upon swallowing • Begins weaning from bottle/breast • Primarily uses cup; often able to take 2 to 3 sips consecutively • Straw introduced
13 to 24 months	• Eats a variety of solid food textures • Varied lip movement during chewing; cleans food from lips • Lip closure with minimal to no spillage of food or liquid from the mouth • Demonstrates controlled/sustained bite on hard solid • Diagonal rotary chewing and movement of the bolus occurs across midline during chewing (closer to 24 months) • Dissociation of tongue and jaw movements
24 to 36 months	• Circular rotary chewing • Self-feeding with utensils

Adapted from Arvedson & Brodsky (2002) and Morris & Klein (2000).

swallowing treatment plan. Lastly, clinicians must not forget that parents or caregivers serve as essential team members in the feeding and swallowing evaluation and the treatment programs (Homer, 2003).

It is essential that the team of professionals coordinate the evaluation and treatment process to ensure an accurate diagnosis and treatment of the disorder. Clinicians are strongly encouraged to seek out and access other professionals to ensure that a complete picture of the child's feeding and swallowing abilities and needs are obtained.

Bearing in mind that the approach and focus of the evaluation may vary depending on the age and developmental abilities of the child, medical diagnosis, evaluation setting, or reason for referral, every evaluation should start with thorough medical, developmental, and feeding histories and an oral-peripheral examination. During the initial stages of the evaluation

Table 14-5. Differences in the Anatomy of the Oropharyngeal Swallow Mechanism in Infants and Older Children

Infants	*Toddlers/Older Children*
Tongue fills the oral cavity	As mouth grows larger, tongue sits on the floor of the mouth
Fatty sucking pads (fatty tissue within buccinator muscles) are present in the cheeks to aid in sucking	The fatty sucking pads of the cheeks dissipate as the buccinator muscles of the cheeks develop for chewing
Small mandible in comparison to maxilla	Mandible and maxilla become relative in size
Teeth are absent	Teeth are present
Oropharynx is not defined	Oropharynx and pharynx become separate due to growth of structures
Soft palate and epiglottis are in close proximity	Hyoid, epiglottis, and larynx descend creating greater distance between soft palate and epiglottis
Larynx is superior and anterior (closer to base of tongue) with limited movement	Range of movement of the larynx during swallowing increases

Adapted from Arvedson & Brodsky (2002) and Wolf & Glass (1992).

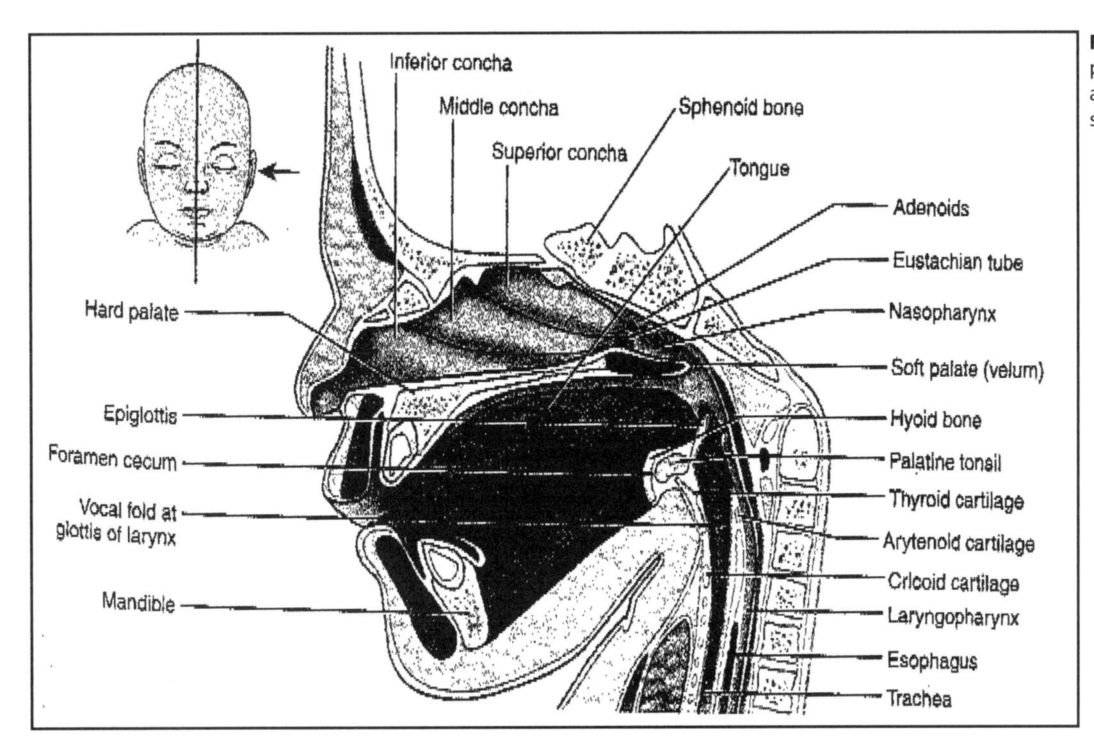

Figure 14-3. Oral, pharyngeal, laryngeal, and upper esophageal structures of an infant.

process, the clinician should be especially mindful of particular medical diagnoses, the overall neurodevelopmental state of the child, functioning of the GI and respiratory systems, and the role that the parent–child dynamic may be contributing to the feeding and swallowing issue. Once the histories are obtained and the physical examination of the oral-peripheral mechanism is complete, direct assessment of the oral and pharyngeal stages of the swallowing mechanism can occur (either clinically and/or instrumentally; Arvedson, 2008).

Medical History

As feeding and swallowing issues in the pediatric population often derive from a medical etiology, a thorough understanding of specific diagnoses is important. Children with medical diagnoses pertaining to the respiratory, neurological, or gastroenterological systems; those with genetic or craniofacial disorders; and premature infants have an increased incidence of feeding and swallowing impairments (Lefton-Greif & Arvedson, 2007; Miller, 2009; Prasse & Kikano, 2009).

Children with medically complex diagnoses often undergo multiple hospitalizations, surgeries, and invasive procedures. This is clinically significant as many of these children may have missed critical periods of feeding and swallowing development while undergoing and recovering from these interventions, procedures, or illnesses. Furthermore, those events may have prevented appropriate developmental stimulation, resulting in gross/fine motor difficulties, oral motor delays, issues of oral sensitivity, and possible oral aversion, adversely affecting feeding and swallowing skill acquisition (Arvedson, 2006; Bingham, 2009; Delaney & Arvedson, 2008; Mason, Harris, & Blisset, 2005).

Respiratory Disease

Coordination of respiration and swallowing is paramount. Respiratory compromise due to an upper airway pathology or obstruction results in increased incidences of feeding and swallowing difficulty. Haibeck and Mandell (2008) have outlined common diagnoses seen in their aerodigestive clinic and discuss the importance of the interdisciplinary approach to management of these children. They report an increased incidence of feeding, swallowing and GI-based problems in children with **laryngomalacia** (collapse of the supraglottic cartilages upon inspiration), **laryngeal cleft** (defect in the posterior larynx), vocal cord paralysis, tracheostomy, and craniofacial malformation. These structural and/or functional problems directly result in difficulty coordinating respiration and swallowing, which can result in poor airway patency and airway protection during the swallowing process.

Furthermore, other pulmonary issues, such as repeated pneumonias, respiratory tract infections, bronchiectasis, wheezing, or persistent coughing, may be red-flag indicators of oropharyngeal swallow dysfunction, aspiration, or disorders of the GI tract (Boesch et al., 2006; deBenedictis, Carnielli, deBenedictis, 2009; Simon & Collins, 2013).

Gastrointestinal Disorders

It is vital to have a working knowledge of the characteristics and diagnoses of GI disorders associated with feeding and swallowing problems. Additionally, it is essential to be familiar with the treatment and management of these GI pathologies and their connection to achieving and maintaining adequate nutrition and hydration children. The literature describes a strong correlation between GI disorders, oropharyngeal dysphagia, and feeding difficulties. Diagnoses such as gastroesophageal reflux, **eosinophilic esophagitis** (allergic inflammatory disease of the esophagus), **gastric dysmotility** (poor movement of contents though the stomach and intestines), and constipation can result in vomiting, aspiration, food impaction, pain, and discomfort upon eating. Failure to thrive, poor oral intake, food refusal, food selectivity, and oral aversion are often consequences of these GI disorders (Haas & Maune, 2009; Levy et al., 2009; Rommel et al., 2003; Schwarz et al., 2001; Sullivan, 2008).

Neurological Disorders

Neurological function has significant impact on feeding and swallowing abilities in children. Severity of impairment, level of dysfunction, site of lesion, and onset of neurological injury will all play a role in the degree to which feeding and swallowing skills are affected. Children with a history of strokes, brain tumors, neuromuscular disease, and seizure disorders are considered at high risk for dysphagia due to changes in swallow physiology. Various parameters of cognition and overall gross motor function will affect feeding/swallowing skills in these children as well. Typical characteristics of the feeding and swallowing abilities in children with neurological impairment include oral motor difficulties, delayed onset of pharyngeal swallow initiation, difficulty with coordination of oral and pharyngeal stages of swallowing, aspiration, and the inability to meet nutritional needs. Additionally, Arvedson et al. (1994) found that there is an increased risk of silent aspiration, no cough elicited in response to aspiration, seen on videofluoroscopic swallowing studies performed on children with neurological impairment. Her study revealed that 94% of the children who aspirated in their study did so "silently." Weir, McMahon, Taylor, and Chang (2011) demonstrated similar findings with a high association of silent aspiration in children with neurological impairment. Additionally, Lefton-Greif and Arvedson (2007) examined children with unexplained respiratory illness and found that approximately 58% of them were aspirating on thin liquids with aspiration occurring without overt response in 100% of those that were aspirating. Clinicians performing bedside swallow assessments with children should be mindful of the incidence of silent aspiration with particular diagnoses/populations and, therefore, instrumental assessment is indicated.

Genetic and Craniofacial Disorders

Certain genetic syndromes and/or craniofacial disorders such as CHARGE association, Pierre-Robin sequence, cleft lip/palate, Prader-Willi syndrome, and

Down syndrome are characterized and described by structural abnormalities of the oral mechanism, oral motor difficulties, discoordination of swallowing and respiration, and aspiration. These difficulties can result in significant feeding and swallowing dysfunction that might require diet modifications, specialized feeding equipment, feeding techniques, positions, or the provision of tube feedings for the child to attain adequate nutrition and hydration (Cooper-Brown et al., 2008).

Prematurity

Lefton-Greif (2008) reported on an increase in feeding and swallowing problems in the pediatric population overall. She summarized data indicating that one consideration for this may be improved rates of survival of premature infants and the resulting medical complexities these children may exhibit throughout their lifetime. A thorough medical history should include the prenatal course, birth history, and neonatal period. A premature birth can predispose babies and toddlers to feeding and swallowing difficulties well beyond the neonatal period and early infancy due to immature neurological systems, complex comorbid medical diagnoses, oral-sensory deprivation due to prolonged use of tube feedings, and developmental delays (Bingham, 2009; Jadcherla, Wang, Vijayapal, & Leuthner, 2010; Lau, Smith, & Schanler, 2003). Early on, these infants may initially demonstrate stress cues related to feeding attempts; oral phase difficulties (e.g., oral disorganization, a weak suck); and the inability to coordinate sucking, swallowing, and respiration. They may also demonstrate aspiration and physiologic instability during feeding (desaturation, bradycardia, or tachypnea). Over time, feeding and swallowing difficulties may evolve and persist, resulting in limited oral intake, ingestion of only particular types or textures of foods, and feeding refusal behaviors (Thoyre, 2007). Samara, Johnson, Lamberts, Marlow, and Wolke (2010) determined that, at 6 years of age, children who were born prematurely exhibited significantly more feeding and swallowing problems than children born at term due to issues of oral motor dysfunction, hypersensitivity, and behavior.

Developmental History

As discussed, there is an increased incidence of feeding and swallowing dysfunction in children with neurodevelopmental disability. Therefore, the global motor, sensory, and cognitive development of the child and its overall impact on the process of feeding and swallowing should be taken into consideration. Clinicians will find that physical and occupational therapists are invaluable resources during this part of the assessment process to assist in evaluating the child's posture, positioning, overall strength, sensory responses, attention to the feeding task, and regulatory abilities (Arvedson, 2008). Concerns regarding overall motor and sensory development and the role this plays in the feeding and swallowing disorder may prompt the need for more in-depth evaluation and referral to physical and occupational therapy as part of the larger "team" evaluation.

Motor Impairments

Several studies report that children with hyper- or hypotonicity, as is often seen in cerebral palsy, demonstrate a high incidence of oral motor dysfunction, aspiration, and malnutrition (Calis et al., 2008; Cass, Wallis, Ryan, Reilly, & McHugh, 2005; Reilly, Skuse, & Poblete, 1996). Posture and positioning during mealtime will need to be addressed in the child who demonstrates motor dysfunction to promote safe feeding and swallowing. The motoric abilities, posture, and position of a child will greatly influence the range of movement, strength, and function of the oral structures, airway protection, coordination of respiration and swallowing, and the child's ability to self-feed. For example, Larnert and Ekberg (1995) found that children with cerebral palsy who are not properly positioned and exhibited head/neck extension while eating demonstrated an increased risk of aspiration due to an unprotected airway.

Sensory Differences

As feeding and swallowing involves a range of sensory processes, it is not unusual for children with issues related to sensory modulation to demonstrate difficulties with oral motor function, feeding, swallowing, and the mealtime environment. Difficulties encountered by these children may include the following:

- Refusal of foods based on smell, texture, flavor, or appearance
- Gagging
- Overstuffing food in their mouth
- Difficulty eating in a distracting mealtime environment (i.e., noisy school cafeteria)
- Seeking out oral stimulation (chewing on clothing, zippers, etc.)
- Avoiding touch to the face or oral area
- Resistant to intraoral stimulation
- Inability to sit at a table with family or friends who are eating

For children in whom issues of oral sensitivity are part of a larger picture of sensory integration difficulty, the feeding and swallowing skills of these children often improve when the global sensory issues are being addressed in the occupational therapy setting.

For more information on sensory integration disorder and its impact upon feeding and swallowing skills, clinicians may find *Pre-Feeding Skills, Second Edition* (Morris & Klein, 2000) beneficial.

Feeding History

Orally Fed Children

A detailed feeding history will provide the time line of various developmental stages of feeding since birth. This would include whether oral feeding was initiated at birth and if the child was breast or bottle-fed. Type of bottles, nipples, and formulas (or expressed breast milk) provided will be important information to gather. Ages at which a child was introduced to spoon-feeding of purees and table food solids and their reactions to these transitions will also be of interest to the clinician. A child may often demonstrate complications with the transition through one or more of these developmental stages of feeding. For example, many babies and toddlers demonstrate tolerance of bottle or breast feedings, transition well to spoon-feeding of "smooth" baby foods, but then begin to demonstrate a "breakdown" in feeding acceptance and tolerance once table food solids are introduced. The SLP should note the types of textures within the child's repertoire, which are mastered, and which the child encounters difficulty with. Parents may describe a range of food textures within the child's diet including smooth purees, chunky purees, dissolvable solids (e.g., Cheerios [General Mills], Gerber puffs), mashable solids (e.g., banana, avocado), mechanical soft solids (e.g., muffins, French toast, scrambled egg), soft solids (e.g., pasta, rotisserie chicken), and hard solids (e.g., hard breads, meats).

Beyond considerations regarding food texture, children with feeding and swallowing impairments may often demonstrate preference and refusal based on food flavors, colors, shapes, and temperatures. Reports of difficulty tolerating foods based upon texture, flavor, visual appearance, temperature, or the way in which foods are served are usually indicators that there is a sensory component to the child's feeding issues. For example, many children on the autism spectrum demonstrate patterns such as these for food acceptance and refusal. Schreck, Williams, and Smith (2004) reported that these patterns of food refusal and acceptance seen in children with autism are more significant than compared to children without autism.

The willingness of a child to self-feed; the length, frequency, and environment of meals; and the child's demonstration of hunger will also be important information to obtain and aid the clinician in determining if there is feeding and swallowing problem.

Nonorally Fed Children

Nonoral means of nutrition and hydration are provided to the child who is unable to meet and maintain nutritional needs via oral means alone. Tube feedings are provided due to oropharyngeal swallow dysfunction or specific medical conditions (e.g., children with cancer sometimes have tube-feeding placement to ensure appropriate nutrition, hydration, and medication delivery during the period of illness and treatment). Please refer to the adult section of this chapter for a description of various nonoral feeding options. The reasons and rationales for opting for one nonoral feeding option over another will vary depending on a number of factors including the medical needs, diagnosis, and expected duration of nonoral feeding. It is important that clinicians working with this population are familiar with these feeding options, along with advantages and disadvantages of each.

Mason et al. (2005) discussed a number of factors that may interfere in the development of oral feeding in children who are tube-fed. The timing of tube-feeding initiation appears to be an important factor. Tube feedings initiated early on in life may interfere with learning patterns of hunger and satiety, establishing the "mouth–stomach" connection, and a child's overall desire to eat. Additionally, significant oral motor and oral sensory impairments may result due to a lack of oral feeding experience. In situations where tube feedings were initiated early on and remained in place for extended periods of time, oral feeding will be more difficult to attain However, if alternative feeding was initiated later in childhood due to illness or trauma, there will likely be a desire for resumption of oral feeding and preservation of some level of feeding and swallowing skill. Additionally, the method for tube-feeding delivery and tolerance of tube feedings will play a role in the willingness for oral stimulation and oral feeding as discomfort or unpleasant associations with tube feedings may lead to oral aversion. Vomiting or retching either during or immediately after tube feedings can contribute to oral defensiveness and aversive responses in many children with feeding and swallowing impairments (Zangen et al., 2003).

Behavioral Dynamics Related to the Feeding and Swallowing Process

The social and behavioral aspects relating to the feeding process, specifically the dynamics of the parent–child relationship surrounding mealtimes, the child's engagement in the feeding process, and the overall perception of the feeding problem by the family are also an important part of the feeding and swallowing assessment. A number of studies demonstrate feeding difficulties and refusal due to issues in mother–infant attachment and relationships. Silberstein et al. (2009) demonstrated that premature infants showed problematic oral feeding skills, behaviors, and a slower transition to oral feedings due to poorly established mother–infant interactions, decreased infant neurobehavioral functioning, parental intrusiveness/control during the feeding, and difficulties in the exchange or interpretation of early mother–child signals or cues. Additionally, Forcada-Guex, Pierrehumbert, Borghini, Moessinger, and Muller-Nix (2006) examined a variety of parent–child dyads at 6 months and the developmental outcomes of those children at 18 months among term and preterm children. They demonstrated that preterm infants show more behavioral feeding difficulties at 18 months when the parent–child interactions had aspects of intrusiveness and control on the part of the mother. The authors suggest that infants experiencing these types of parent–child interactions are at more risk for developing feeding issues.

Feeding refusal by a child can result in force-feeding, parental stress, loss of parental self-esteem, power struggles, abnormal feeding patterns, use of distraction at meals, extended mealtimes, "dream feeding" (feeding when the infant is in a sleepy state), and problems within the family unit overall (Levy et al., 2009). These types of behavioral feeding problems and patterns hinder the development of a normalized feeding process and result in an emotionally charged and stressful mealtime environment.

Additionally, there is the potential for a variety of maladaptive responses to develop that had been initially learned by the child due to a physiological, oral motor, or sensory-based problem. For example, behaviors such as gagging and vomiting may have been symptoms of a medical (i.e., reflux) or sensory (i.e., hypersensitivity) etiology initially; however, over time, after the initial source of the feeding problem has resolved, the gagging or vomiting behavior may remain. These behaviors may have had previous attention paid to them when they initially occurred, which then promoted persistence of the behavior (Levy et al., 2009).

Oral-Peripheral Examination

As part of the assessment process, an examination of the oral-peripheral mechanism is essential. The oral motor assessment will aid the SLP in determining whether oral motor dysfunction is contributing to feeding and swallowing deficits. Oral motor issues can result in difficulty with bolus formation, manipulation, transit, and control of a variety of liquid and food consistencies. Any breakdown in preparation, collection, and transport of the bolus by the oral structures may result in inability to meet nutritional needs (i.e., weak suck resulting in poor expression of liquid), discomfort upon attempts to swallow (i.e., gagging on solids which have not been properly chewed), and/or loss of control of the bolus into the hypopharynx before its ready to be swallowed (i.e., premature spillage into the hypopharynx resulting in an aspiration event before swallow initiation). Again, developmental considerations should be taken into account when conducting the oral-peripheral examination as the range of movement and function of the oral structures changes with maturation (i.e., lingual lateralization is not a voluntary oral motor movement seen in young infancy). Furthermore, direct assessment of the structures may not be appropriate or possible depending on the developmental language and cognitive abilities of the child.

Direct Assessment of Oral and Pharyngeal Stages of Swallowing

Assessment of the oral and pharyngeal stages of swallowing can be conducted via various clinical and instrumental evaluations. Some of these methods of assessment are similar to those outlined in the adult section of this chapter. Examination of feeding and swallowing function can be conducted with or without food and liquid trials dependent on the child's experience with oral feedings, developmental abilities, and medical status. If liquid and food trials are used, it is important to assess function across a variety of textures as appropriate.

Additionally, it may be beneficial for the clinician to perform a brief trial of diagnostic therapy during the direct feeding observation to determine whether the child is stimulable to any therapeutic processes (i.e., compensatory techniques, posture/positioning changes, behavioral or play-based strategies), which may improve oral motor function, normalize oral sensation, improve airway protection, facilitate acceptance of foods, or reduce undesired mealtime behaviors.

If a feeding and swallowing assessment is conducted with a child who is fed nonorally and is demonstrating respiratory compromise, a medically complex diagnosis, or an altered mental state, the child should be judged to be at high risk for oral trials. The clinician might determine that the child is not appropriate for oral feedings at that time and may defer oral trials during the evaluation. Instead, nonoral means of nutrition/hydration should remain in place with frequent monitoring and reassessment for the appropriateness of oral trials to allow for evaluation of thc oropharyngeal swallow. Clinicians make judgments such as these during the evaluation process based on the child's ability to tolerate and manage his or her own secretions, demonstrate appropriate mental status or cognitive function, and the overall medical fragility and prognosis of the child's condition.

Screening of Esophageal Function

A number of children referred for feeding and swallowing assessments will demonstrate abnormal anatomy and/or function of the esophagus. Therefore, as previously stated, it is important for the clinician to be familiar with these disorders, and their clinical symptomology and radiographic presentations. Although it is not within the scope of the SLP to diagnosis these disorders, findings seen during clinical and instrumental assessments of swallowing may be indicative of the need for referral to a pediatric gastroenterologist and further medical assessment. Refer to Table 14-3 in the adult section of this chapter for further description of assessments designed to evaluate esophageal function.

Key Clinical Interview Questions

Use of a detailed questionnaire addressing all of the parameters for assessment, in addition to a 3- to 5-day food diary filled out by parents or caregivers before the evaluation, is useful in providing the clinician with the necessary information to begin the process of evaluation. Morris and Klein (2000) provided examples of reproducible parent questionnaires to obtain background information, medical history, and feeding skills for the orally fed and tube-fed child. The ASHA (n.d.) Practice Portal website within the clinical area of "Pediatric Dysphagia" provides some nice examples of interview and case history forms and assessment templates. Table 14-6 contains examples of interview questions that are essential to the feeding and swallowing assessment.

Clinical "Bedside" Feeding and Swallowing Assessment

All evaluations of feeding and swallowing should commence with a clinical or "bedside" feeding and swallowing assessment. Once the medical, developmental, and feeding histories are collected, the clinician should conduct an examination of the oral-peripheral examination and then proceed with a direct observation of feeding and swallowing skills as may be appropriate.

Oral-Peripheral Examination

Please refer to Chapter 6 for further details and description regarding the oral motor evaluation. However, for the purposes of the pediatric feeding and swallowing clinical assessment, the following should be examined:

- Facial symmetry
- Mandible strength, stability and structure
- Buccal strength and tone
- Labial range of movement, tone, and strength
- Lingual symmetry, visual appearance, range of movement, tone, and strength
- Hard and soft palate appearance and movement
- Dentition
- Gag reflex (hyper-/hyposensitive)
- Primitive oral reflexes
    - **Rooting reflex** (touch to either corner of the mouth results in turning the head toward touch)
    - **Transverse tongue reflex** (movement of the tongue laterally when the lateral surface has been touched)
    - **Protrusion reflex** (protrusion of the tongue from mouth upon touch to the anterior portion)
    - **Phasic bite reflex** (closing and opening of mandible upon pressure to the gums in the molar area)
- Nonnutritive suck
- Vocal quality, pitch, and volume
- Secretion management (presence of excessive drooling, difficulty swallowing saliva, copious secretions and need for suction in patients with tracheostomy)
- Observation of vital signs and physiologic state during nonfeeding tasks
    - Patterns and sounds of respiration
    - Respiratory/heart rates
    - Oxygen saturation levels

Table 14-6. Sample Interview Questions

Background Information	1. What is the reason for referral for feeding/swallowing evaluation? 2. Who referred your child for evaluation? 3. Has your child ever had a swallowing study before? 4. Who are the people who primarily feed your child?
Medical History	1. Was your child born at term or prematurely? 2. Were there any pregnancy or birth complications? 3. Did your child spend time in a neonatal intensive care unit (NICU) after birth? If yes, what was the course of the NICU stay (e.g., surgeries, tube feedings, intubation)? 4. Does your child have a specific medical diagnosis? 5. Has your child undergone any surgeries? 6. Does your child take any medications? If so, which one(s)? 7. What specialists has your child seen (e.g., gastroenterologist, neurologist, ENT, feeding specialist)? 8. Has your child been diagnosed with reflux or other GI disorder? 9. Does your child experience constipation? 10. Has your child undergone other tests related to feeding and swallowing (e.g., upper GI, endoscopy)?
Nutrition Background	1. What is your child's current weight and height? 2. Has your child experienced weight loss or has been diagnosed with failure to thrive? 3. Does your child have any food allergies or intolerances that you are aware of? 4. What are typical foods or liquids consumed by your child? 5. What is the typical feeding schedule per day?
Develop-mental History	1. At what ages did your child meet developmental milestones (sitting, walking, babbling, single words)? 2. Is there any daily activity beyond feeding or mealtime that your child resists or demonstrates difficulty with? 3. Is your child bothered by food on the hands or face? 4. Does your child tolerate touch of different textures (e.g., sand, grass)? 5. Does your child demonstrate difficulty transitioning from activities throughout the day? 6. Does your child sleep through the night? 7. Does your child demonstrate food preferences or refusal based upon particular food categories, textures, or flavors (e.g., crunchy, mushy, savory, sour, sweet, bland, cold)?
Feeding History	1. How long after birth did oral feeding begin? 2. Was your baby breastfed or bottle-fed? Any past or current problems? 3. If your baby received formula, what formula was used or continues to be used currently? 4. At what age was spoon-feeding of baby foods or pureed food introduced? Any past or current problems? 5. When were table foods or solid food items introduced? 6. Did your child exhibit any difficulties tolerating solid food items? 7. Does your child drink from an open cup, straw, and/or sippy cup? 8. What consistencies of food or liquid does your child currently exhibit the most difficulty with? 9. Please describe the difficulty your child experiences when eating/drinking (e.g., coughing, choking, gagging, turning away, batting at the spoon, vomiting, refusal, throwing food, shortness of breath, chewing difficulty). 10. Do you use coaxing, rewards, distraction with toys or television, or force-feeding during mealtime? Are these techniques helpful? 11. Where do feedings take place? 12. What is the typical length of time to complete a mealtime or feeding?
Nonoral Feeding Information	1. If your child is tube fed, what type of feeding tube does your child have? 2. What is the typical tube-feeding schedule? 3. Are there any problems experienced with the tube feeding?

Direct Feeding and Swallowing Observation

To conduct the feeding and swallowing observation with a child who is fed by mouth, parents are typically asked to bring food items to the evaluation that the child accepts and tolerates without difficulty, as well as a few examples of items that are challenging for the child. Presentation of a number of trials across a variety of textures is essential in obtaining a complete assessment. Oral trials provided should be developmentally and medically appropriate and typically progress from "easy" to "more challenging."

Clinical observations made during the feeding examination will provide the clinician with information regarding parent–child mealtime interaction, the child's overall engagement in the feeding process, oral and pharyngeal stage functions, and airway protection.

Direct Assessment of the Oral Stage

The following items related to oral stage function should be evaluated when conducting the feeding and swallowing observation:

- Willingness to accept placement of utensils, cups, or nipples in the mouth
- Stabilization, function, and control of structures during bottle-feeding, cup or straw drinking, and spoon-feeding
- Strength, rhythm, rate, and coordination of nutritive sucking (infant feeding)
- Oral containment of bolus
- Efficiency and age appropriateness of chewing skills
- Presence or absence of gagging
- Oral transit and propulsion of bolus
- Presence or absence of oral residual

Infants

Assessment of oral stage skills will be dependent on the age and developmental abilities of the child. Certainly, special populations such as infants and certain clinical settings such as the neonatal intensive care unit (NICU) require specialized training. However, when conducting clinical evaluations of feeding and swallowing with neonates and infants, the feeding observation should be focused on the infant's overall state before, during, and after feeding; strength and efficiency of nutritive sucking; and the coordination of sucking, swallowing, and respiration. Impairments in sucking abilities and coordination can result in poor extraction of fluid from the nipple; loss of liquid from the mouth; poor weight gain due to limited intake or increased effort of feeding; aspiration of liquid; or physiological instability that may result in tachypnea, episodes of oxygen desaturation, and, at times, bradycardia (Wolf & Glass, 1992). An excellent resource for further in-depth and specific discussion pertaining to infant feeding and swallowing skills is the text *Feeding and Swallowing Disorders in Infancy: Assessment and Management* (Wolf & Glass, 1992). Additionally, works by Lau and colleagues (Lau, 2015; Lau et al., 2003) discuss the integration of sucking, swallowing, and respiration in infant feeding in detail.

Toddlers and Older Children

Examination of oral phase function during the feeding observation with toddlers and older children will include evaluation of function among an array of food consistencies including smooth or textured purees, soft or hard solids, and liquids. The range of specific oral stage functions to be assessed in this age group may include the following:

- Demonstration of lip closure around the spoon
- Stripping of food from the spoon bowl
- The ability to produce a stable, sustained bite into solid food
- Lateral movement of the tongue to sweep the bolus to the molar area for chewing
- Movement of the bolus across midline
- The presence of rotary diagonal chewing skills (as developmentally appropriate)

Impairments such as restricted movement of the oral structures, holding of the bolus in the mouth, prolonged chewing, increased oral transit times, gagging, and pocketing of material in the anterior or lateral sulci may be observed by the clinician during a feeding observation. These oral stage difficulties may result from oral motor, sensory, behavioral, and/or cognitive impairments exhibited. For example, gagging, one of the most common observations noted in the toddler age group, can be suggestive of reduced mastication skills as the child tries to suck on, rather than chew, the bolus, or mash it between the tongue surface and the hard palate, and attempt to swallow before being properly chewed. However, gagging may also be the result of an oral hypersensitivity to a certain food flavor or texture or a developed behavior as a way of gaining attention or a reaction from a caregiver.

Direct Assessment of Pharyngeal Stage

Skilled clinical observations once the pharyngeal swallow is initiated will provide the clinician with insight about the timing and integrity of the pharyngeal swallow. Assessment of timeliness of pharyngeal swallow onset and completeness of hyolaryngeal elevation and excursion can be determined via palpation of the laryngeal area on the neck. Additionally, noted multiple swallows per bolus may indicate reduced pharyngeal propulsion. Audible gulping, coughing, wetness, or congestion may be suggestive of reduced airway protection. In addition to direct observation, several other measurement parameters may be used during the clinical assessment, as described in the adult section of this chapter. Please refer back to that section for further description of the particular assessments outlined in what follows as they pertain to pediatrics.

Cervical Auscultation

Cervical auscultation can also be used in pediatrics to detect the onset of pharyngeal swallow initiation and make assumptions regarding the adequacy of the pharyngeal swallow. In infants and children, the use of cervical auscultation provides information regarding changes in vocal and breath sounds after the swallow, patterns of respiration and swallowing (especially in infants), and movement of the bolus through the hypopharynx (Arvedson & Brodsky, 2002; Vice, Bamford, Heinz, & Bosma, 1995).

The Three-Ounce Water Test

Suiter, Leder, and Karas (2009) reported the 3-oz water test can be used in the clinical setting as a screening measure to determine the presence of aspiration and appropriateness of an oral diet in children. However, in contrast to this, as noted in the adult section of this chapter, other studies have demonstrated "silent" aspiration with the 3-oz water test, and clinicians should be very cautious of its use, especially with children with complex medical diagnoses.

Blue Dye Testing

Although this test can be used with children (using the same methodology outlined in the adult section of this chapter), Arvedson and Brodsky (2002) do not consider the blue dye test sensitive enough to screen for aspiration in children.

Oxygen Saturation Tests

Morgan, Omahoney, and Francis (2008) found oxygen desaturation to be statistically significant as a marker of dysphagia in children with chronic neurological disability as opposed to children without dysphagia. The authors of this study suggest that use of pulse oximetry and monitoring of oxygen saturation levels may be a useful addition to the clinical bedside assessment.

Red-Flag Indicators of Pharyngeal Difficulty or Decreased Airway Protection

During the clinical bedside feeding and swallowing examination, it is essential that items noted in the child's history that may indicate a swallowing problem, as well as overt signs and symptoms of pharyngeal swallowing difficulty noted during the direct feeding observation, be taken into account. These would include the following:

- Spiking fevers
- Pneumonia or unexplained respiratory disease, repeated respiratory illness
- Frequent upper respiration infections/chronic lung disease
- Diagnosis of a medical condition contributing to increased risk of dysphagia
- Coughing
- Throat clearing
- Vocal quality change
- Modification in normal respiratory pattern (i.e., stridor)
- Reduced coordination of respiration and swallowing
- Gagging
- Vomiting
- Oxygen desaturation, bradycardia, tachypnea
- **Autonomic stress signals** (physiologic responses that the infant is under stress including startling, sweating, yawning, gagging, change color, change in respiration, splaying fingers, closing eyes/"shut down")

All of these should be considered serious pieces of clinical information and automatically prompt strong consideration for an instrumental assessment of swallowing.

Additional Clinical Feeding and Swallowing Assessments

A number of other oral motor, feeding, and swallowing evaluations for use in pediatrics are available to clinicians. These inventories, checklists, and questionnaires (several are summarized in Table 14-7) provide clinicians with further insight into a child's oral

Table 14-7. Additional Assessments of Pediatric Feeding and Swallowing Skills

Assessment	*Age Group/Population*	*Description*
The Schedule for Oral Motor Assessment (SOMA; Reilly, Skuse, Mathisen, & Wolke, 1995)	6 months to 2 years	• Standardized oral-motor scale • Clinician scores movement and function of the oral structures given presentation of a variety of food and liquid consistencies
Pediatric Assessment Scale for Severe Feeding Problems (Crist, Dobbelsteyn, Brousseau, & Napier-Phillips, 2004)	Tube-fed children	• Parent questionnaire with demonstrated validity and reliability • Used with children who are solely tube fed and those who are both tube fed and orally fed • Assesses severity of feeding skills • Allows clinicians to track progress from tube to oral feeding • Attempts to combine assessment across oral motor, oral sensory, nutrition, and behavioral areas
The Early Feeding Skills Assessment (Thoyre, Shaker, & Pridham, 2005)	Preterm infants	• 36-item checklist scored during an entire feeding • Three sections: Oral Feeding Readiness, Oral Feeding Skill, and Oral Feeding Recovery • Examines ability of infant to engage in feeding, organize oral motor functioning, coordinate swallowing and breathing, and maintain physiologic stability
Neonatal Oral Motor Assessment Scale (NOMAS; Palmer, Crawley, & Blanco, 1993)	Neonates	• Examines tongue and jaw movement during nutritive and nonnutritive sucking tasks in premature infants • Classifies movements as normal, disorganized, and dysfunctional
Dysphagia Disorder Survey (Sheppard, Hochman, & Baer, 2014)	Children and adults with developmental disability	• Used to identify and characterize feeding and swallowing disorders in children and adults with developmental delay • Differentiates disordered from functional movement patterns
The Brief Autism Mealtime Behavior Inventory (BAMBI; Lukens & Lincheid, 2008)	Children on the autistic spectrum	• Reliable and valid psychometric tool to measure feeding behaviors uniquely associated with autism • 18-item caregiver scale with questions pertaining to sensory issues related to food and behavior

motor, feeding, and swallowing skills among specific pediatric populations (i.e., premature infants, children with autism, etc.). Assessments such as these may help differentiate between normal and atypical movements or skills and determine the level of impairment and overall impact on function.

Pados, Park, Estrem, and Awotwi (2016) provided an overview of a number of assessment tools that are available for bottle-fed and breastfed infants who are less than 6 months of age. Their review includes a flow sheet to help clinicians select the most appropriate assessment tool. Additionally, Benfer, Weir, and Boyd (2012) provide a review of a number of tools for characterizing oropharyngeal dysphagia in children with cerebral palsy or neurodevelopmental disorders.

Instrumental Assessment of Feeding and Swallowing

The information and observations gathered during the clinical feeding and swallowing evaluation will guide the clinician in the decision-making process regarding the need for instrumental or other formal evaluation measures, referrals to other medical and health professionals, and an appropriate treatment/management plan.

The decision to recommend an instrumental assessment measure is multifactorial and based on the medical history, presentation of feeding and swallowing skills during the feeding observation, parental report, and presentation of overt signs and symptoms of pharyngeal swallowing difficulty. For example, a child with a medical history remarkable for a number of pneumonias or chronic pulmonary issues (e.g., asthma, frequent upper respiratory infections) may warrant further evaluation with an instrumental swallowing assessment despite the absence of overt signs and symptoms of aspiration or pharyngeal swallowing difficulty during the clinical evaluation. In this case, the referral for the instrumental swallowing study is generated due to the suspicion of aspiration as contributing to the child's respiratory disease. With any suspicion that the airway protection is compromised, a referral for an instrumental assessment should be made. The documented incidence of silent aspiration and factors contributing to increased aspiration risk with particular diagnoses or in certain populations should be kept in the forefront when considering referrals for further testing. Instrumental assessments should be conducted whenever possible to rule out any anatomical issues, swallowing impairment, or GI-based disorder before initiating any feeding and swallowing treatment program involving oral motor, sensory, and behavioral modifications

The two primary instrumental assessments of feeding and swallowing are the same for pediatrics as they are for adults: the Videofluoroscopic Swallowing Study (VFSS) and the Fiberoptic Endoscopic Evaluation of Swallowing (FEES). Both studies present with advantages and disadvantages as previously outlined in the adult section of this chapter. Refer back to that section for a description of the studies and more in-depth discussion of the differences between VFSS and FEES. The following information pertains to specific aspects of these studies as they relate to pediatrics.

Pediatric VFSS

Use of VFSS offers clear advantages in the pediatric population. As in adults, it allows for each stage of the swallow to be viewed in its entirety, is noninvasive, and allows a variety of consistencies to be administered. Disadvantages of the study include exposure to x-ray radiation and the chance of limited participation/compliance from the child due to the physical setting of the exam and ingestion of barium products. Recently the literature has discussed the limitations of "matching" consistencies typically fed to infants with those given in VFSS. Variables such as type of thickener used, brand and variety of formula, and temperature of liquid will have an impact on swallow performance and may not closely match what was tested during the swallowing study. For this reason, Stuart and Motz (2009) suggested that, although VFSS provides helpful information regarding swallow physiology, its usefulness for providing accurate diet recommendations may be questioned, particularly for infants. Further investigation is needed to closely match barium consistencies to liquid consistencies provided in treatment. In contrast to adult studies, where use of a specific protocol has been outlined by Jeri Logemann (1998), pediatric studies are best performed and conducted according to an individualized protocol based on the child's age, developmental abilities, information being sought from the evaluation, and level of participation. Administration of the test, order in which consistencies are presented, types of textures tested, bolus size, and bolus presentation can all be manipulated to obtain results that will provide a valid picture of a child's swallowing patterns under "typical" feeding conditions (Arvedson, 2007).

Foods and liquids from the child's home are mixed with barium contrast. Clinicians can become quite creative in "masking" the visual difference of the barium by using white foods (e.g., yogurt, cream cheese, milk) and altering the flavor (e.g., hiding as part of the frosting in an Oreo cookie, adding chocolate syrup). Of course, compliance is generally increased during VFSS if the child is kept hungry for the procedure. Additionally, behavioral interventions such as rewards or distraction can also be helpful. Children should not be brought to radiology for VFSS without clinical examination and some experience with manipulating and swallowing small amounts of liquids and foods.

Necessary information is obtained during VFSS, bearing in mind the importance of minimizing radiation exposure. Studies should be conducted using the ALARA principle (As Low As Reasonably Achievable) where radiation exposure is provided to the lowest achievable dose to gain the diagnostic information needed (Willis, 2004). Type of equipment, use of collimation, lowering the fluoroscopy pulse rate (without compromising diagnostic information), reducing fluoroscopy time, and keeping the fluoroscopy off until the food or liquid is in the child's mouth can help to reduce radiation exposure (Arvedson & Lefton-Greif, 1998).

VFSS assesses all stages of the oropharyngeal swallow mechanism. In children, VFSS allows direct visualization of oral bolus formation, manipulation and propulsion, timeliness of oral transit, closure of the velopharyngeal port, timeliness of pharyngeal swallow initiation, pharyngeal propulsion of the bolus through the oropharynx and hypopharynx, closure of the laryngeal vestibule, elevation and excursion of the hyoid bone and larynx, and opening/relaxation of the UES. Symptoms of physiological swallowing deficits as seen during VFSS may include poor oral containment, reduced mastication, oral residual, premature loss of material into the hypopharynx before pharyngeal swallow initiation, delay in pharyngeal swallow initiation, residue in the hypopharynx after the swallow, nasopharyngeal regurgitation, penetration of food and liquid into the laryngeal vestibule, and aspiration.

For additional details regarding the performance and interpretation of pediatric VFSS, refer to *Pediatric Swallow Studies: A Professional Manual With Caregiver Guidelines* (Arvedson & Lefton-Greif, 1998) and *Interpretation of Videofluoroscopic Swallow Studies of Infants and Children* (Arvedson, 2007). These manuals provide detailed instructions and practice exercises for clinicians.

Pediatric Fiberoptic Endoscopic Evaluation of Swallowing With or Without Sensory Testing

Similar to adults, a flexible fiberoptic endoscope (a small, flexible tube with a light and a lens on the end) is passed through the nose, into the nasal cavity, and down into the oropharynx and hypopharynx. As in VFSS, the child is fed a variety of food and liquid consistencies that are developmentally appropriate. All of the food and liquid items are dyed blue or green so that they will be visible upon swallowing. Leder and Karas (2000) demonstrated that FEES can be routinely used in the diagnosis of dysphagia in children. They reported that FEES was equally as sensitive as VFSS in detecting premature spillage of material, residue, penetration, and aspiration. FEES offers the advantage of no radiation and the ability to study the child in various positions (i.e., side-lying for infants or on a caregiver's lap) compared with VFSS. However, with the pediatric population, this may be a difficult study to complete as compliance might be reduced due to its invasive nature. Furthermore, the study offers incomplete viewing of oropharyngeal swallow function, as all stages of the swallowing process are not visualized. The study allows the view of the pharyngeal and laryngeal structures before and directly after the initiation of the pharyngeal swallow. As in the adult FEES evaluation, the view during the swallow is obstructed due to deflection of the epiglottis and closure of the laryngeal vestibule. Additionally, viewing of the oral stage, coordination between the oral and pharyngeal stages, and movement of the bolus through the upper cervical esophagus is not possible.

Willging and Thompson (2005) reported on the use of FEESST in children. They determined that it can be used in children as safely as it is in adults. Additionally, they discussed use of the evaluation to not only examine swallow function, but to determine the effects of GERD on the larynx and the swallow mechanism as well.

In recent years, there has been increased discussion of the use of FEES with infants. FEES has been found to be beneficial for use in the NICU environment to allow for feeding in typical positions, avoid transport to radiology, and eliminate exposure to radiation during assessment of swallowing. Benefits also include the ability to assess breastfeeding and perform repeat assessments without repeated radiation exposure (Reynolds, Carroll, & Sturdivant, 2016). Willette, Hinkes Molinaro, Thompson, and Schroeder (2016) also discussed the clinical utility of FEES with breastfed infants. These authors describe their procedure to involve "swabbing" the infant's mouth with green food coloring, which mixes with the mother's breast milk once the letdown reflex occurs and allows for the milk to be visualized. Additionally, the authors describe the benefits of structural assessment via endoscopy and the evaluation of the infant's ability to manage secretions and saliva swallows before initiation of oral feeding with FEES.

Differential Diagnosis

Once all necessary clinical and/or instrumental feeding and swallowing assessments as well as evaluations by other feeding and swallowing team professionals (e.g., GI workup, occupational therapy evaluation) have been completed, an accurate diagnosis may be delineated. Because of the interacting and "layering" effect of the different disorder components, it is often challenging to finalize a clear and definitive diagnosis in the area of pediatric feeding and swallowing. As was discussed in the introduction to this section of the chapter, feeding and swallowing disorders in children can be due to a wide range of etiologies (e.g., complex medical issues, oral motor problems, oropharyngeal swallowing impairment, global sensory or motor components), each playing a role in the development and the persistence of the disorder. To assign a diagnosis of oral or pharyngeal swallowing impairment and ignore the other contributory components of that child's medical history or global developmental issues would be limiting in portraying a truly accurate and complete diagnosis and treatment plan for the child's feeding and swallowing problem.

To illustrate the dynamic nature of the disorder, a child may be referred to the feeding and swallowing team for feeding refusal, vomiting, and poor weight gain. Upon GI examinations, the diagnosis of eosinophilic esophagitis (EoE) may be determined. Furthermore, through the assessments of the other feeding and swallowing team members such as the SLP, occupational therapist, and psychologist, the child was found to exhibit oral motor delay and global sensory impairments, and learned "undesired" behavioral responses to feeding. The oral motor, sensory, and behavioral components of the feeding and swallowing disorder may have derived from food avoidance and "missed opportunities" for feeding skill development due to the discomfort, pain and vomiting associated with EoE. However, in this situation, it is not realistic to assign the diagnosis of EoE solely as the etiology of the feeding and swallowing problem. The oral motor, sensory and behavioral factors are all contributors to the persistence or maintenance of the feeding problem at this point as well. If the EoE is resolved, food refusal and limited oral intake will likely persist without proper identification and treatment of these additional components. Many times, health care professionals who are not properly trained in the area of feeding and swallowing issues may have the tendency to assign one causation (e.g., "It is behavioral") without proceeding with all the proper investigative channels to determine comorbidities and other possible contributing factors to the child's feeding and swallowing problems.

Finally, in determining the presence of a feeding and swallowing disorder through the process of differential diagnosis, it is imperative to recognize and distinguish between problematic feeding patterns and "normal" age-appropriate picky eating and feeding refusal patterns. All toddlers go through periods of feeding refusal, decreased oral intake, missed meals, food selectivity, and food jags (when a child is "stuck" on a food for a certain period of time). These things occur due to a slow down in growth around 2 years of age, exerting the children's increased independence and increased mobility. It is important not to over-pathologize the typical pattern feeding issues that may be demonstrated by a child. When conducting the feeding assessment, for example, clinicians may find answers to questions regarding the length of meals, parental stress associated with mealtime, recent weight gain and growth, respiratory difficulties, and patterns and types of food refusal (e.g., does the child just refuse green vegetables but eat a variety of all other foods) helpful in teasing out normal from problematic patterns of eating (Arvedson, 2006, 2008).

The clinician should culminate the feeding and swallowing evaluation with clearly outlined impressions of the oropharyngeal swallow impairment or feeding difficulty and the characteristics of the disorder (e.g., oral motor delay, reduced hyolaryngeal excursion and elevation, oral hypersensitivity). Furthermore, recommendations regarding the appropriateness of an oral diet, safe food and liquid consistencies, feeding strategies (posture/positioning, bolus delivery methods, meal schedule, equipment, etc.), the need for feeding/swallowing treatment, or other consultations with specialists/team members all need to be delineated. Clinicians should be keenly aware of the impact that their recommendations may have on the patient's overall medical status, quality of life, ability to maintain adequate nutrition and hydration, and functionality of implementing the proposed feeding techniques and strategies in the child's daily life.

Sample Case History

L.T. is a 19-month-old male referred for evaluation due to limited acceptance of oral intake and dependence on G-tube feedings for his primary source of nutrition and hydration. Medical history is remarkable for **tracheoesophageal fistula**, weak left vocal cord, congenital heart defect, significant gastroesophageal reflux disease and reduced esophageal motility. L.T. is status post G-tube placement with a Nissen fundoplication around 3 months of age. Because of persistently slow weight gain/growth, retching with occasional vomiting, and pain or discomfort associated with increased tube-feeding volume and rate, he is followed closely by gastroenterology. He demonstrates developmental delays requiring physical, occupational, play, vision, and speech-language therapies. L.T. demonstrates resistance and crying upon attempts to seat him in his highchair. Additionally, his parents report that refusal, gagging, and coughing occur when small amounts of oral feeding (formula via bottle or puree on spoon) are fed. Reportedly, intake improves slightly if they use television as a distraction. He uses a pacifier for sleep and throughout the day. Vocal quality is hoarse, with decreased volume and respiratory support.

Selected Assessments With Rationale

- Clinical Feeding and Swallowing Assessment
  - Medical, Developmental, and Feeding Histories: Gathering in-depth and thorough histories is important in this case given L.T.'s medical diagnoses, documented delays, and lack of oral feeding experience. Clear understanding of each of his medical diagnoses and their impact on feeding and swallowing abilities and behaviors is essential.
  - Oral-Motor Examination: This will be performed as a component of the complete feeding and swallowing evaluation to determine current strength, and range of motion of the oral structures for oral feeding.
  - Direct Feeding Observation: This will be performed to assess L.T.'s willingness to accept oral trials in preparation of a possible instrumental assessment. If any trials are accepted, one can assess oral stage function, and observe parent–child interactions and child behaviors during the feeding.
- Instrumental Assessments
  - Videofluoroscopic Swallowing Study: Performed to obtain objective evaluation of oropharyngeal swallow function. Of particular interest will be L.T.'s ability to protect the airway during swallowing given the presence of vocal cord weakness and reports of "coughing" during oral feeding trials. This is chosen over FEES due to its less invasive nature and allowance for visualization for all of the stages of the swallow.
  - Other Related Instrumental Assessments ordered by the GI and ENT members of the feeding/swallowing team:
    - Barium esophagram and nuclear scintigram: to determine overall functioning of the GI tract with specific focus on the integrity of the Nissen Fundoplication and gastric motility due to difficulties with tolerating increased volume/rate of tube feeds and episodes of vomiting.
    - Flexible endoscopy: performed by the ENT to determine current functional status of the left vocal cord.

Instructional Writing Rubric (Clinical and/or Instrumental Assessment of Feeding and Swallowing)

☐ Introductory Statement
  - Provide an introductory statement to include which assessments were conducted (clinical and/or instrumental), age of child, and reason for referral. For example: "A clinical and videofluoroscopic assessment of feeding and swallowing was performed on this 19-month-old male. The child was referred for evaluation due to coughing and gagging during feeding."

☐ Medical and Developmental History
  - In paragraph form, outline medical and developmental histories, therapies the child is receiving currently, previous tests performed that are pertinent to the feeding and swallowing evaluation, and other concerns.

☐ Feeding History
  - Provide relevant feeding history information. Depending on the age of the child and feeding/swallowing issues, this may include feeding progression since birth or from the onset of the feeding and swallowing problem. In this section, include information on nonoral feedings provided to the child (as applicable).

☐ Testing Performed
  - Outline which assessments were performed and the findings of each. For example, this diagnostic report may surmise findings from the oral-peripheral examination, direct feeding observation, and videofluoroscopic swallowing assessment. This section should include findings regarding the oral and pharyngeal stages of swallowing and signs or symptoms of swallowing difficulty. Additionally, for the videofluoroscopic assessment, the clinician will need to include the protocol for assessment including seating position of the child, radiographic view (i.e., lateral view), and the types and presentation of food and liquid consistencies. For example: "L.T. was seated upright in a toddler feeding seat. A lateral view was taken. Trials of thin liquid and puree were impregnated with barium and provided via syringe and spoon."

- ☐ Impressions
  - Provide a diagnosis based on the testing results. Outline the level of impairment (i.e., mild, moderate), characteristics of the disorder or physiological impairments seen during the instrumental assessment and the "symptoms" of these deficits. For example: "L.T. presents with a moderate-to-severe oropharyngeal dysphagia characterized by oral motor impairment, delay in pharyngeal swallow initiation, reduced hyolaryngeal elevation, and closure of the laryngeal vestibule. These deficits resulted in aspiration of thin liquids." or "L.T. presents with a significant oral sensorimotor feeding disorder characterized by oral motor impairments and oral hypersensitivity. This has resulted in delayed acquisition of age-appropriate mastication skills and difficulty transitioning to solid foods." This section should also include the functional impact of the disorder as well as contributory and maintaining factors of the disorder.
- ☐ Recommendations
  - In this section, summarize recommendations based on the assessment, including appropriate food/liquid consistencies, specific recommendations for oral intake (e.g., amounts, schedule, etc.), and safe feeding strategies or precautions (e.g., appropriate seating position during oral intake, rate of intake, bolus size delivered, particular feeding equipment, etc.). Additionally, provide recommendations regarding the need for therapy, specific goals or outcomes to be addressed in treatment, and referrals to other specialists.

Sample Report

Identifying Information

Client's Name: L.T. **Date of Evaluation**:

Address: *(street)* **Phone**:

(city, state, zip code)

Date of Birth:

Diagnosis:

Referred by: Dr. John Smith, Pediatric Gastroenterologist

Reason for referral: Dependence on G-tube feedings, refusal of oral feedings

Background Information

L.T., a 19-month-old boy, was seen for a clinical and videofluoroscopic assessment of feeding and swallowing. The child was accompanied to the evaluation by his mother.

Medical and Developmental Histories

L.T. was born prematurely at 32 weeks of gestation. Medical history is remarkable for tracheoesophageal fistula, weak left vocal cord, congenital heart defect, frequent upper respiratory infections requiring antibiotics, significant gastroesophageal reflux disease, and reduced esophageal motility. Approximately 1 month ago, L.T. underwent examination with a pediatric otolaryngologist, which revealed persistent left vocal cord weakness with right vocal cord compensation. L.T. is status post G-tube placement with Nissen fundoplication around 3 months of age. Before that, he was fed via nasogastric and orogastric tubes. Prevacid is currently the only medication taken.

L.T. receives developmental therapies through the Early Intervention program. He currently receives physical, occupational, play, vision, and speech-language therapies at home. Speech-language therapy is provided 5 times weekly for 30 minutes.

Feeding History

L.T. demonstrates poor tolerance of tube feedings. Often, retching, gagging, and crying in pain are seen with increased rate or volume of tube feeding. On rare occasions, a small amount of emesis has occurred. Currently, L.T. receives 800cc of Alimentum formula (Similac) at a delivery rate of no more than 50cc/hour. He demonstrates pain, discomfort, and gagging if the rate is increased.

Oral feeding acceptance is limited. Oral feeding is attempted three times daily. Typically, L.T. is offered a small amount of formula via bottle, rice cereal, or jarred baby food fruit or vegetables by spoon. Dissolvable solids (i.e., Gerber puffs) have been offered as well with limited acceptance. On occasion, L.T. will accept a limited amount of formula (i.e., < 10cc) or a few teaspoons of cereal/baby food, or mouth a piece of fruit placed in a "safe feeder" netting; however, the majority of times, he refuses all trials. Distraction with toys or television appears to increase intake. L.T.'s mother reported that L.T. sits at all family meals whenever possible and she has requested that all caretakers eat in front of L.T. and provide for a model of positive interaction with food.

Feeding refusal behaviors seen at mealtime include refusal to sit in the high chair, refusal to open the mouth, throwing food, crying, gagging, turning away, and back arching.

Testing

Oral-Peripheral Examination

Cursory observation of the oral-peripheral mechanism revealed all structures to be intact. A spontaneous smile was observed. Overall range of motion, strength, and tone of the oral structures appears adequate. Lingual protrusion and retraction were noted during vocal play; however, lateralization of the tongue was not seen during spontaneously. The clinician made several attempts to perform intraoral examination with oral motor tools; however, L.T. repeatedly refused to open the mouth when approached and turned away. Mouthing of toys was not noted during this evaluation. L.T. was observed to maintain a pacifier throughout the session with minimal willingness to remove it from his mouth. Secretion management was within normal limits. Vocal quality was judged to be hoarse. The behaviors observed during attempts to perform an intraoral examination are suggestive of a degree of heightened oral sensitivity.

Feeding Observation

L.T. was seated in a toddler-feeding seat and fed by his mother. He was presented with small amounts of baby food applesauce on a spoon, cheese puffs, and formula in a bottle with a standard nipple. Upon presentation of the bottle, L.T. immediately turned away in refusal and continued to resist despite repeated attempts with coaxing and distraction with toys. He allowed the spoon containing a small amount of applesauce to be placed at his lips; however, minimal mouth opening was observed. His mother "pushed" the spoon into his mouth, resulting in L.T. arching the back to pull away from the spoon. A small amount of puree was swallowed after prolonged holding of the bolus in his mouth. Approximately 50% of the bolus was pushed out of his mouth with his tongue. An immature oral stage of swallowing pattern was observed, primarily evidenced by sucking and tongue protrusion through the lips upon swallowing. Small pieces of Gerber puffs were placed in front of L.T. on the tray. He was observed to "sweep" the items onto the floor. He allowed his mother to place a small piece into his mouth. He appeared to suck on the piece of food in an attempt to soften it and prepare for swallowing. Lingual lateralization or manipulation of the bolus away from the midline of the tongue was not noted. An episode of gagging with quick recovery was observed. Shortly after the gag, the small piece of food was pushed out of the mouth.

Videofluoroscopic Assessment of Swallowing

A videofluoroscopic assessment of swallowing was conducted. L.T. was seated in a Tumble Form feeding seat; a left lateral view was taken. Trials of thin liquid, nectar-thick liquid, and smooth baby food puree (Stage I jarred foods) were impregnated with barium and administered.

Oral bolus formation, manipulation, and propulsion were reduced for all consistencies characterized by reduced acceptance of oral trials, anterior spillage of bolus from mouth, spreading of the bolus throughout the oral cavity, slow oral transit, piecemeal deglutition, and premature spillage of material into the hypopharynx before pharyngeal swallow initiation. Thin liquid and thick liquid trials were delivered via syringe due to difficulty with acceptance of a bottle.

Initiation of the pharyngeal swallow was timely with the majority of trials. Upon triggering of the pharyngeal swallow, pharyngeal propulsion/stripping of bolus was mildly reduced as small amounts of valleculae residue were noted. This appeared to clear with a second swallow initiated spontaneously. The bolus moved through the UES into the upper cervical esophagus with ease.

Hyolaryngeal elevation and closure of the laryngeal vestibule were within normal limits for nectar thick liquids and puree consistencies as there were no occurrences of penetration or aspiration. However, for small amounts of thin liquids swallowed, intermittent trace aspiration was noted. A cough reflex was elicited in response with the majority of trials. The cough was judged to be nonproductive as clearance of the aspiration was not seen.

Impressions

L.T. exhibits a significant oral sensorimotor feeding disorder characterized by oral hypersensitivity, feeding aversion, delayed oral motor skills for feeding, and feeding refusal behaviors. Additionally, a mild-to-moderate oropharyngeal swallowing impairment is present, characterized by oral phase deficits, reduced pharyngeal propulsion of bolus, and reduced closure of the laryngeal vestibule. Deficits resulted in trace aspiration of thin liquids.

Recommendations

It is suggested that L.T. continue to receive G-tube feedings as his primary source of nutrition and hydration at this time. Initiation of outpatient feeding therapy services is strongly recommended.

Additionally, it is suggested that the family continue attempts at small oral feedings of puree and nectar-thick liquids as L.T. will allow and tolerate. It is important to provide positive oral feeding experiences and opportunities for food exploration. This can be achieved by providing positive models of eating and interaction with food, inclusion at family meals, and play or sensory exploration with food (encourage touch, smell, tasting). Additionally, oral sensorimotor stimulation may be provided with oral motor tools to facilitate normalization of intraoral sensation and development of age-appropriate oral motor skills. In an attempt to shape appropriate feeding behaviors, suggest providing verbal and/or positive contingent reinforcements for desirable mealtime behaviors. Undesired behaviors should be ignored.

Continued follow-up with pediatric gastroenterology for management of G-tube feedings is recommended as L.T. continues to experience retching, vomiting, pain, and discomfort with G-tube feedings.

The results and recommendations of this assessment were discussed with L.T.'s parents who expressed understanding. Thank you for this referral.

____

(Name and credentials)
Speech-Language Pathologist

Practice Exercise: Second Case History

Read the following case history and decide which assessment tools as well as any other relevant medical assessments that may be beneficial should be used. Write a list of appropriate evaluations with the rationale as to why these particular assessments were selected.

D.M. is an 11-month-old boy referred for poor weight gain/growth, feeding refusal, and difficulty transitioning to age-appropriate puree and solid foods. He presented as an alert, engaged baby. D.M. was born prematurely at 34 weeks of gestation. Feeding history is remarkable for initial difficulty latching onto the breast and acceptance of oral feedings. Medical history is remarkable for suspected reflux in earlier infancy (as the baby demonstrated frequent vomiting), but the pediatrician was resistant to a trial of reflux medication. Over several months, D.M. has experienced minimal weight gain and is now classified as "failure to thrive." Weight and height are well below expectations and are unable to be charted on the normal growth curve. He is primarily fed expressed breast milk via bottle or breastfeeds. At 6 months of age, his mother introduced puree foods with limited success; she discontinued trials and reattempted 1 and 2 months later with the same result. Upon presentation of the spoon, D.M. typically accepts one or two trials. Gagging is seen intermittently. He appears to dislike touching wet foods and does not like food on his face. He typically turns away in refusal, bats at the spoon, keeps his lips tightly closed, throws food on the floor, or begins to cry. First solids such as Cheerios or crackers/cookies have been introduced, but D.M. reportedly demonstrates "no interest" and throws these items on the floor. D.M. accepts water from an open cup or sippy cup. His mother reports D.M. frequently coughs when drinking from the cup or on occasion during bottle and breastfeeding.

Summary

SLPs play an important role in diagnosing, treating, and managing feeding and swallowing disorders in children and adults. For students and new clinicians in the field, a solid understanding of the incidence of feeding and swallowing problems, anatomy and physiology of the oropharyngeal swallow mechanism, associated medical diagnoses, and overall complexity of feeding and swallowing process is essential before embarking on evaluation and intervention. Clinical decisions made during and after the assessment process should be grounded in the knowledge that feeding and swallowing issues have a far-reaching impact on the patient's overall health, nutritional status, social-cognitive development or well-being, and the family unit as a whole. Clinicians are reminded that working collaboratively with other professionals, specialists, and caregivers is essential in order to maximize outcomes regardless of the setting of clinical practice. Bearing these considerations in mind, SLPs can greatly contribute to the diagnosis and management of these patients and provide support to both the patient and the primary caregivers as they face the difficulties associated with feeding difficulty and oropharyngeal dysphagia.

Glossary

Achalasia: Primary esophageal dysmotility; often incomplete relaxation of the lower esophageal sphincter, which may result in retention of food and, at times, regurgitation of the food hours later.

Anterior faucial arches: Structural arches that separate the mouth from the pharynx.

Aspiration: The misdirection of foreign material (food, liquid, or gastric contents) into the lungs.

Autonomic stress signals: Physiologic responses that the infant is under stress including startling, sweating, yawning, gagging, change color, or change in respiration, among others.

Cervical auscultation: Listening to the sounds of the swallow on the neck with a stethoscope lateral to the cervical vertebrae.

Cervical osteophyte: Bony overgrowth affecting one or more of the cervical vetebra(e), which may interrupt the easy flow of foods and liquids through the pharynx and cervical esophagus.

Dehydration: Having insufficient fluids in the body to maintain a healthy level of fluids in body tissues.

Eosinophilic esophagitis: Allergic inflammatory disease of the esophagus in which a large number of eosinophils (a white blood cell found in the immune system that helps fight infection) is present, resulting in pain, nausea, vomiting, food impaction, and dysphagia.

Extubation: Removal of an airway tube used for breathing that has been placed through the larynx into the trachea.

Failure to thrive: Poor weight gain and growth in early infancy/childhood; weight usually falls below the third percentile on the normal growth charts.

Gastric dysmotility: Abnormal or slowed movement of the contents of the stomach and gastrointestinal tract.

Gastroesophageal reflux disorder: Food or liquid travels up from the stomach back into the esophagus.

Gastrostomy tube (G-tube): Feeding tube surgically placed into the stomach.

Intubation: The placement of a tube through the larynx and into the trachea to supply respiratory support; often used short term for critically ill patients; can be attached to a ventilator.

Laryngeal cleft: Defect in the posterior larynx; classified based on severity. A Type I cleft, in which there is an interarytenoid defect with an intact cricoid cartilage, is the most common (Haibeck & Mandell, 2008).

Laryngomalacia: Common pediatric laryngeal disorder characterized by a collapse of the supraglottic laryngeal cartilages upon inspiration, decreased laryngeal sensation, and stridor.

Laryngopharyngeal reflux (LPR): Backflow of stomach contents into the laryngopharynx. Multiple synonyms are used including reflux laryngitis, laryngeal reflux, and supraesophageal reflux.

Malnutrition: Poor nourishment of the body. May be due to poor oral intake, not eating healthy foods, impaired digestive system, or poor absorption of nutrients.

Mastication: To chew, grind, or crush food with the teeth to prepare food for swallowing.

Nasogastric tube (NG-tube): Small tube inserted through the nasal cavity, through the pharynx, though the esophagus, and into the stomach.

Nasopharyngeal regurgitation: Regurgitation of food or liquid into the velopharyngeal port and into the nasal cavity.

Oral aversion: Refusal to eat or allow touch to the mouth or perioral area.

Orogastric tube (OG-tube): Small tube inserted through the oral cavity, through the esophagus, and into the stomach.

Oxygen desaturation: A decrease in the fraction of the hemoglobin molecules in a blood sample that are saturated with oxygen. Normal saturation is usually 95% to 100%.

Penetration: Passage of material from the oropharynx, into the laryngeal airway entrance (laryngeal vestibule), to the level on/or above the true vocal cords.

Percutaneous endoscopic gastrostomy (PEG): G-tube that is placed endoscopically.

Percutaneous endoscopic jejunostomy (PEJ or J-tube): Feeding tube that is inserted into the second part of the small intestine known as the *jejunum*.

Peristalsis: Alternating contraction and relaxation of the esophagus and the intestines to propel material through the digestive system.

Phasic bite reflex: Closing and opening of mandible upon pressure to the gums in the molar area.

Pneumonia: An acute infection and inflammation that often begin in the bronchioles and spread through the lung tissues. Efficient exchange of oxygen and carbon dioxide is compromised, affecting the patient's health (Ashford, 2005).

Protrusion reflex: Protrusion of tongue from mouth upon touch to the anterior portion.

Pulse oximetry: Sensor (usually attached to the finger or toe) applied to the skin that measures pulse rate and the percentage of oxygenated hemoglobin.

Rooting reflex: Touch to either corner of the mouth results in turning the head toward the touch.

Sensory integration dysfunction: Difficulty with processing of sensory information received from the senses.

Silent aspiration: Absence of coughing in response to aspiration.

Total parenteral nutrition (TPN): Nutrition/hydration is delivered through a central venous catheter when the gastrointestinal tract cannot be used for medical reasons.

Tracheoesophageal fistula (TEF): Abnormal fistula (hole) in the soft tissue common wall between the trachea and esophagus. A TEF allows some material entering the esophagus to flow back into the trachea. It is often located at the level of the first and third thoracic vertebrae.

Transverse tongue reflex: Movement of the tongue laterally when the lateral surface has been touched.

Upper esophageal sphincter (UES): The UES is a tonically contracted group of skeletal muscles separating the pharynx from the esophagus. The major muscle of this sphincter is the cricopharyngeus muscle that is contracted except when food, liquid, or saliva is swallowed (Murry & Carrau, 2006). When swallowing, the UES relaxes during the pharyngeal propulsion and stripping of the bolus into the cervical esophagus.

Valleculae: Lateral recesses (spaces) at the base of the tongue on each side of the epiglottis.

Zenker's diverticulum: An outpouching of the pharyngeal mucosa at the level of the UES. The diverticulum often protrudes between the fibers of the cricopharyngeal muscle and the inferior constrictor muscle. During oral intake, ingested food may collect in it, and when a swallow occurs, backflow of material into the pharynx may occur. The patient may report coughing or choking when swallowing or recurrent respiratory infections.

References

American Speech-Language-Hearing Association. (n.d.). Practice portal. Retrieved from http://www.asha.org/practice-portal/

American Speech-Language-Hearing Association. (2016). Scope of practice in speech-language pathology. Retrieved from http://www.asha.org/policy/SP2016-00343/

Antonios, N., Carnaby-Mann, G., Crary, M., Miller, L., Hubbard, H., Hood, K., . . . Silliman, S. (2010). Analysis of a physician tool for evaluating dysphagia on an inpatient stroke unit: The modified Mann Assessment of Swallowing Ability. *Journal of Stroke and Cerebrovascular Diseases, 19*(1), 49-57.

Arvedson, J. (2006, May 16). Swallowing and feeding in infants and young children. *GI Motility Online.*

Arvedson, J. (2007). *Interpretation of videofluoroscopic swallow studies of infants and children. A study guide to improve diagnostic skills and treatment planning.* Gaylord, MI: Northern Speech Services.

Arvedson, J. (2008). Assessment of pediatric dysphagia and feeding disorders: Clinical and instrumental approaches. *Developmental Disabilities Research Reviews, 14*, 118-127.

Arvedson, J., & Brodsky, L. (2002). *Pediatric swallowing and feeding, assessment and management* (2nd ed.). Canada: Singular.

Arvedson, J., & Lefton-Greif, M. (1998). *Pediatric videofluoroscopic swallow studies.* San Antonio, TX: Communication Skill Builders.

Arvedson, J., Rogers, B., Buck, G., Smart, P., & Msall, M. (1994). Silent aspiration prominent in children with dysphagia. *International Journal of Pediatric Otorhinolaryngology, 28*, 173-181.

Ashford, J. R. (2005). Pneumonia: Factors beyond aspiration. *Swallowing and Swallowing Disorders (Dysphagia), 14*, 10-16.

Aviv, J. E., Kaplan, S. T., Thomson, J. E., Spitzer, J., Diamond, B., & Close, L. G. (2000). The safety of flexible endoscopic evaluation of swallowing with sensory testing (FEESST): An analysis of 500 consecutive evaluations. *Dysphagia, 15*(1), 39-44.

Aviv, J. E., Kim, T., Sacco, R. L., Kaplan, S., Goodhart, K., Diamond, B., & Close, L. (1998). FEESST: A new bedside endoscopic test of the motor and sensory components of swallowing. *Annals of Otology, Rhinology Laryngology, 107*, 378-387.

Aviv, J., Murry, T., Zschommler, A., Cohen, M., & Gartner, C. (2005). Flexible endoscopic evaluation of swallowing with sensory testing: Patient characteristics and analysis of safety in 1,340 consecutive examinations. *The Annals of Otology, Rhinology Laryngology, 114*, 173-176.

Aviv, J., Spitzer, J., Cohen, M., Ma, G., Belafsky, P., & Close, L. (2002). Laryngeal adductor reflex and pharyngeal squeeze as predictors of laryngeal penetration and aspiration. *The Laryngoscope, 112*, 338-341.

Benfer, K. A., Weir, K .A., & Boyd, R. N. (2012). Clinimetrics of measures of oropharyngeal dysphagia for preschool children with cerebral palsy and neurodevelopmental disabilities: A systematic review. *Developmental Medicine Child Neurology, 54*, 784-795.

Bingham, P. (2009). Deprivation and dysphagia in preterm infants. *Journal of Child Neurology, 24*, 743-749.

Boesch, R. P., Daines, C., Willging, J. P., Kaul, A., Cohen, A. P., Wood, R. E., & Amin, R. S. (2006). Advances in the diagnosis and management of chronic pulmonary aspiration in children. *European Respiratory Journal, 28*, 847-861.

Calis, E., Veugelers, R., Sheppard, J., Tibboel, D., Evenhuis, H., & Penning, C. (2008). Dysphagia in children with severe generalized cerebral palsy and intellectual disability. *Developmental Medicine and Child Neurology, 50*, 625-630.

Cass, H., Wallis, C., Ryan, M., Reilly, S., & McHugh, K. (2005). Assessing pulmonary consequences of dysphagia in children with neurological disabilities: When to intervene? *Developmental Medicine and Child Neurology, 47*, 347-352.

Cooper-Brown, L., Copeland, S., Dailey, S., Downey, D., Petersen, M., Stimson, C., & Van Dyke, D. C. (2008). Feeding and swallowing dysfunction in genetic syndromes. *Developmental Disabilities Research Reviews, 14*, 147-157.

Crist, W., Dobbelsteyn, C., Brousseau, A., & Napier-Phillips, A. (2004). Pediatric assessment scale for severe feeding problems: Validity and reliability of a new scale for tube-fed children. *Nutrition in Clinical Practice, 19*, 403-408.

Daniels, S., & Huckabee, M. L. (2008). *Dysphagia following stroke.* San Diego, CA: Plural.

deBenedictis, F. M., Carnielli, V. P., & deBenedictis, D. (2009). Aspiration lung disease. *Pediatric Clinic North America, 56*, 173-190.

Delaney, A., & Arvedson, J. (2008). Development of swallowing and feeding: Prenatal through first year of life. *Developmental Disabilities Research Reviews, 14*, 105-117.

Dodrill, P., & Gosa, M. M. (2015). Pediatric dysphagia: Physiology, assessment and management. *Annals of Nutrition & Metabolism, 66*(5), 24-31.

Forcada-Guex, M., Pierrehumbert, B., Borghini, A., Moessinger, A., & Muller-Nix, C. (2006). Early dyadic patterns of mother-infant interactions and outcomes of prematurity at 18 months. *Pediatrics, 118*, 107-114.

Goodrich, S., & Walker, A. (2008). Clinical swallow evaluation. In R. Leonard & K. Kendall (Eds.), *Dysphagia assessment and treatment planning* (2nd ed.). San Diego, CA: Plural.

Groher, M. (1997). *Dysphagia: Diagnosis and management* (3rd ed.). Boston, MA: Butterworth- Heinemann.

Groher, M. (2010a). Esophageal disorders in dysphagia. In M. Groher & M. Crary (Eds.), *Dysphagia: Clinical management in adults and children* (pp. 126-145). Maryland Heights, MO: Mosby-Elsevier.

Groher, M. (2010b). Ethical considerations. In M. Groher & M. Crary (Eds.) *Dysphagia: Clinical management in adults and children* (pp. 308-320). Maryland Heights, MO: Mosby-Elsevier.

Groher, M., & Crary, M. (2010). *Dysphagia: Clinical management in adults and children*. Maryland Heights, MO: Mosby-Elsevier.

Haas, A., & Maune, N. (2009). Clinical presentation of feeding dysfunction in children with eosinophilic gastrointestinal disease. *Immunology and Allergy Clinics of North America, 29*, 65-75.

Haibeck, L., & Mandell, D.L. (2008). The aerodigestive clinic: multidisciplinary management of pediatric dysphagia. *Perspectives on Swallowing and Swallowing Disorders (Dysphagia), 17*, 101-109.

Homer, E. (2003). An interdisciplinary team approach to providing dysphagia treatment in the schools. *Seminars in Speech and Language, 24*, 215-234.

Jadcherla, S. R., Wang, M., Vijayapal, A. S., & Leuthner, S. R. (2010). Impact of prematurity and comorbidities on feeding milestones in neonates: A retrospective study. *Journal of Perinatology, 30*, 201-208.

Langmore, S. (2001). *Endoscopic evaluation and treatment of swallowing disorders*. New York, NY: Thieme Medical.

Langmore, S., Skarupski, K., Park, P., & Fries, B. (2002). Predictors of aspiration pneumonia in nursing home residents. *Dysphagia, 17*, 298-307.

Larnert, G., & Ekberg, O. (1995). Positioning improves the oral and pharyngeal swallowing function in children with cerebral palsy. *Acta Paediatrica, 84*, 689-692.

Lau, C. (2015). Development of suck swallow mechanisms in infants. *Annals of Nutrition & Metabolism, 66*(suppl 5), 7-14.

Lau, C., Smith, E. O., & Schanler, R. J. (2003). Coordination of suck-swallow and swallow respiration in preterm infants. *Acta Paediatrica, 92*, 721-727.

Leder, S. (1996). Comment on Thompson-Henry and Braddock: The modified Evan's blue dye procedure fails to detect aspiration in the tracheostomized patient. *Dysphagia, 11*(1), 80-81.

Leder, S. B., & Karas, D. E. (2000). Fiberoptic endoscopic evaluation of swallowing in the pediatric population. *The Laryngoscope, 110*, 1132-1136.

Leder, S., & Suiter, D. (2010, March). Presentation at the Dysphagia Research Society Annual Meeting, San Diego, CA.

Lefton-Greif, M. A. (2008). Pediatric dysphagia. *Physical Medicine and Rehabilitation Clinics of North America, 19*, 837-851.

Lefton-Greif, M., & Arvedson, J. (2007). Pediatric feeding and swallowing disorders: State of health, population trends, and application of the international classification of functioning, disability, and health. *Seminars in Speech and Language, 28*, 161-165.

Levy, Y., Levy, A., Zangen, T., Kornfeld, L., Dalal, I., Samuel, E., & Boaz, M. (2009). Diagnostic clues for identification of nonorganic vs. organic causes of food refusal and poor feeding. *Journal of Pediatric Gastroenterology and Nutrition, 48*, 355-362.

Logemann, J. (1993). *Manual for the videofluoroscopic study of swallow* (2nd ed.). Austin, TX: Pro-Ed.

Logemann, J. (1998). *Evaluation and treatment of swallowing disorders*. Austin, TX: Pro-Ed.

Logemann, J., Veis, S., & Colangelo, L. (1999). A screening procedure for oropharyngeal dysphagia. *Dysphagia, 14*(1), 41-51.

Lukens, C., & Linscheid, T. (2008). Development and validation of an inventory to assess mealtime behavior problems in children with autism. *Journal of Autism and Developmental Disorders, 38*, 342-352.

Mann, G. (2002). *MASA: The Mann Assessment of Swallowing Ability*. Clifton, NY: Thompson Learning.

Martin-Harris, B., Brodsky, M. B., Michel, Y., Castell, D. O., Schleicher, M., Sandidge, J., . . . Blair, J. (2008). MBS measurement tool for swallow impairment-MBSImp: Establishing a standard. *Dysphagia, 23*, 392-405.

Martin-Harris, B., & Jones, B. (2008). The videofluoroscopic swallowing study. *Physical Medicine and Rehabilitation Clinics of North America, 19*, 769-785.

Martino, R., Maki, E., & Diamant, N. (2014). Identification of dysphagia using the Toronto Bedside Swallowing Screening Test (TOR-BSST): Are 10 teaspoons of water necessary? *International Journal of Speech Language Pathology, 16*, 193-198.

Mason, S., Harris, G., & Blisset, J. (2005). Tube feeding in infancy: Implications for the development of normal eating and drinking skills. *Dysphagia, 20*, 46-61.

McHorney, C. A., Bricker, D. E., Kramer, A. E., Rosenbek, J. C., Robbins, J., Chignell, K. A., . . . & Clarke, C. (2000). The SWAL-QOL outcomes tool for oropharyngeal dysphagia in adults: Conceptual foundation and item development. *Dysphagia, 15*, 115-121.

McHorney C. A., Robbins J., Lomax, K., Rosenbek, J. C., Chignell, K., Kramer, A. E., & Bricker, D. E. (2002). The SWAL-QOL and the SWAL-CARE outcomes tool for oropharyngeal dysphagia in adults: III. Documentation of reliability and validity. *Dysphagia, 17*, 97-114.

Miller, C. (2009). Updates on pediatric feeding and swallowing problems. *Current Opinions in Otolaryngology & Head & Neck Surgery, 17*, 194-199.

Miller, C., Burklow, K.A., Santoro, K., Kirby, E., Mason, D., & Rudolph, C. D. (2001). An interdisciplinary team approach to the management of pediatric feeding and swallowing disorders. *Children's Healthcare, 30*, 201-218.

Morgan, A. T., Omahoney, R., & Francis, H. (2008). The use of pulse oximetry as screening assessment for paediatric neurogenic dysphagia. *Developmental Neurorehabilitation, 11*, 25-38.

Morris, S., & Klein, M. (2000). *Pre-feeding skills: A comprehensive resource for mealtime development* (2nd ed.). Austin, TX: Pro-Ed.

Murry, T., & Carrau, R. (2006). *Clinical management of swallowing disorders*. San Diego, CA: Plural.

Pados, B. F., Park, J., Estrem, H., & Awotwi, A. (2016). Assessment tools for evaluation of oral feeding in infants younger than 6 months. *Advances in Neonatal Care, 16*, 143-150.

Palmer, M., Crawley, K., & Blanco, I. (1993). Neonatal Oral-Motor Assessment Scale: A reliability study. *Journal of Perinatology, 13*, 28-35.

Perlman, A., & Schulze-Delnieu, K. (1997). *Deglutition and its disorders: Anatomy, physiology, clinical diagnosis and management*. San Diego, CA: Singular.

Prasse, J., & Kikano, G. (2009). An overview of pediatric dysphagia. *Clinical Pediatrics, 48*, 247-251.

Reilly, S., Skuse, D., Mathiesen, B., & Wolke, D. (1995). The objective rating of oral motor functions during feeding. *Dysphagia, 10*, 177-191.

Reilly, S., Skuse, D., & Poblete, X. (1996). Prevalence of feeding problems and oral motor dysfunction in children with cerebral palsy: A community survey. *Journal of Pediatrics, 129*, 877-882.

Reynolds, J., Carroll, S., & Sturdivant, C. (2016). Fiberoptic endoscopic evaluation of swallowing: A multidisciplinary alternative for assessment of infants with dysphagia in the neonatal intensive care unit. *Advances in Neonatal Care, 16*(1), 37-43.

Robbins, J., Coyle, J., Rosenbek, J., Roecker, E., & Wood, J. (1999). Differentiation of normal and abnormal airway protection during swallowing using the penetration-aspiration scale. *Dysphagia, 14*, 228-232.

Rommel, N., DeMeyer, A.M., Feenstra, L., & Veereman-Wauters, G. (2003). The complexity of feeding problems in 700 infants and young children presenting to a tertiary care institution. *Journal of Pediatric Gastroenterology and Nutrition, 37*, 75-84.

Rosenbek, J. C., Robbins, J. A., Roecker, E. B., Coyle, J. L., & Wood, J. L. (1996). A penetration-aspiration scale. *Dysphagia, 11*, 93-98.

Samara, M., Johnson, S., Lamberts, K., Marlow, N., & Wolke, D. (2010). Eating problems at age 6 years in a whole population sample of extremely preterm children. *Developmental Medicine and Child Neurology, 52*, 16-22.

Sandidge, J. (2009). The Modified barium swallow impairment profile (MBSIm): A new standard physiologic approach to swallowing assessment and targeted treatment. *ASHA Perspectives on Swallowing and Swallowing Disorders, 18*, 117-122.

Schreck, K., Williams, K., & Smith, A. (2004). A comparison of eating behaviors between children with and without autism. *Journal of Autism and Developmental Disorders, 34*, 433-438.

Schwarz, S. M., Corredor, J., Fisher-Medina, J., Cohen, J., & Rabinowitz, S. (2001). Diagnosis and treatment of feeding disorders in children with developmental disabilities. *Pediatrics, 108*, 671-676.

Sheppard, J. J., Hochman, R., & Baer, C. (2014). The Dysphagia Disorder Survey: Validation of an assessment for swallowing and feeding function in developmental disability. *Research in Developmental Disabilities, 35*, 929-942.

Sherman, B., Nisenboum, J., Jesberger, B,. Morrow, C., & Jesberger, J. (1999). Assessment of dysphagia with the use of pulse oximetry. *Dysphagia, 14*, 152-156.

Shipley, K., & McAfee, J. (2009). Assessment in speech-language pathology: A resource manual (4th ed.). *Clifton Park, NY: Delmar Cengage Learning, 475*.

Silberstein, D., Geva, R., Feldman, R., Gardner, J., Karmel, B., Rozen, H., & Kuint, J. (2009). The transition to oral feeding in low-risk premature infants: Relation to infant neurobehavioral functioning and mother-infant feeding interaction. *Early Human Development, 85*, 157-162.

Simon, M., & Collins, M. S. (2013, December). The pediatric lung and aspiration. *ASHA SIG 13, Perspectives on Swallowing and Swallowing Disorders, 22*, 142-154.

Smith, C., Logemann, J., Colangelo, L., Radmaker, A. W., & Pauloski, B. R. (1999). Incidence and patient characteristics associated with silent aspiration in the acute care setting. *Dysphagia, 14*, 1-7.

Stuart, S., & Motz, J. M. (2009). Viscosity in infant dysphagia management: Comparison of viscosity of thickened liquids used in assessment and thickened liquids used in treatment. *Dysphagia, 24*, 412-422.

Suiter, D., Leder, S., & Karas, D. (2009). The 3-ounce (90-cc) water swallow challenge: A screening test for children with suspected oropharyngeal dysphagia. *Otolaryngology-Head and Neck Surgery, 140*, 187-190.

Sullivan, P., (2008). Gastrointestinal disorders in children with neurodevelopmental disabilities. *Developmental Disabilities Research Reviews, 14*, 128-136.

Thoyre, S. M. (2007). Feeding outcomes of extremely premature infants after neonatal care. *Journal of Obstetric, Gynecologic, and Neonatal Nursing, 36*, 366-375.

Thoyre, S., Shaker, C., & Pridham, K. (2005). The Early Feeding Skills Assessment for Preterm Infants. *Neonatal Network, 24*(3), 7-16.

Vandenplas, Y., Rudoloph, C.D., DiLorenzo, C., Hassall, E., Liptak, G., & Mazur, L. (2009). Pediatric gastroesophageal reflux clinical practice guidelines: Joint recommendations of the North American Society for Pediatric Gastroenterology, Hepatology, and Nutrition (NASPGHAN) and the European Society for Pediatric Gastroenterology, Hepatology, and Nutrition (ESPGHAN). *Journal of Pediatric Gastroenterology and Nutrition, 49*, 498-547.

Vice, F. L., Bamford, O., Heinz, J. M., & Bosma, J. F. (1995). Correlation of cervical auscultation with physiological recording during suckle-feeding in newborn infants. *Developmental Medicine and Child Neurology, 37*, 167-179.

Weir, K. A., McMahon, S., Taylor, S., & Chang, A. B. (2011). Oropharyngeal aspiration and silent aspiration in children. *Chest, 140*, 589-597.

Willette, S., Hinkes Molinaro, L., Thompson, D. M., & Schroeder, J. W. (2016). Fiberoptic examination of swallowing in the breastfeeding infant. *Laryngoscope, 126*, 1681-1686.

Willging, J. P., & Thompson, D. (2005). Pediatric FEESST: Fiberoptic endoscopic evaluation of swallowing with sensory testing. *Current Gastroenterology Reports, 7*, 240-243.

Willis, C. E. (2004). The ALARA concept in pediatric CR and DR: Dose reduction in pediatric radiographic exams—a white paper conference executive summary. *Pediatric Radiology, 34*, 162-164.

Wolf, L. S., & Glass, R. P. (1992). *Feeding and swallowing disorders in infancy: Assessment and management*. Tucson, AZ: Therapy Skill Builders.

Yorkston, E., Miller, R. & Strand, E. (2004). *Management of speech and swallowing in degenerative diseases* (2nd ed.). Austin, TX: Pro-Ed.

Zangen, T., Ciarla, C., Zangen, S., Di Lorenzo, C., Flores, A., Cocjin, J., . . . Hyman, P. E. (2003). Gastrointestinal motility and sensory abnormalities may contribute to food refusal in medically fragile toddlers. *Journal of Pediatric Gastroenterology and Nutrition, 37*, 287-293.

Additional Recommended Reading

Cherney, L. R. (1994). *Clinical management of dysphagia in adults and children*. Gaithersburg, MD: Aspen Publishers.

Corbin-Lewis, K., Liss, J. M., & Sciortino, K. L. (2004). *Clinical anatomy and physiology of the swallow mechanism*. Clifton Park, NY: Thompson Delmar Learning.

Dikeman, K., & Kazandjian (2002). *Communication and swallowing management of tracheostomized and ventilator-dependent adults*. San Diego, CA: Singular Publishing Company.

Golper, L. (2009). *Medical speech-language pathology: A desk reference* (3rd ed.). San Diego, CA: Singular.

Groher, M., & Crary, M. (2010). *Dysphagia: Clinical management in adults and children*. St. Louis, MO: Mosby Elselvier.

Leonard, R., & Kendall, K. (2008). *Dysphagia assessment and treatment planning: A team approach*. San Diego, CA: Plural Publishing.

Murray, J. (1998). *Manual of dysphagia assessment: Assessment in adults*. San Diego, CA: Singular Publishing Group

Shaker, R. (2013). *Manual of diagnostic and therapeutic techniques for disorders of deglutition*. New York, NY: Springer Publisher.

Shaker, R. (2013). *Principles of deglutition: A multidisciplinary text for swallowing and its disorders*. New York, NY: Springer Publisher.

Sonies, B. C. (Ed.). (2002). *Dysphagia: A continuum of care*. Gaithersburg, MD: Aspen Publishers.

Swigert, N. (2007). *The source for dysphagia* (3rd ed.). Austin, TX: Lingui Systems.

VanDahm, K., & Sparks-Walah, S. (2002). *Tracheostomy tubes and ventilator dependence in adults and children.* Austin, TX: PRO-ED.

Yorkston, K., Miller, R., & Strand, E. (2003). *Management of speech and swallowing in degenerative diseases.* Austin, TX: PRO-ED.

Cookbooks for Patients With Dysphagia

Buttaro, T. M., Trybulski, J., Polgar-Bailey, P., & Sandberg-Cook, J. (2016). *Primary care: A collaborative practice* (5th ed.). St. Louis, MO: Mosby.

Larson, J. (2016). *Group home cookbook* (3rd ed.). New York, NY: Page.

Weihofen, D., Robbins, J., & Sullivan, P. *Easy to swallow, easy to chew cookbook: Over 150 tasty and nutritious recipes for people who have difficulty swallowing.* New York, NY: Houghton Mifflin Harcourt.

Website Resources

ASHA Practice Portal: Adult and Pediatric Dysphagia content areas: www.asha.org/practice-portal/

American Board of Swallowing & Swallowing Disorders: www.swallowingdisorders.org/

Dysphagia Café: https://dysphagiacafe.com/

Dysphagia: Nestlé Health Science: https://www.nestlehealthscience.com/health-management/gastro-intestinal/dysphagia

Dysphagia Research Society: www.dysphagiaresearch.org/

Dysphagia Resource Center: https://wp.dysphagia.com/

Feeding Matters: www.feedingmatters.org

GI Motility Online: www.nature.com/gimo/

National Foundation of Swallowing Disorders: swallowingdisorderfoundation.com/

Pediatric Feeding Association: http://pedsfeeds.com/

Special Interest Division 13 (ASHA): https://www.asha.org/SIG/13/

Dysphagia Assessments

Bedside Evaluation of Dysphagia (BED)

Clinical Observational Dysphagia Assessment (CODA)

Dysphagia Evaluation Protocol

Mann Assessment of Swallowing Ability

Quick Assessment for Dysphagia

Swallowing Ability and Function Evaluation (SAFE)

15

Assessment of Accent

Dalia Elbaz-Pinto, MS, CCC-SLP, TSSLD and Laurie Michaels-Wilde, MS, CCC-SLP, TSSLD

Key Words

- accent
- accent modification (or reduction)
- African American Vernacular English
- allophones
- articulation
- Asian American speech
- communication difference
- communication disorder
- contrastive features
- dialect
- discourse
- ethnographic interviews
- figurative language
- fluency
- foreign accent
- Formal Standard English
- Informal Standard English
- intelligibility
- International Phonetic Alphabet
- metalinguistic awareness
- morpheme
- morphology
- morphosyntax
- noncontrastive features
- phonetic placement
- pragmatics
- prosodic features
- regional accent
- Russian-Influenced English
- semantics
- Spanish-Influenced English
- Standard American English
- syntax

An **accent** is a particular way that speech is pronounced by people who speak the same language. In the United States, our population is considered to be a "melting pot," or a conglomeration of diverse racial, ethnic, and cultural backgrounds. Because of the vast array of languages spoken, we frequently speak with or listen to various accents on a daily basis. Correspondingly, the term **dialect** is defined "as a neutral label to refer to any variety of a language which is shared by a group of speakers" (Wolfram & Schilling-Estes, 2006, p. 2). In other words, if you speak a language, you are speaking a dialect of that language. It should be noted that an accent is the way the speech actually sounds, whereas a dialect denotes a variation of the language itself. A **regional accent** is a variation in dialect of the same language based on a specific geographic region. For instance, a person who lives in Texas may sound quite different from someone residing in New York, despite the fact that they are both speakers of the same language. Even though both speakers communicate in the same language (i.e., English), their dialects are not the same. A

Stein-Rubin, C., & Fabus, R. *A Guide to Clinical Assessment and Professional Report Writing in Speech-Language Pathology, Second Edition (pp 381-411).*

foreign accent refers to the speech of a person from another country whose primary language was or remains a language other than **Standard American English** (SAE). For instance, a person who was raised speaking Spanish and learned English later in life may sound different from a native-born American whose predominant language is English (American Speech-Language-Hearing Association [ASHA], 2017).

For the purposes and scope of this chapter, we will primarily discuss accent reduction as it pertains to the adult population, who may electively pursue an evaluation or may be referred by a university speech screening or his or her place of employment. To investigate the role that speech-language pathologists (SLPs) play with school-age children, we refer you to the seminal works of Adgar, Wolfram, & Christian (2007); Cheng (1995); Paul (2007); and Roseberry-McKibben (1995).

The conception that one dialect is "standard" and that the rest are "nonstandard" is one that is ubiquitous and crucial for us, as speech and language professionals, to understand. In terms of **Formal Standard English**, the norms are outlined for us by accepted sources of authority, such as educational textbooks on grammar and usage, acknowledged writers, and language educators. When analyzing most people's speech, we can glean that not many Americans use speech that is completely consistent with Formal Standard English. Thus, **Informal Standard English** is a term used to describe the more colloquial way of speaking that is still deemed to be "standard." This incongruence makes it difficult for us to clearly define what is meant by *Standard American English*, the term commonly used to refer to the dialect that appears to be prevalent in North America.

Given the preliminary information, the initial questions you may ask are the following: "What is it about a speaker's dialect that makes it standard or nonstandard?" and "How do we decide what is consistent with SAE and what is not?" According to Wolfram and Schilling-Estes (2006), listeners tend to judge speakers as "nonstandard" when their speech differs dramatically in grammatical structure from what is conventionally considered to be the norm. Hence, the use of stigmatized grammatical structures, such as double negatives (e.g., "We don't need no help") and conflicting verb agreement patterns (e.g., "They's good") would likely classify an individual's speech pattern as "nonstandard." Later in this chapter, we will learn that the use of these syntactic structures is not erroneous per se, but rather characteristic of another regional or cultural dialect. Our definition of SAE is one that takes into account both formal and informal standard English as well as society's notions of acceptable forms of speech.

Although SAE is often perceived as the prevalent dialect, it is a vital part of our humanity and professional ethics that we honor and value the rich diversity of cultures of human beings. Consonant with this, it is incumbent on us to respect all dialects equally. Moreover, a particular dialect is a direct representation of the social, cultural, and historical background of its speakers and is thought to strengthen and unify the social network of its communicators. Unequivocally, no one dialect is superior to another based on linguistics. Correspondingly, individual dialects are neither right or wrong nor good or bad; they are merely different. No speaker is at a disadvantage or less equipped to function expressively or cognitively based on his or her dialect.

For our purposes as diagnosticians of speech and language, and according to ASHA (2003), accents are deemed to be a **communication difference** rather than a **communication disorder**. A communication difference refers to the use of a rule-governed language system that deviates from the language used by the mainstream culture, whereas a disorder indicates a discrepancy in expected linguistic skills based on a person's age and developmental stage (Paul, 2007). A person's accent does not in any way indicate a deficit in speech or language. It is merely a variation in the way that the speech sounds (Saad & Polovoy, 2009). Thus, we must acknowledge that no particular dialect is better than another (Adgar et al., 2007). In fact, according to the ASHA's most recent Position Statement regarding this issue, "no dialectal variety of American English is a disorder or a pathological form of speech or language. Each dialect is adequate as a functional and effective variety of American English" (ASHA, 2003).

Now that we have established the parameters of SAE, the meaning of dialect, and ASHA's position on addressing accent, several inquiries may come to mind. The first may be, what would prompt individuals with a dialectic influence on their spoken English to seek the assistance of a speech/language pathologist to assess and possibly modify their accent?

There are various types of clients that may wish to receive accent modification therapy, including non-native English speakers, speakers who want to diminish a regional accent, employees and professionals who desire to enhance their communication skills, and actors who have to learn a novel accent for a role (ASHA, 2017).

Although many individuals take pride in their accents, as a symbol of their backgrounds, many believe that their accents, in one or more ways, adversely affect their daily lives. An accent may affect a speaker's **intelligibility**, or clarity of speech, and ability to be understood by others. As a result, other individuals may have difficulty understanding the message that a speaker with an accent different from his or her own is trying to convey. Sikorski (2005) noted that the term comprehensibility is generally preferred within the teachers of English to speakers of other languages (TESOL) community of professionals. Intelligibility measurements and/or rating scales are objective; they are quantifiable by transcription accuracy (Munro & Derwing, 1994). However, the companion component, comprehensibility, "denotes listeners' perceptions of understanding as measured by listeners' scalar rating of how easily they understand speech" (Trofimovich & Isaacs, 2012, p. 906.)

Aligned with this perspective, individuals with accents have frequently related that they feel powerless and frustrated in a variety of communicative contexts. These situations include, although are not limited to, circumstances that require individuals with accents to assert themselves; to be understood on the telephone; to attempt to explain pertinent information to a professional (e.g. physician, attorney, accountant, teacher); or to interact in social, educational, and employment settings.

As mentioned earlier, one of the contexts in which individuals with foreign accents frequently express a variety of communicative constraints is in social situations. Typically, native English speakers may request that others with accents reiterate what was previously said to clarify their intended message. This recurring interaction promotes embarrassment in the speaker and often leads to diminished self-confidence and self-perception with regard to their communicative efficacy. Ultimately, their diminished intelligibility often promotes these individuals to avoid social situations, exacerbating their loneliness and isolation.

In the university setting, clients with accented English report that they hesitate to speak in class. Moreover, they may withhold responses despite knowing the correct answer. This avoidance of expressing themselves in the classroom environment may result from one or a combination of factors. One constraint in self-expression is the client's self-consciousness that they sound "different" from or do not "speak English as well as" the milieu. The second obstacle to class participation is due to the adverse reaction of their classmates. The responses of their peers may not necessarily be vocal, but nonverbal, such as through facial expression and body language. The third reason that individuals with accent may avoid participating in class may be due to their instructor's reaction or attitude. For example, a classroom instructor may request repeated clarification or even verbally comment on the student's accent, thereby embarrassing or humiliating the student. Moreover, oral presentations assignments are a cause of more pronounced anxiety than for native English speakers. The resulting anxiety may compound the student's pronunciation differences and further diminish their speech clarity.

A foreign accent may impact upon an individual's life in the domains such as socialization, educational advancement, and job performance (ASHA, 2017). Due to one or more of the aforementioned reasons, there are individuals who independently seek **accent modification** or **accent reduction** to modify or alter their accent, usually in an attempt to conform to SAE. Hence, the majority of clients who seek assessment and plausible treatment of accent are self-referred due to personal concerns.

In addition to self-referred clients, individuals with foreign or cultural accents may be referred for accent assessment and modification. Corporate offices may require that accent modification services be pursued by their employees to increase their speech clarity. Similarly, university departments may have students undergo accent modification as part of their conditions of acceptance into or continuation in a higher education program (McLeod, 2007). In these situations, although the original decision may not be the student's, once introduced to the process, the individuals are generally interested and motivated to partake in the services we have to offer (Schmidt & Sullivan, 2003).

What is our role as SLPs in a communication domain that is not connected with disorder? Starting in the late 1990s, clinicians in our field began to contemplate the implications of the increase in non-native English speakers within our client population (Schmidt & Sullivan, 2003). Because of the increased prevalence of clients with accented English in recent years, it is apparent that there is considerable probability that speech clinicians will service non-native English speakers at some point in their careers. Therefore, it is imperative that graduate students as well as clinicians become educated and informed themselves in this area of increasing client population.

As speech and language professionals, it is not our place to dissuade or encourage people who wish to alter their accents. Rather, our role is to work with such individuals to ensure that they are able to communicate as efficaciously as possible, so long as that is aligned with the client's personal goal. As clinicians, it is important to bear in mind that this is not about us and adopt a client-centered approach where we place the client's perspective and agenda at the forefront of our evaluative and therapeutic regime (see Chapter 2 for further discussion). It is within our scope of practice to assess and treat individuals who electively pursue accent modification. Part and parcel of our role in the diagnosis and therapeutic intervention is the ability to help the client acquire proficiency in the second dialect while maintaining the integrity of his or her first dialect. In this way, accent modification differs dramatically from the other topics covered in this book. Because the issue at hand is initially one of aesthetics, such services are typically not covered by insurance, as there are no underlying medical or cognitive concerns.

Bearing that in mind, assessment of accent remains somewhat of a gray area in terms of the SLP's ethical responsibility. Because this is not a speech-language disorder but rather a matter of elocution, it is still ambiguous for where to draw the line on assessment and treatment. There is no generally accepted diagnostic protocol for accent modification clients. Evaluative aspects that are included in an assessment many vary from one clinician to another and from facility to facility. They range from solely assessing phonetic inventories, **morphosyntax**, and **prosodic features** of speech to including additional areas of assessment such as **semantics**, comprehension, and **figurative language** (Schmidt & Sullivan, 2003).

In the case of accent reduction, the individual essentially electively wishes to modify his or her accent. Based on ASHA's position statement, discussed at the onset of this chapter, it remains questionable whether it is under our jurisdiction, as speech-language professionals, to address other aspects of the client's communication. On the other hand, there are aspects of communication that intertwine with phonetic pronunciation and influence both the client's comprehension and transmission of his or her intended message. These additional assessment areas may include the prosodic features (intonation, timing, and stress) of speech as well as the client's rate and degree of articulatory excursion. As such, SLPs differ widely in terms of what they include in their diagnostic assessment of accent. Moreover, in addressing our ethical role as communication professionals, are we assuming appropriate responsibility when we choose to eliminate the observation and reporting on other aspects of communication?

The following examples may serve to further clarify the previous point. If an individual seeks our services for accent and exhibits a dysphonia, are we to assess accent, given that accent modification does not encompass aspects of pathology? Moreover, what are the implications for neglecting to refer the client to the appropriate medical resource as well as to address something that may be a medical or even life-threatening issue? To further illustrate this point, during the course of the evaluation, a client may exhibit behavior that indicates difficulty with receptive or expressive language independent of his or her accent. Perhaps the client is struggling with reading comprehension significantly affecting his schoolwork. Are we in best service to the client if appropriate assessments or referrals are not made which could perhaps lead to additional educational support as well as benefit the client's academic and social functioning?

The preceding points resonate with the premise in Chapter 2 on counseling—that the clinician must consistently adhere to the client's agenda. In line with this, a sensitive and collaborative (clinician and client) interview provides opportunities to ask questions, obtain the client's perspective, and allow the client to make decisions about his or her personal goals. Often, as a result of this interchange, the additional factors realized and owned by the client, when presented with the opportunity, may alter or expand his or her goal.

This brings us home to the art segment of our profession, which is often thought to be a combination of art and science. If we are able to illuminate the big picture for our clients, then we succeed in empowering them to make informed decisions about their goals. Is our responsibility fulfilled when we withhold information about a client's oral and written communication skills, or is using our clinical intuition and insight part of the process of addressing the whole person? These are questions that require additional exploration.

Considering the previously mentioned ideas, we present information in this chapter on accent assessment from the perspective of "more is more" rather than "less is more." Therefore, in addition to the basics of accent assessment, we endeavor to offer the reader information on additional or "other" assessment areas in the sections to follow.

Specific Parameters for Assessment

Assessment is one of the most significant tasks a clinician will perform. It is the foundation from where all treatment goals are derived. Assessment is used to evaluate the client's spoken language through both standardized and non-standardized measures.

As previously mentioned, one unresolved ethical question is whether the clinician should solely evaluate and treat the client's intelligibility or whether the clinician should assess the client comprehensively by examining all areas of speech and language to rule out the possibility of a language disorder. It seems as though more research is needed to clarify this dilemma (Schmidt & Sullivan, 2003). Due to the uncertainty that remains regarding this quandary, we leave it up to the discretion of the clinician to make that determination. It should be noted that it appears as though evaluating the various aspects of speech and language would be helpful to the clinician in terms of establishing a differential diagnosis and determining if a client's dialectal variations are a result of a difference vs. a disorder. In our opinion, the assessment of accent should evaluate the client's difference from SAE in the following areas:

- **Phonetic placement** for sounds in words, sentences, and connected speech. Phonetic placement consists of the individual's placement of the articulators for specific speech sounds in different contexts. To assess this aspect of speech, we used the **International Phonetic Alphabet** (IPA), an alphabet designed to represent the sounds of the world's languages to provide a universal method of phonetic transcription (Small, 1999). (Refer to Chapter 7 for an inventory on IPA vowels and consonants.) We typically analyze dialectically influenced speech through classification of phonological processes or patterns (Paul, 2007). We look for consistent variant patterns and compare these phonological differences with what is expected for that dialect and for speakers of SAE.
- Prosodic features (stress, intonation, phrasing, linking, and rate) are the larger linguistic units, elements occurring across segments, that can alter the meaning of the message (Bauman-Waengler, 2008). Certain dialects lend themselves to limited articulatory excursions and rapid speech rate in their native language. This often generalizes to their pronunciation and prosody in spoken English.
- **Morphology** refers to the structure, classification, and relationship of **morphemes** (the smallest meaningful unit or form in a language.
- **Syntax** (word order and sentence structure) during oral and written expression. Syntax is the architecture of phrases, clauses, and sentences.

Additional parameters include the following:

- Semantics (vocabulary knowledge and use) during oral and written expression. While assessing semantic knowledge and use, it is imperative to consider the client's culture and possible lack of linguistic exposure.
- **Metalinguistic awareness** (the ability to think about and reflect on language). This includes figurative language (nonliteral language to include the comprehension and use of idiomatic expressions, humor, puns, proverbs, metaphors, and similes). Clients who present with dialects may have difficulty with figurative language skills, which can affect their ability to follow conversation, monologue, and reading, and to communicate with others.
- Presence of speech-language problems in primary language (e.g., receptive and/or expressive language disorder)
- Vocal parameters (vocal quality, pitch, intensity, and resonance) during conversational speech. Vocal parameters can affect overall speech intelligibility and assessment of these parameters may indicate a possible underlying problem (nodules, polyps, etc.).

  It is noteworthy that some individuals with dialectic influence on their spoken English speak in a low vocal volume, conceivably as a result of low self-confidence in their English communication skills.
- **Fluency** (the smoothness or flow of sounds, syllables, words, and phrases in connected speech) is another parameter that can be assessed informally.

Please refer to Chapters 7, 10, 12 and 13 for a detailed explanation on the elements of articulation, language, voice, and fluency.

We can use the parameters of assessment to analyze a client's accent compared with SAE. Let us now examine in detail the expected speech and language characteristics of dialects commonly spoken in the United States that differ from SAE. It is beyond the scope of this chapter to provide an inventory and analysis of the influence of all foreign accents on spoken English. Therefore, we provide you with the accented speech patterns of the speakers of the most frequently occurring dialects, including **African American Vernacular English**, **Spanish-Influenced English**, **Asian American Speech**, and **Russian-Influenced English**, that seek accent assessment and modification services.

Differences Between Standard American English and Other Dialects of American English

As mentioned earlier in the chapter, many perceive SAE as the preferred dialect. It is typically employed by governmental institutions and the media. However, various other dialects are commonly spoken across the country depending on the cultural, ethnic, geographic, or social setting. It is important to note that a dialect is a rule-governed linguistic system that will most likely have an impact on the language form of the individual's spoken English in predictable ways. By analyzing the phonemic systems of various dialects other than SAE, we can assess particular sounds that the client has difficulty pronouncing in accordance with SAE. Similarly, when comparing grammatical structures of other dialects with those acceptable in SAE, we may see marked differences. Furthermore, the parameters of accent assessment may include more than a phonetic/phonemic inventory. To determine the variables that impact on speech clarity, one must take a closer look at the client's accented speech and examine the prosodic elements such as intonation, timing, and stress that provide the utterance with its melodic contour (see the following section for an inventory of expected patterns of morphosyntax on the spoken English of individuals with accent).

When assessing an individual with a foreign accent who wishes to modify or reduce his or her accent, diagnosticians should consider the specific preceding parameters to complete a comprehensive assessment. An individual who wishes to modify his or her accent may choose to alter these elements of their speech to increase intelligibility and align their speech more closely with the spoken English of their surroundings. By comparing and contrasting these aspects of phonology, prosody, and morphosyntax, we will gain insight in selecting goals for the accent reduction process. Let us take a closer look at several major dialects frequently spoken in the United States.

African American Vernacular English

African American Vernacular English (AAVE) is a social dialect spoken by many people of African descent residing in the United States. The development of this dialect is related to the history of the migration of these individuals from Africa to the southern United States that began in the 1600s (Small, 1999). We must acknowledge that not all African American people use this dialect to communicate, nor is this dialect confined to this population. Some speakers of AAVE may speak using this particular dialect at all times. Others may opt to code-switch depending on the situation; in other words, they may select which dialect they use (AAVE or SAE) based on the educational, professional, or social environment.

AAVE is a rule-governed dialect of SAE that has previously been labeled an assortment of names to include Black English, Ebonics, and Black English Vernacular (Hollie, 2001).

Phonological Characteristics of AAVE

AAVE can be typified by phonological patterns that impact on the production of certain phonemes. These patterns encompass omission or substitution of the medial and final consonant in a word, reduction of consonant clusters in final position, omission of unstressed initial phonemes or syllables, raising of vowels, and simplification of diphthongs (Pearson, Velleman, Bryant, & Charko, 2009; Small, 1999). Table 15-1 provides a summary of the abovementioned phonological features. The reader is referred to Chapter 7 for a detailed explanation regarding the phonological patterns discussed in Table 15-1.

Morphosyntactic Characteristics of AAVE

In addition to the aforementioned variations in phonology, there are various morphosyntactic features that are typical of AAVE. These features include the omission of the copula, the lack of the past tense marker *-ed*, the absence of possessive *'s*, irregular verb form usage, the absence of the plural *-s* marker, the use of negation, and the inflection of "be" (Bland-Stewart, 2005). Although these features signify a difference rather than a deficit, omission of structures considered necessary as per SAE could potentially hinder the clarity of the message or alter its meaning. See Table 15-2 for a detailed explanation of morphosyntactic differences noted in AAVE.

Semantic Features of AAVE

Some lexical items are specific to AAVE or have even been integrated into SAE over time from their use in AAVE (e.g., funky, rap). Other words have particular implications in AAVE and often may transfer to mainstream use as well (e.g., the use of "all that" to imply "excellent," "dude" to signify a person; Paul, 2007).

Table 15-1. Phonological Features of African American Vernacular English

Type of Phonological Difference	*Explanation*	*Examples*
Omission or substitution of consonant in medial or final position	Final stop deletion—final /d/ or /t/ may be omitted	/bæt/ (bat) → /bæ/
	Final nasal deletion—nasals in final position are omitted, and the preceding vowel is nasalized	/fin/ (fin) → /fi/
	Liquid deletion—deletion of middle and final /r/ and /l/	/starfiʃ/ (starfish) → /stafiʃ/ /hɛlp/ (help) → /hɛp/ /wɪl/ (will) → /wɪ/
	Substitution of final /n/ for /ŋ/	/wɪnɪŋ/ (inning) → /wɪnɪn/
	Devoicing of final stops—voiced consonants in the final position are devoiced	/fid/ (feed) → /fi:t/
	Stopping—when voiced fricatives are replaced by voice stops (Wolfram, 1994)	/ɪznt/ (isn't) → /ɪdnt/ /ðɛm/ (them) → /dɛm/
	Place of articulation change for /ð/ and /θ/	/bɛrθde/ (birthday) → /bɛrfde/ /mɔʊθ/ (mouth) → /mɔʊf/
Reduction of consonant clusters in final position	When the consonant cluster in the final position of a word share the same voicing pattern (i.e., both voiced or voiceless), the consonant cluster is reduced (Small, 1999).	/faɪnd/ (find) → /faɪ/ /kwɛst/ (quest) → /kwɛs/
Omission of unstressed initial phonemes and syllables	The initial unstressed (or weak) phoneme or syllable may be deleted.	/biniθ/ (beneath) → /niθ/ /əmʊŋ/ (among) → /mʊŋ/
Vowel raising	The vowel /e/ may be produced as /i/ when the preceding nasal consonant is /n/. Thus, the vowels /e/ and /i/ sound the same.	/ɛni/ (any) → /ɪnɪ/ /mɛn/ (men) → /mɪn/
Diphthong simplification	Diphthongs are simplified and transform into a monophthong, or just one vowel sound.	/raɪm/ (rhyme) → /ram/ /flɔʊr/ (flower) → /flar/

Adapted from Bland-Stewart (2005), Paul (2007), Small (1999), and Wolfram (1994).

Table 15-2. Morphosyntactic Features of AAVE

Type of Morphosyntactic Difference	*Examples in AAVE*	*Usage as per SAE*
Zero copula—deletion of the verb "be" and its variants	"He a good man"	"He **is** a good man"
Lack of the past tense marker *–ed*	"Yesterday he cook breakfast"	"Yesterday he cook**ed** breakfast"
Absence of possessive *–s*	"Here is Deb coat"	"Here is Deb**'s** coat"
Irregular verb form usage	"She knowed the material"	"She **knew** the material"
Absence of plural *–s* marker	"You have five cookie"	"You have five cookie**s**"
Omission of third-person singular	"She go to school"	"She go**es** to school"
Use of negation: Permissible to use "ain't" Multiple negation	"I ain't going" "I don't want no food"	"I **am not** going" "I don't want food"
Inflection of be (to denote habitual state)	"We be sleep"	"We **sleep** all the time"
Comparative and superlative markers differences	"badder" "most stupidest"	"more bad" "most stupid"

Adapted from Bland-Stewart (2005), Goldstein (2000), and Paul (2007).

Pragmatic Differences in AAVE

Because AAVE is a dialect that is culturally based, social norms vary from SAE as well. Silence is often employed in AAVE when a speaker is confronted with an unfamiliar situation or when an invasive question is posed. Indirect eye contact is considered proper listening behavior, particularly for children or people of lower status; speakers of SAE may consider this behavior to be inappropriate. Moreover, asking personal inquiries regarding a novel acquaintance's family or career is frequently thought of as rude, while an SAE speaker may ask such questions in an attempt to be gregarious. Additionally, interruption is acceptable, and the conversation is usually dominated by the most aggressive speaker, whereas turn-taking rules in SAE provide each speaker with ample time to convey his or her message. Lastly, narrative style in AAVE is more associational than based on a central theme, as SAE narratives are. AAVE narratives are derived from comments made in association with the previous statement as opposed to SAE narratives that are all based on a common subject matter (Paul, 2007).

Prosodic Features of AAVE

In AAVE, most stress differences involve the primary stress placement being moved to the initial syllable (e.g., "po'lice" instead of "poli'ce"). Furthermore, AAVE intonation often includes a higher pitch range, and a "falsetto" register is sometimes employed, particularly by males (Bernthal & Bankson, 1994).

Spanish-Influenced English

Spanish-Influenced English (SIE) is a term used to denote a dialect used by speakers whose primary language is Spanish and thus speak a dialect of English that is influenced by Spanish. Individuals of Hispanic descent constitute the largest minority group in the United States. Spanish is also considered to be the second most spoken language in our country (Perez, 1994). It is imperative for us to analyze SIE because it is highly likely that we will work with individuals who use this dialect. To address accent modification or to distinguish between a language difference or disorder (particularly with youngsters), we must compare and contrast elements of SIE across the areas of phonology, syntax and morphology, semantics, and **pragmatics** (Paul, 2007; Perez, 1994; Small, 1999).

Phonological Characteristics of SIE

SIE can be classified by phonological differences that alter the way in which particular phonemes are produced. The phonemic system of Spanish differs from that of English, affecting the speech of people who communicate using SIE. The English consonants /v/, /θ/, /ð/, /z/, and /ʒ/ are not present in Spanish (Perez, 1994). At times, **allophones**, or variant productions of phonemes, will occur (e.g., the fricative /th/ occurs in Spanish only as an allophone of the voiced stop /d/; Small, 1999). Additionally, there are allophonic variants in production of consonants when contrasting SIE and SAE (e.g., voiceless stops such as /p, t, and k/) are not aspirated in Spanish. Table 15-3 outlines these salient phonological features.

Take note that the aforementioned phonological patterns may or may not be observed in SIE. Not all speakers of this dialect will exhibit these differences, and variable patterns may be displayed depending on the context. In addition to the preceding phonological differences, there are several interferences that cause alterations in vowel production as well. The diminished vowel inventory causes confusion among Spanish American speakers, and often similar American English vowels are substituted for one another. Spanish includes only five vowels (/ɑ/, /i/, /ɛ/, /u/, and /ɵ/), whereas English comprises at least 15 vowels. In addition to adjacent vowel substitutions, monopthongization may occur where diphthongs are reduced to a single vowel. Central diphthongs (e.g., /ɛr/) are usually pronounced with a trill (Perez, 1994).

Some vowel differences include:

- /e/ → /ɛ/ /mek/ (make) → /mɛk/
- /æ/ → /ɑ/ /pæk/ (pack) → /pɑk/
- /ʊ/ → /u/ /gʊd/ (good) → /gud/

Other vowel confusions are not predictable based on interference, such as /u/ → /ʊ/ (as in room becomes /rʊm/). See Perez (1994) for more detailed examples.

Morphosyntactic Characteristics of SIE

Morphosyntactic features typical of speakers of SIE include the following (Paul, 2007; Roseberry-McKibbin, 1995):

- Omission of the regular past tense *–ed* (e.g., "Last week he walk")
- Omission of regular third-person singular marking (e.g., "he wonder")
- Inconsistent use of possessive markers (e.g., "the book of my sister"; "the boy hat")
- Omission of the plural /s/ marker (e.g., "two book")
- Omission of articles (e.g., "I go to house")

Table 15-3. Phonological Features of Spanish-Influenced English

Type of Phonological Difference	*Explanation*	*Examples*
Stopping	/θ/ in English is changed to /t/ in SIE	/bɛrθ/ (birth) → /bɛrt/
	/ð/ in English is changed to /d/ in SIE	/ðɛm/ (them) → /dɛm/
	/v/ in English is changed to /b/ in SIE	/væn/ (van) → /bæn/
Voicing	/s/ in English can be changed to /z/ in SIE (in prevocalic position)	/sɪp/ (sip) → /zɪp/
Devoicing	/z/ in English is often changed to /s/ in SIE (usually in postvocalic position)	/zu/ (zoo) → /su/
	/dʒ/ in English can be changed to /tʃ/	/dʒɛm/ (gem) → /tʃɛm/
Affrication of fricatives	/ʃ/ in English is changed to /tʃ/ in SIE	/ʃu/ (shoe) → /tʃu/
Affrication of glide	/j/ in English can be changed to /dʒ/ depending on the context	/ju/ (you) → /dʒu/
Deaffrication	/dʒ/ in English often becomes /j/ in SIE	/dʒok/ (joke) → /jok/
	/tʃ/ in English can be changed to /ʃ/	/tʃuz/ (choose) → /ʃuz/
Nasal velarization	/n/ in English becomes /ŋ/	/bæn/ (ban) → /bæŋ/
Consonant cluster reduction	Consonant clusters may be reduced in initial or final position of a word	/stɛp/ (step) → /tɛp/ /dɛsk/ (desk) → /dɛs/
Epenthesis	Addition of the schwa vowel (usually preceding /s/ initial consonant clusters)	/skul/ (school) → /əskul/
Unstressed syllable deletion	Weak syllables are omitted	/ɛksplen/ (explain) → /plen/

Adapted from Bleile (2004), Goldstein (2000), Paul (2007), Perez (1994), and Small (1999).

- Omission of subject pronouns (e.g., "Jan is home. Got sick")
- Adjectives after nouns (e.g., "the book red")
- Adverbs in improper order (e.g., "She eats slowly her food")
- More is used as a comparative marker instead of *-er* (e.g., "She is more taller")
- Inconsistent use of negatives in various contexts (no may be used instead of not or don't)

Semantic Features of SIE

There are several semantic differences when comparing SIE with SAE. According to Paul (2007), letter, number, and color words often receive less emphasis among SIE speakers compared with speakers of Standard American English. Names and labels for objects and people are stressed in parent–child interactions. Because of such semantic distinctions, it is conceivable that individuals are exposed to different items based on their respective cultures (Kester & Gorman, 2010).

Pragmatic Characteristics of SIE

Pragmatic differences exist that can alter the dynamic between a speaker of SIE and a speaker of SAE. For instance, speakers of SIE allow for closer personal space during conversation than speakers of SAE. People engaging in conversational **discourse** also tend to use physical gestures during their dialogue more than speakers of SAE. Additionally, direct eye contact is often avoided because it is considered a signal of inattentiveness, whereas it has the opposite implication in SAE (Paul, 2007).

Prosodic Features of SIE

Spanish is considered a syllable-timed language, which denotes that there is a recurrence of syllables rather than stress at intervals. Thus, stressed syllables in Spanish are not much longer in duration than unstressed syllables, whereas this is not the case in SAE. Additionally, pitch does not modulate as much in Spanish as it does in English, causing the pitch range for speakers of SIE to be more limited than it is for speakers of SAE. Utterances also begin at a lower pitch in SIE (McLeod, 2007).

Table 15-4. Phonological Features of Asian American Speech

Type of Phonological Difference	*Explanation*	*Examples*
Final consonant deletion	The consonant in the final position of a word is often omitted	/gɛt/ (get) → /gɛ/
Substitution	/r/ can be changed to /l/	/rɛd/ (red) → /lɛd/
	/l/ can be changed to /r/	/æktuəli/ (actually) → /æktuəri/
Stopping	/θ/ can be changed to /t/	/θæt/ (that) → /tæt/
	/ð/ can be changed to /d/	/ðo/ (though) → /do/
	/v/ can be changed to /b/	/væn/ (van) → /bæn/
	/f/ can be changed to /p/	/fæt/ (fat) → /pæt/
Deaffrication	/tʃ/ can be changed to /ʃ/	/tʃer/ (chair) → /ʃer/
Consonant devoicing	/v/ can be changed to /f/	/stov/ (stove) → /stof/
	/z/ can be changed to /s/	/noz/ (nose) → /nos/
	/g/ can be changed to /k/	/flæg/ (flag) → /flæk/
	/d/ can be changed to /t/	/pæd/ (pad) → /pæt/
	/b/ can be changed to /p/	/vaɪb/ (vibe) → /vaɪp/
Consonant cluster reduction	Consonant clusters are reduced	/skrim/ (scream) → /skim/ /tren/ (train) → /ten/
Epenthesis	Addition of the schwa vowel	/blu/ (blue) → /bəlu/
Vowelization	Substitution of a vowel for a liquid phoneme	/foɚk/ (fork) → /fɑk/
Vowel raising	/ʊ/ may be changed to /u/	/bʊk/ (book) → /buk/
Vowel lowering	/e/ may be changed to /ɛ/	/snek/ (snake) → /snɛk/
	/i/ may be changed to /ɪ/	/lif/ (leaf) → /lɪf/

Adapted from Goldstein (2000), Paul (2007), and Roseberry-McKibben (1995).

Asian American Dialect

Asian/Pacific Islanders comprise a large percentage of immigrants coming to the United States today (Cheng, 1994). The term *Asian American* refers to cultural groups who come from China, Japan, Korea, India, Vietnam, Thailand, Cambodia, Laos, and various Pacific Islands. Individuals who constitute this group of "Asian Americans" may speak various languages, all of which can affect Asian American speech (Chan & Lee, 2004).

Phonological Differences of Asian American Speech

Asian American speech may be characterized by distinctions in phonology that affect the way that particular phonemes are produced. Because Asian languages have open (consonant-vowel) rather than closed (consonant-vowel-consonant) syllables, final consonants are often deleted in Asian American speech. Consonant blends are also rare in many Asian languages, precipitating the tendency to simplify consonant clusters in Asian American speech. Furthermore, the /r/ and /l/ phonemes are in the same phonemic category, which may cause confusion in Asian dialects of English. Table 15-4 lists prominent phonological features that are commonly observed in Asian American speech.

Note that information presented in Table 15-4 is based on research about typical differences observed in Asian American speakers. There is no implication that every feature is consistently exhibited in the same manner.

Morphosyntactic Differences of Asian American Speech

When analyzing the differences between SAE and Asian American speech, we can outline key distinctions between the two in the areas of morphology and syntax. These salient differences include, but are not limited to, the following (Cheng, 1987; Goldstein, 2000; Owens, 2007; Paul, 2007):

- "Be" verbs may be omitted or inflected inaccurately (e.g., "I coming"; "I is coming")
- Past tense marker *-ed* may be omitted (e.g., "He walk to school yesterday") or doubly marked (e.g., "He didn't saw her")
- Present tense marker may vary (e.g., "She go home"; "They eats food")
- Past participle can be unmarked (e.g., "I have drink"), overgeneralized (e.g., "She has wented")
- Noun–verb agreement may be inappropriate (e.g., "She have"; "I goes")
- Plurals containing quantifiers may be omitted (e.g., "three book")
- Subject-object confusion may be present (e.g., "Him coming")
- Possessive marking may vary (e.g., "him hat"; "it's the girl shirt")
- Demonstrative pronouns may vary (e.g., "those girl")
- Double marking for negatives may be present (e.g., "I didn't see nothing"; "She don't have no work")
- Markers may be simplified (e.g., "She no like")
- Omission or overgeneralization of articles (e.g., "she sang song"; "She go to the home")
- Auxiliary verb is not reversed (e.g., "You are coming?"; "she is going now?")
- Auxiliary may be omitted (e.g., "You want food?"; "he not go there")
- Copula may be omitted (e.g., "She eating supper")
- Difficulty with using prepositions (e.g., "We go store")
- Omission of conjunctions (e.g., "She you go now"; "My sister I went")
- Comparatives may vary (e.g., "more smarter"; "bestest friend")
- Word differences, to include adjectives following nouns (e.g., "house new"), possessives following nouns (e.g., "book yours"), subject–verb–object order (e.g., "She gave out them")

These distinctions may or may not be present when analyzing the morphology and syntax of the Asian American speaker. It is integral to compare and contrast these features of language during the assessment process, bearing in mind that such differences can be indicative of typical patterns observed across Asian American speech rather than reflective of a deficit in morphosyntax of the speaker.

Semantic Patterns Observed in Asian American Speakers

Semantic word knowledge, use, and interpretation may differ dramatically in Asian American speakers. Speakers of Asian-influenced English will often misunderstand speakers of SAE because they tend to take statements literally and may not understand the implications of a speaker's intended message. For instance, an Asian American speaker may interpret the phrase "Do you have the time?" in a literal sense and respond, "Yes, I do" whereas the conventional SAE connotation is for the listener to provide the actual time (e.g., "It is four o'clock"; Cheng, 1995). Thus, Asian American speakers may present with difficulty understanding colloquialisms and idiomatic language (Paul, 2007). Addressing these issues may or may not be within the scope of therapeutic intervention depending on the needs and expectations of the particular client.

Pragmatic Differences in Asian American Speakers

Because of the influence of their cultural and social background, Asian American speakers may display differences in the area of pragmatics compared with speakers of SAE. First, laughter may signify shyness as opposed to humor, which is the implication in SAE. Feelings and emotions are not overtly expressed; Asian American speakers often present with a flat affect and do not modify their facial expressions to reflect their internal emotions. Many speakers of this dialect may appear physically composed despite being frustrated or upset. When being reprimanded, one typically maintains silence and lowers his or her eyes. Moreover, social status is of great value and is established on the basis of age, marital status, and profession. Asian American speakers may pose questions on these facts to novel acquaintances to form appropriate social order among conversationalists. Elders and professionals are regarded as having significant stature and command respect. It is deemed impolite to say no, particularly to individuals of high social stature (Paul, 2007). Children are expected not

Table 15-5. Phonological Features of Russian-Influenced English

Type of Phonological Difference	*Explanation*	*Examples*
Final consonant devoicing	The consonant in the final position of a word is often devoiced (produced as a voiceless phoneme)	/stov/ (stove) → /stof/ /noz/ (nose) → /nos/
Voicing	Voiceless phonemes can be produced as their voiced counterparts, particularly in initial position.	/pɪg/ (pig) → /bɪg/
Alveolarization	Dental sounds (e.g., /θ,ð/ can be replaced by alveolar sounds /d,z/)	/θɛm/ (them) → /zɛm/ /wɪθ/ (with) → /wɪz/ /ðɪs/ (this) → /dɪs/
Velarization	Glottal /h/ can be produced as velar fricative /x/	/het/ (hate) → /xɛt/ /hɛlo/ (hello) → /xɛlo/
Stopping	/θ/ can be changed to /t/	/θɪn/ (thin) → /tɪn/
Substitution	/ŋ/ becomes /v/	/pɪŋk/ (pink) → /pɪnk/
Labialization	/v/ becomes /w/, depending on the context	/vækjum/ (vacuum) → /wækjum/
Frication	/w/ becomes /v/, depending on the context	/wɪtʃ/ (witch) → /vɪtʃ/

Adapted from Bleile (2004) and Small (1999).

to behave rambunctiously; they are expected to remain quiet and are discouraged from participating vivaciously in the classroom setting. Direct eye contact is generally avoided, and repeated head nodding is used during discourse (Cheng, 1987). As clinicians, we must acknowledge and respect these differences and take them into account when conducting assessment and intervention services (Cheng, 1995).

Prosodic Differences of Asian American Speech

Many Asian languages are monosyllabic in nature, which can impact Asian dialects of English. The speech of Asian Americans can sound staccato-like and may mimic telegraphic speech. Stress may also be misplaced compared with expected stress markers in SAE. Additionally, most Asian languages are tonal; changes in prosody reflect semantic information rather than classifying sentence types (e.g., declarative vs. interrogative) or expressing a communicative message, as they do in English. Therefore, Asian Americans may have difficulty with SAE intonational patterns, which could be cause for misinterpretation (Paul, 2007).

Russian-Influenced English

Much like the dialects already discussed, Russian-Influenced English (RIE) possesses distinct features that differ dramatically from SAE. This dialect is often employed by immigrants from Eastern Europe, particularly from Russia.

Phonological Differences in RIE

The Russian consonant system differs significantly from that of SAE. In Russian, all stop consonants are unaspirated; thus, Russian speakers of English may produce voiceless stops without aspiration. An unaspirated voiceless stop in the initial position of a word may also sound voiced (e.g., "tune" → /dun/). In Russian, voiced stops do not occur in the final position of a word. Therefore, voiced stops and fricatives in the final position may be changed to their voiceless cognates (e.g., "rags" → /ræks/). Moreover, the following consonants in English do not exist at all in Russian: /ð, θ, w, ŋ/. The phonemes /h/ and /v/ can also be difficult for speakers of RIE. In addition, Russian has only five vowels (i.e., /i/, /ɛ/, /ɑ/, /u/, /o/) and only one diphthong (i.e., /aʊ/ ; Small, 1999). Because of this limited vowel inventory, Russian speakers learning to speak English may present with difficulty with vowel production. Refer to Table 15-5 for an outline of phonological differences between SAE and RIE.

As per Small (1999), vowel differences can include, but are not limited to, the following:

- /ɪ/ → /i/ /pɪt/ (pit) → /pit/
- /ʊ/ → /u/ /lʊk/ (look) → /luk/
- /æ/ → /ɛ/ /ræt/ (rat) → /rɛt/
- /ɔ/ → /o/ /cɔt/ (caught) → /cot/
- /ʌ/ → /ɑ/ /gʌm/ (gum) → /gɑm/

Morphosyntactic Features of RIE

In addition to the phonological distinctions already noted, there are key morphosyntactic differences that can be highlighted in RIE. These differences may include the following:

- Inappropriate use of the articles "a" and "the" (e.g., "He was smart guy"; "After the invention of a barbed wire")
- Inconsistent use of the possessive marker 's (e.g., "Kathy book"; "President Day")
- Inconsistent use of third-person regular present tense (e.g., "Now he say thank you")
- Difficulty with subject–verb agreement (e.g., "My mother have a snake")
- Difficulty with word order and sentence structure (e.g., "Bad attitude person had")

Prosodic Differences in RIE

In the Russian language, stress typically falls on every word in a sentence with the exception of articles and conjunctions. Therefore, intonation of RIE is perceptually "flat" when compared with SAE (Bleile, 2004).

Key Clinical Interview Questions

The evaluation process includes both formal and informal measures to obtain a comprehensive picture regarding the client's functioning. Qualitative measures should also be included in assessments before accent improvement programs. Self-evaluation before and throughout the program is essential to positive improvements. Data from qualitative self-evaluations in a long-term study at the University of Missouri Accent Modification and Pronunciation Program from 2006 to 2013 revealed the following:

> Ongoing review of their [participants] concerns could assist in the instructors' ability to: (a) clearly demonstrate to (thus, motivate) participants the rationale behind certain target choices and practice strategies, (b) measure outcomes more objectively against participants' post-program self-ratings, and (c) maintain and/or increase motivation and d) increase recommendations. (Fritz & Sikorski, 2013, pp. 118-126)

First and foremost, it is integral to gather background information so you can gain insight as to how an accent affects a client's daily life. **Ethnographic interviews** help speech-language professionals develop an understanding of the client's perceptions, desires, and expectations. We attempt to learn about the cultural values of the client and his or her family without considering our preconceived notions about cultural, ethnic, or racial ideas. By understanding the perspectives of clients and their families, we are enhancing the efficaciousness of the clinician–client relationship (Westby et al., 2003). Refer to Chapters 1 and 2 for additional information on the pivotal role of the family in the therapeutic relationship and in its outcome.

> Cultural generalizations are never true of all individuals. One must refrain from creating assumptions about individuals or families based on general cultural, ethnic, or racial information. It is helpful to learn about the cultural values of the individual and his or her family through techniques such as ethnographic interviewing. Understanding the views of clients and their families often determines the success of clinical interactions. (Westby et al., 2003, p. 4)

Establishing a clinical relationship with any client can be a challenging task. Many clients find it hard to divulge personal information to a stranger, even if that stranger comes from the same cultural background. When the client and clinician represent different cultures, the ability to establish a clinical relationship becomes even more troublesome. However, this does not imply that a relationship cannot be formed. It is the clinician's responsibility to be sensitive to cultural differences and have a vast knowledge of multicultural deviations. Individuals from many cultures (i.e., Native Americans, Asians) find it difficult and unnatural to share personal information with unfamiliar people. An interview setting may be extremely uncomfortable for them, and the clinician must be sensitive to these cultural beliefs and should not impose upon the client the necessity to answer all personal questions at the initial interview. It may be necessary to have more than one interview session to establish rapport and make the client more comfortable with providing the requested personal information (Haynes & Pindzola, 2008).

When conducting ethnographic interviews, clinicians should keep the following principles in mind (Westby et al., 2003):

- Pose open-ended questions rather than questions yielding a simple yes–no response.
- Recast what the client says by reiterating the client's exact words; do not attempt to paraphrase or interpret.

- Sum up the client's statements to provide him or her with the opportunity to correct you if you have misunderstood something that was said.
- Avoid asking multiple consecutive questions and/ or multipart questions.
- Avoid leading questions in order to not sway the client toward a particular response.
- Avoid asking "why" questions because such questions often sound judgmental and may influence the client to become defensive or skeptical.

In addition, conducting a client interview will ultimately assist the evaluator in selecting appropriate tests necessary to determine goals of remediation that are specific to the client's particular needs. Clinicians should collect relevant background information, such as the length of time that the client has lived in the United States, the amount of exposure to the English language, and the degree to which accented speech impinges upon speech intelligibility. These factors will also help the evaluator make a determination about assessment and plausible intervention.

Interview Questions

Opening Questions

- What brings you here today?
- What was the stated purpose of the evaluation (e.g., university or work-related requirement)?
- How do you feel about the recommendation for an assessment of your accent (if applicable)?
- What are your concerns about your speech, language, or communication skills?
- What are you hoping or expecting to learn from this evaluation?

Language History

- When did you arrive in this country?
- At what age(s) did you learn or acquire each language?
- In which order did you learn or acquire each language?
- How long have you been in the United States?
- Is there a family history of speech, language, or hearing difficulties? Explain.

Educational History

- Where were you educated?
- In which language was your formal school education?
- When were you introduced to English?
- In what ways were you introduced to English (through education, literature, et cetera).
- How would you describe yourself as a student?

Language Use

Home Setting

- What family members or friends reside in your current home?
- What language(s) do you speak predominantly in the home and with whom?
- How much time do you spend communicating with each person?

Social Settings

- Who do you communicate with outside of your home?
- In what social and/or leisure activities do you engage?
- In what language(s) do you communicate in social settings?
- In which situations do you find communicating in English most difficult?
- What is your preferred language for watching television, listening to music, and reading newspapers or books?

Occupation

- What is your job description?
- What is your work schedule?
- What language(s) do you use at work?
- Do others understand you when you speak?
- How much time do you spend communicating verbally in each language?
- How much time does your job require you to read and/ or write in a particular language?
- How would working on your English communication skills affect your job in particular and your overall life in general?

Formal Assessment Measures

When conducting a comprehensive assessment of accent, as in all areas of speech and language, diagnosticians rely on formal tests to provide them with valid and reliable information about the client's communicative functioning. To date, there is a paucity of formal tests for the assessment of accent modification in adult nonnative English speakers.

Table 15-6. Accent Modification Assessment Measures

Test, Author (Year)	*Ages*	*Test Description*
The Compton Phonological Assessment of Foreign Accent (COMPTON; Compton, 2002)	Adult	Comprehensive analysis of how a person's speech production varies from SAE
Proficiency in Oral English Communication (POEC; Sikorski, 2016a)	Adult with moderate English language skills and at least a seventh-grade vocabulary level	Measures articulation, intonation, auditory discrimination, language (optionally provides content for a complete language sample and a pragmatics rating scale)
POEC Screen (Sikorski, 2016b)	Adults, low/intermediate + English language skills	Verbal and auditory limited survey for SAE sound and intonation variation rules

The standardized assessment measures used for this population are typically criterion-referenced as opposed to norm-referenced. As noted in Chapter 4 norm-referenced instruments refer to a standardized comparison of an individual's performance with that of a larger group, called a *normative group*. Norm-referenced tests help determine how a client performs in relation to the "average." Conversely, criterion-referenced tests do not attempt to compare a client's performance to that of other individuals. Rather, they measure what a client can and cannot do in relation to a predetermined criterion (Shipley & McAfee, 2009). For a more in-depth explanation of standardized assessment, to include norm- and criterion-referenced measures, we refer the reader to Chapter 4 of this text.

Clinically, it is more relevant for the speech clinician to acquire information about the client's functioning relative to his or her dialect as opposed to comparing ability to a group of other individuals. Therefore, for the purposes of the assessment of accent, criterion-referenced measures allow the clinician to determine what specific phonemes, or speech sounds, the client has in his or her repertoire. Refer to Table 15-6 for a brief overview of the most commonly used formal assessment measures in this area.

Compton Phonological Assessment of Foreign Accent

One of the most widely publicized and commonly used accent modification assessment instruments is the criterion-referenced COMPTON (Compton, 2002). A comprehensive analysis of a foreign-born client's speech production patterns can be achieved using the COMPTON assessment battery. This tool requires the client to complete word-production, sentence-production, spontaneous reading, imitation, and spontaneous conversational tasks. The clinician uses IPA transcription to analyze the phonological patterns produced by the client during specific tasks (see Chapter 7 for an explanation of the IPA system).

The COMPTON has been based on samples obtained from more than 300 individuals from 25 language backgrounds. Compton and Hutton (1980) have found that the accented sounds of English are not an arbitrary conglomeration of speech errors, but rather they consist of a system of pronunciation patterns that are generated by the speaker's native language.

The COMPTON is divided into six components. Part I is a background information form that is filled out by the client. Part II comprises a stimulus word list that provides a phonetic sample of each initial and final consonant, consonant blend, vowel, and diphthongs commonly occurring in SAE. Each sound is sampled a minimum of two times, and each word is tested twice (once in isolation and once in context) to evaluate the consistency of the client's phonetic productions. Part III contains a form for transcribing the client's variant productions in spontaneous speech. Part IV is an oral reading passage to help analyze the client's pronunciation while reading aloud. Part V is a phonetic transcription of the oral reading passage that should be used as a response form for documenting the client's inaccurate productions. Lastly, Part VI is a pattern analysis that helps consolidate the data from Parts II, III, and V so that particular patterns are outlined.

While administering the COMPTON, it is essential that the diagnostician use a tape recorder or video recorder, with the client's consent. This audio-visual recording will aid with the transcription of the client's speech and allow for clarification of missed or unintelligible spontaneous responses.

Following administration of the COMPTON, the clinician may then identify which phonemes to implement into the client's therapy regimen. Phonemes that are the most stimulable, and potentially have the greatest impact on increasing speech intelligibility, should be addressed at the onset of therapy. Please refer to the COMPTON Pronouncing English as a Second Language (COMPTON P-ESL) Program for more information on establishing treatment goals and resources for therapeutic techniques (www.ajcomptonpesl.com).

Proficiency in Oral English Communication

The POEC (Sikorski, 2016a) is an assessment measure that can objectively evaluate a foreign or regional accent. As per the publisher of this measure, standardization as either norm- or criterion-referenced has not yet been established for this diagnostic tool.

The POEC includes six subtests that allow the clinician to assess the client's speech patterns across different contexts (words, sentences, auditory discriminations, spontaneous speech samples). The POEC also measures intonational skills (word level stress and pitch changes, message level stressed words and global inflections, and stress and pitch changes demanded by conversational exchanges). By analyzing the client's responses, the clinician can measure the client's prosodic features of language. Another unique element of the POEC is its pragmatic rating scale that assesses eye contact, facial expressions, gestures, and turn-taking skills (on a 4 to 1 scale; 4 = appropriate and 1 = inappropriate).

For administration of the POEC, the clinician is responsible for documenting the client's observed intonation patterns, specific to rising–falling inflection, and word-level and message-level stress and response variations (Sikorski, 2016a). The clinician's task further encompasses documenting the client's variant productions across single words, sentences, and spontaneous conversational speech via IPA narrow transcription. After administration of this assessment measure, the examiner will be able to determine how the client's foreign or regional accent affects speech intelligibility and comprehensibility and to design a program that meets the desired communication goals.

POEC Screen, Second Edition (Sikorski, 2016b) is a screening and/or placement tool for English language output rules, such as phonological variation rules as well as stress and pitch rules for word and extended speech. Again, using the definitions for comprehensibility and intelligibility given earlier, this tool is primarily a comprehensibility instrument because it weights issues that impact native English "understanding as measured by listeners' scalar rating of how easily they understand speech" (Trofimovich & Isaacs, 2012, p. 906). The POEC Screen results are compiled to yield an Auditory Score and a Verbal Score. It contains auditory discrimination subtests for sound and intonational issues as well as verbal performance subtests for vowel, consonant, and intonational allophonic rules of American English. An optional Verbal Performance Test can be examiner-rated on a three-point scale for the categories of Articulation, Intonation, Language Skills, and Voice/Nonverbal Skills.

Supplementary Articulation Tests

As per a survey compiled by Schmidt and Sullivan (2003), some university programs and SLPs utilize supplementary measures of assessment to evaluate **articulation** skills. Such evaluation tools are not normed for accent modification assessment (e.g., The Fisher–Logemann Test of Articulation [F-LTAC; Fisher & Logemann, 1971]; Arizona Articulation Proficiency Scale [Fudala, 2001]). See Schmidt and Sullivan (2003) for a complete list of these instruments.

Accent and Concurrent Disorder

For the purpose of this chapter, the test descriptions include measures for clients who present as accent modification clients in the absence of a language disorder. If a language disorder is suspected, further evaluation of language skills is warranted. There are several formal assessment tools that allow for a more elaborate evaluation of receptive and expressive language that include, but are not limited to, semantic, syntactic, morphologic, and figurative language skills. In a case where a language disorder may be an underlying issue concomitant with the client's accent, the following guidelines should be considered:

- Determine whether you are testing to assess comprehension of the English language or whether you are testing language skills in the client's native language. If the latter is the case, there are several formal assessment measures that have normative data for different languages. The clinician must be fluent in the client's native language, or have a suitable interpreter, in order to administer and properly score a formal test.
- If you are testing to assess the client's comprehension of the English language, formal assessment measures that have been standardized on the English-speaking population should be administered, interpreted, and reported informally.

Refer to the influential works of Goldstein (2000), Owens (2007), Paul (2007), and Shipley and McAfee (2009) for additional information on bilingual assessments of receptive and expressive linguistic skills.

Advantages and Disadvantages of Formal Assessment Measures

Before initiating a foreign accent modification program, clinicians should determine the specific areas of speech that need to be modified. Formal assessment provides information that allows the evaluator to objectively analyze a person's dialect in comparison to SAE. By using formal instruments, clinicians are equipped with the tools necessary to gather information with regard to the client's phonological system and the extent to which these speech patterns influence SAE phoneme production.

There are several advantages to using formal assessment measures when these tests are administered and analyzed by qualified professionals. Formal tests are objective and test administration is typically efficient (Shipley & McAfee, 2009). In the case of the client who presents with an accent, formal measures allow the clinician to compare the client's speech production to the expected SAE targets. This allows the speech clinician to determine the specific sounds that are present or absent in the client's phonetic repertoire of SAE. The speech diagnostician may then refer to this foundational information for further qualitative analysis and for purposes of therapeutic intervention.

Although formal tests have an important and integral role in the assessment of accent, standardized instruments present with inherent limitations. Although formal measures allow for the clinician to objectively identify a client's strengths, weaknesses, error patterns, and phonological variations from SAE, naturalistic speech context becomes compromised for the structure. For example, formal assessment instruments provide structured tasks such as reading words, generating a corresponding phrase, and reading sentences. Informal assessment provides the examiner with a client's functional use of language in a more social, conversational, and relaxed framework. When assessing a client's speech in a more naturalistic context, a client may exhibit patterns that were not discernable during formal evaluation measures.

Therefore, to examine the client's abilities in varied contexts and to include oral reading and conversational discourse, informal assessment is crucial. Once assessment information is gathered from formal and informal testing, the clinician should then compare the results of both types of assessments for alignment or discrepancies.

Because there is limited access to date for assessment materials for the evaluation of the linguistic components of communication for second-language learners, other measures are significantly relied on to provide us with additional information about the client's morphosyntactic skills, semantic knowledge and use, and metalinguistic abilities. (A commonly used bilingual language assessment for lexical–semantic knowledge is the Bilingual Verbal Abilities Test; Munoz-Sandoval, Cummins, Alvarado & Ruef, 1998).

Both formal and informal measures have distinct advantages in the evaluation of individuals with dialectic influence on their spoken English. Therefore, to obtain a comprehensive depiction regarding the client's overall functioning with regard to speech and language speech, it is important that speech diagnosticians integrate the two procedures in the assessment of accent.

Informal Assessment Measures

Informal assessments are an invaluable component of the evaluation process. Coupled with formal scores, they allow the speech clinician to obtain a comprehensive view of the client's presenting problem or concerns. Informal tools provide the diagnostician with a more accurate portrayal about the client's functioning in a variety of contexts. Informal instruments allow the clinician flexibility and autonomy with respect to modifying administration procedures. Such measures are more dynamic in their assessment because they allow the clinician the authority to repeat or alter instructions or to probe further in a specific area. Scoring and interpretation of findings are left up to the discretion of the examiner (ASHA, 2004). The clinician is also at liberty to provide prompting to assess the client's stimulability for plausible intervention.

This section primarily focuses on assessment of accent modification with regard to articulation (the motor process involved in planning and executing sequences of sounds that result in speech), intelligibility, and prosody. It then briefly touches on evaluation of the linguistic components of morphosyntax, semantics, pragmatics, and metalinguistics for purpose of comparison to what is expected in the client's dialect. For a more in-depth discussion of evaluation procedures with regard to receptive and expressive language, the reader is referred to Chapter 10.

Aspects of Informal Assessment for Evaluation of Accent

Informal measures could include, but are not limited to, a hearing screening, oral-peripheral exam, analysis of a speech sample, reading passages, writing samples, and informal rating scales, which are explained next (Shipley & McAfee, 2009):

- Audiological screening is indicated to rule out the possibility of hearing loss. If the client does not hear the pure tone at any of the designated frequencies, results are not within functional limits, and a complete audiological evaluation is recommended (see Chapter 5 for additional information).
- An oral-peripheral examination is an important component of a complete speech and language evaluation. Its overall function is to identify or rule out structural and/or functional factors that could be impacting the client's speech intelligibility and phoneme production (see Chapter 6 for detailed guidelines).
- Following identification of problematic phonemes, it should be noted that before production training ensues, it is imperative that the clinician perform auditory perception testing. The appraisal of auditory perceptual skills has been used with clients who present with phoneme production difficulties. Inaccurate speech sound discrimination has been inconsistently linked to production differences (Bauman-Waengler, 2008). Auditory discrimination testing evaluates the client's ability to discriminate between the target phoneme and other sounds, including the misarticulated sounds used by the client. If the client is able to adequately discriminate the targeted sound, than production training can begin. If the client is unable to discriminate the target sound with the inaccurate production, then sensory-perceptual training should take precedence before the clinician begins the accent reduction regime (Bauman-Waengler, 2008).
- Speech samples can supply valuable information about a client's articulation, language (semantic, morphosyntactic, pragmatic), and prosodic features. There are various types of discourse (spoken or written communication) that the speech clinician may analyze, such as (a) conversational, (b) expository, and (c) narrative.
    - A conversational discourse sample can be obtained by instructing the client to discuss familiar topics such as favorite foods, family, friends, or extracurricular activities. This type of discourse may need prompting questions and may not elicit syntactic complexity. If the clinician is unable to assess lexical knowledge and use with this type of discourse, requesting an additional expository and/or narrative discourse sample is warranted.
    - An expository discourse sample can be elicited by instructing the client to explain or describe a specific topic. For example, the clinician can ask the client to explain specific rules of a sport, procedures, cause-and-effect relationships, or compare-and-contrast relationships. Expository discourse provides an unambiguous topic that allows the client to narrow his or her focus and provide precise details increasing in length and complexity.
    - A narrative discourse can be obtained by requesting that the client "tell a story" either by recounting an event or retelling previously read text. A narrative discourse will include motion and action words to describe a series of events. If the client is having difficulty verbalizing a story, pictorial prompts may be used to educe oral expression.

Refer to Chapter 10, which elucidates the various types of discourse.

Although a conversational speech sample is included in the COMPTON and POEC, we suggest an additional spontaneous speech sample, in a naturalistic context, to elicit a more representative sample of the client's speech sound production. Obtaining a more complete inventory of the client's phoneme production may reveal which sounds in English that are nonexistent in the person's native language and can display which sounds or words, across two languages, are not utilized in the same way.

The use of speech samples provides the clinician with the opportunity to examine the client's phonemic inventory from a different perspective. In connected speech, each word is not pronounced individually; connected words are pronounced differently depending on the influence of neighboring sounds that immediately precede or follow them (Peña-Brooks & Hegde, 2007). Hence, a contextual speech sample of connected discourse allows us to examine the effects of coarticulation, or the rapid overlapping movements of the articulators on a client's speech (Small, 1999). In addition, speech samples help clinicians evaluate the client's prosodic features of speech (stress, intonation, phrasing, linking words and phrases, and rate).

Moreover, a speech sample enables the clinician to assess the client's morphosyntax (linguistic units that have morphology and syntax properties). The clinician can examine morphosyntactic variant productions (e.g., omission of the plural *-s* marker), and compare the possible alterations in their grammatic inventory to that of SAE. For example, a clinician may note the omission of articles (e.g., "She sang song") in the speech sample of an Asian American speaker. Furthermore, the speech sample may be further analyzed for semantic accuracy and diversity (lexical knowledge and use) obtaining a sense of the client's receptive and expressive vocabulary. In addition, the speech diagnostician can assess at the client's speech sample to gain information about the client's pragmatics (appropriate social language use) by paying attention to his conversational ability, use of eye-contact (which may be culturally based), metalinguistic skills such as use of figurative language.

Tasks to Obtain a Speech Sample

- Informal conversation
- Answering various open-ended questions
- Reading aloud from a newspaper, magazine, or short story
- Paraphrasing information that was orally or auditorily presented
- Describing a favorite movie or television show
- Describing an activity or event (self-initiated or using contextual or sequential pictures)

Reading Samples

A reading passage allows the clinician to obtain information during oral reading specific to the client's articulation, voice, fluency, and decoding abilities (Shipley & McAfee, 2009). Oral reading allows the clinician to further evaluate articulatory abilities in a range of positions and contexts. Moreover, while engaged in oral reading tasks, the diagnostician can evaluate prosodic features to include variation in vocal inflection and intonation, pausing and phrasing, and alterations in word and sentence stress. Reading passages may be used to informally assess articulation and prosodic features during a structured activity. To refer back to the client's prosodic pattern for analysis, it is important, given verbal consent, to tape record the client's oral reading.

Resources for Oral Reading Passages

- A passage from a favorite magazine related to the particular client's interests
- "Grandfather Passage" (Darley, Aronson, & Brown, 1975)
- "Rainbow Passage" (Fairbanks, 1960).
- A portion of the Declaration of Independence. (refer to Shipley and McAfee [2009] for complete transcript)
- "Arthur the Rat," a standard passage used by dialectologists because it purportedly contains all the phonemes in Standard American English (Refer to the Dictionary of American Regional English to locate this passage: http://dare.wisc.edu/audio/arthur-the-rat.)
- "Comma Gets a Cure: A Diagnostic Passage for Accent Study" (see Appendix 15-A.)

Additional Resources for Oral Reading

In addition to the aforementioned reading passages, clinicians may use portions of standardized tests informally to obtain diagnostic information about the client's decoding and comprehension skills. When a selected excerpt of a formal test is employed, it is considered to be part of informal assessment in the diagnostic report. Correspondingly, when a test is standardized on a particular population (e.g., ages 3 to 21 years), and the client does not fall into that criterion (e.g., he is 25 years old), a clinician may administer the test informally to gain qualitative information about the client's functioning. The following standardized tests may be used informally with the accent modification client:

- Select passages from the Gray Oral Reading Tests-4 (GORT-4; Wiederholt & Bryant, 2001)
- Select passages from the Stanford Diagnostic Reading Test-4 (SDRT-4; Karlsen & Gardner, 1995)

Additional Assessment Measures

In addition to evaluation of articulation and prosodic features of speech, areas of language should be informally assessed as well. Individuals who pursue accent modification therapy may wish to address linguistic aspects of their speech to help them communicate with others more effectively. Clients often wish to work on their accent to assist their performance with regard to school or profession. Assessing language in speakers of foreign accent is often reflective of the client's experience and or exposure with regard to SAE.

Gaps in comprehension, understanding of idiomatic expressions, variations in pragmatic norms, and differences in written expression may impact a client's ability to relate to others in his or her educational, professional, and/or social environment. Thus, it is suggested that clinicians informally evaluate basic areas of language as part of a comprehensive assessment.

Assessment of Comprehension Skills

In addition to evaluating the client's oral reading, it is worthwhile to screen the client's comprehension skills. To examine other modalities, the diagnostician may get a sense of the client's receptive skills by presenting a listening comprehension task.

- Select portions (specific questions in relation to oral reading passages) of the GORT-4 (Wiederholt & Bryant, 2001)
- Select portions (specific questions in relation to oral, silent, and listening passages) of the SDRT-4 (Karlsen & Gardner, 1995)
- Understanding Spoken Paragraphs subtest of the Clinical Evaluation of Language Fundamentals-4 (CELF-4; Semel, Wiig, & Secord, 2003).
- Refer to Reading Comprehension Cards, Level 2, at https://www.linguisystems.com/products/product/display?itemid=10505

Assessment of Figurative Language

The speech-language professional should informally evaluate the client's knowledge and use of figurative language, or the ability to interpret language in a non-literal way. Because of particular cultural and/or social backgrounds, some clients may have limited exposure to figurative language.

- Figurative Language and Non-literal Language subtests from the Comprehensive Assessment of Spoken Language (CASL; Carrow-Woolfolk, 1999)
- Refer to www.superduperinc.com: Figurative Language: A comprehensive program, Second Edition (Gorman-Gard, 2008).
- Refer to Spotlight on Reading and Listening Comprehension Level 2: Figurative Language (https://www.linguisystems.com/products/product/display?itemid=10505)
- Figurative language cards provide an engaging way of exploring idioms, proverbs, similes, metaphors, and clichés (These cards could be adapted for assessment and treatment purposes; available at www.proedinc.com.)

Assessment of Pragmatic Skills

During conversational discourse, the speech clinician can informally evaluate the client's eye contact, gestures, and facial expressions. Note the client's topic maintenance and turn-taking skills. While considering these factors, it is imperative to bear in mind the previously mentioned dialectal characteristics with regard to pragmatics. (See "Differences Between Standard American English and Other Dialects of American English" earlier in the chapter for details on pragmatic features of particular dialects.)

- Refer to the Pragmatics Profile of the CELF-4 (Semel et al., 2003)
- Pragmatic Judgment subtest of the CASL (Carrow-Woolfolk, 1999)

Assessment of Writing Skills

A writing sample allows the clinician to analyze the client's ability to organize and generate cohesive ideas for written expression. Through this analysis, the clinician can determine whether the client demonstrates appropriate sentence length and structure, syntactic ability, grammatical complexity, and lexical knowledge. An informal rubric system can be used to document the presence or absence of specific expository elements. This rubric (Table 15-7) can be used at the onset of therapy and then yearly to assess progress. Key writing elements are listed in Table 15-8.

Assessment of the Client's Self-Perception of Linguistic Skills

An informal rating scale can be used to assess the client's self-perception of his or her accent and how it affects activities of daily living. The client's self-awareness is a key element to a successful therapy regime. If the client is unaware or unwilling to accept correction, the intervention's success will be significantly affected. A client's self-rating of his or her communicative skills provides the speech clinician with access to his or her attitude and motivation.

Following is a sample informal rating scale.

Language Skills

Using a scale from 1 to 10; 10 = excellent skills

How would you rate your skill to verbally communicate in each language?

Native Language ______________________

1. ___ Socially, with friends or family
2. ___ In class, answering or asking questions, giving a presentation
3. ___ At work, with colleagues or with clients

Table 15-7. Rubric for Assessment of Writing Skills in Adults

	4	*3*	*2*	*1*	*Total*
Content	Writing sample presents with meaningful content, relevant supporting details, and unity.	Writing sample includes some meaningful content, supporting details, and unity.	Writing sample includes minimal meaningful content, supporting details, and unity.	Writing sample includes no meaningful content, supporting details, or unity.	
Language Use	Writing sample has 0 article, phrase, or verb form errors.	Writing sample has no more than two article, phrase, or verb form errors.	Writing sample has no more than six article, phrase, or verb form errors.	Writing sample has more than 10 article, phrase, or verb form errors.	
Vocabulary	Age-appropriate vocabulary noted throughout written expression.	Some age-appropriate vocabulary noted throughout written expression.	Minimal age-appropriate vocabulary noted throughout written expression.	No age-appropriate vocabulary noted throughout written expression.	
Mechanics	Mastery of conventions including spelling, capitalization, commas, punctuation, and conventional structures.	Writing sample has no more than two errors in each: spelling, capitalization, commas, punctuation, and conventional structures.	Writing sample has no more than six errors in each: spelling, capitalization, commas, punctuation, and conventional structures.	Writing sample has more than 10 errors in each: spelling, capitalization, commas, punctuation, and conventional structures.	
Total ___					

Adapted from Carrow-Woolfolk (1996).

Table 15-8. Key Writing Elements

Language Use

- Articles: a, an, the
- Phrases: Prepositional phrases, gerunds, infinitives
- Verb form: Subject–verb agreement

Content

- Meaningful content: Developed main idea related to topic posed by clinician
- Supporting details: Details that elaborate on and support the main idea
- Unity: Sentences are in sequence, connect to each other and reinforce the main idea

Mechanics

- Spelling, capitalization, commas, and punctuation (end of sentence as well as internal)

Conventional structures

- Different types of written expression are formatted correctly including: letter writing, paragraphs and various expository texts.

Vocabulary

- Age-appropriate lexical knowledge and usage

Adapted from Carrow-Woolfolk (1996).

4. ___ Incidentally, asking a question at a store or for directions, etc.
5. ___ How would you rate your literacy skills in each language?
6. ___ Reading and writing a letter, email, or text
7. ___ Reading a newspaper, magazine, or book (for pleasure/recreational reading)
8. ___ Reading a school textbook or assignments
9. ___ Writing a class required paper or assignment

English Language

1. ___ Socially, with friends or family
2. ___ In class, answering or asking questions, giving a presentation
3. ___ At work, with colleagues or with clients
4. ___ Incidentally, asking a question at a store or for directions, etc.
5. ___ How would you rate your literacy skills in each language?

6. ___ Reading and writing a letter, email, or text
7. ___ Reading a newspaper, magazine, or book (for pleasure/recreational reading)
8. ___ Reading a school textbook or assignments
9. ___ Writing a class required paper or assignment

Differential Diagnosis

As mentioned previously, this chapter is primarily focused on assessing foreign accents in adults. When conducting a comprehensive evaluation, it is imperative that we take into account all aspects of articulation and language to make an accurate assessment of the client's skills and overall functioning. For the purpose of differential diagnosis, we must keep in mind whether our findings are indicative of a communication difference as opposed to a communication disorder (see introductory section to this chapter for a more elaborate explanation of these terms).

To aid in differential diagnosis, clinicians must familiarize themselves with the particular dialect of their client and should refer to **contrastive** and **noncontrastive features** of that dialect to make an accurate diagnosis (Bland-Stewart, 2005). The clinician should be able to recognize and differentiate contrastive features (features unique to a particular dialect) vs. noncontrastive features (features shared with SAE) to distinguish a dialectal speaker with a disorder from a typical dialectal speaker. An individual may employ contrastive features consistent with his or her dialect; however, this does not suggest an articulation or language disorder. Conversely, if the client uses a specific dialect but exhibits difficulties in use of the features shared with SAE, then a clinician may suspect a language disorder. For instance, if we have a client who is a speaker of AAVE, we would want to differentiate whether the linguistic deficits noted are a characteristic of that dialect. If a speaker of AAVE exhibited the use of multiple negation (e.g., "I don't got no money"), we can discern that such a morphosyntactic difference is typical of AAVE speakers. However, if this client demonstrated inappropriate use of pronouns (such as referring to a female as "he"), that might be a diagnostic indicator that there are underlying linguistic deficits that are not attributable to the client's dialect. Therefore, noncontrastive features are more diagnostically relevant in determining differences vs. deficits.

We, as clinicians, may access important insight about the client's functioning from information obtained through the client interview. Clients may report difficulties with auditory retention, comprehension, short-term memory, and word retrieval. As diagnosticians, we must probe the client to determine whether these deficits occur in their native language as well, which may suggest difficulties that surpass merely a dialectical difference. If a deficit is suspected, and the client agrees, we may opt to follow up with additional assessment in the client's native language as well. Additional remedial referrals, such as to English as a Second Language classes, may be warranted in certain instances.

Correspondingly, we must use our clinical savvy to distinguish whether deficits in language are merely a result of exposure or if there is a problem with processing, comprehending, and formulating language that is separate from the client's accent. When informally assessing metalinguistic ability by providing the client with idiomatic expressions and logical abstract thinking tasks, we need to decipher whether the client presents with difficulty due to lack of exposure as opposed to lack of age-appropriate comprehension skills. In this chapter, the focus is on clients who present with foreign accents in the absence of linguistic deficits. If a clinician finds that a client plausibly exhibits breakdowns in language in addition to displaying features of a particular dialect, as noted earlier, further testing should ensue.

The following sections encompass a sample case history, a rationale for using particular assessment measures, a template to guide you with writing formal and informal sections, a model report, and a novel case history for practice. By familiarizing yourself with these guidelines and examples, you will equip yourself with the knowledge and skills required to write a comprehensive, well-written diagnostic report that accurately portrays the client's strengths, weaknesses, and potential abilities.

Case History for Sample Report

K.E. is a 24-year-old woman who was referred for a complete speech and language assessment as a result of failing a required university screening due to diminished intelligibility, reportedly resulting from the influence of an Asian accent. K.E.'s medical history was unremarkable, and no significant family history of speech or language disorders was reported. K was born and raised in China and immigrated to the United States in 2003. She currently resides at home with her mother, father, and younger sister. K reported that her native language is Chinese, which is the predominant language spoken at home. K was first introduced to English in China when she was in grade school. She took ESL classes at Brooklyn College before enrolling as a full-time student to prepare herself for college. She currently speaks English solely at school, on a consistent basis. She noted that she is often fearful of participating in class or expressing her opinion in English because of self-consciousness about her accented speech. She is currently a full-time student and plans to eventually pursue a master's degree. K expressed a desire to ameliorate her intelligibility by improving pronunciation, vocabulary, and prosody.

Assessment Tool Selection and Rationale

- The clinical interview provides information to the evaluator regarding why the client is seeking this evaluation. It is integral to learn about the client's language background and to obtain an idea about the client's perception of his speech.
- The audiological screening rules out hearing loss that could potentially hinder a client's speech perception and production.
- The oral-peripheral mechanism examination assists in ruling out any plausible structural or functional anomalies that could affect the client's speech.
- The COMPTON was selected as a formal criterion-referenced test to provide an overview of the client's articulatory abilities in various positions and contexts. The COMPTON is also a useful tool for devising therapy goals.
- The POEC Screen was chosen to measure the client's auditory discrimination skills at the word and sentence levels. By using both the COMPTON and POEC Screen, diagnosticians can compare results and decipher whether findings from these two assessment tools are aligned.
- Articulation was informally evaluated via oral reading and spontaneous conversational interaction. By listening to the client's oral reading and conversational discourse, the evaluator can assess the client's overall intelligibility and prosodic features (e.g., pausing and phrasing, vocal inflection and intonation, and word and sentence stress).
- Linguistic skills were informally assessed via oral reading, a reading comprehension task, spontaneous speech sample, and analysis of figurative language. These tasks help the clinician evaluate reading comprehension, verbal expository skills, morphosyntactic features of language, semantic abilities, metalinguistic skills, and pragmatic abilities. The clinician can analyze these elements of language to determine whether they are characteristic of the client's particular dialect and reflect a difference rather than a disorder. Additionally, if the client is interested in pursuing therapy, he or she may desire to improve any inconsistencies in such areas to enhance intelligibility and potentially increase performance in educational, social, and/or professional domains (McLeod, 2007).

Rubric for Pertinent Sections of a Diagnostic Report

❑ For formal assessment: Introductory statement to include the name of the complete name of the test (underlined) and in abbreviated form in parenthesis (not underlined)

Example: Speech sound production was formally assessed through administration of the Compton Phonological Assessment of Foreign Accent (COMPTON) and Proficiency in Oral English Communication, Screening Version (POEC Screen).

❑ Test construct (cite what the test purports to measure)

Example: The COMPTON is a criterion-referenced instrument that assesses initial and final consonants, consonant blends, vowels, and diphthongs at the word, sentence, paragraph, and spontaneous speech levels.

Example: The POEC Screen is an instrument that measures the client's auditory discrimination skills at both the word and sentence levels.

❑ Elicitation procedures (describe where appropriate)

Example: For the COMPTON, the client is instructed to read target words aloud and verbally incorporate each word in a spontaneous sentence.

- ☐ General qualification of results in paragraph form (derived scores from formal test where applicable; qualitative analysis of variant patterns)

  Example: Formal assessment measures revealed inconsistent vowel and consonant substitutions in all assessed levels, dialectical in nature, and characteristic of Asian American speakers. These deviations in speech production indicated a difference in pronunciation, rather than a disorder. A combination of syllable structure and substitution processes were noted; see Table 1, Analysis of Phonological Processes. Vowel production consisted of various vowel alterations; see Table 2, Analysis of Vowel Alterations.

  Example: Results of the POEC Screen were essentially aligned with those derived from the COMPTON. K achieved a percentile score of 77, and exhibited specific difficulty discriminating between voiced and voiceless sounds.
- ☐ General qualification of results or analysis of variant productions in table form

Table 1. Analysis of Phonological Processes

Target Word	*Client's Response*	*Phonological Process*
/stov/	/stof/	Devoicing
/brið/	/brif/	
/ʃuz/	/sus/	
/wɪtʃ/	/wiʃ/	Deaffrication
/kedʒ/	/kæʒ/	

See the Sample Report for more detailed tables relevant to the case history.

- ☐ Intelligibility (note this is generally included in the informal section of the report)

  Example: Intelligibility deteriorated in connected discourse, seemingly due to the effects of coarticulation, restricted prosody, limited articulatory range of motion, restricted vocabulary, and deviations in language form.
- ☐ Additional observations and interpretation of findings: Discuss error consistency across different tasks presented. In the case of the accent modification client, it is important to mention difference vs. disorder.

Sample Report Based on Case History

Patient Information

Client: K.E. Date of Evaluation: 12/29/09
Address: *(street)* Phone number:
(city, state, zip code)
Date of Birth: 11/29/1985
Diagnosis: Foreign Accent

I. Reason for Referral

K.E. is a 24-year-old female Brooklyn College student who was seen for a complete speech and language evaluation on December 29, 2009. She was referred to the speech clinic upon failing a required university speech screening due to diminished intelligibility, reportedly resulting from the influence of an Asian accent.

II. Tests Administered/Procedures

- Client Interview
- Hearing Screening
- Oral Peripheral Mechanism Examination
- Compton Phonological Assessment of Foreign Accent (COMPTON)
- Proficiency in Oral English Communication, Screening Version (POEC Screen)
- Informal assessment of articulation and language skills

III. Background Information

Medical/Health History

K.E.'s medical history was unremarkable. She is not currently taking any prescription medications. No significant family history of speech or language disorders was reported.

Family/Social History

K was born and raised in China and immigrated to the United States in 2003 with her family. She currently resides at home with her mother, father, and younger sister. K reported that her parents made the decision to relocate to the United States for employment opportunities; her mother currently works as a waitress in a restaurant and her father is currently employed in the construction industry.

K reported that her native language is Chinese, and it is the only language spoken at home. She speaks predominantly Chinese with family and friends and explained that she feels more at ease conversing with people who speak in her native language. Thus, K speaks English solely in school, on a regular basis. The client noted that her pronunciation difficulties in English impede upon her ability to communicate efficiently. Similarly, K explained that she is least confident speaking in front of a class because she has been ridiculed as a result of her pronunciation differences. She noted that her fear of participating in class further contributes to feelings of isolation at the college. The client further conveyed that due to her pronunciation differences, she avoids expressing her opinion in English.

K was first introduced to the English language in China, when she was in grade school, where her classroom teachers reportedly taught "English vocabulary." However, the client noted that she learned how to speak fluent English in 2003, when she immigrated to the United States. To prepare herself for the college admission process, she enrolled in ESL courses at Brooklyn College. When questioned about her goals in improving spoken English, she conveyed the desire to improve her pronunciation, vocabulary, and prosody.

K expressed that she does not engage in social ventures and prefers spending time with her mother. The client's hobbies and interests include watching science fiction movies and listening to music.

Educational History

K is currently a full time student at Brooklyn College and is pursuing a bachelor's degree in business. She expressed a desire to continue her education and pursue a master's degree, although she is undecided about a specific career pursuit.

Therapeutic History

The client has no previous history of speech or language therapy.

IV. Clinical Observations

Behavior

K presented as a pleasant, polite, and bright young woman who participated amenably in the assessment process. She was motivated to improve her pronunciation, vocabulary knowledge, and prosody. K expressed that improving her pronunciation would maximize her opportunities for graduate school admission and ensuing employment. Furthermore, she conveyed that improving her articulation skills would improve the quality of her daily life and enhance her feeling of connection in her current society.

Hearing Screening

The client failed a hearing screening administered at 25 dB HL and 1000 Hz in the right ear. Therefore, a complete audiological evaluation is recommended.

Oral-Peripheral Examination

An oral-peripheral examination was conducted to determine the structural and functional integrity of the speech mechanism. The examination revealed normal facial symmetry and intact oral structures, adequate for speech production. Normal dental occlusion was observed. Informal assessment of velopharyngeal movement for /a/ phonation suggested appropriate function. K maintained air in the oral cavity upon resistance, confirming velopharyngeal movement, labial, and buccal strength. Informal assessment of diadochokinetic rate for /pʌtʌkʌ/, in isolation and in sequence, was appropriate. Lingual mobility for elevation, depression, and lateralization was mildly labored but was essentially within normal limits. In addition, a normal swallowing pattern was noted.

Speech and Articulation

Formal Assessment

Speech sound production was formally assessed through the administration of the COMPTON and POEC Screen.

The COMPTON is a criterion-referenced instrument that assesses initial and final consonants, consonant blends, vowels, and diphthongs at the word, sentence, paragraph, and spontaneous speech levels. The client is instructed to read target words aloud and verbally incorporate each word in a spontaneous sentence.

Formal assessment measures revealed inconsistent vowel and consonant substitutions in all assessed levels, dialectical in nature, and characteristic of Asian American speakers. These deviations in speech production indicated a difference in pronunciation, rather than a disorder. A combination of syllable structure and substitution processes were noted; see Table 1, Analysis of Phonological Processes. Vowel production consisted of various vowel alterations; see Table 2, Inventory of Vowel Alterations.

The POEC Screen is a diagnostic tool that measures the client's auditory discrimination skills at both the

Table 1. Analysis of Phonological Processes

Target Word	*Client's Response*	*Phonological Process*
/stov/ /brið/ /ʃuz/ /noz/ /twɪnz/ /θrɛd/ /dʒɑb/	/stof/ /brif/ /sus/ /nos/ /twims/ /flɛt/ /dʒɑp/	Devoicing
/wɪtʃ/ /kedʒ/	/wiʃ/ /kæʒ/	Deaffrication
/θʌ/ /ðʌoz/ /dʒus/	/dʌ/ /dos/ /dus/	Stopping
/foɤk/	/fɑk/	Vowelization
/frɑg/ /skræm/ /foɤk/	/fɑ/ /skæm/ /fɑk/	Cluster reduction
/lif/ /glʌv/ /blɑks/ /splæʃ/ /rɛkʌmɛnd/ /æktjuʌli/	/rif/ /grov/ /brɑ/ /spʌræʃ/ /lɛkʌmɛnd/ /æktjuʌri/	Substitution
/dɑg/ /slaɪd/ /flæg/ /zɪpkod/ /blɑks/	/dɑ/ /slaɪ/ /fræ/ /zipko/ /brɑ/	Final consonant deletion

word and sentence levels. Results of the POEC Screen were essentially aligned with those derived from the COMPTON. K achieved a percentile score of 77 and exhibited specific difficulty discriminating between voiced and voiceless sounds. Variant productions exhibited were consistent with those typical of Asian American speech.

Informal Assessment

Articulation was informally assessed through a variety of linguistic contexts to include oral reading and spontaneous conversational interaction. Results of informal testing were essentially aligned with those derived from the COMPTON and POEC Screen. It is noteworthy that intelligibility deteriorated in connected discourse, seemingly due to the effects of coarticulation,

Table 2. Inventory of Vowel Alterations

Target Word	*Client's Response*	*Phonological Process*
/wɪtʃ/ /twɪnz/ /lʊk/ /bʊk/	/wiʃ/ /twims/ /luk/ /buk/	Vowel raising
/sket/ /kedʒ/ /pɪg/ /drʌm/ /tɔɪ/	/skæt/ /kæʒ/ /pɛg/ /drɑm/ /taɪ/	Vowel lowering
/glʌv/ /pʊt/	/grov/ /put/	Vowel backing
/klaʊn/ /jɔn/ /mæp/	/krʌm/ /jʌm/ /mʌp/	Vowel centralization

restricted prosody, limited articulatory range of motion, restricted vocabulary, and deviations in language form.

Suprasegmental features of speech were characterized by limited variation in vocal inflection and intonation, deficient phrasing and pausing, and alterations in word and sentence stress. K's prosody was compromised by a staccato-like rhythm, and she tended to end the majority of her utterances with rising inflection. All of the aforementioned components were typical and consistent with Asian American speech and suggest a speech difference rather than a disorder.

Language

Informal Assessment

Informal assessment of linguistic skills included a spontaneous speech sample, oral reading, a reading comprehension task, and analysis of figurative language.

To informally assess oral reading comprehension, K was instructed to read a passage aloud. K accurately summarized the main idea and included relevant details. Thus, the client demonstrated good reading comprehension skills.

While summarizing the passage, the client exhibited morphosyntactic patterns characteristic of bidialectism, to include the following: omission of the article "the" ("Go to store"); deletion of regular past tense marker *-ed* (e.g., "I graduate"); omission of the plural *-s* marker (e.g., "I have two dog"); and omission of the copula (e.g., "She eating"). These differences in language form were consistent with an Asian-influenced dialect.

With regard to semantic skills, K exhibited a limited receptive–expressive vocabulary. She was unfamiliar with the meaning of the following common words: cage, crib, thread, and swing. The examiner informally evaluated figurative language skills by presenting common American idiomatic expressions and proverbs. Assessment of figurative language suggested a limited working knowledge of English idioms and proverbs, seemingly due to a lack of exposure rather than deficits in metalinguistic ability.

Pragmatic skills for conversational and social interaction skills were appropriate.

K maintained adequate eye contact and displayed adequate topic maintenance and turn-taking skills throughout the evaluation.

Voice and Vocal Parameters

Subjective analysis suggested normal vocal volume and quality. Prosody reflected limited variation in vocal inflection and intonation resulting in a monotone pitch pattern. In addition, K tended to use a rising vocal inflection at the ends of utterances. However, prosodic pattern in connected discourse was consistent with Asian American speech.

Fluency

Fluency was judged to be within normal limits during conversation. There were limitations in phrasing and pausing, and speech rhythm was characterized by a staccato-like rhythm, consistent with Asian American speech.

V. Clinical Impressions

K.E. is a 24-year-old female university student who pursued this evaluation as a result of failing a required college speech screening. She was pleasant and cooperative throughout the evaluation. She presented with several speech and language differences that were dialectal in nature and characteristic of Asian American speakers. Her articulation variations were characterized by phonological patterns to include a combination of syllable structure and substitution processes. Prosodic features were consistent with dialectical differences and were characterized by inappropriate word and sentence stress, inappropriate pausing and phrasing, a lack of inflectional variation resulting in a monotonous intonation pattern, and a rising intonation at the ends of utterances. Articulation and prosodic differences contributed to a mildly reduced intelligibility. Receptive and expressive language skills were characterized by morphosyntactic differences, a limited semantic inventory, and difficulty with figurative language. K's language form was consistent with that of Asian American speakers. Prognosis, with intervention, is good due to the client's high level of motivation and stimulability.

VI. Recommendations

A. Accent modification is recommended to commence once per week, with emphasis on the following:

1. To increase intelligibility, K will:
   - Increase articulation skills in Standard American English by remediation of the following phonological processes:
     - Stopping for fricatives
     - Deaffrication for affricates
     - Final consonant deletion
     - Devoicing
     - Cluster reduction
     - Substitution /r/ → /l/, /l/ → /r/
   - Increase Standard American English production of the following vowels /ɪ/, /ʊ/, /e/, /ʌ/, and diphthongs /ɔɪ/ and /aʊ/. Therapy should progress in a hierarchy from isolation, to monosyllabic words, phrases, and connected speech.
   - Improve suprasegmental features of speech by:
     - Producing appropriate rising and falling inflections in phrases and sentences
     - Increasing use of appropriate pausing and phrasing
     - Increasing appropriate placement of word and sentence stress
2. To increase working knowledge of correct grammatical structures, K will:
   - Produce articles (i.e., the, a) in sentences, paragraphs, structured spontaneous speech, and spontaneous speech
   - Encode correct usage of morphosyntactic structures (e.g., plurals, possessives, copula)

B. K failed a hearing screening administered at 25 dB HL and 1000 Hz in the right ear. Therefore, a complete audiological evaluation was recommended.

____

(Name of clinician or clinical supervisor and credentials)

Speech-Language Pathologist

Practice Exercise

Read the case history that follows. Your task is to select, identify, and describe specific formal and informal assessment measures for this client. Be sure to explain a rationale as to why you chose these particular tools to help you complete a comprehensive diagnosis.

D.P., a 25-year-old man, was seen for a complete speech and language evaluation secondary to personal concerns regarding diminished intelligibility reportedly resulting from the influence of an Eastern European dialect. Medical history is remarkable for a history of hypertension. No family history of speech or language disorders was reported. D.P. was born and raised in Russia and immigrated to the United States 3 years ago. He currently resides with his mother, who is employed as a home attendant. Currently, D.P. uses English and Russian on an equal basis, depending on the context and the communication partners involved in the discourse. D.P. was introduced to the English language in middle school, and upon arriving in the United States, he enrolled in ESL courses at his university. D.P. is currently pursuing a bachelor's degree in business and stated that he aspires to earn his law degree and become a tax attorney. D.P. expressed a desire to improve his pronunciation and grammar in English because he feels that it is impeding his academic performance, social interactions, and future career opportunities.

Summary

This chapter has discussed how to complete a comprehensive diagnosis of a client with accented speech. Such clients may be referred by an employer or school/university, or they may self-refer due to personal wishes to improve speech intelligibility. We learned about the significance of conducting a client interview in obtaining the linguistic background of the client as well as ascertaining the client's self-perceptions and expectations. To make a complete diagnosis, we must use formal tests in conjunction with informal procedures and an extensive client interview. It is our responsibility to analyze the client's speech and language and determine whether discrepancies are a result of a language difference or disorder. This information will ultimately provide a basis for the clinician to establish a differential diagnosis and will be helpful in devising treatment goals should the client decide to pursue therapeutic intervention.

Appendix 15-A

Comma Gets a Cure: A Diagnostic Passage for Accent Study

by Jill McCullough & Barbara Somerville

Edited by Douglas N. Honorof

Well, here's a story for you: Sarah Perry was a veterinary nurse who had been working daily at an old zoo in a deserted district of the territory, so she was very happy to start a new job at a superb private practice in north square near the Duke Street Tower. That area was much nearer for her and more to her liking. Even so, on her first morning, she felt stressed. She ate a bowl of porridge, checked herself in the mirror and washed her face in a hurry. Then she put on a plain yellow dress and a fleece jacket, picked up her kit and headed for work. When she got there, there was a woman with a goose waiting for her. The woman gave Sarah an official letter from the vet. The letter implied that the animal could be suffering from a rare form of foot and mouth disease, which was surprising, because normally you would only expect to see it in a dog or a goat. Sarah was sentimental, so this made her feel sorry for the beautiful bird.

Before long, that itchy goose began to strut around the office like a lunatic, which made an unsanitary mess. The goose's owner, Mary Harrison, kept calling, "Comma, Comma," which Sarah thought was an odd choice for a name. Comma was strong and huge, so it would take some force to trap her, but Sarah had a different idea. First she tried gently stroking the goose's lower back with her palm, then singing a tune to her. Finally, she administered ether. Her efforts were not futile. In no time, the goose began to tire, so Sarah was able to hold onto Comma and give her a relaxing bath.

Once Sarah had managed to bathe the goose, she wiped her off with a cloth and laid her on her right side. Then Sarah confirmed the vet's diagnosis. Almost immediately,

> she remembered an effective treatment that required her to measure out a lot of medicine. Sarah warned that this course of treatment might be expensive—either five or six times the cost of penicillin. I can't imagine paying so much, but Mrs. Harrison—a millionaire lawyer—thought it was a fair price for a cure.

Glossary

Accent: A particular way that speech is pronounced by people who speak the same language.

Accent modification or accent reduction: Refers to services designed to modify or alter an individual's accent, usually in an attempt to conform to Standard American English.

African American Vernacular English (AAVE): A term used to refer to a rule-governed social dialect often used by African Americans and others.

Allophones: Variant productions of phonemes.

Articulation: The motor process involved in planning and executing sequences of sounds that result in speech.

Asian American speech: A term used to refer to a dialect employed by cultural groups who come to the United States from China, Japan, Korea, India, Vietnam, Thailand, Cambodia, Laos, and various Pacific Islands.

Communication difference: The use of a rule-governed language system that deviates from the language used by the mainstream culture.

Communication disorder: A discrepancy in expected linguistic skills based on a person's age and developmental stage.

Contrastive features: Elements of a particular dialect that are specific to that dialect and are not shared with Standard American English, thus making them in contrast with SAE.

Dialect: Any variety of language employed by a group of speakers (Wolfram & Schilling-Estes, 2006).

Discourse: Spoken or written communication.

Ethnographic interviews: Interviews that take into account the client's cultural background without considering preconceived notions about cultural, ethnic, or racial ideas. These interviews help speech-language professionals develop an understanding of the client's perceptions, desires, and expectations.

Figurative language: The ability to understand and use language in nonliteral ways.

Fluency: The smoothness or flow of sounds, syllables, words, and phrases in connected speech.

Foreign accent: The speech of a person from another country whose primary language was or still remains a language other than SAE.

Formal Standard English: A dialect generally used in the United States where the norms are outlined for us by accepted sources of authority, such as grammar and usage books, acknowledged writers, and language educators.

Informal Standard English: A term used to describe the more colloquial way of speaking that is still deemed to be "standard" in the United States.

Intelligibility: Clarity of speech and ability to be understood by others.

International Phonetic Alphabet (IPA): An alphabet used to represent the sounds of the world's languages that was designed as a universal method of phonetic transcription.

Metalinguistic awareness: The ability to think about and reflect on language.

Morpheme: The smallest meaningful unit or form in a language.

Morphology: The structure, classification, and relationship of morphemes.

Morphosyntax: Linguistic units that have morphology and syntactical properties.

Noncontrastive features: Elements of a dialect that are shared with SAE and therefore are not in contrast with SAE.

Phonetic placement: The individual's placement of the articulators for specific speech sounds in different contexts.

Pragmatics: Refers to social language use.

Prosodic features: Stress, intonation, phrasing, linking, and rate which are the larger linguistic units which can alter the meaning of what is said.

Regional accent: A variation in dialect of the same language based on a specific geographic region.

Russian-Influenced English (RIE): A term used to refer to a dialect used by speakers who emigrated from Eastern Europe, particularly Russia.

Semantics: Vocabulary knowledge and use.

Spanish-Influenced English (SIE): A term used to denote a dialect used by speakers whose primary language is Spanish and thus speak a dialect of English that is influenced by Spanish.

Standard American English (SAE): The term commonly used to refer to the dialect that appears to be prevalent in America. It is the basis of comparison by which we can measure differences in speech and language with regard to various foreign dialects.

Syntax: Word order and sentence structure during oral and written expression. Syntax is the architecture of phrases, clauses, and sentences.

References

Adgar, C. T., Wolfram, W., & Christian, D. (2007). *Dialects in schools and communities* (2nd ed.). Mahwah, NJ: Erlbaum.

American Speech-Language-Hearing Association. (2003). Technical Report: American English dialects. *ASHA Supplement 23*. Rockville, MD: Author.

American Speech-Language-Hearing Association. (2004). Preferred practice patterns for the profession of speech-language pathology. Retrieved from https://www.asha.org/policy/PP2004-00191/

American Speech-Language-Hearing Association. (2017). Accent modification. Retrieved from https://www.asha.org/public/speech/development/Accent-Modification

Bauman-Waengler, J. (2008). *Articulatory and phonological impairments: A clinical focus* (3rd ed.). Boston, MA: Allyn & Bacon.

Bland-Stewart, L. (2005, May 3). Difference or deficit in speakers of African American English? What every clinician should know ... and do. *The ASHA Leader Online*. Retrieved from http://leader.pubs.asha.org/article.aspx?articleid=2278382

Bernthal, J. E., & Bankson, N. W. (1994). *Child phonology: Characteristics, assessment, and intervention with special populations*. New York, NY: Thieme Medical Publishers.

Bleile, K. M. (2004). *Manual of articulation and phonological disorders: Infancy and adulthood* (2nd ed.). Clifton Park, NY: Thomson Delmar Learning.

Carrow-Woolfolk, E. (1996,). *Oral and Written Language Scales [OWLS] Written Expression Scale*. Circle Pines, MN: American Guidance Service.

Carrow-Woolfolk, E. (1999). *Comprehensive Assessment of Spoken Language*. Circle Pines, MN: American Guidance Service.

Chan, S., & Lee, E. (2004). Families with Asian roots. In E.W. Lynch and M.J. Hanson (Eds.), *Developing cross-cultural competence* (3rd ed., pp. 219-298). Baltimore, MD: Brookes.

Cheng, L. (1987). Cross-cultural and linguistic considerations in working with Asian populations. *American Speech-Language-Hearing Association, 29*(6), 33-41.

Cheng, L. (1994). Asian/Pacific students and the learning of English. In J. E. Bernthal & N. W. Bankson (Eds.), *Child phonology: Characteristics, assessment, and intervention with special populations* (pp. 255-279). New York, NY: Thieme Medical.

Cheng, L. (1995). Service delivery to Asian/Pacific LEP children: A cross-cultural framework. In D. T. Nakanishi & T. Y. Nashida (Eds.), *The Asian-American educational experience: A source book for teachers and students*. New York, NY: Routledge.

Compton, A. J. (2002). *Compton Phonological Assessment of Foreign Accent*. San Francisco, CA: Carousel House.

Compton, A. J. & Hutton, S. (1980). *Phonetics for children's misarticulations*. San Francisco, CA: Carousel House.

Darley, F. L., Aronson, A. E., & Brown, J. R. (1975). *Motor speech disorders*. Philadelphia: W.B. Saunders.

Fairbanks, G. (1960). *Voice and articulation drillbook* (2nd ed., pp 124-139). New York: Harper and Row.

Fisher, H., & Logemann, J. (1971). *The Fisher-Logemann Test of Articulation Competence (F-LTAC)*. Boston, MA: Houghton Mifflin Co.

Fritz, D., & Sikorski, L. (2013). Efficacy in accent modification services: Quantitative and qualitative outcomes for Korean speakers of American English. *Perspectives on Communication Disorders and Science in Culturally and Linguistically Diverse Populations, 20*, 118-126.

Fudala, J.B. (2001). *Arizona Articulation Proficiency Scale* (3rd ed.). Torrance, CA: Western Psychological Services.

Goldstein, B. (2000). *Cultural and linguistic diversity resource guide for speech-language pathologists*. San Diego, CA: Thomson Delmar Learning.

Gorman-Gard, K. A. (2008). *Figurative language: A comprehensive program* (2nd ed.). Greenville, SC: Super Duper Publications.

Haynes, W. O., & Pindzola, R. H. (2008). *Diagnosis and evaluation in speech pathology* (7th ed.). Boston, MA: Allyn & Bacon.

Hollie, S. (2001). Acknowledging the language of African American students: Instructional strategies. *The English Journal, 90*(4), 54-59.

Karlsen, B., & Gardner, E. (1995). *Stanford Diagnostic Reading Test* (4th ed.). San Antonio, TX: Psychological Corporation.

Kester, E. S., & Gorman, B. K. (2010). Spanish-influenced English: Typical semantic and syntactic patterns of the English language learner. Retrieved from http://studylib.net/doc/8237268/spanish-influenced-english

McLeod, S. (2007). *The international guide to speech acquisition*. Clifton Park, NY: Thomson Delmar Learning.

Munoz-Sandoval, A. F., Cummins, J., Alvarado, C. G., & Ruef, M. L. (1998). *Bilingual Verbal Ability Tests*. Itasca, IL: Riverside Publishing.

Munro, M. J., & Derwing, T. M. (1994). Foreign accent, comprehensibility, and intelligibility in the speech of second language learners. *Language Learning, 49*, 285-310.

Owens, R. (2007). *Language development: An introduction* (7th ed.). Boston, MA: Allyn & Bacon.

Paul, R. (2007). *Language disorders from infancy through adolescence: Assessment and intervention* (2nd ed.). St. Louis, MO: Mosby.

Pearson, B. Z., Velleman, S. L., Bryant, T. J., & Charko, T. (2009). Phonological milestones for African American English-speaking children learning mainstream American English as a second dialect. *Language, Speech, and Hearing Services in Schools, 40*, 229-244.

Peña-Brooks, A., & Hegde, M. N. (2007). *Assessment and treatment of articulation and phonological disorders in children*. Austin, TX: Pro-Ed.

Perez, E. (1994). Phonological differences among speakers of Spanish-Influenced English. In J. E. Bernthal & N.W. Bankson (Eds.), *Child phonology: Characteristics, assessment, and intervention with special populations* (pp. 245-254). New York, NY: Thieme Medical.

Roseberry-McKibbin, C. (1995). *Multicultural students with special language needs*. Oceanside, CA: Academic Communication Associates.

Saad, C., & Polovoy, C. (2009). Differences or disorders? In the 1980s, research focused on culturally and linguistically diverse populations. Retrieved from http://www.asha.org/Publications/leader/2009/090505/090505d

Schmidt, A. M., & Sullivan, S. (2003). Clinical training in foreign accent modification: A national survey. *Contemporary Issues in Communication Science and Disorders, 30*, 127-135.

Semel, E., Wiig, E., & Secord, W. (2003). *Clinical evaluation of language fundamentals* (4th ed.). San Antonio, TX: Psychological Corporation.

Shipley, K., & McAfee, J. (2009). *Assessment in speech-language pathology: A resource manual* (4th ed.). Clifton Park, NY: Delmar Cengage Learning.

Sikorski, L. (2005). *Mastering effective English communication: The vowel system of American English.* Tustin, CA: LDS & Associates.

Sikorski, L. (2016a). *Proficiency in Oral English Communication: An assessment battery of accented oral English* (6th ed.). Tustin, CA: LDS & Associates.

Sikorski, L. (2016b). *Proficiency in Oral English Communication POEC Screen* (2nd ed.). Tustin, CA: LDS & Associates.

Small, L. (1999). *Fundamentals of phonetics: A practical guide for students.* Needham Heights, MA: Allyn & Bacon.

Trofimovich, P., & Isaacs, T. (2012) Disentangling accent from comprehensibility. *Bilingualism: Language and Cognition, 15*, 905-916.

Westby, C., Burda, A., & Mehta, Z. (2003). Asking the right questions in the right ways: Strategies for ethnographic interviewing. *The ASHA Leader, 8*(8), 4-5, 16-17.

Wiederholt, J., & Bryant, B. (2001). *Gray Oral Reading Tests* (4th ed.). Austin, TX: Pro-Ed.

Wolfram, W. (1994). The phonology of a sociocultural variety: the case of African American Vernacular English. In J. E. Bernthal & N. W. Bankson (Eds.), *Child phonology: Characteristics, assessment, and intervention with special populations* (pp. 227-244). New York, NY: Thieme Medical.

Wolfram, W., & Schilling-Estes, N. (2006). *American English: Dialects and variation* (2nd ed.). Malden, MA: Blackwell.

Financial Disclosures

Beryl T. Adler has no financial or proprietary interest in the materials presented herein.

Dr. Diana Almodóvar has no financial or proprietary interest in the materials presented herein.

Dr. Rochelle Cherry has no financial or proprietary interest in the materials presented herein.

Dr. Naomi Eichorn has no financial or proprietary interest in the materials presented herein.

Dalia Elbaz-Pinto has no financial or proprietary interest in the materials presented herein.

Dr. Baila Epstein has no financial or proprietary interest in the materials presented herein.

Dr. Renee Fabus has no financial or proprietary interest in the materials presented herein.

Dr. Elizabeth E. Galletta has no financial or proprietary interest in the materials presented herein.

Dr. Felicia Gironda has no financial or proprietary interest in the materials presented herein.

Charles Goldman has no financial or proprietary interest in the materials presented herein.

Dr. Gail B. Gurland has no financial or proprietary interest in the materials presented herein.

Patricia Kerman Lerner has no financial or proprietary interest in the materials presented herein.

Dr. Susan Longtin has no financial or proprietary interest in the materials presented herein.

Dr. Klara Marton has no financial or proprietary interest in the materials presented herein.

Laurie Michaels-Wilde has no financial or proprietary interest in the materials presented herein.

Susanna Musayeva has no financial or proprietary interest in the materials presented herein.

Dr. Dorothy Neave-DiToro has no financial or proprietary interest in the materials presented herein.

Dr. Adrienne Rubinstein has no financial or proprietary interest in the materials presented herein.

Dr. Natalie Schaeffer has no financial or proprietary interest in the materials presented herein.

Dr. Liat Seiger-Gardner has no financial or proprietary interest in the materials presented herein.

Naomi Shualy has no financial or proprietary interest in the materials presented herein.

Cyndi Stein-Rubin has no financial or proprietary interest in the materials presented herein.

Tina M. Tan has no financial or proprietary interest in the materials presented herein.

Amy Vogel-Eyny has no financial or proprietary interest in the materials presented herein.

Index